Volume 1

General Knowledge

EUROPEAN FEDERATION OF NATIONAL ASSOCIATIONS
OF ORTHOPAEDICS AND TRAUMATOLOGY

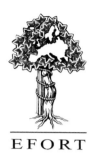

EFORT

SURGICAL TECHNIQUES
in
Orthopaedics and Traumatology

Coordinated by Professor Jacques Duparc

Honorary Chairman, Orthopaedic Department, Hôpital Bichat, Paris, France

Volume 1

General Knowledge

Associate Editor

Roger Lemaire

ELSEVIER

Paris, Amsterdam, New York, Oxford, Shannon, Tokyo

SURGICAL TECHNIQUES
in
Orthopaedics and Traumatology

Coordinated by Professor Jacques Duparc

In this collection:

1. General Knowledge   ISBN 2-84299-414-0

2. Spine   ISBN 2-84299-415-9

3. Shoulder   ISBN 2-84299-416-7

4. Arm, Forearm and Elbow   ISBN 2-84299-417-5

5. Wrist and Hand   ISBN 2-84299-439-6

6. Pelvic Ring and Hip   ISBN 2-84299-440-X

7. Femur and Knee   ISBN 2-84299-441-8

8. Lower Leg, Ankle and Foot   ISBN 2-84299-442-6

8 volume collection (full set)   ISBN 2-84299-443-4

Also available: the prestigious 4 volume Hardbound Package. Attractive loose-leaf binders allow continual updating. Includes quarterly updates and Internet access to the full text articles. For further information, please contact Editions Scientifiques et Médicales Elsevier or see: www.surgical-techniques-efort.com or www.elsevier.fr.

© 2003 Éditions scientifiques et médicales Elsevier SAS. Tous droits réservés. All rights reserved
23, rue Linois, 75724 Paris cedex 15, France
http://www.elsevier.fr – http://www.surgical-techniques-efort.com

Printed by SGIM, 10, rue du Parc, Parc Industriel Euronord, 31150 Bruguières, France

Bookbinding by Atenor, 11, rue de Lutèce, 78500 Sartrouville, France

Imprimé par SGIM, 10, rue du Parc, Parc Industriel Euronord, 31150 Bruguières, France

Façonnage par Atenor, 11, rue de Lutèce, 78500 Sartrouville, France

Dépôt légal N° : 03-555 - Janvier 2003   ISBN : 2-84299-414-0

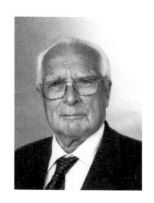

Preface

First and above all, this collection dedicated to surgical techniques in orthopaedics and traumatology is truly European.

It is published under the auspices of the European Federation of National Associations of Orthopaedics and Traumatology (EFORT), which at present groups 35 national associations. The creation of EFORT in 1992 resulted from the wish to form a European orthopaedic community. This has been made all the more important by the need to organise and standardise the training and qualifications of all European orthopaedists, according to the requirements and advice of the orthopaedic section of the European Union of Medical Specialists (UEMS).

Over the past 30 years, Europe has reclaimed its position among the leaders in the development of orthopaedics and traumatology. There has been a great deal of creativity. Among the many new contributions, we can mention the progress in osteosynthesis techniques due to the intramedullary nailing developed by Küntscher and the methods of internal fixation for fractures invented and developed mainly in Switzerland. The development of total joint replacement in the United Kingdom has revolutionised our field. Mention must also be made of the original ideas of Ilizarov, which were introduced and developed by the Italian School. We should add the Swedish National Survey of Hip and Knee Arthroplasties, initiated by the late Goran Bauer and continued by Peter Herberts, and the contributions to treatment of spinal pathology by R. Roy Camille and J. Dubousset of France. The above list is far from complete and will grow as new advances are made.

There is no doubt that Europe has an important role to play in the future of orthopaedics and traumatology.

This extraordinary growth and the development of increasingly sophisticated techniques in our field has made teaching and training more arduous. It has been suggested that the knowledge required by a general orthopaedic surgeon has increased 40 times over the past 40 years.

For all these reasons, EFORT decided to publish a collection covering the surgical techniques for all aspects of locomotor pathology in adults and children, without excluding non-operative treatment.

Thanks to the Editorial Board of EFORT, I have the honour - and also the very heavy responsibility - to be Editor of this work. For such a task, a large team was necessary, the members of which are listed at the end of this preface.

The collection is divided into eight sections, each under the responsibility of one or more Associate Editors. They have played an important part in selecting and contacting the contributing authors, in reviewing and coordinating the manuscripts. I must warmly thank these Associate Editors, who have accepted to undertake this additional work along with their surgical practice. They have played an essential role in its creation and publication.

The first section, "General Knowledge", is devoted to the general problems encountered in the practice of orthopaedic surgery: anaesthesia, prevention of deep venous thrombosis and infection, bone grafts, etc. The seven sections that follow concern the anatomical sites: the spine; shoulder; arm, elbow and forearm; hand and wrist; hip and pelvis; femur and knee; lower leg, ankle and foot.

It must be emphasised that this collection does not represent the work of a single group, school or institution, but rather results from the contributions of specialists and leaders in their fields throughout Europe. This explains its diversity. This collection is naturally written in English, which, as John Goodfellow put it, is the "new Esperanto" permitting scientific communication.

Each article must be considered as a separate entity and can be read without referring to the others. This has lead to some unavoidable overlapping, which we have tried to reduce to a minimum.

Most of the articles are devoted mainly to the surgical techniques themselves, which are described step by step and copiously illustrated. Variations of the techniques are discussed, as well as complications and clinical results. Some articles devote more discussion to the indications when this is necessary for the choice of treatment.

In general, the articles largely cover current orthopaedic practices. Most of these have already been widely tested by the orthopaedic community. Nevertheless, some articles discuss newer techniques, such as meniscal allograft transplantation, computerised pedicular screw fixation, video-assisted anterior approach to the spine, etc. It seems appropriate to include these new techniques which are already known to a large public but which have not yet been tested by time.

There are now two presentations of this collection. The first is the prestigious 4-volume, loose-leaf Hardbound Package which includes quarterly updates and access to the articles on Internet. The second, this edition, is divided into eight paperback volumes which may be purchased separately, allowing the specialised orthopaedic surgeon to select those parts of the collection devoted to his daily activities.

Many thanks to the editorial team at Elsevier - Sylvie Vercken, Agnès Brunel, Evelyne Lambert and Annabel Courage. I cannot too deeply express my appreciation to Gregg Colin for her assistance in the preparation of the manuscripts. Without her help, this publication would not have been possible.

Most of all, I would like to thank the authors and the Associate Editors who have contributed their time and their expertise to create this publication.

Jacques Duparc
Editor

The aim of EFORT, the European Federation of National Associations of Orthopaedics and Traumatology, is to promote science and education in the field of orthopaedics and traumatology.

The EFORT collection "Surgical Techniques in Orthopaedics and Traumatology", first published in 2000, was therefore a major step forward in demonstrating the great variety of European orthopaedic techniques.

Thanks to the unstinting work of Professor J. Duparc and the entire editorial board, in the short time since this collection has been launched it has attained a place in all the major European libraries. The next important step is the introduction of the new paperback edition. This will allow our orthopaedic colleagues who have specialised in a specific field to focus on one or several topics in which they are particularly interested.

On behalf of EFORT, I also want to thank the publisher, Elsevier, who accepted to join us in this editorial adventure to enhance orthopaedic operative techniques in Europe.

Nikolaus Böhler
President
European Federation of National Associations
of Orthopaedics and Traumatology (EFORT)

Patronage Committee

EFORT Jacques Duparc, Michael A R Freeman, Erwin Morscher, Otto Sneppen, Paolo Gallinaro, Nikolaus Böhler

UEMS Rafael Esteve de Miguel, Marc Speeckaert

Scientific Committee

Jacques Duparc, George Bentley, Henri Dorfmann, John Kenwright, Roger Lemaire, Frantisek Makai, Antonio Navarro, Panayotis N Soucacos, Nikolaus Böhler, Joachem Eulert, Frantz Langlais, Lars Lidgren, Pier Giorgio Marchetti, Wolfhart Puhl, Tibor Vízkelety

Editor

Jacques Duparc, MD, Professor
Honorary Chairman of Orthopaedic Department
Hôpital Bichat
Paris, France

Associate Editors

1. General Knowledge

Roger Lemaire, MD
Professor and Chairman
Department of Orthopaedic and Trauma Surgery
University Hospital
Liège, Belgium

2. Spine

Claus Carstens, MD
Head of Department
Paediatric Orthopaedics
Orthopaedic Hospital, University of Heidelberg
Heidelberg, Germany

Alain Deburge, MD
Professor, Department of Orthopaedics and Traumatology
Hôpital Beaujon
Clichy, France

3. Shoulder

Mario Randelli, MD
Professor
Istituto Clinico Humanitas
Milan, Italy

Jens-Ole Søjbjerg, MD, Professor
Department of Orthopaedics
University Hospital of Aarhus
Aarhus, Denmark

Jón Karlsson, MD, PhD
Department of Orthopaedics
Sahlgrenska University Hospital/Östra
Göteborg, Sweden

4. Arm, Forearm and Elbow

Norbert Gschwend, Prof Dr med
Orthopaedic Department
Schulthess Klinik
Zurich, Switzerland

Piet M. Rozing, MD
Department of Orthopaedic Surgery
Leiden University Medical Center
Leiden, The Netherlands

5. Wrist and Hand

Jean-Yves Alnot, MD, Professor
Chief of Orthopaedic Department
Upper Limb and Nerve Surgery Unit
Hôpital Bichat
Paris, France

Panayotis Soucacos, MD, FACS
Professor and Chairman
Department of Orthopaedic Surgery
University of Ioannina School of Medecine
Ioannina, Greece

6. Pelvic Ring and Hip

André Kaelin, MD
Paediatric Orthopaedic Unit
Hôpital des Enfants
Geneva, Switzerland

Erwin Morscher, MD, Professor
Felix Platter Hospital
Basel, Switzerland

Pär Slätis, MD, Professor
Orthopaedic Hospital of the Invalid Foundation – Helsinki
Grankulla, Finland

Roberto Giacometti Ceroni, MD
Istituto Galcazzi
Milan, Italy

7. Femur and Knee

Paul Aichroth, MD, MS FRCS
Emeritus Consultant Orthopaedic Surgeon
Knee Surgery Unit, The Wellington Hospital
London, United Kingdom

John Fixsen, MA, M.Chir, FRCS
Department of Orthopaedic Surgery
Great Ormond Street Hospital for Chidrren
London, United Kingdom

René Verdonk, MD, PhD
Department of Orthopaedic Surgery
Ghent University Hospital,
Ghent, Belgium

Ate Wymenga, MD
Knee Reconstruction Unit
Sint Maartenskliniek
Nijmegen, The Netherlands

8. Lower Leg, Ankle and Foot

Tomás Epeldegui Torre, MD, PhD
Hospital Nino Jesus
Madrid, Spain

Nikolaus Wülker, MD, Professor
Orthopaedic Department
Orthopädische Klinik und Poliklinik
Tubigen, Germany

Table of Contents
Volume 1 - General Knowledge
Surgical Techniques in Orthopaedics and Traumatology

Participating Authors
Volume 1 - General Knowledge
Surgical Techniques in Orthopaedics and Traumatology

Operating theatre

P Gallinaro
EM Brach del Prever

Abstract. – *The design and organisation of the operating theatre are fundamental in decreasing surgical complications and improving the quality of work. The "5D law" is still a good strategy: Discipline, Design, Devices, Defence mechanism of the patient, Drugs. The first three of these are discussed herein. Discipline remains the critical factor, as its lack may decrease the efficacy of others. Of new relevance is the organisation of the operating block and its relationship with surgical complications. Designing the operating theatre must be a multidisciplinary task, involving architects, engineers, surgeons and nurses who work in the operating theatre, and microbiologists. Ventilation is essential for both infection control and the comfort of personnel and patients. There are no existing methods that reduce air contamination to zero. Conventional ventilation with positive pressure, 30-40 air exchanges per hours and HEPA filters are often enough to ensure good results, if correctly associated with the other 5D rules. Ultraclean air, operating rooms with laminar-airflow require bacteriological sample analysis and whole body exhaust-ventilated suits. The separation of elective orthopaedic surgery from trauma and septic surgeries is of vital importance. To identify the priorities in improving the operating theatre, work safety risk analysis may be used. Analysis of time and financial support, identification of risk in the operating room, evaluation of the value of the damage eventually caused by the risk factor absence, analysis of probabilities that the damage will take place in the absence of the risk factor may be used to decide how, when and if to modify the operating theatre.*

Keywords: operating theatre, operating theatre design, hand scrubbing, ventilation, HEPA (high efficiency particulate) filter.

Introduction

The operating theatre is the heart of any hospital. There, patients spend the most critical time of their hospital stay and the surgical team spends a considerable portion of its life. Patients, doctors and nurses alike must feel comfortable; modern facilities must be made available in an environment designed to lower the risk of infection for both the patient and the surgical team. Many hospitals are centuries old, in Italy, as in other European countries. Even if their operating theatres have been rebuilt or refurbished, the global structure of the hospital remains old and difficult to clean properly, thus representing a weak link in the chain of combat against infection. However, there is no technology - clean air, ultraclean air, occlusive staff garments or hoods with an exhaust system - which can substitute for good, effective and rapid

Paolo Gallinaro, Director, First Orthopaedic Clinic.
Elena Maria Brach del Prever, Associate Professor.
Universita degli Studi di Torino, Dipartimento di Traumatologia, Ortopedia e Medicina del Lavoro, Torino, Italy.

surgery. The well-known rule of the 5 Ds [15] is still the key-stone in the strategy to fight infection: 1. Discipline, 2. Design, 3. Devices, 4. Defence mechanism of the patient, 5. Drugs. The first three of these are the subject of this article; the discussion of item 1 is not extended to preparation of the patient.

Discipline

Discipline is a critical factor, as lack of it may decrease the efficacy of others. Discipline concerns both personnel and patients, regardless of hierarchy, sex and job. Human skin bacteria are both residents (deep in the skin) and transients (in the superficial skin layers due to temporary contamination). They can contaminate the environment by direct contact, when touching something or someone, and by airborne contamination, by the release of hundreds of thousands of small skin desquamative particles into the air from all over the body (particularly from the groin, axilla, and scalp) when making movements. Some of these particles are a colony-forming

unit (CFU) or bacteria carrying particles (BCP) which settle on the room surfaces and may contaminate the surgical wound, surgical instruments, gloves, etc. The percentage of BCP in the air depends both on the ventilation characteristics and on discipline; the mathematical relationships between the influencing factors are discussed elsewhere in this chapter.

The following behavioural rules should be considered. Their scientific relevance has been tested and reported in many papers, sometimes with contradictory results. Unfortunately, surgical infection is multifactorial and it is difficult to scientifically demonstrate the relevance of each single factor. Hilary Humphreys, in a letter to the Lancet [11], emphasises the relevance of all these rules to influence, above all, our way of thinking and our behaviour. She gives as an example the red line which usually separates the dirty from the clean zone. She suggests that the colour of the line should be changed to amber, indicating "pause", to induce staff to think about what they are doing, and not simply to stop.

HAND WASHING AND SCRUBBING

Mechanical fretting removes the transient bacteria; detergent, useful to dissolve the dirt, facilitates the mechanical action by including transient bacteria in the emulsion. Before entering the operating block, all staff must wash their hands with a detergent for at least 20 seconds, paying particular attention to interdigital spaces and nails, in order to eliminate as much as possible of the transient bacteria on the hands. For the chemical reaction of large spectrum bactericidal products (such as povidone-iodine and chlorhexidine) to take place, they must remain in contact with the skin for at least two minutes. Legendary sequential ritual manoeuvres have developed in an effort to fill these two minutes. The chemical reaction and mechanical fretting must be recognised as the scientific basis for surgical scrub time; the "chemical" time is also necessary for the surgical preparation of the patient's skin.

DRESS, MASK AND HOOD

Clothes must be dedicated and designed to minimise BCP dispersion from the contaminating skin zones: the blouse is closed at the neck, elasticised fabrics close the arm; the trousers are closed at the ankle. A bright colour can be used as a marker to identify any undisciplined personnel who do not change garments before leaving the operating block [5]. Traditional cotton clothing allows both wet strike-through contamination and free egress of bacteria; in addition, the weave becomes enlarged after multiple washings [16]. Non-woven impermeable clothes are effective in protecting both the personnel and the patient, but could expose the personnel to stressful concentrations of humidity and heat [19]. The use of head-gear is recommended for personnel working around the surgical table [12]. The hood should leave no hair exposed. The mask retains bacteria expelled from the mouth and nose. Although its use has been debated in some papers [20], it is mandatory, especially with prosthetic surgery, to decrease the risk of contamination of personnel [29]. The use of completely machine-washable plastic boots and clogs is advisable, even if their efficacy in controlling bacterial floor contamination is controversial [22]; however, waterproof shoes decrease personnel contamination and are a "discipline factor", modifying behaviour.

STERILE GOWNS AND DRAPES

Gowns must completely cover the back, with a lateral double closure. The choice of disposable non-woven cloth must take into account very different physical characteristics, which have different performances both in decreasing contamination and in improving personnel comfort. Cotton allows wet strike-through contamination, making direct contact with non-sterile underwear; this could release many small particles into the air, but their role in airborne contamination is controversial [10, 14]. However, reduction in air contamination is not always reflected in minor wound contamination [28]. Whole body exhaust ventilated suits are mandatory in an ultraclean operating room with laminar flow [30], and advisable in a conventionally-ventilated clean theatre during prosthesis implants [1, 13].

GLOVES

Two pairs of gloves is a good rule, although not synonymous with a significantly-decreased infection risk either for patient or surgeon [3, 6, 26]. Outer latex gloves are perforated more often than inner gloves and the number of punctures increases when operations last longer than three hours. It is a good rule to periodically change the outer glove. The use of cotton cloth gloves seems to decrease the punctures of the inner latex gloves [6, 26].

SURGICAL TEAM

There are two different ways of managing nursing staff: a nurse may always work with the same team, or nurses may be interchangeable. The choice of a dedicated and steady team [21] is advisable, as only a well-trained team can reduce surgical times, thus decreasing airborne contamination risk. Non-specialised and non-dedicated personnel, lacking perfect familiarity with the surgical instruments, timing and the surgeon's preferences, will prolong surgical times, increasing movement in and out of the room, which may lead to poor surgery. Two specialised interchangeable nurses are needed: one attending to instruments, the other to their preparation. If the operating block is in a teaching hospital, the presence of surgical and nursing students must be planned, placing the students beside a more experienced tutor.

At this point, the term "atraumatic surgery" must be introduced; it may seem a "nonsense" word, but it well describes the rapid, effective, good surgery that only a good team can ensure. Schaefer and Helmreich [27] reported on "the importance of human factors in the operating room", and recommended training and educating surgical teams using "Medical Resource Management", a protocol adapted from that used in aviation. They conclude that recognising the importance of human factors in medical work will allow cost-effective high-quality health care.

Music in the operating theatre could also improve surgery: it has been demonstrated [31] that familiar music reduces stress and improves staff performance... if the staff all have the same musical tastes!

ORGANISATION AND RESPONSIBILITY FOR THE OPERATING BLOCK

All the aforementioned rules, culminating with formation of the surgical team, require centralised organisation and responsibility, as well as co-ordination of hospital policies and economic choices; these cannot be limited to the operating block alone. The operating team must be selected on the basis of specific training and learning of maintenance and discipline protocols; other criteria must be excluded. Therefore, it follows that the surgeon's liability, when the unfortunate outcome is an infection, is highly debatable. When the surgeon is a simple manual operator, working in a badly-organised block where maintenance, servicing and ventilation controls are not routinely scheduled and performed, the responsibility should be shifted to the hospital management.

Design

Designing operating theatres is commonly seen as the job of specialised architects and engineers. Surgeons and nurses, i.e. those who will eventually work there, are seldom involved in the projects. The results may sometimes be quite unsatisfactory, as shown by Holton [7], who also advocates the involvement of the microbiologist for effective monitoring of theatre commissioning and upgrading [8]. In the authors' experience, mistakes are quite frequent, especially in the lack of medical supervision. We have seen brand-new theatres with swinging doors, instead of automatic sliding doors, corridors and passages so narrow as to be a problem for large patients with multiple external fixation devices, and toilets near the operating room. The most frequent deficiencies concern the ventilation system and are difficult to detect: continuous monitoring of positive pressure is rarely seen; maintenance and servicing are often not performed on schedule ... when a schedule does indeed exist! We have seen filters fitted back to front, poor final cleaning, poor sealing of ventilation ducting, poor or no sealing of windows. Even double-glazing needs to be silicon-sealed, as wind pressure may be higher than the positive pressure of clean air in the operating room. We have also seen some curious technical choices which are not optimal from a cost-effective point of view: Italian marble for the wash-basins in Germany and German stainless steel basins in Italy!

GENERAL DESIGN RULES

■ *Where to place the operating room?*

The best location is a less congested area of the hospital, not too far from the intensive care unit or the laboratory. Should the operating room be underground or at the top of the building? Although underground theatres eliminate the problem of perfectly-sealed double-glazing, working in such an environment may be psychologically distressing. Being able to look outside, while waiting for the next operation and having a cup of tea or coffee, is a relaxing factor. Furthermore, when the operating block is on the top floor, it is easier to have a dedicated ventilation system [9].

■ *Entry to the operating room*

Patients

Patients must be moved from the wards by means of dedicated lifts, reserved strictly for this purpose. The bed is stopped at the border between the "dirty" and "clean" area. Transfer to the clean area is preferably done by the aid of a "tapis roulant", working without any manual aid; the transfer window remains open just long enough for transfer. The patient, covered only with a disposable paper gown and wearing a standard head cover, is transferred to a stretcher or directly to the operating bed which is then moved to the anaesthesia room. Be sure when choosing such a system that your hospital beds are not longer than the pass-through! Nevertheless, the transfer area is a controversial choice. If the aim is prevention of floor bacterial contamination, dedicated trolleys which are regularly washed (especially the wheels!) seem more comfortable and effective; if the aim is to restrict the access to essential persons, the transfer area is mandatory [9]. A recent paper demonstrated the benefits, in terms of increased efficiency and reduced manual handling, of accompanied walking of unpremedicated patients into the operating theatre [32].

Personnel

Male and female dressing rooms with enough space to lock clothing and shoes must be available. This is the most contaminated area and should be in negative pressure with the clean area. The presence of one or two simple sinks for hand washing before leaving the dressing room is a must. Enough toilets and showers should also be available. To avoid walking bare foot, disposable plastic bags can be used to reach the clean area where clean boots or clogs are ready.

■ *Special design features*

Special features, such as one-way doors, will discourage staff from by-passing procedures and ensure they follow the correct way to enter the clean area. However, wide emergency exits must be planned as escape routes, as well as to allow passage of large and heavy machines, such as a C-arm image intensifier. Obviously, this machine should not be moved outside the operating department unless absolutely necessary (servicing, for example).

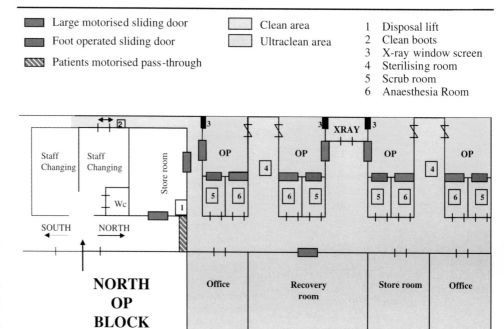

Legend:
- ▭ Large motorised sliding door
- ▭ Foot operated sliding door
- ▨ Patients motorised pass-through
- ▢ Clean area
- ▢ Ultraclean area

1 Disposal lift
2 Clean boots
3 X-ray window screen
4 Sterilising room
5 Scrub room
6 Anaesthesia Room

1 *Lay-out of an ideal operating block, very similar to the one now in use at the Centro Traumatologico Ortopedico of Turin.*

Significant quantities of waste material are produced by an orthopaedic operating room, especially if disposable garments are used. All of this used material is to be considered contaminated and should be disposed of through a dedicated pathway which does not interfere with the clean areas.

CONVENTIONAL OPERATING ROOM DESIGN

The preparation room should allow at least three people to scrub at the same time, while anaesthesia is induced in a near-by room (and not in the theatre!). A glass wall might allow for some "silent" communication. The orthopaedic operating room needs to be large enough to allow for at least two teams operating on the same patient, a traction bed and C-arm intensifier, i.e. no less than 5 x 7 m. The height of the ceiling must allow mounting of the ventilation system. Extra space must be left if vertical laminar air flow is to be mounted. On the contrary, extra horizontal space must be considered in the case of horizontal laminar air flow, which is less expensive, but also dangerous if not properly used [25], and no longer advisable (see Addendum). The door should be large and slide horizontally to avoid air turbulence and to allow transfer of beds or machines. A swinging door is not acceptable in this area. Electrically-driven doors (easily passing to "manual"), which close automatically, avoid the risk of a door left open; the switch should be foot-operated. X-rays can be handed from outside using an X-ray screen hinged like a window opened from outside, while a well-sealed glass keeps this "opening" closed from inside. Walls, floor and ceiling should be as smooth as possible with rounded corners. When choosing the type of floor, the type of beds to be used must be considered, i.e. old and

heavy or new. Modern beds, such as the ones with a pillar fixed to the floor, are compatible with the usual plastic flooring without risk of damage, as they have large, wide wheels. Stainless steel covered walls may be ideal, but are also quite expensive. The ceiling must be capable of supporting the extra weight of any heavy equipment to be hung, which allows easy cleaning of the floor. The proposed layout (*fig 1*) of an arrangement of up to eight theatres is very similar to the one now in use at the Centro Traumatologico Ortopedico of Turin. The need for separate clean and dirty corridors was not accepted. "This requirement was based on beliefs and theories that have not been vindicated by subsequent experience, and separate clean and dirty corridors are no longer a design requirement." [4]

Another controversial issue is the theatre sterile supply unit (TSSU) or the central sterile supply department (CSSD). The hospital management is obviously in favour of the CSSD for economic reasons; however orthopaedic surgeons do not always agree: " ...several hospitals hire orthopaedic sets for procedures that require specific instruments" [4].

NON-CONVENTIONAL OPERATING ROOMS

In the last two decades, specialised industries have optimised construction of operating rooms by using pre-built modules. Construction time is reduced as is the risk of "mistakes". The project is adapted to the bare area that the hospital has chosen for the operating suite, and the theatres are built and purchased "key in hand", ready for use. A new proposal is to place multiple enclosures with vertical laminar air flow in a large area, without walls; this allows easy movements of personnel and patient, without risk of contaminating the clean enclosures. Special equipment is available for sterilisation of the operating bed and the patient's bed.

GENERAL HOSPITALS WITH COMMON THEATRE SUITES FOR ALL TYPES OF SURGERY

Special problems arise in connection with the dangerous presence of urological, colorectal and other surgery where the consequences of infection are not so catastrophic as in orthopaedic surgery. The problems are not only technical (i.e. connected to the need to avoid contamination from dirty to clean areas) and the most dangerous and common contamination concerns the habits and discipline of the staff, including anaesthesiologists. The operating room dedicated to bone and joint surgery should be in the least congested area and should never be used for other surgical activities. Due to the dangerous proximity of other theatres not dedicated to clean orthopaedic surgery, a ultraclean air ventilation system might be preferable to conventional operating rooms.

SPECIALISED HOSPITALS FOR ORTHOPAEDICS AND TRAUMA

The special problems which arise here concern trauma and septic surgery. More than 30 years' experience in such a hospital leads to the following statement: trauma surgery should not interfere with elective and planned orthopaedic surgery. The best solution is to have dedicated operating rooms in the emergency department working day and night. In this case, having three operating rooms, one can be dedicated to emergency surgery, including hip fractures in the elderly, one is reserved for neurosurgical emergencies, and the third for delayed trauma surgery. Conventional ventilation with high efficiency particulate filters (HEPA filters) and positive pressure may be sufficient. The general lay-out of this operating suite does not differ from the dedicated elective surgery suite; the anaesthesia induction room is particularly essential in trauma surgery to prepare the injured patient, who frequently comes directly from the emergency side, in the correct way. The operating suites for elective orthopaedic surgery should be located far from the emergency department. Although expensive, the optimal choice is the non-conventional theatre with multiple laminar air flow enclosures. Six theatres with conventional ventilation (i.e. positive pressure, 30-40 air exchanges per hour and HEPA filters) can also be acceptable, provided that design and devices are optimised and discipline is respected. One extra operating room dedicated to septic surgery in strict proximity to the septic department, as far away as possible from emergency and elective surgery rooms,

should be available. Operating room and instrument decontamination, including the X-ray image intensifier, after each septic operation is obtained by means of accurate washing and correct ventilation through HEPA filters.

Devices

VENTILATION

Ventilation is necessary for staff comfort and to clean the air of the operating room micro-environment and eliminate the airborne BCP which enter with the patient and personnel. Clearly, even the most sophisticated and expensive system will never cut air contamination down to zero; furthermore, costs rise with air quality. The zero infection rate is not only expensive, but also an impossible dream. This can be translated into mathematical formulas: "I" infection rate as a function of "P" number of persons in the operating room, "T" operating time and "V" ventilation (number of air exchanges per hour): $I = PxT/V$.

■ *Conventional ventilation*

External air is pre-filtered to around 80% and then pumped to the operating room through HEPA filters. The exchange rate is rather low, 20-30 times per hour, and in operational conditions, the BCP/m^3 may exceed 100. When the system is off, the BCP/m^3 can rise to over 1,000, depending on the number of people in the room. Filtered air distribution is quite critical, the main problems being turbulence and noise. Frequent control of the pre-filters and final HEPA filters is essential. Even with efficient pre-filtration, the HEPA filters must be changed periodically. An excellent and easy way to check the filters is continuous measurement of positive pressure, using instruments mounted in the theatre. When the initial 20 mm H_2O of positive pressure increases to 35-40 or more, it is time to change. If the system is efficient and a positive pressure of 16-20 mm H_2O is maintained, even such conventional ventilation can be acceptable for orthopaedic surgery, with an infection rate around 1%, provided that the 5D rules are respected. Routine microbiological sampling should not be necessary, unless there is evidence of filter leakage [2]. On the contrary, bacteriological sampling analysis is mandatory in ultraclean theatres [10]. Ultraviolet radiation has limited indications [17].

■ *Clean air and ultraclean air rooms*

A greenhouse enclosure with vertical laminar air flow was first used by John Charnley, where a positive pressure area of unidirectional air flow allows for a change rate of 400 times or more per hour of air filtered through HEPA filters. This maintains

very low BCP/m^3 levels, i.e. less than 20 at the periphery of the clean area, less than 10 at 30 cm from the operating field. If hoods with a body exhaust system are also used, with occlusive garments, even lower BCP/m^3 levels can be reached, i.e. less than 1 BCP/m^3 at the operating field and less than 10 at the periphery of the enclosure. Clinical results are good [18], but the global costs of such a system are high (purchase cost, servicing and power consumption) and a 0.5-1% decrease in infection rate hardly justifies these costs. Furthermore, demonstration of the factors able to further reduce the incidence of infection to below 0.5% would mean a study population exceeding 10,000 in each group [16]. One last consideration: pumping air means to heat it, as anybody pumping the tyres of a bicycle knows; to maintain 20-21° C and 50% humidity requires the installation of quite powerful conditioning machines. Exposed to this air flow at a speed of 1m/second, the patient's tissues are usually dried and must be very frequently irrigated; this factor might also contribute to decreasing the infection rate: "dilution is solution for pollution...", provided the surgeon knows and prevents the risk of self contamination [23].

■ *European and American Standards*

At the time of writing (1998), some European countries have fixed standards for the ventilation and maximum acceptable BCP/m^3 concentrations [24]. In some countries, such as Italy, only the physical parameters of air have been fixed, i.e. the number of exchanges per hour, positive pressure HEPA filters, temperature and humidity. Furthermore, to date, there is no standardised method to evaluate and classify conventional, clean or ultraclean air operating rooms. Even the terminology is controversial: BCP (airborne bacteria carrying particles) or CFU (colony forming units)? In the USA, the American Academy of Orthopaedic Surgeons has proposed its own classification according to the number of CFU/ft^3, different from the Federal Standard 209E of 1992. Class 1 corresponds to 1 CFU/ft^3 (35/m^3), class 5 corresponds to 5 CFU/ft^3 (175/m^3), and class 20 corresponds to 20/ft^3 (700/m^3). The European Community has not yet worked out rules to be endorsed by all countries. According to the American Academy, at least 3 classes of operating rooms should be considered, ranging from the ultraclean room to the conventional one.

POWER SUPPLY

Electrical power tools connected to the main supply have been largely replaced by compressed air tools. The latter usually need no less than 8 Atm of pressure to work correctly. However, some high speed drills need higher pressures, and it does not seem acceptable to bring gas cylinders close to the operating room. No exhaust gas (air or nitrogen) coming from these tools may remain in the operating room. These gases, along with the anaesthesia gases, must be aspirated outside through special pipes. Pressurised nitrogen might be preferable as it is dry and sterile. Heavy-duty battery driven tools have also been proposed, but have not found general acceptance, even if no surgeon has ever published anything on the benefits of battery or electric power versus pneumatic power. Now, it has been suggested to move away from air power, as these instruments require more maintenance, and may cause unsterile air emission on the sterile field. In addition, their speed is not as variable as that of electric tools, and their power is lower.

An electrical supply must have different voltages, from 24 Volts to power an electrical operating bed to 117 Volts if US-made instruments are used. The standard 220 Volts is the main supply for the majority of European electrical instruments, while a three-phase 400 Volt supply is needed for some powerful lasers. Experience shows the electrical supply is often insufficient for all equipment routinely used in modern orthopaedic surgery. Here is a short list of the most common instruments and facilities which require a power supply, either electrical or pneumatic:

– aspirators (at least three: two for surgery, one for anaesthesiology);

– electrocoagulator and bipolar electrocoagulator;

– VCR, cold light and pulse pump for arthroscopy;

– C-arm image intensifier;

– infusion pumps;

– blood cell saver;

– operating computer-assisted surgery microscope and TV screen;

– outlets for headlights and TV cameras;

– equipment to heat the patient or transfusion fluids;

– at least two pressurised gas outlets and a spare one, necessary when two teams are operating simultaneously on the same patient;

– "viva voce" phone;

– computer terminal;

– at least 2 vacuum outlets;

– water outlet.

A total of 15 to 20 power supply outlets is not to be considered exaggerated, even if not all the aforementioned instrumentation will ever be used at the same time. Anaesthesiology equipment is not considered, as it is usually mounted and power-supplied in one single hanging unit.

Finally, it should not be forgotten that now all instruments must be European Community registered and that very strict safety regulations exist in the EEC for all electrical equipment and outlets. Non-compliance may be considered a criminal offence, for which the physicians may also be held responsible.

Conclusion

At this point a surgeon may well ask: all this is correct, but what can I do in practice in my hospital, where, for example, no ventilation system exists and reality differs from the rules?

Risk for personnel and patients will always be present, in operating rooms as in other environments, and can never be zero. The problem is to quantify the risks and determine how they could be lowered. We suggest adopting the method of risk analysis, now mainly used in work safety evaluations. This consists of the following steps: 1) identification of risk factors (R); 2) analysis of the value of the damage (D) eventually caused by the risk factor absence; 3) analysis of the probabilities (P) that the damage will take place, in the absence of the risk factor. The last two steps could be quantified with a relative value, ranging from 1 to 5. With this same method, the discipline or sliding automatic doors and all other risk factors can be analysed, obtaining the relative R values. The priorities for intervention in each hospital will be identified according to the R analysis list, providing that there is a standard risk analysis for comparison. The risk analysis must eventually be compared with the financial supports and time limits. Ideally, without financial and time limits, all rules listed in the text could be applied; in practice, an operating block cannot remain closed for long periods, as the public service cannot be interrupted, and financial resources are never unlimited. Choices must be made, and that is why the risk analysis is mandatory. It is possible that the surgeons and the management of an older hospital will decide that the only possible intervention to improve the operating theatre is the training and information of personnel, because no time or financial support are available, and the risk values are acceptable (for example, because in the operating room only minor hand surgery is performed). On the contrary, if prosthetic surgery is to be performed, the risks would be *very high, and therefore it would be mandatory to modify, for example, the ventilation system.*

Addendum

A warm and grateful thank you to P. Bartolozzi, G. Bentley, M.A.R. Freeman, R. Ganz, R. Giacometti Ceroni, J. Harms, I. Kempf, F. Langlais, P.G. Marchetti, E. Morscher, G. Peretti, W. Puhl.

The following three questions have been put to a restricted number of colleagues and friends, and their answers have been of great help:

– Have you had any influence in building or renovating your operating rooms?

– In your opinion, which are the wrong choices and which are the right ones?

– If you had a new operating room, how would you like it to be?

All agreed that the surgeon should be involved in the planning from the beginning, but only if he has enough experience to formulate the requirements. Unfortunately, only a few were in fact involved and in most cases only partially; their influence in the decision-making seems to have been proportional to their hierarchical level at the time of planning. The need for a separate theatre dedicated to septic cases is felt to be of the utmost importance, as is the separation between elective orthopaedic surgery and trauma. The movement of the anaesthesiologists in different (more or less clean) areas seems to be a common problem. Another common complaint is that the air-conditioning plant is not powerful enough to face extreme conditions on very hot days. Lack of space is also a common complaint: some of the instruments must be stored inside the theatres, which is absolutely unacceptable. The problem of space will increase further with telesurgery. As to laminar air flow, experience with horizontal flow is widely considered to be negative. Vertical flow, even if considered the best option in combination with good theatre technique, conventional modern clothing and antibiotic prophylaxis, seems to be a real must only or especially in teaching hospitals. Among the European surgeons collaborating in this small inquiry, only one has claimed that his operation facilities are optimal, without any defect or failure, and has stated he could not ask for anything better.

References ➤

References

[1] Ahl T, Dalen N, Jörbeck H, Hoborn J. Air contamination during hip and knee arthroplasties. Horizontal laminar flow randomised versus conventional ventilation. *Acta Orthop Scand* 1995 ; 66 : 17-20

[2] Babb JR, Lynam P, Ayliffe GA. Risk of airborne transmission in an operating theatre containing four ultraclean air units. *J Hosp Infect* 1995 ; 31 : 159-168

[3] Dodds RD, Barker SG, Morgan NH, Donaldson DR, Thomas MH. Self protection in surgery: the use of double gloves. *Br J Surg* 1990 ; 77 : 219-220

[4] Essex-Lopresti M. Operating theatre design. *Lancet* 1999 ; 353 : 1007-1010

[5] Gallinaro P. La difesa delle infezioni in sala operatoria. Significato della ristrutturazione del complesso operatorio del CTO. Torino : Giornale dell'Accademia di Medicina, 1981 : 1-19

[6] Hester RA, Nelson CL, Harrison S. Control of contamination of the operative team in total joint arthroplasty. *J Arthroplasty* 1992 ; 7 : 267-269

[7] Holton J, Ridgway GL. Commissioning operating theatres. *J Hosp Infect* 1993 ; 23 : 153-160

[8] Holton J, Ridgway GL, Reynoldson AJ. A microbiologist's view of commissioning operating theatres. *J Hosp Infect* 1990 ; 16 : 29-34

[9] Humphreys H. Infection control and the design of a new operating theatre suite. *J Hosp Infect* 1993 ; 23 : 61-70

[10] Humphreys H. Theatre air and operating conditions. *J Hosp Infect* 1995 ; 31 : 154-155

[11] Humphreys H, Lewis D, Reeves D. Why isolate theatre suites? *Lancet* 1991 ; 337 : 178

[12] Humphreys H, Russel AJ, Marshall RJ, Ricketts VE, Reeves DS. The effect of surgical theatre head-gear on air bacterial counts. *J Hosp Infect* 1991 ; 19 : 175-180

[13] Humphreys H, Stacey AR, Taylor EW. Survey of operating theatres in Great Britain and Ireland. *J Hosp Infect* 1995 ; 30 : 245-252

[14] Jalovaara P, Puranen J. Air bacterial and particle counts in total hip replacement operations using non-woven and cotton gowns and drapes. *J Hosp Infect* 1989 ; 14 : 333-338

[15] Joubert JD. Conception des blocs opératoires [2e éd]. Cahiers antipollution. COMIPRIM Lyon : 1980

[16] Learmonth ID. Prevention of infection in the1990s. *Orthop Clin North Am* 1993 ; 24 : 735-741

[17] Lidwell OM. Ultraviolet radiation and the control of airborne contamination in the operating theatre. *J Hosp Infect* 1994 ; 28 : 245-248

[18] Lidwell OM, Elson RA, Lowbury EJ, Whyte W, Blowers R, Stanley SJ et al. Ultraclean air and antibiotics for prevention of postoperative infection. A multicenter study of 8,052 joint replacement operations. *Acta Orthop Scand* 1987 ; 58 : 4-13

[19] Lotens WA, Van DeLinde FJ, Havenith G. Effects of condensation in clothing on heat transfer. *Ergonomics* 1995 ; 38 : 1114-1131

[20] Mitchell NJ, Hunt S. Surgical face masks in modern operating rooms: a costly and unnecessary ritual? *J Hosp Infect* 1991 ; 18 : 239-242

[21] Nercessian OA, Joshi RP. General principles of surgical technique. In : Callaghan JJ, Rosenberg AG, Rubash HE eds. The adult hip. Philadelphia : Lippincott-Raven, 1998 : 951-958

[22] Perceval A. Theatre overshoes and operating theatre floor bacterial counts *J Hosp Infect* 1991 ; 19 : 283-284

[23] Quebbeman EJ, Telford GL, Hubbard S, Wadsworth K, Hardman B, Goodman H et al. Risk of blood contamination and injury to operating room personnel. *Ann Surg* 1991 ; 214 : 614-620

[24] Sacchi E. Stato dell'impiantistica di climatizzazione in sale operatorie ad alto rischio di infezioni. *Minerva Ortop Traumatol* 1998 ; 49 : 91-118

[25] Salvati EA, Robinson RP, Zeno SM, Koslin BL, Brause BD, Wilson PD Jr. Infection rates after 3175 total hip and total knee replacements performed with and without a horizontal unidirectional filtered air-flow system. *J Bone Joint Surg Am* 1982 ; 64 : 525-535

[26] Sanders R, Fortin P, Ross E, Helfet D. Outer gloves in orthopaedic procedures. *J Bone J Surg Am* 1990 ; 72 : 914-917

[27] Schaefer HG, Helmreich RL. The importance of human factors in the operating room. *Anesthesiology* 1994 ; 80 : 479

[28] Scheibel JH, Jensen I, Pedersen S. Bacterial contamination of air and surgical wounds during joint replacement operations. Comparison of two different types of staff clothing. *J Hosp Infect* 1991 ; 19 : 167-174

[29] Smith RC, Mooar PA, Cooke T, Sherk HH. Contamination of operating room personnel during total arthroplasty. *Clin Orthop* 1991 ; 271 : 9-11

[30] Taylor GJ, Bannister GC. Infection and interposition between ultraclean air source and wound. *J Bone Joint Surg Br* 1993 ; 75 : 503-504

[31] Thompson JF, Kam PC. Music in the operating theatre. *Br J Surg* 1995 ; 82 : 1586-1587

[32] Turnbull LA, Wood N, Kester G. Controlled trial of the subjective patient benefits of accompanied walking to the operating theatre. *Int J Clin Pract* 1998 ; 52 : 81-83

Anaesthesia and analgesia in orthopaedic surgery

B Remy
M Lamy

Abstract. – *Regional anaesthesia either alone or in combination with general anaesthesia can be performed in orthopaedic surgery. The pain experienced after major orthopaedic surgery is among the most intense postoperatively. It is now recognised that pain can have a considerable influence, usually negative, on recovery from these physiological perturbations. The quality and timing of the pain is that of an inflammatory source. The concept of pre-emptive and balanced analgesia is now recognised. Opioid agonists, non steroidal anti-inflammatory drugs (NSAIDs), local anaesthetics and inhibitors of excitatory amino acid neurotransmission (NMDA antagonists) may be used for the management of acute pain in orthopaedic surgery.*

Keywords: anaesthesia, analgesia, local anaesthesia, regional anaesthesia, general anaesthesia.

Introduction

Anaesthesia for orthopaedic surgery is one of the most varied to be found. Both general anaesthesia (GA) and regional anaesthesia (RA) can be used for this type of surgery. A pre-anaesthetic consultation is the ideal moment to discuss the advantages and disadvantages of the various forms of anaesthetic with the patient. The critical factors in making the decision for or against a given technique are the patient's wishes, his or her medical history, and the experience of the anaesthesiologist.

Regional anaesthesia

Surgery itself induces a series of reactions in the body, including an endocrinal and a metabolic response corresponding to a stress reaction [18, 33, 41].

Epidural anaesthesia can attenuate the response to surgical stress. The time course of postoperative pain is improved, allowing for earlier ambulation. This may be associated with a shorter hospital stay, a reduced incidence of complications (especially cardiopulmonary) [37], and improved cognitive function. Regional anaesthesia reduces blood loss and may

Bernadette Remy, M.D.
Maurice Lamy, M.D.
Department of Anaesthesia and Intensive Care Medicine, University Hospital of Liège, Domaine Universitaire du Sart Tilman - B35, 4000 Liège, Belgium.

prevent thromboembolism. It can be applied to a wide variety of orthopaedic surgical procedures involving the hips, pelvis and distal lower extremities.

EPIDURAL ANAESTHETIC TECHNIQUE

The Tuohy needle (either 17 or 18G) is perfectly adapted to this technique. The patient can be either seated or in the lateral decubitus position, depending on the proposed surgery, the patient's habits, and the experience of the anaesthesiologist. In the lumbar area, the most frequently used interspaces are L2-L3 and L3-L4 [15]. A catheter is inserted five centimetres into the epidural space. A test dose of three millilitres of 1% lidocaine with adrenaline (1/200,000) is injected via the catheter to elicit signs of a sensory-motor block in the lower extremities, or of an intravenous placement of the catheter. The anaesthetic itself is started with the injection of a bolus of 10 ml of 0.5% bupivacaine (Marcaine®) or 0.5% ropivicaine (Naropin®) [5, 12]. Both these agents produce anaesthesia with a rapid onset and a duration of approximately 200 minutes. In order to increase the duration of the sensory block, either opioids (Fentanyl®, Sufentanil®) and/or α_2-mimetic (clonidine) [11, 26, 27] can be added.

TECHNIQUE OF SPINAL ANAESTHESIA

Spinal anaesthesia is the most common regional anaesthetic technique applied to orthopaedic surgery. Several types of spinal

needles are available on the market; the choice of needle will depend, among other factors, on the patient's age. In our hospital, we always use small gauge needles (25 or 27G) with pencil points for young adults. These needles are associated with a reduced incidence of post-dural puncture headache. For patients older than 70 years, we use 22 gauge needles.

Local anaesthetic can be injected as a "single shot", with the needle withdrawn after the injection, or continuously via a catheter placed in the subarachnoid space. A continuous technique allows more precise control of the duration and of the extension of the spinal block, using repeated small doses of local anaesthetic. Improved haemodynamic tolerance to the spinal block can result from use of a catheter technique. It should be noted, however, that because of the prolonged exposure of nervous tissue to the local anaesthetic, medullary toxicity can result [19]. This usually takes the form of a cauda equina syndrome, with an estimated incidence of 1 in 1000 spinal anaesthetics.

Bupivacaine is the most frequently used local anaesthetic. When single boluses are injected, we administer the following mixture: 4 ml hyperbaric 0.5% bupivacaine, with 5 μg Sufentanil® and 150 μg clonidine. Three ml of this solution is injected. The latency of action is approximately five to ten minutes. The duration of the anaesthetic varies between 180 and 480 minutes. After the anaesthetic agent is injected, the upper level of the block is monitored. Extension of the block is usually finished after 30 minutes, but later changes in the level can occur.

When continuous spinal anaesthesia is planned, we either use plain hyperbaric 0.5% bupivacaine, at an initial dose of 1.5 ml, followed by "top-ups" of 1 ml when the block begins to regress or on emergence of postoperative pain, or the same mixture mentioned above.

TECHNIQUE OF SEQUENTIAL SPINAL-EPIDURAL ANAESTHESIA

This technique has been available for several years. It combines epidural analgesia with spinal anaesthesia [6, 36]. It involves a single puncture with a Tuohy needle used as an introducer for the spinal needle. Combining these two techniques allows the fast onset of sensory and motor blockade, the use of low doses of intrathecal anaesthetic (with fewer haemodynamic modifications), and continuation of postoperative analgesia via the epidural catheter. The local anaesthetics used, and their doses, are similar to those seen in the previously discussed techniques (spinal and epidural anaesthesia and analgesia). Complications of regional anaesthesia are severe hypotension, cardiac arrest [1, 24, 25], pain with placement of the block, risk of infection, injury to blood vessels (haematoma) or nerves, allergy and medullary toxicity [2].

TECHNIQUE OF REGIONAL BLOCKS

Regional techniques can provide preoperative pain relief, anaesthesia and analgesia intraoperatively and postoperative pain relief.

■ *Shoulder and upper extremity*

The choice of block depends on the site of surgery [42, 45]. A nerve stimulator is used with an appropriate insulated needle. In our institution, we administer 20 ml of 1% lidocaine and 20 ml of 0.5% bupivacaine. Sufentanil (10 μg) [44] and clonidine (150 μg) [43] can be added for increased effect and longer duration. Forty ml of 0.5% ropivacaine may also be used. The principal indication for interscalene block is surgery of the proximal upper extremity. Supraclavicular block can be applied to any surgical procedures. The main indication for axillary block is surgery of hand and wrist (*fig 1*). Intravenous regional anaesthesia can be applied to any procedure distal to the elbow, provided its expected duration is one hour or less and it allows for placing a small intravenous catheter in the distal vein on the dorsum of the hand. The volume injected is 3 mg/kg of 1% lidocaine or prilocaine.

■ *Lower extremity regional anaesthesia*

For the lower extremity, it is now common practice to use the "3 in 1" block which will block the lumbar plexus including the

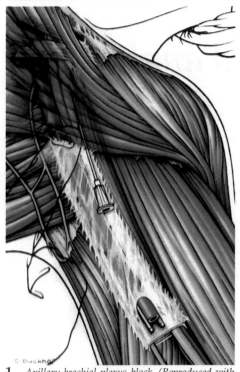

1 *Axillary brachial plexus block. (Reproduced with permission from Scott DB. Techniques of regional anaesthesia. New York : MediGlobe, 1989 : 1-224).*

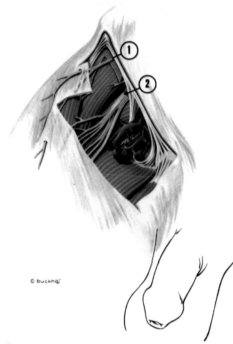

2 *"3 in 1" lumbar plexus blocks. 1. Lateral cutaneous nerve of the thigh; 2. femoral nerve. (Reproduced with permission from Scott DB. Techniques of regional anaesthesia. New York : MediGlobe, 1989 : 1-224).*

femoral, obturator and lateral cutaneous nerves. Combined femoral-sciatic nerve blocks are effective for lower extremity surgery (*fig 2*). Ankle block can be selected for surgery of the foot distal to the malleoli, especially in patients too sick for central block regional techniques. This block is ideally suited to outpatient surgery of the foot or toes (*fig 3, 4*). Caudal block is performed in children.

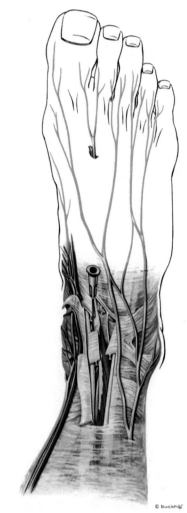

3 *Deep peroneal nerve block. (Reproduced with permission from Scott DB. Techniques of regional anaesthesia. New York : MediGlobe, 1989 : 1-224).*

Local anaesthesia

Local anaesthesia is a simple technique. It can be used for mildly painful surgery (knee arthroscopy, median nerve neurolysis, removal of minor orthopedic hardware, etc.). Local anaesthesia permits residual analgesia and short term hospitalisation. It is particularly suitable for day cases.

Local anaesthetics employed are lidocaine or prilocaine. Bupivacaine is used for arthroscopic surgery of the knee. Vasoconstrictors, particularly epinephrine, are frequently added to local anaesthetic solutions to prolong the duration of anaesthesia and reduce blood levels.

The most common potential source of toxicity when local anaesthesia is used is accidental intravascular injection. Cardiotoxicity and neurotoxicity may occur quickly. Allergic reactions are exceptional but can be lethal. Careful monitoring of the patient must be continuously provided in cases managed with local anaesthesia.

General anaesthesia

General anaesthesia can be used for all surgical indications. Newer agents,

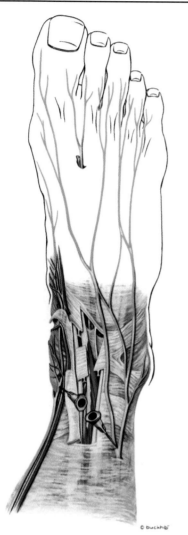

4 *Superficial peroneal and saphenous nerve block. (Reproduced with permission from Scott DB. Techniques of regional anaesthesia. New York : MediGlobe, 1989 : 1-224).*

characterised by short half-lives with rapid onset and offset of activity, probably improve the quality of the anaesthetic delivered. The advantages of GA are improved patient comfort in the perioperative period and rapid onset of effect. The disadvantages of this form of anaesthesia are related to its morbidity (which probably does not exceed 0.3%), to the respiratory depression which inevitably occurs, to the problem of postoperative nausea and vomiting (PONV), and that of difficult endotracheal intubation, especially frequent in patients with rheumatoid arthritis (who have a high incidence of atlanto-axial subluxation), or with ankylosing spondylitis, with decreased mobility of the cervical spine.

Blood sparing techniques

Many orthopaedic procedures (for example, total hip arthroplasty, scoliosis, arthrodeses, etc.) are associated with blood loss that is great enough to justify use of blood sparing techniques. Those most often used include

controlled hypotension, autologous predonation of blood, normovolaemic haemodilution, and recovery of blood shed into the surgical field. Various pharmacological methods for reducing transfusion requirements are also available. These include antifibrinolytics such as aprotinin (Trasylol®, 1 million IU as a loading dose, followed by 500,000 IU/h continuous infusion) and tranexamic acid (Exacyl®, 10 to 15 mg/kg as a single bolus at the start of surgery). Erythropoietin can be administered to increase the patient's red cell volume prior to operation. This drug requires several weeks to show its full effects. This is especially useful for Jehovah's Witnesses. It is given intravenously at a dose of 200 units/kg for three days, followed by 150 units/kg subcutaneously twice weekly for two weeks. It is always given in association with iron supplements (100 mg elemental iron/d) and folic acid (15 mg/d).

Deep venous thrombosis prophylaxis

Administration of low molecular weight heparin (LMWH) compounds significantly reduces the incidence of thromboembolic complications after orthopaedic surgery [17]. Prophylaxis with LMWH does not appear to increase the incidence of spinal bleeding when central nervous system blocks are used, provided that an interval of 10 to 12 hours has elapsed between administration of the LMWH and puncture. This same interval should be observed prior to removing an epidural or spinal catheter. The subsequent dose of LMWH should not be given until at least four hours after either puncture [46].

Postoperative analgesia

Pain is defined as an unpleasant sensory and emotional experience associated with real or potential tissue damage, or described as such [28, 29]. The pain experienced after major orthopaedic surgery is among the most intense seen postoperatively. It is noted at rest, with marked increases during mobilisation as well as during reflex muscular spasm. It is generally short-lived, with a maximum three to six hours postoperatively, decreasing to 36 hours. Consumption of major analgesics is almost nil after two days [38]. The concept of preemptive analgesia is to initiate treatment for pain before the painful stimulus is applied so as to prevent or reduce the subsequent pain experience [30, 40]. Administration of analgesics before the nociceptive stimulus is more effective than after it. The practice of balanced analgesia involves the use of several medications and techniques, each of which acts at a different site in the origin and transmission of postoperative pain [8, 21]. The goal is to improve the quality of the

analgesia. Balanced analgesia promotes an opiate sparing effect (which can be as much as 30% to 70% according to published studies) and reduces the incidence and intensity of secondary effects (which include nausea, vomiting, sedation, respiratory depression induced by opiates, motor block and orthostatic hypotension induced by regional analgesic techniques).

The most frequent analgesic combinations used are:

– combinations of non opiate analgesics (nonsteroidal anti-inflammatory drugs, paracetamol);

– opiates combined with non-opiate analgesics;

– local anaesthetics administered with opiates and/or α_2 adrenergic agonists by either local infiltration or by central neural blocks (epidural or spinal) or peripheral nerve blocks (brachial plexus, "3 in 1" block).

PERIPHERAL ANALGESICS

■ *Non-anti-inflammatory analgesics*

The antipyretic analgesics, including paracetamol and its precursor propacetamol (Prodafalgan®, which is available for intravenous injection) play an increasingly important role in the treatment of postoperative pain [9]. Their analgesic potency can be compared to that of aspirin. The absence of gastrointestinal, renal, and coagulation effects place these compounds on the front line for this indication, either alone or combined with opiates and/or a regional anaesthetic technique [13, 23]. Excellent tolerance allows systematic administration every six hours. Doses are reduced, or the medication avoided, in patients with hepatic insufficiency. Several preparations are available for oral administration which combine paracetamol with aspirin and/or a mild opiate (codeine, dextropropoxyphen). These are useful when parenteral analgesics are to be discontinued after the first few hours postoperatively.

■ *Non-steroidal anti-inflammatory drugs (NSAIDs)*

The NSAIDs reduce both the inflammatory reaction as well as the oedema seen postoperatively. After major orthopaedic surgery, the NSAIDs have a ceiling effect, and are not sufficient by themselves [21]. These drugs must be administered with caution, if at all, to patients with renal insufficiency, active gastric or duodenal ulcers, or allergies. The most frequently used NSAIDs for postoperative analgesia are diclofenac (Voltaren®), ketoprofen (Rofenid®), indomethacin (Indocid®), ketorolac (Toradol®), and acetylsalicylic acid. These can be administered by oral, rectal, intramuscular, and intravenous routes.

OPIATES

■ *Patient-controlled analgesia (PCA)*

The opiates are major analgesics [3, 4]. The administration of opiates via a specialised PCA apparatus can be extremely useful. The patient can self-administer small boluses of opiate according to his needs [22, 48]. These pumps can also be used to self-administer local anaesthetic (with or without adjuvant medications) into an epidural catheter. Most pumps can also be programmed to provide a baseline continuous infusion. Numerous studies have shown that such infusions do not improve the quality of analgesia and increase overall opiate consumption, with a consequent rise in the incidence of side effects. In order to use PCA, the patient must be able to understand the technique, be sufficiently awake to operate the button, and must not have any physical hindrances which prevent him from using the machine. The technique is applicable to children, starting at approximately six to seven years of age [14]. Only the patient must push the button requesting analgesic (this is especially important with children). Most teams caring for paediatric patients add a baseline infusion to the PCA for the first 24 to 36 hours.

■ *Tramadol (Contramal®, Dolzam®)*

Tramadol is an analgesic with combined opioid agonist and monoamine re-uptake blocker properties [16, 35]. Tramadol's affinity for μ opioid receptors is 600 times weaker than that of morphine. This results in two clinically useful properties: a virtual absence of respiratory depression [20, 47], and a very low risk of tolerance [32, 34]. The most frequently noted side effects are nausea, vomiting, headache, and dizziness [7]. Analgesic effects start less than one hour after oral administration and reach a peak at two to three hours. The duration of effect is approximately six hours. Tramadol can be administered intravenously (50 to 200 mg q 8 h), via PCA (0.35 to 0.5 mg/kg/h), epidurally (100 mg/dose), intra-articularly (10 mg), by mouth (50 to 200 mg q 8 h) with good results.

INHIBITORS OF EXCITATORY AMINO ACID NEUROTRANSMISSION

Ketamine and MgSO$_4$ are two NMDA antagonists [10]. The intravenous administration of ketamine or MgSO$_4$ before surgery can reduce the doses of morphine, local anaesthetics and NSAIDs [39, 49]. 0.1 mg/kg ketamine during the preoperative period is prescribed for reducing phantom pain after amputation [31].

Conclusion

Major progress in anaesthesia has improved the comfort and the security of both the patient and surgeon. The decision for one anaesthetic technique (general or regional anaesthesia) is indicated by the surgical technique, the intensity of pain and the emotional behaviour of the patient. Optimal results in pain relief may be achieved by several treatments such as systemic NSAIDs, opioids and clonidine. Patient controlled analgesia and regional anaesthesia improve the patient's outcome.

References

[1] Auroy Y, Bargues L, Samii K. Épidémiologie des complications des anesthésies locorégionales. Paris : MAPAR édition, 1998 : 129-140

[2] Auroy Y, Narchi P, Messiah A, Litt L, Rouvier B, Samii K. Serious complications related to regional anaesthesia, results of a prospective survey in France. *Anesthesiology* 1997 ; 87: 479-486

[3] Basbaum A, Fields H. Endogenous pain control systems: brainstem spinal pathways and endorphin circuitry. *Annu Rev Neurosci* 1984 ; 7 : 303-338

[4] Besson JM, Chaouch A. Peripheral and spinal mechanisms of nociception. *Physiol Rev* 1990 ; 87 : 67-186

[5] Brown DL, Carpenter RL, Thompson GE. Comparison of 0,5% Ropivacaine and 0,5% bupivacaine for epidural anaesthesia in patients undergoing lower-extremity surgery. *Anesthesiology* 1990 ; 72 : 633-636

[6] Carrie LE, O'Sullivan GM. Subarachnoid bupivacaine 0.5% for cesarean section. *Eur J Anesthesiol* 1984 ; 1 : 275-283

[7] Cossmann M, Wilsmann KM. Effect and side effects of tramadol. *Therapiewoche* 1987 ; 37 : 3475-3485

[8] Dahl JB, Rosenberg J, Dirkes WE, Mogensen T, Kehlet H. Prevention of postoperative pain by balanced analgesia. *Br J Anaesth* 1990 ; 64 : 518-520

[9] Delbos A, Boccard E. The morphine sparing effect of propacetamol in orthopaedic postoperative pain. *J Pain Symptom Manage* 1995 ; 10 : 279-286

[10] Dickenson AH. A cure for wind up: NMDA receptor antagonists as potential analgesics. *Trends Pharmacol Sci* 1990 ; 11 : 307-309

[11] Eisenach JC, Lysak SZ, Viscomi CM. Epidural clonidine analgesia following surgery: phase I. *Anesthesiology* 1989 ; 71 : 640-646

[12] Erichsen CJ, Sjövall J, Kehlet H, Hedlund C, Arvidsson T. Pharmacokinetics and analgesic effect of ropivacaine during continuous epidural infusion for postoperative pain relief. *Anesthesiology* 1996 ; 84 : 834-842

[13] Fowler PD. Aspirine, paracetamol and non steroidal anti-inflammatory drugs. A comparative review of side effects. *Med Toxicol* 1987 ; 2 : 338-366

[14] Gaukroger PB, Chapman MJ, Davey RB. Pain control in paediatric burns - the use of patient controlled analgesia. *Burns* 1991 ; 17 : 396-399

[15] Gauthier-Lafaye P. Précis d'anesthésie loco-régionale. Paris : Masson, 1985 : 1-336

[16] Gentili ME, Estebe JP. Utilisation clinique du tramadol. Paris : MAPAR édition, 1998 : 233-241

[17] Gogarten W. Regional anaesthesia and thromboembolism prophylaxis / anticoagulation. *Anaesth Intensive Med* 1997 ; 12 : 623-628

[18] Goschke H, Bar E, Girard J, Leutenbergyer A, Niederer W, Oberholzer M et al. Glucagon, insulin, cortisol and growth hormone levels following major surgery: their relationship to glucose and free-fatty acid elevation. *Horm Metab Res* 1978 ; 10 : 465-470

[19] Horlocker TT, McGregor DG, Matsushige DK, Chantigian RC, Schroeder DR, Besse JA, and the perioperative outcomes group. Neurologic complications of 603 consecutive continuous spinal anaesthetics using macrocatheter and microcatheter techniques. *Anesth Analg* 1997 ; 84 : 1063-1070

[20] Houmes RJM, Voets MA, Erdmann W, Lachmann B. Efficacy and safety of tramadol versus morphine for moderate and severe postoperative pain with special regard to respiratory depression. *Anesth Analg* 1992 ; 74 : 510-514

[21] Joris J. Les associations thérapeutiques. In : Brasseur L, Chauvin M, Guilbaud G éd. Douleurs, bases fondamentales, pharmacologie, douleurs aiguës, douleurs chroniques, thérapeutique. Paris : Maloine, 1998 : 243-251

[22] Joris J, Sferlazza A, Van Erck J, Lamy M. Patient controlled analgesia with opiate is not significantly influenced by programmation choice of narcotics, and combination with a minor analgesic. *Reg Anesth* 1992 ; 17 (suppl 3) : 153

[23] Koch-Weser J. Nonsteroidal inflammatory drugs. *N Engl J Med* 1980 ; 303 : 189-195

[24] Lambert LA, Lambert DH, Strichartz GR. Irreversible conduction block in isolated nerve by high concentrations of local anaesthetics. *Anesthesiology* 1994 ; 80 : 1082-1093

[25] Liguori GA, Sharrock NE. Asystole and severe bradycardia during epidural anaesthesia in orthopaedic patients. *Anesthesiolgy* 1997 ; 86 : 250-257

[26] Mendez R, Eisenach JC, Kashtan K. Epidural clonidine analgesia after cesarian section. *Anesthesiology* 1990 ; 73 : 848-852

[27] Mensink FJ, Kozody R, Kehler CH, Wade JG. Dose response relationship of clonidine in tetracaine spinal anaesthesia. *Anesthesiology* 1987 ; 67: 717-721

[28] Merskey H. Classification of chronic pain. Descriptions of chronic pain syndromes and definitions of pain terms. *Pain* 1986 ; 24 (suppl) : S1-S225

[29] Merskey H, Bogduk N. Classification of chronic pain. Descriptions of chronic pain syndromes and definitions of pain terms. Seattle : IASP Press, 1994

[30] Motsch J, Graber E, Ludwig K. Addition of clonidine enhances postoperative analgesia from epidural morphine: a double-blind study. *Anesthesiology* 1990 ; 73 : 1067-1073

[31] Olsson G, Berde C. Neuropathic pain in children and adolescents. Refresher Course Syllabus, 1993 : 53-66

[32] Osipova NA, Novikov GA, Beresnev VA, Loseva NA. Analgesic effect of tramadol in cancer patient with chronic pain: a comparison with prolonged action morphine sulfate. *Curr Ther Res* 1991 ; 50 : 812-821

[33] Oyama T. Endocrine response to general anaesthesia and surgery. Endocrinology and the anesthetist. Amsterdam : Elsevier, 1983 : 1-22

[34] Preston KL, Jasinski DR, Testa M. Abuse potential and pharmacological comparison of tramadol and morphine. *Drug Alcohol Depend* 1997 ; 27 : 7-17

[35] Raffa RB, Friderichs E, Reimann W, Shank RP, Cod EE, Vaught JL et al. Opioid and non opioid components independently contribute to the mechanism of action of tramadol and "atypical" opioid analgesic. *J Pharmacol Exp Ther* 1992 ; 260 : 275-285

[36] Rawal N, Schollin J, Wesström G. Epidural versus combined spinal epidural block for caesariean section. *Acta Anaesthesiol Scand* 1988 ; 32 : 61-66

[37] Renaud B, Brichant JF, Clergue F, Chauvin M, Leron JC, Viars P. Ventilatory effects of continuous epidural infusion of fentanyl. *Anesth Analg* 1988 ; 67 : 971-975

[38] Rosencher N, Barré J, Eyrolle L. Anesthésie pour prothèse totale de hanche. In : 37e congrès national d'anesthésie et de réanimation et Xes journées franco-québécoises. Conférences d'actualisation SFAR. Paris : Masson, 1995 : 291-304

[39] Royblat L, Korotkoruchko A, Klatz J, Glazer M, Greemberg L, Fischer A. Postoperative pain: the effect of low dose ketamine in addition to general anaesthesia. *Anesth Analg* 1993 ; 77 : 1161-1165

[40] Scherpereel PH. Prévention de la douleur postopératoire. *Doul Analg* 1993 ; 3 : 75-79

[41] Scherpereel PH. Réactions endocriniennes et métaboliques à la chirurgie: modifications liées aux techniques anesthésiques. In : 38e congrès national d'anesthésie et de réanimation. Conférences d'actualisation SFAR. Paris : Elsevier, 1996 : 317-328

[42] Scott DB. Techniques of regional anaesthesia. New York : Medi Globe, 1989 : 1-224

[43] Singelyn FJ, Dangoisse M, Bartholomée S, Gouverneur JM. Adding clonidine to mepivacaine prolongs the duration of anaesthesia and analgesia after axillary plexus block. *Reg Anesth* 1992 ; 17 : 148-150

[44] Stein C. Peripheral mechanisms of opioid analgesia. *Anesth Analg* 1993 ; 76 : 182-191

[45] Tetzlaff J. Clinical orthopaedic anaesthesia. London : Butterworth-Heinemann, 1995 : 1-406

[46] Tryba M. Low molecular weight heparins and heparinoids, risks and benefits. The FDA alert. Refresher Course lectures. ESA, 1999 : 77-81

[47] Vickers MD, O'Flaherty D, Szekely SP, Read M, Yoshizumi J. Tramadol: pain relief by an opioid without depression of respiration. *Anaesthesia* 1992 ; 47 : 291-296

[48] White PF. Patient controlled analgesia. In : Brown DL ed. Problems in anaesthesia: perioperative analgesia. Philadelphia : JB Lippincott, 1988 : 339-350

[49] Wilder-Smith O, Hoffman A, Borgeat A, Rifat K. Fentanyl or magnesium analgesic supplementation of anaesthesia: effect on postoperative analgesic requirements. [abstract]. *Anesthesiology* 1992 ; 77 : A208

The pneumatic tourniquet

JP Estebe

Abstract. – The pneumatic tourniquet is widely used in orthopaedic surgery to achieve a bloodless surgical field, to minimise blood loss and to aid in identification of vital structures. However, its use is known to cause many adverse effects. Tourniquet pain is one well-known phenomenon. Another adverse effect, which is probably underestimated, is a secondary injury induced by ischaemia-reperfusion, which could end in the "no reflow phenomenon". The risk of deep venous thrombosis, pulmonary embolism and infection is also increased. Knowledge of the contraindications and the possible consequences will improve the safety of using the pneumatic tourniquet. The electronic tourniquet controller system must be checked regularly. The widest curved cuff adapted to the application site must be selected. Exsanguination should be performed by gravity. The tourniquet is inflated to the arterial occlusion pressure plus 50 to 75 mm Hg. Safe tourniquet application must be less than one hour. When a longer duration is anticipated, a reperfusion period of at least 10 minutes may be initiated within 45 to 60 minutes of ischaemia. Release of the tourniquet prior to haemostasis and closure is preferable. After tourniquet deflation, the patient's vascular status must be evaluated.

Keywords: pneumatic tourniquet, shape, pressure, duration, adverse affects, shear forces, pain, ischaemia-reperfusion, venous thrombosis, infection.

Introduction

The first recorded use of a tourniquet was by a Roman surgeon in the second century A.D. In 1817, a French surgeon, Jean-Louis Petit, described his device for haemostasis which he named the "tourniquet". The pneumatic tourniquet was introduced by Harvey Cushing in 1904 as an adjunct for surgery of the extremities. The pneumatic tourniquet is now widely used to achieve a relatively bloodless surgical field, minimise blood loss, aid in identification of vital structures, and expedite the surgical procedure. However, its use is known to cause many adverse effects and knowledge of possible consequences will help to increase the safety of tourniquet use.

Jean-Pierre Estebe, M.D., Ph.D., Department of Anaesthesia, Intensive Care and Pain Clinic, CHRU of Rennes, Orthopaedic Research Laboratory (Pr Frantz Langlais), Service d'Anesthésie Réanimation Chirurgicale 2, Hôpital Hôtel Dieu, 35000 Rennes, France.

Recommended practices

INDICATIONS, CONTRAINDICATIONS

Several relative contraindications for the use of a tourniquet have been reported in the literature, including severe atherosclerotic disease, severe crush injuries and diabetes mellitus. Tourniquet use is generally discouraged in patients who carry the sickle-cell gene, but if optimal acid-base status and oxygenation are maintained throughout the procedure, it may be safe for such patients. Severe brain injury must be considered as a relative contradiction. Proven or suspected deep venous thrombosis (DVT), the presence of calcified vessels, rheumatoid arthritis and other collagen-vascular diseases associated with vasculitis are also relative contraindications. When a tumour is present, a tourniquet may be used only if it is positioned proximal to the tumour and at a distance from it.

The main indication must not be the haemostatic effect of the tourniquet, as this is not the only technique available to obtain a bloodless field. Step-by-step haemostasis and pharmacological vasoconstriction may also be used. Simultaneous bilateral tourniquets must be avoided. If it is necessary to use bilateral tourniquets, their application should be alternated.

TECHNICAL GUIDELINES

All studies suggest that recommendations for safe tourniquet use should be based on the degree of neuromuscular injury beneath the cuff rather than distal to it. Manual and mechanical systems with non-electronic regulation of pressure must be avoided. A programme of periodic inspection of electronic devices with indicators and alarms must be instituted to avoid over- or under-pressurisation (the chosen pressure must be maintained to within 5% of a set value). Policies and procedures for the use of a pneumatic tourniquet should be written, reviewed annually, and readily available. Whenever there is a major or minor problem, a full investigation must be carried out promptly.

■ Tourniquet application site

Usually the pneumatic tourniquet is applied at the most proximal site of the extremity. When this is not surgically necessary, it could be beneficial to apply the tourniquet at a lower site: at the forearm [23], wrist [21], calf [36] or forefoot [14]. Digital tourniquet use [46] has been much discussed, as it could

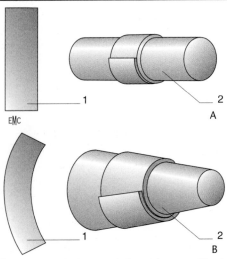

1 *A. A straight (rectangular) tourniquet provides the optimal fit on a cylindrical limb. 1. Straight cuff; 2. cylinder.*
B. Curved tourniquets are best for conical limbs. 1. Curved cuff; 2. cone.

compromise the vascular status of a finger. A tourniquet at the calf must be positioned at a distance from the fibular head (i.e. mid-calf) to avoid injury to the common peroneal nerve.

■ *Tourniquet shape*

A straight tourniquet cannot fit a limb of conical shape, particularly in patients with large and conical thighs (*fig 1*). A wide cuff is much more effective in the occlusion stage than a narrow cuff and is painless when pressure is limited to the lowest effective pressure. Conversely, a wide cuff proves to be more painful if "standard" pressure is applied [11]. The widest curved cuff appropriate to the size of the extremity must be chosen (i.e. more than 5 cm and 9 cm for the upper and the lower limb, respectively) and must be connected to an integrated cuff inflation system.

■ *Tourniquet padding*

To reduce skin damage due to shearing stresses, wrinkle-free padding of the tourniquet is essential. To avoid chemical burns beneath the tourniquet, it must be excluded from the operative field with a self-adhesive plastic drape before skin preparation. The tourniquet cuff should not be rotated to a new position after it has been applied (shearing forces from rotating a cuff may damage underlying tissues).

■ *Limb exsanguination*

Limb exsanguination before tourniquet inflation is usually accomplished by mechanical means. Such devices (Esmarch bandage, Rhys-Davies exsanguinator) increase the risk of disseminating a tumour or infection or the risk of DVT. Exsanguination of the limb by elevation is an effective, safe and easy procedure. It is slightly less effective than a mechanical

procedure, but it permits better visualisation of superficial vessels than complete exsanguination, allowing better haemostasis [33]. To achieve maximal exsanguination in the upper limb, it is recommended to elevate the arm at 90° for 5 minutes [57]; in the lower limb, it is recommended to elevate the leg at 45° for 5 minutes without arterial compression [58], while limb preparation (e.g. disinfecting and draping) is being performed.

■ *Pressure*

Better than opting for an arbitrary pressure (350 mm Hg for the lower extremity and 250-300 mm Hg for the upper extremity), the arterial occlusion pressure (AOP) must be determined before application of a tourniquet. Lowering the inflation pressure to the minimal value necessary to achieve an effective arrest of blood flow distal to the tourniquet cuff should increase the safety of these systems. First of all, the AOP must be determined in the clinical situation (i.e. under anaesthesia) based on the loss of arterial pulse (ultrasonic Doppler, pulse oximeter, photoplethysmograph). The AOP depends on the size of the tourniquet used. The AOP is inversely proportional to the ratio of the tourniquet cuff to the limb circumference and could be in the subsystolic range when this ratio is above 0.5 [16]. A tourniquet pressure is then set at AOP plus 50 to 75 mm Hg. The tourniquet pressure may be adjusted during surgery according to changes in blood pressure (i.e. increase in arterial pressure). If the AOP is not determined, the tourniquet pressure used could be 75 to 100 mm Hg above systolic arterial pressure. Insufficient pressure (i.e. below arterial pressure) could induce venous congestion (venous tourniquet), which is easily recognised during surgery, particularly in the case of an incorrect tourniquet shape and size for athletic or obese patients. Calcified, non-compressible arteries may be another cause of tourniquet failure.

■ *Duration*

The "safe" duration of tourniquet ischaemia remains controversial. It has been reported that tourniquet application longer than 60 minutes increases the risk of complications after arthroscopy [49]. On the other hand, it has been demonstrated that three hours of continuous ischaemia will not produce generalised irreversible damage in healthy (non-traumatised) muscle, although it will result in widespread sublethal injury to cells. Based on recent human and animal investigations [44], the recommended period of tourniquet ischaemia is about one hour.

If tourniquet use must exceed one hour for surgical reasons, it is common practice to deflate the tourniquet intermittently in an attempt to minimise the ischaemic damage. Such reperfusion periods must be longer than 10 minutes. It has been suggested that

hourly reperfusion could decrease muscle dysfunction, but it has also been demonstrated that a reperfusion interval after two hours of ischaemia tends to exacerbate muscle injury (in [13]). Recognition of the fact that reperfusion may initiate pathological reactions that increase the injury sustained by ischaemic tissue has important clinical implications. Based on physiological data, it seems that reperfusion is deleterious due to an ischaemia-reperfusion injury when ischaemia of skeletal muscle lasts longer than one hour. When tourniquet application is not anticipated to be more than one hour, the inflation period must be continued until the end. When the time required is expected to be longer than one hour, a reperfusion period could be initiated within 45 to 60 minutes of ischaemia. Tourniquet inflation time should be kept to a minimum; the surgeon should be informed of this duration at frequent, predetermined intervals (e.g. every 30 minutes during the first hour, then every 15 minutes).

■ *Release*

The release of the tourniquet prior to haemostasis and closure allows reduction of tourniquet application time and a period of reperfusion (i.e. oedema) before bandage or cast application, thus reducing the risks linked to the increase in intracompartmental pressure, as compared to applying the dressing before tourniquet release (in [13]). Deflation should be quick to prevent the capillary bleeding which occurs when deflation is carried out slowly.

To reduce the risk of haematoma when there is a haemostasis defect, it is still common practice to apply a compression bandage prior to deflation of the tourniquet and to leave it for a few minutes after deflation. However, it is necessary to take into account the risk of raising the intracompartmental pressure. A splint or split plaster cast for two days should be preferred to a circumferential plaster cast. Reinflation of the tourniquet in order to apply a compressive dressing after haemostasis following tourniquet release seems to increase the postoperative bleeding [31] as well as the risk of DVT migration. Careful monitoring of the vascular status of the limb (i.e. distal pulses and capillary refill) is required in the early postoperative period to detect any vascular compromise.

Tourniquet deflation frequently occurs near the end of a surgical procedure. The ventilatory and haemodynamic effects and the release of anaesthetic drugs which have been sequestered by the pneumatic tourniquet cause transient changes (physiological, pharmacokinetic and pharmacodynamic) which are of limited clinical importance in a healthy patient. However, in critical patients (i.e. brain injury), the anaesthesiologist must be informed before release of the tourniquet (in [13]).

■ *Prophylactic antibiotics*

Parenteral prophylactic antibiotics must be administered 10-20 minutes before tourniquet inflation, as the tourniquet isolates the operative site from the systemic circulation (in [13]). After inflation of the tourniquet, antibiotics and anaesthetic drugs (i.e. neuromuscular blocking agents) may not reach the exsanguinated limb. If the tourniquet has been inflated, regional intravenous injection of antibiotics would be a good alternative [20]. Additional doses are not warranted after tourniquet release if the tourniquet application time is less than two hours.

■ *Prevention*

Local hypothermia by cold gel packs reduces the metabolic demands. A decrease in temperature could reduce ischaemic and anoxic degeneration, but hypothermia is clinically difficult to perform without adverse general effects (in [13]). Administration of an inhibitor of endothelial xanthine oxidase (allopurinol) or a radical scavenger (vitamin E) could decrease oxidative stress and the occurrence of oedema in postischaemic skeletal muscle. To reduce microvascular reperfusion injury following tourniquet ischaemia in striated muscle, buflomedil could be used [35]. Pretreatment with inosine attenuates the local and systemic pro-inflammatory response associated with tourniquet use. Regional limb heparinisation is not effective in reducing the embolic phenomena after pneumatic tourniquet release [15].

Topical application of an anaesthetic cream (EMLA® cream) is as effective as semicircular subcutaneous anaesthesia in preventing tourniquet pain [54]. In order to efficiently reduce pain following arthroscopy, intra-articular injection of local anaesthetics must be performed 10 minutes before tourniquet deflation to allow fixation of local anaesthetics before the washout period of tourniquet release (in [13]). Preoperative intravenous injection of a small dose of ketamine could prevent an increase in systemic arterial pressure during tourniquet inflation. Regional anaesthesia is better than general anaesthesia to decrease the consequences of tourniquet pain such as arterial hypertension (in [13]).

Local effects

EFFECTS ON MUSCLE

Local complications result both from tissue compression beneath the cuff and tissue ischaemia beneath the cuff and distally. Skin, muscles, nerves and vessels may be damaged by the mechanical pressure of the tourniquet, as a result of sagittal forces causing compression, and axial forces (due to the uneven distribution of pressure under the cuff) causing stretching [34, 47] (*fig 2*).

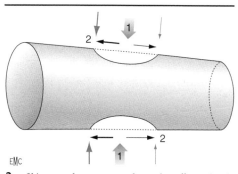

2 *Skin, muscles, nerves and vessels suffer under the tourniquet due to mechanical pressure, with both sagittal forces responsible for compression (1) and axial forces due to uneven pressure distribution responsible for stretching (2).*

Clinically relevant conclusions are difficult to draw from animal studies because muscle tissue in small animals is much more sensitive to ischaemia than is human muscle. Recently, an animal cuff design (curved cuff) has allowed determination of the magnitude and distribution of tissue pressures caused by tourniquet compression similar to those recorded in previous human studies. This has allowed better interpretation of the experimental results. In summary, it has been clearly demonstrated that compression injury by the tourniquet results in a more significant loss of functional strength, contractile speed and fatigability than tourniquet-induced ischaemia (in [13]). Skeletal muscle may be severely affected, even during relatively short periods of ischaemia-compression, and this might facilitate the development of muscle atrophy during immobilisation after orthopaedic surgery. The occurrence of electromyographic abnormalities has been noted systematically during and after tourniquet use, and these may persist for up to six months [30]. In animal studies, it was demonstrated that tourniquet compression injury results in more significant loss of functional strength and contractile speed than tourniquet ischaemia. After anterior cruciate ligament reconstruction, the amount of quadriceps amyotrophy after tourniquet use was significantly greater than that observed without tourniquet use [37]. Cases of rhabdomyolysis or compartment syndrome have been reported after a tourniquet was left inflated for long periods (more than 4 hours), but also for shorter periods (45 to 120 min) [19, 41, 48].

EFFECTS ON NERVES

Especially at higher levels of inflation, tourniquet-induced neurological injuries due to shear forces are relatively common, and frequently paralysis occurs transiently at a subclinical level (in [13]). In animal studies, it has been clearly demonstrated that nerve injury is more pronounced beneath the cuff than distal to it (i.e. a combination of ischaemia and direct mechanical deformation). In a single electromyography laboratory, 35 cases of tourniquet paralysis

were recorded within a 3 year period [40]. It was also demonstrated in an animal study that the hyperaemic flow response in nerve is more prolonged than in muscle during reperfusion. Limb dysfunction during ischaemia and reperfusion may be largely the result of axonal or neuromuscular junction injury or both [28].

EFFECTS OF REPERFUSION

Despite the frequent use of the tourniquet during surgery on limbs, it remains difficult to identify manifestations of the resulting ischaemia/reperfusion in man. Animal model studies, however, have shown that tourniquet use might be associated with significant ischaemia/reperfusion injury. Signs of primary injury have been observed immediately after one hour of tourniquet application; secondary injury represents a progression of cell injuries despite reperfusion. This secondary injury could end in the "no reflow phenomenon". Leukocytes play a significant role in this no reflow phenomenon: adhesion in post-capillary venules, microvascular barrier disruption and oedema formation (in [13]). Tourniquet release is associated with an immediate 10% increase in limb girth, due to refilling of the vessels and hyperaemia. Oedema following ischaemia and reperfusion results in an increase in intra-compartmental pressure in the reperfusion injury. Also, over the first postoperative day, the limb girth has been noted to increase to 150% as compared to the initial limb girth.

Described in 1951, the "post-tourniquet syndrome" combines weakness, stiffness, oedema, dysaesthesia and pain. These symptoms may be wrongly attributed to surgical trauma or to lack of patient motivation.

Systemic effects

PAIN

A number of mechanisms have been cited to explain tourniquet pain (i.e. ischaemic pain, compression pain). Pain tolerance in studies on volunteers was around 20 to 30 minutes [11]. In addition to local explanations (in [13]), sensitisation of the central nervous system may also represent another factor of pain. Animal studies have shown evidence of expansion of the receptive field of nociceptor neurons in response to tourniquet pain [9]. Tourniquet pain is increased when hyperalgesia (e.g. traumatic injury) is present [6]. After tourniquet deflation, other types of pain (a warming sensation, quickly turning into an aching sensation of burning), are associated with limb reperfusion [11]. The factors that incite the ischaemic nerves to spontaneously discharge and cause paraesthesias upon reperfusion are not known.

Postoperative pain control is important for optimal recovery from surgery. In a randomised study, pain scores were often lower in groups without tourniquet use [38, 39, 53], or the pain scores were similar [22] but never higher than in tourniquet groups. This may explain delayed functional recovery following surgery [17, 56].

RISK OF THROMBOSIS

The increase in the risk for DVT following tourniquet use is much debated. Following knee arthroscopy, the incidence of DVT diagnosed using contrast venography was around 18% one week after surgery [10]. In that study, the risk of DVT was significantly increased among patients who had a tourniquet applied for more than 60 minutes. It was demonstrated by an increase in circulating markers of thrombosis that DVT begins during tourniquet inflation and this increase in marker levels persisted after tourniquet deflation [45]. On the other hand, tourniquet application may increase fibrinolysis [2]. This could be caused by release of anti-clotting factors from the surgical site, increasing the risk of hemarthrosis after arthroscopy [8].

RESPIRATORY RISKS

■ *Risk of embolism*

Fatal or near-fatal pulmonary embolism was first reported after use of the Esmarch bandage and/or tourniquet inflation in orthopaedic surgery. It was also subsequently reported after deflation of the tourniquet [4]. A significant correlation was noted between the amount of emboli and duration of tourniquet application [18]. These emboli occur in all patients within 1 minute of tourniquet release. It was suggested that the pulmonary embolism occurring during orthopaedic surgery might result from fat embolism caused by invasion of the medullary cavity [15]. In patients undergoing intramedullary guided total knee arthroplasty, it was found that the emboli (in blood aspirated from the femoral vein of the operated limb after tourniquet release) could consist of fresh thrombus and not necessarily of fat [42] or cement [4]. Air emboli were also occasionally noted after tourniquet release (in [13]). The amount of emboli in patients undergoing invasive surgery (e.g. knee replacement) was extremely large compared with that in non-invasive surgery (e.g. diagnostic arthroscopy) [18]. Even in the absence of a patent foramen ovale, cerebral microembolism frequently occurs (60%) upon tourniquet release (probably through the opening of recruitable pulmonary vessels) [50]. In summary, compared with total knee replacement (TKR) without a tourniquet, tourniquet use places patients at a 5.33-fold greater risk of having large emboli [42]. Obviously, the risk of embolism is increased in the case of a one-stage bilateral total knee arthroplasty (TKA).

However, the rate of DVT and pulmonary embolus appears to be less after knee surgery than after hip surgery, which is probably related to the rapid mobilisation of patients following knee surgery.

■ *Physiological respiratory response*

There is a 25% increase in CO_2 production resulting from metabolic acidosis due to acid metabolites washed from the ischaemic area (in [13]). This increase depends on the duration of tourniquet inflation and on the muscle mass involved (e.g. it is greater in a lower limb). The difference between the pulmonary elimination of CO_2 and the arterial CO_2 pressure was increased, probably due to a reduction in pulmonary blood flow caused by the emboli [18]. Acute lung injury could be observed after limb reperfusion (increased microvascular permeability, sequestration of neutrophils, and generation of free oxygen radicals) (in [13]).

CARDIOVASCULAR RISKS

Tourniquet application also has significant effects on the cardiovascular system. The mean arterial pressure increases progressively after tourniquet inflation (26%). After a transitory hypotension upon deflation, which may be dangerous in elderly patients and in patients having lost much blood during the operation, the mean arterial pressure returns to basal values. Due to activation of the sympathetic nervous system, the cardiac index increases immediately after tourniquet inflation (18%), and a further increase (40%) occurs five minutes after tourniquet deflation. Postoperative hypovolaemia may be observed after tourniquet deflation, due in part to haemorrhage at the surgical site but mostly to a combination of reactive vasodilatation and increased microvascular permeability in the entire reperfused limb during the first hour. K+ intoxication in tourniquet shock in rats is the principal cause of cardiac death (in [13]).

NEUROCEREBRAL RISKS

Some case reports have shown a dramatic decrease in cerebral perfusion in head injury patients. This change was accompanied by a dangerous increase in intracranial pressure, due mainly to a simultaneous increase in CO_2 production upon release of the tourniquet and a decrease in systemic blood pressure; this could lead to a severe reduction in cerebral perfusion pressure with potentially disastrous consequences in patients with brain injury (in [13]). During general anaesthesia, hyperventilation after tourniquet deflation could prevent an increase in cerebral blood flow velocity in trauma patients without head injury [27]. In patients who are breathing spontaneously (under regional anaesthesia), changes in oxygen consumption were noted to rapidly return to the baseline [51].

RISK OF INFECTION

A review focusing on infectious complications of arthroscopy (0.01%-0.48%) has suggested that risk factors include prolonged tourniquet application [3]. The first explanation for this is the systemic inflammatory response to tourniquet use in extremity surgery. Various animal studies have demonstrated a transient neutrophil and monocyte activation after tourniquet ischaemia, which translates into enhanced neutrophil transendothelial migration with a potential for tissue injury [55]. In a randomised study, it was demonstrated that wound hypoxia during total knee replacement was greater in the tourniquet group than in the control group without tourniquet [7, 43]. These findings may have clinical relevance with respect to wound healing and the development of wound infection. Similar findings occurred in a prospective study on internal fixation of fractures of the distal part of the fibula [32]. Various results suggest that xanthine oxidase and others mediators (e.g. nitrite) released from the ischaemic limb on reperfusion induced polymorphonuclear neutrophil activation (in [13]).

As an indication of the potential power of this neutrophil activation inducing a respiratory burst (or oxidative stress), activation of neutrophils was used in an animal model to develop a multi-organ failure (in [13]). This model of tourniquet shock may be easily obtained with two tourniquets applied simultaneously on the two lower limbs of the animal.

BLEEDING RISKS

In randomised studies, tourniquet use during TKA did not reduce total blood loss [1, 24, 52, 56]. Similar findings were made regarding plating of tibial fractures [43]. The benefit of surgical haemostasis after tourniquet release is still under debate [5, 26, 59]. The risk of having a poor cement bone interface in cemented arthroplasty without tourniquet use may also be debated, but this has never been demonstrated.

Arterial complications after total knee arthroplasty are rare, but the sequelae can be disastrous (e.g. vascular reconstruction or amputation). The use of a tourniquet during TKA in the presence of peripheral arterial disease or ipsilateral peripheral arterial reconstruction has been implicated in subsequent arterial complications.

VALUE OF TOURNIQUET USE FOR IDENTIFICATION AND VISUALISATION OF ANATOMICAL STRUCTURES

When studies were randomised, the operating time and intraoperative technical difficulties were found to be similar for arthroscopic surgery performed with or without a tourniquet [22, 27, 52, 53]. Only one study demonstrated a slightly better visualisation in the tourniquet group, whereas the operative time did not differ between groups [29]. All of these studies concluded that the use of a pneumatic tourniquet is not necessary to perform arthroscopic surgery. Similar results were reported for TKR [56], plating of tibial fractures [43] and fixation of fibula fractures [32].

EFFECTS ON TEMPERATURE

An increase in core temperature during tourniquet inflation was reported in adult and paediatric studies [12], with the greatest changes in patients who were actively warmed (i.e. in paediatric surgery). After tourniquet release, the core temperature decreased rapidly but transiently (maximal decrease 10 minutes after tourniquet deflation). It then showed a secondary increase [12]. It is possible that the tourniquet plays a role in the increased postoperative temperature in orthopaedic surgery. It must be remembered that tourniquet ischaemia may initiate a reaction similar to malignant hyperthermia.

Conclusion

In conclusion, the combination of these different complications could explain the prolonged hospitalisation time and delayed return to work observed in the tourniquet group compared to the group without tourniquet in various randomised studies [32, 43]. A cost-benefit analysis would obviously have implications for health-care management. The pneumatic tourniquet is a useful tool to achieve a bloodless field in some orthopaedic surgery, but it carries a risk of adverse effects. It is necessary to weigh the advantages and disadvantages before deciding to use a tourniquet. To minimise its side effects, the tourniquet must be used within the framework of a strict procedure, with well-adapted and regularly checked equipment.

Annex - Recommended protocol for pneumatic tourniquet use

1. Check equipment; use an electronic tourniquet controller system.

2. Ensure that the patient has no contraindication to pneumatic tourniquet use and that there is an indication for tourniquet use.

3. Parenteral antibiotics must be administered 10-20 minutes before tourniquet inflation.

4. Use the widest curved cuff appropriate to the application site.

5. Apply a stockinette on the operative limb.

6. Apply the tourniquet snugly over the padding. Exclude the tourniquet from the operative field with a self-adhesive plastic drape before skin preparation.

7. Measure the arterial occlusion pressure (AOP).

8. Exsanguinate the extremity by gravity.

9. Inflate the tourniquet to AOP plus 50 to 75 mm Hg or, if AOP was not measured, 75 to 100 mm Hg greater than systolic blood pressure.

10. Palpate the distal artery to ensure absence of pulse.

11. Tourniquet duration must be below one hour. When the duration is not anticipated to be more than one hour, the inflation period must be continued until the end of tourniquet application. When tourniquet time is anticipated to be longer than 1 hour, a reperfusion period of at least 10 minutes may be initiated within 45 to 60 minutes of ischaemia.

12. Release of the tourniquet prior to haemostasis and closure is preferable.

13. The cuff may be deflated in one step.

14. After deflation, monitoring of the vascular status must be carried out.

15. A temporary bandage or split plaster cast must be applied for the first two postoperative days.

References

[1] Abdel-Salam A, Eyres KS. Effects of tourniquet during total knee arthroplasty: a prospective randomised study. *J Bone Joint Surg Br* 1995 ; 77 : 250-253

[2] Aglietti P, Baldini A, Vena LM, Abbate R, Fedi S, Falciani M. Effect of tourniquet on activation of coagulation in total knee replacement. *Clin Orthop* 2000 ; 371 : 169-177

[3] Babcock HM, Matava MJ, Fraser V. Postarthroscopy surgical-site infections: review of the literature. *Clin Infect Dis* 2002 ; 34 : 65-71

[4] Berman A, Parmet JL, Harding SP, Israelite GL, Chandrasekaran K, Horrow JC et al. Emboli observed with use of transesophageal echocardiography immediately after tourniquet release during total knee arthroplasty with cement. *J Bone Joint Surg Am* 1998 ; 80 : 389-396

[5] Burkart BC, Bourne RB, Rorabeck CH, Kirk PG, Nott L. The efficacy of tourniquet release in blood conservation after total knee arthroplasty. *Clin Orthop* 1994 ; 299 : 147-152

[6] Byas-Smith MG, Bennett GJ, Gracely RH, Max MB, Robinovitz E, Dubner R. Tourniquet constriction exacerbates hyperalgesia-related pain induced by intradermal capsaicin injection. *Anesthesiology* 1999 ; 91 : 617-625

[7] Clarke MT, Longstaff L, Edwards D, Rushton N. Tourniquet-induced wound hypoxia after total knee replacement. *J Bone Joint Surg Br* 2001 ; 83 : 40-44

[8] Coupens SD, Yates CK. The effect of tourniquet use and hemovac drainage on postoperative hemarthrosis. *Arthroscopy* 1991 ; 7 : 278-282

[9] Crews JC, Cahall MA. An investigation of the neurophysiologic mechanisms of tourniquet-related pain: changes in spontaneous activity and receptive field size in spinal dorsal horn neurons. *Reg Anesth Pain Med* 1999 ; 24 : 102-109

[10] Dermers C, Marcoux S, Ginsberg JS, Laroche F, Cloutier R, Poulin J. Incidence of venographically proved deep vein thrombosis after knee arthroscopy. *Arch Intern Med* 1998 ; 158 : 47-50

[11] Estebe JP, Le Naoures A, Chemaly L, Ecoffey C. Tourniquet pain in a volunteer study: effect of changes in cuff width and pressure. *Anaesthesia* 2000 ; 55 : 21-26

[12] Estebe JP, Le Naoures A, Malledant Y, Ecoffey C. Use of a pneumatic tourniquet induces changes in central temperature. *Br J Anaesth* 1996 ; 77 : 786-788

[13] Estebe JP, Malledant Y. Pneumatic tourniquets in orthopaedics (review article). *Ann Fr Anesth Réanim* 1996 ; 15 : 162-167

[14] Finsen V, Kasseth AM. Tourniquets in forefoot surgery: less pain when placed at the ankle. *J Bone Joint Surg Br* 1997 ; 79 : 99-101

[15] Giachino AA, Rody K, Turek MA, Miller DR, Wherrett C, Moreau G et al. Systemic fat and thrombus embolization in patients undergoing total knee arthroplasty with regional heparinization. *J Arthroplasty* 2001 ; 16 : 288-292

[16] Graham B, Breault MJ, McEwen JA, McGraw RW. Occlusion of arterial flow in the extremities at subsystolic pressures through the use of wide tourniquet cuff. *Clin Orthop* 1993 ; 286 : 257-261

[17] Gutin B, Warren R, Wickiewicz T, O'Brien S, Altchek D, Kroll M. Does tourniquet use during anterior cruciate ligament surgery interfere with postsurgical recovery of function? A review of the literature. *Arthroscopy* 1991 ; 7 : 52-56

[18] Hirota K, Hashimoto H, Kabara S, Tsubo Y, Sato Y, Ishihara H et al. The relationship between tourniquet time and pulmonary emboli in patients undergoing knee arthroscopic surgeries. *Anesth Analg* 2001 ; 93 : 776-780

[19] Hirvensalo E, Tuominen H, Lapinsuo M, Heliö H. Compartment syndrome of the lower limb caused by a tourniquet: a report of two cases. *J Orthop Trauma* 1992 ; 6 : 469-472

[20] Hoddinott C, Lovering AM. Regional prophylactic antibiotic in knee arthroplasty. *J Bone Joint Surg Br* 1993 ; 75 : 157-158

[21] Hodgson AJ. The wrist tourniquet: an alternative technique in hand surgery. *J Hand Surg Am* 1994 ; 19 : 341-342

[22] Hooper J, Rosaeg OP, Krepski B, Johnson DH. Tourniquet inflation during arthroscopic knee ligament surgery does not increase postoperative pain. *Can J Anaesth* 1999 ; 46 : 925-929

[23] Hutchison DT, McClinton MA. Upper extremity tourniquet tolerance. *J Hand Surg Am* 1993 ; 18 : 206-210

[24] Iorio R, Healy WL. Tourniquet use during total knee arthroplasty did not reduce total blood loss. *J Bone Joint Surg Am* 2001 ; 83 : 1282

[25] Johnson DS, Stewart H, Hirst P, Harper NJ. Is tourniquet use necessary for knee arthroscopy? *Arthroscopy* 2000 ; 16 : 648-651

[26] Jorn LP, Lindstrand A, Toksvig-Larsen S. Tourniquet release for hemostasis increases bleeding. A randomised study of 77 knee replacements. *Acta Orthop Scand* 1999 ; 70 : 265-267

[27] Kadoi Y, Ide M, Saito S, Shiga T, Ishizaki K, Goto F. Hyperventilation after tourniquet deflation prevents an increase in cerebral blood flow velocity. *Can J Anaesth* 1999 ; 46 : 259-264

[28] Kinoshita Y, Monafo WW. Limb ischemia and reperfusion relationship of functional recovery to nerve and muscle blood flow. *J Trauma* 1994 ; 36 : 555-561

[29] Kirkley A, Rampersaud R, Griffin S, Amendola A, Litchfield R, Fowler P. Tourniquet versus no tourniquet use in routine knee arthroscopy: a prospective, double-blind, randomized clinical trial. *Arthroscopy* 2000 ; 16 : 121-126

[30] Kokki H, Vaatainen U, Miettinen H, Parviainen A, Kononen M, Partanen J. Tourniquet-induced changes in arthroscopic anterior cruciate ligament reconstruction: a comparison of low and high-pressure tourniquet systems. *Ann Chir Gynaecol* 2000 ; 89 : 313-317

[31] Lotke PA, Farall VJ, Orenstein EM, Ecker ML. Blood loss after total knee replacement. *J Bone Joint Surg Am* 1991 ; 73 : 1037-1040

[32] Mafulli N, Testa V, Capasso G. Use of a tourniquet in the internal fixation fractures of the distal part of the fibula. *J Bone Joint Surg Am* 1993 ; 75 : 700-703

[33] Marshall PD, Patil M, Fairclough JA. Should Esmarch bandages be used for exsanguinations in knee arthroscopy and knee replacement surgery? A prospective trial of Esmarch exsanguination versus simple elevation. *J R Coll Surg Edinburgh* 1994 ; 39 : 189-195

[34] McLaren AC, Rorabeck CH. The pressure distribution under tourniquets. *J Bone Joint Surg Am* 1985 ; 67 : 433-438

[35] Menger MD, Steiner D, Pelikan S, Messner K. Buflomedil hydrochloride attenuates tourniquet-induced microvascular reperfusion injury in striated muscle. *Int J Microcirc Clin Exp* 1994 ; 14 : 296-302

[36] Michelson JD, Perry M. Clinical safety and efficacy of calf tourniquets. *Foot Ankle Int* 1996 ; 17 : 573-575

[37] Nicholas SJ, Tyler TF, McHugh MP, Gleim GW. The effect on leg strength of tourniquet use during anterior cruciate ligament reconstruction: a prospective randomized study. *Arthroscopy* 2001 ; 17 : 603-607

[38] Ömerroglu H, Günel U, Biçimoglu A, Tabak AY, Uçamer A, Güney Ö. The relationship between the use of tourniquet and the intensity of postoperative pain in surgically treated malleolar fractures. *Foot Ankle Int* 1997 ; 18 : 798-802

[39] Ömerroglu H, Uçamer A, Tabak AY, Güney O, Biçimoglu A, Günel U. The effect of using a tourniquet on the intensity of postoperative pain in forearm fractures. *Int Orthop* 1998 ; 22 : 369-373

[40] On AY, Ozdemir O, Aksit R. Tourniquet paralysis after primary nerve repair. *Am J Phys Med Rehabil* 2000 ; 79 : 298-300

[41] Palmer SH, Graham G. Tourniquet-induced rhabdomyolysis after total knee replacement. *Ann R Coll Surg* 1994 ; 76 : 416-417

[42] Parmet JL, Horrow JC, Berman AT, Miller F, Pharo G, Collins L. The incidence of large venous emboli during total knee arthroplasty without pneumatic tourniquet use. *Anesth Analg* 1998 ; 87 : 439-444

[43] Salam AA, Eyres KS, Cleary J, El-Sayed HH. The use of a tourniquet when plating tibial fractures. *J Bone Joint Surg Br* 1996 ; 73 : 86-87

[44] Sapega AA, Heppenstall BR, Chance B, Sin Park Y, Sokolow D. Optimizing tourniquet application and release times in extremity surgery. *J Bone Joint Surg Am* 1985 ; 67 : 303-314

[45] Sharrock NE, Go G, Sculco TP, Ranawat CS, Maynard MJ, Harpel PC. Changes in circulatory indices of thrombosis and fibrinolysis during total knee arthroplasty performed under tourniquet. *J Arthroplasty* 1995 ; 10 : 523-528

[46] Shaw JA, Demuth WW, Gillespy AW. Guidelines for the use of digital tourniquets based on physiological pressure measurements. *J Bone Joint Surg Am* 1985 ; 67 : 1086-1090

[47] Shaw JA, Murray D. The relationship between tourniquet pressure and underlying soft-tissue pressure in the thigh. *J Bone Joint Surg Am* 1982 ; 64 : 1148-1152

[48] Shenton DW, Spitzer SA, Mulrennan BM. Tourniquet-induced rhabdomyolysis. *J Bone Joint Surg Am* 1990 ; 72 : 1405-1406

[49] Sherman OH, Fox JM, Snyder SJ, Del Pizzo WD, Freidman MJ, Ferkel RD et al. Arthroscopy: "no problem surgery"? An analysis of complications in two thousand six hundred and forty cases. *J Bone Joint Surg Am* 1986 ; 68 : 256-265

[50] Sulek CA, Davies LK, Enneking K, Gearen PA, Lobato EB. Cerebral microembolism diagnosed by transcranial Doppler during total knee arthroplasty. *Anesthesiology* 1999 ; 91 : 672-676

[51] Takahashi S, Mizutani T, Sato S. Changes in oxygen consumption and carbon dioxide elimination after tourniquet release in patients breathing spontaneously under epidural anesthesia. *Anesth Analg* 1998 ; 86 : 90-94

[52] Tetro AM, Rudan JF. The effects of a pneumatic tourniquet on blood loss in total knee arthroplasty. *Can J Surg* 2001 ; 44 : 33-38

[53] Tibrewal SB. The pneumatic tourniquet in arthroscopic surgery of the knee. *Int Orthop* 2001 ; 24 : 347-349

[54] Tschaikowsky K, Hemmerlind T. Comparison of the effect of EMLA and semicircular subcutaneous anaesthesia in the prevention of tourniquet pain during plexus block anaesthesia of the arm. *Anaesthesia* 1998 ; 53 : 382-403

[55] Wakai A, Wang JH, Winter DC, Street JT, O'Sullivan RG, Redmond HP. Tourniquet-induced systemic inflammatory response in extremity surgery. *J Trauma* 2001 ; 51 : 922-926

[56] Wakankar HM, Nicholl JE, Koka R, D'Arcy JC. The tourniquet in total knee arthroplasty: a prospective randomised study. *J Bone Joint Surg Br* 1999 ; 81 : 30-33

[57] Warren PJ, Hardiman PJ, Woolf VJ. Limb exsanguination. I. The arm: effect of angle of elevation and arterial compression. *Ann R Coll Surg Engl* 1992 ; 74 : 320-322

[58] Warren PJ, Hardiman PJ, Woolf VJ. Limb exsanguination. II. The leg: effect of angle of elevation. *Ann R Coll Surg Engl* 1992 ; 74 : 323-325

[59] Widman J, Isacson J. Surgical hemostasis after tourniquet release does not reduce blood loss in knee replacement. A prospective randomised study of 81 patients. *Acta Orthop Scand* 1999 ; 70 : 268-270

Prevention and treatment of infection in orthopaedic surgery and traumatology

Walenkamp GH

Abstract. – *The incidence of postoperative infections in orthopaedics is mainly the result of contamination of the wound during the trauma or the operation. Prevention of infection includes efforts to increase the patient's own immune status as well as to decrease the bacterial load in wounds. The most effective prophylactic measure is systemic antibiotics for 24 hours: in total hip prostheses it provides a 75% reduction in infection rate. In combination with antibiotic-loaded cement and a clean air installation in the operating theatre, the infection rate following total hip replacement can be reduced to 0.2%.*
In the treatment of early postoperative infections, it is most important to avoid delay in starting treatment, providing adequate antibiotic treatment and, if necessary, early debridement of the infected haematoma, leaving stable implants in situ.
In chronic osteomyelitis, staged operative debridement is the main treatment, and antibiotics are supportive: locally and, if necessary, also systemic. The infection should be treated first and reconstruction not begun when healing is inappropriate.
Infected arthroplasties with early postoperative infections can be debrided with the prosthesis in situ and treated with antibiotics. In late infections, all prosthetic components and bone cement must be removed. Reimplantation should only be performed when healing is appropriate, which may require months without a prosthesis in order to observe the healing process.

© 2000, Editions Scientifiques et Médicales Elsevier SAS. All rights reserved.

Keywords: infection, prevention, treatment, infected arthroplasty, osteomyelitis, operating theatre.

Introduction

This chapter will discuss infections in orthopaedic surgery and traumatology, briefly named orthopaedics. It will focus on prevention and treatment of iatrogenic infections, and mainly osteomyelitis and prosthesis infections.

PREVALENCE AND INCIDENCE OF ORTHOPAEDIC INFECTIONS

The prevalence of all kinds of infection in hospitalised patients in 14 European countries ranges from 3 to 21%, with a mean of 8.4%. However, in prevalence studies, new as well as old infections are counted. There is a wide variation, because in prevalence studies the number of infections is determined over a very short time period. The incidence of all hospital infections is about 5%, and these infections are mainly caused by bacteria. In these cases, 45% of the patients have a urinary infection, 29% a wound infection, 19% pneumonia, 2% sepsis (positive blood cultures), and 6% another kind of hospital infection. About 10% of the patients with a hospital infection die during the infection, and 1% because of the infection [16, 17].

The incidence of wound infections after trauma, as well as after clean and dirty elective operations, depends on the degree of contamination of the wound during the operation. In so-called "clean" wounds, the postoperative wound infection rate in large series is about 2%. After "dirty" operations (for example, where there is pus), the infection rate rises to about 40% [3].

Results of infection surveys of orthopaedic operations confirm these data [10, 21, 35]. Risk factors in clean surgery are, for example, diabetes, rheumatoid arthritis, use of immunosuppression, hip surgery and the use of implants. Infections of open fractures are due to contamination during the trauma, or to extended exposure during the treatment. When infection occurs, the infective organism could be identified in the initial cultures from the open wound in 66% [29].

PATHOPHYSIOLOGY OF ORTHOPAEDIC INFECTIONS

Infection of a wound will occur when bacterial contamination is high enough: the minimum infective dose. In experimental studies, such a dose appeared to be 2-8 million organisms of *St. aureus* when intradermally injected into healthy volunteers. However, when a foreign body (a stitch) was introduced, the minimum infective dose was reduced 10,000 times [5].

The extensive use of biomaterials in orthopaedics requires a better understanding of the pathophysiology of musculoskeletal sepsis, especially the molecular mechanisms. Microbial adhesion to inert substrates causes colonisation of biomaterials and damaged tissues. This microbial adhesion is caused by chemical bonding of bacterial extracapsular structures to the surface of implant or bone [15]. Bacteria and substrates are anionic and repel each other. Dipoles of the surface molecules, however, create electromagnetic "VanderWaals" forces, and bacterial cells and biomaterials will bond. A strong connection is now created by fimbriae and exopolysaccharides *(fig 1)*.

A biofilm consists of exopolysaccharide polymers produced by the bacteria, and

Geert H.I.M. Walenkamp, M.D., PhD, Associate Professor, Department of Orthopaedic Surgery, Academic Hospital Maastricht, Postbox 5800, 6202 AZ Maastricht, The Netherlands.

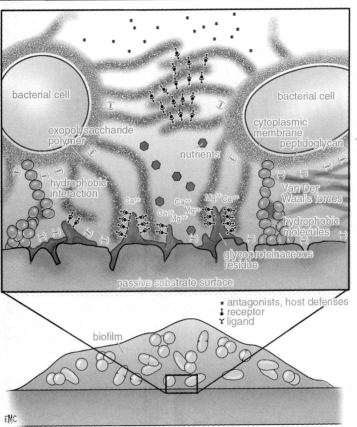

1 *Mechanism of bacterial adhesion on a passive substrate (prosthesis, sequestrum). (Redrawn with permission from Gristina AG et al. Adherent bacterial colonization in the pathogenesis of osteomyelitis.* Science *1985 ; 228 : 990-993. Copyright 1985 American Association for the Advancement of Science.)*

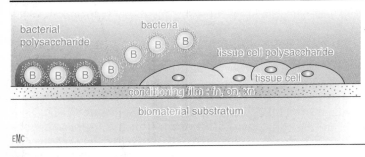

2 *"The race for the surface". (Redrawn with permission from Gristina AG, Barth E, Webb LX. Microbial adhesion and the pathogenesis of biomaterial centered infections. In: Gustilo RB ed. Orthopaedic infections. Diagnosis and treatment. Philadelphia: WB Saunders, 1989 : 325.)*

varies with local conditions and bacterial species [34]. The biofilm protects bacteria against several mechanisms of host defence and antibiotics, and serves as an adhesive mechanism for the bacteria on a passive substrate, with the help of proteins such as fibronectin, osteonectin, fibrogen, collagen and others. Devitalised bone can act as the passive substrate, but also all biomaterials such as heart valves, endotracheal tubes, Hickman catheters, and joint prostheses. It appears that in the case of biomaterials containing polymers, the principal isolate is *St. epidermidis*, and *St. aureus* is mainly found in conjunction with metals, compromised tissues, surgical wounds and bone infections. At the time of implantation, a biomaterial will attract cells to its surface, due to free energy sites. These sites will be bound within a few hours by either the patient's own host tissue cells or by bacteria: the "race for the surface" [14] *(fig 2)*.

Once the biofilm with bacteria is formed, it creates a micro-environment of its own, regarding pH, ions and nutrients; the germs multiply and the infection is established.

In conjunction with the adverse effects of relative hypoxia of the tissues in chronic osteomyelitis, this mechanism of adhesion and biofilm protection may be an explanation for the ability of bone infections to remain dormant for very long periods, the ineffectiveness of antibiotic treatment in the presence of dead bone and biomaterials, and the pathogenicity of low-virulence organisms such as *St. epidermidis* and some anaerobes [27]. Another mechanism could explain why orthopaedic infections can be difficult to heal and relapse years later. *St. aureus* especially can form small colony variants (SCV). These SCV can persist in endothelial cells, and they cause persistent and antibiotic-resistant infections in humans [32].

Bone resorption in infection is induced by cytokines that stimulate osteoclasts, and by direct resorptive effects by inflammatory cells such as macrophages and granulocytes. In osteomyelitic bone, the prostaglandin activity appears to be 5-30 times higher than in normal bone. In septic arthritis, cartilage destruction seems to be caused mainly by

the release of destructive enzymes by the synovium, but in addition, focal adherence and invasion of bacteria into the cartilage results in destruction of the integrity of the cartilage with loss of collagen and proteoglycan [27].

Prevention of postoperative infections

The need for and the effectiveness of prophylactic measures can be assessed when postoperative infection rates are known. All orthopaedic clinics should therefore have an adequate registration system. However, such a registration is only helpful when it provides reliable information; it is more dangerous to draw conclusions from incorrect data than to have no registration. Several useful software programmes are available. To obtain a postoperative infection percentage, a denominator and numerator must be available to construct this percentage.

The hospital financial administration is mostly used to create the denominator: all operations performed. When several operations during the same operative session are performed, one of them should to be chosen as the main operation which is registered. The numerator must be found by registration of the healing of the wounds of all patients. In addition, those where no infection occurred must be registered to be sure that no infections have been missed. Such a registration is only possible with the active involvement of the surgeons themselves. Only when 90% of the wounds have been evaluated can a registration system provide reliable information. Total hip replacement is a good operation for estimating the quality of operative work in a clinic, because it is a standardised and clean operation, which, in many clinics, is performed on a large scale. In an optimal situation, the postoperative infection rate of primary hips should be no higher than 0.5%, including high-risk patients. If the percentage is higher, thorough analysis should be carried out as to the cause of the high infection percentage - for example, checking the bacteriological quality of the air in the operating theatre.

PATIENT FACTORS

Patient factors that may increase the risk for postoperative infections in clean operations are: advanced age, a high ASA classification, diabetes (up to 10.7%), obesity (13.5%) and malnutrition (16.6%) [3]. Rheumatoid arthritis was not found to be related to higher infection rates in total hip replacement [42]. Most of these patient factors cannot be influenced. In elective surgery, patients may try to reduce obesity, but this will mostly not be effective. Malnutrition, as reflected by reduced serum albumin, is also related to higher infection rate, but is especially seen in patients with acute problems, such as hip fractures, and can only be corrected postoperatively by supplementary nutrition. Studies on the immune responses in osteomyelitis patients seem to indicate that immunoglobulins do not increase despite infection [1]. The phagocytic activity is also diminished. The amounts of T-cells and helper T-cells are decreased [31]. Improving the immune response by vaccination has been tried for many years, but without evident success. Studies are now ongoing on vaccine therapy [26].

The preoperative hospital stay seems to be a risk factor, but this is apparently due to confusion in the studies: there is no relationship in otherwise healthy patients, and a strong relationship in patients with co-morbidity. Therefore, the infection rate is increased not so much due to the long preoperative stay itself, during which colonisation of the patient with hospital germs may increase the risk for wound infection, but rather due to other pathological conditions also present in the patient, and which are the reason for long preoperative hospital treatment.

Some studies suggest that patients with St. aureus colonisation of the nose are prone to a higher risk, and that preoperative prophylactic therapy with an anti-staphylococcal ointment could reduce the risk [11]. In orthopaedic surgery, however, this is not yet proved.

An important preventive measure is preoperative care of the patient's skin, to reduce its bacterial load. Measures that can be applied are washing, shaving and disinfection.

Washing the skin with disinfecting soap is only necessary in patients who are hospitalised preoperatively for more than 2-3 days. Special soap containing 4% chlorhexidine has to be used repeatedly. There is evidence that this will reduce the degree of colonisation of the skin.

Removal of hair from the operation area is necessary mainly for practical surgical reasons, to avoid any hairs getting into the wound. There is no evidence that hair removal is necessary for infection prevention. In fact, more bacteria live in the follicles of the hairs than on the hairs themselves. Shaving may even have a negative effect on wound infection rates. Shaving the skin with a knife produces small skin lesions which facilitate bacterial growth. The longer these lesions exist, the heavier the skin colonisation and the more the risk increases for postoperative wound infection. Therefore, if shaving is done, it should be done as soon before the operation as possible. Better methods are the use of hair-clippers or depilatory cream because they leave the skin more intact.

Disinfection of the skin is performed immediately preoperatively, in the operation theatre. The most effective disinfectants are 1% iodine in 70% alcohol or 0.5% chlorhexidine in 70% alcohol (ethanol or isopropanolol). The advantage of chlorhexidine is that it sticks to the skin, which makes it effective for six hours. The effectiveness is decreased by soap, not by blood. Iodine also kills bacterial spores. Some clinics therefore apply towels with iodine to the area some hours preoperatively. Povidone-Iodine is iodine in water. Solutions of 0.1-10% are used as a disinfectant, especially in wounds or on mucous membranes.

Systemic antibiotics

Antibiotic prophylaxis has been widely used in orthopaedics since the 1970s. It has proved to be very effective in reducing deep as well as superficial postoperative infections. In total hip surgery, reduction is about 75%. In closed fracture surgery, antibiotic prophylaxis claims a reduction of the infection rate of 5% to less than 1%, and the mean risk reduction for deep infection in closed fractures is 2.8% (95% CI: 1.3-4.3%) [12].

In recent years, the duration of the prophylaxis has gradually decreased to one day. A large study investigated the possibility of using only one dose in total hip replacements. This study did not find a significant difference between one dose of cefuroxim and one day [42]. However, this particular study also did not prove that there was no difference; the trend of the study was even that prophylaxis with only one dose was two times less effective compared with prophylaxis for one day. Other studies indicate that a one-dose regimen can be worse, because an antibiotic may not have the appropriate pharmacokinetics. The minimal inhibitory concentrations for the causative bacteria must be exceeded throughout the period during which the wound is open, and the antibiotic should therefore have a half-life that is long enough [12]. It therefore appears, at the present time, that it is safer to stay on a schedule of 24 hours of prophylaxis in orthopaedic surgery.

The choice of the antibiotic used for prophylaxis should be based on the expected causative bacteria. If biomaterials are implanted, the antibiotic must have bactericidal effect against St. aureus and St. epidermidis. Many authors therefore advise a first generation cephalosporin or a penicillin active against β-lactamase-producing bacteria, such as flucloxacillin. In arthroplasty, anaerobic bacteria may play an important role in low-grade infections; therefore, they should also be covered: metronidazol should be added, or amoxycillin-clavulanic acid should be administered.

The prophylaxis must be given intravenously and not later than half an hour before the operation starts. In case of a bloodless field with an Esmarch bandage, the antibiotic must be given at least 10 minutes before the bandage is applied. If antibiotics are given to prevent a relapse of infection after an operation on a formerly infected bone, then the antibiotic must also cover the causative germ of the former infection.

Systemic antibiotic prophylaxis is indicated in orthopaedics when the risk of an infection is relatively high, or when an infection is likely to result in serious consequences:

- implantation of joint replacement prostheses;

- osteotomies and arthrodeses of large bones or joints;

- hip operations;

- spondylodeses;

- operations lasting longer than 2 hours;

- operations in patients with decreased immunity.

If bacteriological samples must be taken, as in prosthesis revisions, then the antibiotic must be given only after deep tissues have been taken for bacteriological evaluation.

ANTIBIOTIC-LOADED BONE CEMENT

A number of antibiotics have been admixed to various bone cements: many combinations are possible. However, a combination should only be used if adequate test results are available showing that the antibiotic is well-released from the cement. The release of the antibiotic from the bone cement is a diffusion process in which antibiotics are exchanged against water. The centre of an antibiotic-loaded bone cement block still has the same antibiotic concentration after several years: the release is only from a few millimetres of the superficial layer of the cement. The antibiotic must be water-soluble to diffuse into a haematoma. Because of the temperature elevation during the polymerisation of the cement, the antibiotic must also be heat-stable. Several other prerequisites are important in choosing the antibiotic (table I). Tetracycline, chloramphenicol and polymyxin are not released from bone cement, and cephalosporins are poorly released. If gentamicin is chosen, Palacos® has the best release and is therefore the best choice as cement. New antibiotic-cement combinations are available with tobramycin, clindamycin and vancomycin.

The release of the antibiotic results in a relatively high antibiotic concentration in the tissues immediately around the cement, but diffusion throughout the rest of the body is low, resulting in antibiotic concentrations in the serum that are too low to be measured, and with no toxic side effects. The antibiotic concentration in the exudate, as present in the joint space of the prosthesis, varies widely in the literature. This can be explained by variation in the surface of bone cement that comes into contact with the haematoma.

Table I. – Prerequisites for antibiotics for effective use in bone cement.

heat stable
water soluable
small volume
little mechanical influence
not toxic
broad spectrum
bactericidal
low MIC and MBC
low resistance rate
low allergy rate

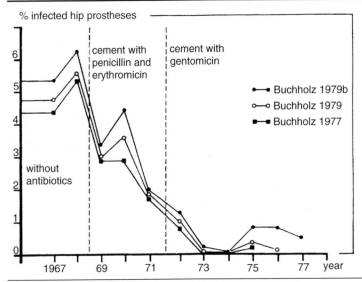

3 *The effect of admixing antibiotics in bone cement, as reflected by the infection percentages of primary THR. The graph shows the increasing infection percentages with increasing follow-up by Buchholz, as published in three consecutive publications* [36].

In animal experiments, the evidence for prophylaxis is well-documented. The antibiotic-loaded bone cement (ABC) protects not only against peroperative contamination, but also against postoperative haematogenous infection. Gentamicin was found to effectively prevent the haematogenous infection of a cement plug in a rat tibia with *St. aureus*, *Pseudomonas*, *Proteus* and group G *Streptococcus* when bacteria were i.v-injected half an hour after the operation, but not when the injection was administered 6 weeks postoperatively [6]. In a knee arthroplasty model in the rat, protection could also be proved, and lasted for only 6 weeks [2]. However this period of 6 weeks may be just as important as the peroperative and early postoperative period: in these early postoperative weeks, patients often have urinary infections, pneumonia and decubitus.

The clinical use of antibiotic-loaded bone cement started in 1969 when Buchholz used it as a prophylactic measure in primary total hip arthroplasty. After penicillin and erythromycin, he has successfully used gentamicin since 1972 (fig 3). The reduction of the infection rate in primary hip replacement in his clinic was confirmed by others: in non-randomised cohort studies, the reduction was from 3-6% to about 1%. This is confirmed in the Swedish Hip Register study on almost 150,000 total hip prostheses: gentamicin-containing Palacos® had the most pronounced association with the prevention of infection, with a risk ratio of 0.61 (CI 0.50-0.74%) [25]. An interesting finding in the register is that antibiotic-loaded bone cement is also associated with a reduced rate of aseptic loosening. It is probable that this is related to non-recognised low-grade infections due to false negative peroperative cultures, or to an absence of cultures. In a large randomised study of 1688 total hip arthroplasties, Josefsson found a significant reduction of deep infection using gentamicin-containing cement. The reduction was still significant at follow-up at 2 and 5 years, but no more at the 10-year follow-up [19]. In the Norwegian Arthroplasty Register, it was shown that the lowest probability of revision for infection of a total hip was found in patients who received systemic antibiotics in combination with antibiotic-loaded cement. This benefit was highest in the first and second postoperative year. If only systemic antibiotics were used, the risk was 4.3 times higher [8]. Also in the Swedish Total Hip Register, the cost-benefit analysis of prophylaxis in almost 150,000 total hips showed that the best and most cost-effective combination was antibiotic-loaded bone cement in combination with systemic antibiotics [30].

In conclusion, antibiotic-loaded bone cement was found to be effective in in-vitro studies, in animal experiments as well as in clinical, randomised and cohort studies. There is no evidence that using gentamicin-loaded bone cement is related to an increased incidence of multiresistant *St. epidermidis*, with high resistance to gentamicin. It seems wise, however, not to routinely use vancomycin-admixed bone cement in the near future, not even in clinics where gentamicin resistance is common. Vancomycin and other last resort drugs should never be used in routine prophylaxis, since they are needed for therapy.

OPERATING THEATRE (OP): GENERAL MEASURES

The postoperative infection rate of clean wounds depends largely on contamination of the wound during operation. Of the bacteria in a clean wound, 98% came from the air in the OP, and 2% from the patient. Bacteria in the OP do not float free in the air, but are carried by particles of varying sizes, mainly skin cells of the individuals present. An individual sheds about 10^9 skin cells per day. These have an average size of 20 µm, with about 7% having a size of less than 7 µm [40]. One in every 100-5000 cells carries bacteria.

The size of the bacteria-carrying particles is over 3 µm, with an average of 12-14 µm. The larger particles with bacteria that enter the wound fall directly downward from the heads of the surgical team, while the smaller ones follow the air stream and thus contaminate the wound or the surgical team's instruments and hands. Bacteria found in the wound have entered via the air of the OP in 30%, and via hands and instruments in 70%. These, however, are contaminated via the OP air as well.

There are two important conclusions possible from the above-mentioned. First, the air in the OP has a decisive role in the contamination of the wound and in prophylaxis of wound infection. Second, the main sources of the contamination are the workers in the OP, more specifically the bacteria on their skin cells. This is confirmed by the relationship found in several studies between the concentration of bacteria in the air and:

– the number of persons present in the OP;

– the activity of these individuals (highest during start and end of operation);

– the use of occlusive operation gowns;

– the use of helmets ("aspiration suit");

– the use of an "ultra-clean air" installation.

Several relationships between infections and increased wound contamination are in fact related to prolonged exposure to the air contamination in the OP, depending on the time needed for the operation (especially more than 2 hours).

More bacteria in the air results in more bacterial contamination of the wound [41], and more bacteria in the wound results in more wound infections [5]. However, the direct relationship between the air contamination and the postoperative wound infection rate could only be proved in a large, multicenter study [22].

The above-mentioned relationship between air contamination and wound infection is the reason why general measures that reduce the bacterial load of the OP air are effective and indicated:

– reduce the number of people in the OP;

– have them wear proper head cover and masks;

– have them reduce their movements, walk slowly, not too close to the tables;

– have them speak only if necessary, and not loudly;

– make certain their clothes reduce the shedding of their skin scales;

– be aware that persons with skin diseases should not work if they have increased shedding, or have *St. aureus* skin infections;

– be aware that instruments should only be exposed to the OP air when the air contamination is reduced (after preparing the patient).

An important factor is the reduction of shedding. Good clothing systems can reduce the airborne bacterial counts 5-10 times. Clothes with an open structure are not at all capable of preventing bacterial dispersion: ordinary cotton is woven with a pore size > 80 μm, so all bacteria on skin scales can pass easily. Reduction of the pore size is possible when the fabric is very tightly woven, or when the clothes are made of semi-impermeable or impermeable material. When these clothes are used as a gown over cotton clothing, they provide no reduction. Because the material is impermeable to air, skin debris is pumped out from the suit neck opening. These materials should be used as a suit with effective seals at the neck, trousers and waist; in that case, they are 1,000 times more effective than open cotton clothing [40]. Unfortunately, such a design is uncomfortably warm. When air exhaust systems are used under impermeable gowns, the heat may be reduced, as well as the dispersion of skin scales carrying bacteria.

AIR HANDLING SYSTEMS IN THE OPERATION THEATRE

The role of the air handling system is to supply the OP with sterile and fresh air, and also to take away the air with pollution: narcotic gases as well as particles with bacteria. Not all air handling systems can fulfil these tasks well. Broadly speaking, there are two systems: mixing and non-mixing systems.

In the older mixing systems, fresh, clean air is introduced into the OP room with the objective of reducing the contamination of the air by dilution (*fig 4*). It appears that there is no additional effect when more than 20 times the content of an OP is refreshed. In a regular OP of 100 m³, this results in an air supply of 2,000 m³/h. This is therefore the amount of air introduced into most of the OPs formerly built in the Netherlands. Instructions for architects and the budgets were based on this calculation. However, this kind of mixing system provides no special directing of the air towards the OP table, and is not designed to remove germs away from the OP field. The airflow is also turbulent.

In non-mixing systems, the insufflated air itself is used to drive away the polluted air (*fig 5*). These systems deliver sterile laminar flow, directed to the wound, and must be

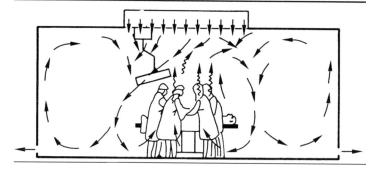

4 *Mixing type OP air handling system: the system is not capable of directing the airstream from clean to contaminated zones* [37].

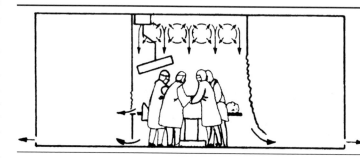

5 *Non-mixing type OP air handling system: clean air does not mix with contaminated air, but is able to push it away, in this case with the help of curtains and laminar flow* [37].

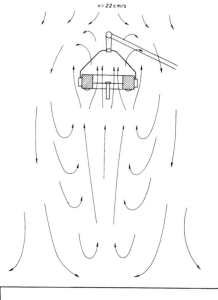

6 *OP-lamps must be designed to minimise the obstruction of the downward air flow, and to produce minimal convection warmth* [37].

AB = antibiotics
UCA = Ultra Clean Air enclosure
VS = ventilated suits

7 *Relationship of reduction of postoperative deep infections of THR by several prophylactic measures* [22].

capable of taking away shed contaminated particles to the outlet openings. It has been proved that downflow laminar systems are more effective than horizontal flow systems, often used in rebuilding situations. The OP lamp forms the most important obstruction for an effective downflow, and the heat produced also causes an upward convection force (*fig 6*). Therefore, in practice, the downflow speed of the air must be about 30-45 cm/sec at the plenum, and the best temperature is 19° C. To maintain the downflow as long as possible, side walls hung from the ceiling around the plenum can be used. For practical reasons, these walls are usually not less than about 2 meters high, so as to be higher than individuals and, for example, the image intensifier. In the well known "greenhouse" (according to Charnley-Howorth or Weber-Meierhans), these walls come down to 10 cm above the floor. In such ultra-clean air installations, large volumes of air are used, up to 12.000 m³/h, with up to 600 exchanges per hour. In optimal situations these air systems are combined with "body exhaust suits": impermeable gowns and helmets, suctioning the air away. In such an operating environment, the infective bacterial dose of the wound via hands, instruments and air is reduced to the absolute minimum.

The reduction of the deep postoperative infection rate in primary total hips is 50% with an ultra-clean air installation, and also 50% with a body exhaust suit. Because these reductions act independently of one another, in combination they provide a reduction of 75%. In combination with the 75% reduction of infection provided by systemic antibiotics, the infection rate can be reduced from 3.4% to 0.2% (*fig 7*) [22]. The same calculation has been made by Persson et al, based on data

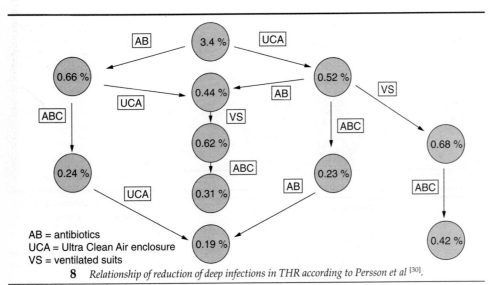

AB = antibiotics
UCA = Ultra Clean Air enclosure
VS = ventilated suits

8   *Relationship of reduction of deep infections in THR according to Persson et al* [30].

Treatment of orthopaedic infections

EARLY POSTOPERATIVE WOUND INFECTIONS

Early postoperative infections are due to contamination:

– Preoperative: in case of open fractures, especially when necrotic tissues are left in the wound.

– Peroperative: mostly from shedding with *St. aureus* or *St. epidermidis* spread by air in the operation theatre during the operation.

– Postoperative contamination: when wound secretion permits the introduction of bacteria via the wound in case of improper wound care, especially when large haematomas are formed.

The result of treatment largely depends on time elapsed since the operation - which is often too long, for two reasons. First, the diagnosis is often difficult to make, because operation and haematoma result in many similar, aspecific symptoms. Waiting can provide some evidence about this differential diagnostic problem. Second, surgeons are as biased when judging their own work as anyone else. In case of a possible infection, they must admit to imminent failure concerning the operation, and telling this to the patient is a problem. A process of unconscious denial may result in not diagnosing a probable infection. The diagnosis may be postponed by these factors, and therefore the therapy delayed. Although this is dangerous, often the therapy is half-hearted and therefore not effective - for example, a week of oral antibiotics.

In the case of suspected wound infection in the early postoperative period, the first concern is to culture the causative bacteria: if pus can be collected, a syringe is filled and sent to the laboratory. If a wound secretes, then the skin is disinfected, and a swab introduced into the wound, if necessary after removal of one of the stitches. The treatment choice at that moment is between:

1. waiting and deciding later;

2. starting antibiotic therapy only;

3. re-operating: debridement, then starting antibiotics.

In case of obvious symptoms, such as high fever and large haematomas, operative debridement should be performed. Antibiotics will not sufficiently penetrate pus and haematomas, and the bacterial load of the contamination must be reduced. All necrotic tissue, pus and haematomas must be removed, extensive lavage done, and eventually local antibiotics (resorbable or not) placed in the wound. After deep specimens have been taken for culture, intravenous treatment with antibiotics is started. In the first days, a broad spectrum

from almost 150,000 total hips as registered in the Swedish National Register (*fig 8*). In addition, they were able to evaluate the influence of antibiotic-loaded cement, and to calculate the costs of the various prophylactic measures. When the costs of hip revision are also taken into account, the most cost-effective strategy of prophylactic measures can be calculated. The best combination appeared to be gentamicin-loaded bone cement in combination with systemic antibiotics (as in the Josefsson study), which resulted in a reduction of the postoperative infection percentage from 3.4% to 0.24%. The use of ultra-clean air in combination with antibiotic-loaded bone cement and systemic antibiotics further reduced the risk to 0.19%. This percentage is comparable with the percentage in the Lidwell study, where ultra-clean air and ventilated suits were used (see figures 7 and 8). In their calculations, the extra costs of such a sterile enclosure depend on the number of total hips implanted a year: from USD 157 for 100 THR/year to USD 66 for 250 THR/year [30]. There is no good explanation as to why, in their study, ventilated exhaust suits always had a negative influence when combined with any other prophylactic measure.

The quality of the air in an OP can be measured using several methods. The technical equipment is tested by measuring the air velocity at the plenum (30-45 cm/sec) and on the level of the OP table (about 25 cm/sec). The pattern of streaming of the air can be checked with smoke: the stream must be downward and laminar. This test cannot be performed during an operation; the heat of an OP lamp and the convection of the warmth generated by active surgeons must be simulated. The technical check also includes particle measurement at the plenum and control of the temperature of the air introduced (19° C). These tests should be done once or twice a year, and when there are problems. Filters must be tested (DOP test) and renewed if necessary. The bacteriological quality of the OP air is expressed as the

number of colony-forming units per cubic metre (CFU/m^3). The measurement is possible using slit samplers: these instruments suction a certain amount of air and direct it along Petri dishes which are cultured in the bacteriology laboratory. There is no standardised method, but measurements should be done during an actual operation, near the wound and the surgeon. Petri dishes must be placed, because the larger particles are not taken by the air stream but simply sedimented downwards from the heads and bodies of the surgical team.

In OPs where operations more prone to infection are performed, such as for prostheses and hip fractures, the standard for the bacteriological quality of the air should be < 10 CFU/m^3 during the operations. Other types of operations, including day care treatment, can best be performed in an OP air with a contamination of not more than 100 - 200 CFU/m^3, if cost-efficiency is a matter of concern.

It is important to give attention to the prophylactic measurements in the OP itself, because that is the most causative approach to postoperative infections. It is much better to avoid contamination than to combat it later with the help of antibiotics. Because all prophylactic measures reduce the infection rate independently, the choice in prosthesis implantation could include the following:

1. always using systemic antibiotics;

2. optimising the OP air handling system (downflow, laminar, clean) and clothing;

3. using antibiotic-loaded bone cement (ABC), if:

– most of the germs in the hospital are susceptible to gentamicin loaded bone cement, and

– no ultra-clean air system is available.

If an ultra-clean air system is available, using plain bone cement without antibiotic admixture can be considered.

Table II. – Classifications for osteomyelitis.

Buckholz	aetiology
Cierny/Mader	extent + host resistance
Ger	wound characteristics
Gordon	bone damage and loss
Kelly	aetiology and region
Waldvogel	aetiology
Weiland	extent of infection

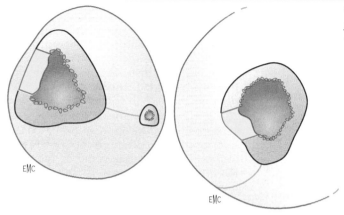

9 *Best places in tibia and femur for windows used for intramedullary debridement* [38].

antibiotic (combination) should be used, such as amoxycillin-clavulanic acid with aminoglycosides. When the result of the culture is known, the appropriate antibiotic with a smaller spectrum can then be administered.

CHRONIC OSTEOMYELITIS

There are several classifications of osteomyelitis (*table II*), none of which seem to apply to all types of osteomyelitis. Chronic osteomyelitis is characterised by relapses after long periods of apparent healing. Relapses have been described after decades, and are not rare when a formerly infected bone is reoperated years later. The chronic infection may vary in activity, and patients with chronic osteomyelitis often have only slight secretion with the absence of any pain. The bone is mostly sclerotic with changes in structure due to the infection and sometimes to multiple operations. The infection may become quiescent or heal, either due to treatment or spontaneously. Relapses have a typical sequence: after a period of relative quiescence without complaints, a relapse results in an increasing amount of oedema and secretion. The stowing of secretion results in increasing pressure, which causes pain and fever up to the moment that the secretion finds its way out, mostly via the old fistula. Local factors influence the course of this typical pattern, regarding the pressure needed and the levels of pain and fever reached in relation to the secretion. Treatment of chronic osteomyelitis is indicated when:

– the chronic secretion hinders (is profuse, emits odour, is a psychological problem);

– the infection is too active, with soft tissue induration;

– progressive bone lysis is present;

– relapses occur too often;

– joint prostheses or heart valves prone to haematogenous infection are present.

■ *Conservative treatment*

Conservative treatment may be indicated when surgical treatment seems to be exhausted, as regards the capacity of the patient or the doctor, and extensive surgery or amputation is refused or contraindicated. In these patients, antibiotics can be given lifelong to suppress the activity of the infection. This is possible with relatively non-toxic antibiotics that can be given orally.

However, most of these patients will not want to be treated lifelong, and advanced age in itself is not a contraindication to extensive surgical treatment, considering that immune capacity will decrease with age. These patients will usually be treated by "supervised neglect": incision of abscesses via an old fistula and short-term antibiotic treatments to suppress the clinical manifestations of the infection.

■ *Operative treatment: debridement*

Operating is necessary to remove infected and non-vital tissue: granulation tissue, abscesses, sequestra and other sclerotic less viable bone, as well as all kinds of foreign bodies. All these tissues harbour bacteria that is either not or poorly accessible to antibiotics and host defence. Preoperative imaging should have localised not only the infection but also these less vital tissues and should give information about the topography and accessibility of the infection. Most informative is filling the fistula with methylene blue. This should be done by the surgeon himself the day before operation, instead of during or immediately before the operation: in that case the blue will colour too much healthy tissue during the operation. The dye must be injected with pressure, causing the same pain as during stowing of secretion. During the 12-24 hours before the operation, the superfluous dye will be lost and the granulation tissue of fistula and abscess wall is coloured selectively. Following the methylene blue tissue during operation in this way is often much more helpful than elaborate preoperative imaging with frequent false positive and aspecific findings [38].

Giving preoperative antibiotics may hinder peroperative identification of a causative germ. Therefore, antibiotics are generally not started before deep cultures have been taken.

The operation should preferably be done with an Esmarch bandage without exsanguinating the limb ("Blutsperre", "blood blocking"). This avoids the invasion of infective products into the blood during compression. Leaving some blood in the limb also makes it easier to check the viability of the tissues.

Complete debridement is often only possible via a cortical window. This window should not weaken the bone too much, and must avoid the linea aspera in the femur and important cristae, such as the three cristal rims of the tibia (*fig 9*). If these can be kept, the strength of the bone will not be decreased too much if sharp edges which form stress risers have also been avoided. Therefore, the osteotomy of the window is predrilled and the edges rounded off. Intra-osseous sequestra and granulation tissue are removed. A thickened cortex is reduced to a normal thickness with a chisel or, better, with a high speed burr. The cortex of the window is not replaced and the defect needs no special reinforcement if the debridement is well-performed. If it has weakened the bone too much, a bone graft must be done. Intra-medullary infections after an empyema or infected nail are debrided by drilling the medullary canal with intra-medullary reamers to remove small circular sequestra. Such debridement by reaming is more effective when a small window is made in the distal metaphysis to remove the debris. Debridement must be radical to promote healing of the infection, but this results in large defects that must be reconstructed. One of the usual causes for non-healing is a fear of this radical therapy because the surgeon has insufficient experience in reconstruction: the skills for reconstruction define how radical the debridement can be. There is a parallel with oncology surgery. At this moment, a reconstruction can be performed in larger defects with the help of two techniques. Regarding bone, larger resections can be made because very large defects can be treated by bone transport (Ilizarov technique, segment transport): the osteomyelitic bone is widely resected and healthy bone is transported by external fixators. The disadvantage is the long amount of time it takes, plus the long learning curve for the surgeon. Regarding soft tissues, tissue transfers with free flaps can create a vital soft tissue cover for scarred, chronically infected limbs. Microvascular surgery and other techniques of plastic surgery can transplant muscle, possibly with full thickness skin and also parts of bone.

■ Stability

Implants must be removed if possible, together with non-vital tissues. They are left in place only when they are needed for fixation of a fracture or osteotomy. In that case, the infection is treated as usual with debridement and antibiotics, and the implant is removed after consolidation. Such cases must always be regarded as low-grade infected and, even in the absence of infection symptoms, be re-debrided when the implant is removed. Stability is often said to be absolutely necessary for the healing of an infection. This statement reflects, however, more a clinical experience than experimentally proved evidence. Two animal experiments studied the relationship between infection and stability. It was proved that consolidation can occur in a sheep tibia despite infection [33]. In a rabbit tibia, it was proved that in case of serious instability the infection is more severe, and also that consolidation occurs despite infection [9].

Therefore, an infection may heal despite instability, but the clinical experience is that, especially in the diaphyseal region, stability is needed to obtain a dry wound. Stability helps, but there is no need to achieve absolute rigidity. Infected hips can heal very well despite the instability of a Girdlestone situation. The advantages of stability must be weighed against the disadvantages of an implant. In most cases, the application of an external fixator is therefore the best solution.

The use of an intramedullary nail despite infection has been described by Papineau [28]. This use of intramedullary nails in osteomyelitis has increased since the introduction of interlocking screws. There is, however, a considerable risk that the infection, not yet healed, will spread along the entire length of the nail and result in an abscess distally. As when another internal osteosynthesis is used to stabilise an infected bone, such cases must be regarded as low-grade infected, even when no signs of infection are evident. The bed of the hardware must be debrided and possibly locally treated when the nail is removed.

■ Local antibiotic treatment

Following debridement, the area is still more or less heavily contaminated with bacteria, and must be sterilised. Antibiotics and antiseptics can be used. Since 1977, growing experience has been obtained with gentamicin-impregnated beads of polymethyl-methacrylate (PMMA, bone cement) [20]. These beads of 4.5 mm diameter exchange their gentamicin content with the water in the surrounding haematoma and tissues. This diffusion process builds up a high local gentamicin concentration in 2-3 days in the haematoma and tissues around the beads. The gentamicin concentration can reach values that are 10-100 times higher than needed to stop the bacterial growth (MIC, minimal inhibitory

concentration) or to kill them (MBC, minimal bactericidal concentration). However, this high concentration is limited in time and distance. The concentration decreases to below MIC values after 2-3 weeks. At a distance of 2-3 centimetres from the beads, the concentration will often decrease too much to be effective.

Too low, subinhibitory concentrations of gentamicin can develop when the beads are left in place. Although no increased resistance to gentamicin could be found in Klemm's clinic, the formation of intracellular-persistent bacteria in the form of SCVs (small colony variants) may be caused by beads [4], and can result in relapses.

The bacteriology laboratory gives a clinician the sensitivity to gentamicin of an identified germ by the abbreviations S (= sensitive), I (= intermediate sensitive) or R (= resistant). These characterisations are nonetheless determined by the values that can be achieved in the tissues when antibiotic treatment is given systemically, and in local treatment, the concentrations are much higher. Therefore, to know if an infection can be treated by local gentamicin treatment, the antibiogram of the cultures must specify what the MIC for gentamicin of the causative germ is. When this MIC value is arbitrarily below the value of 100 µg/ml the infection can be treated with gentamicin PMMA beads; otherwise other antibiotics have to be mixed into bone cement by hand, or a suction drainage system has to be applied.

Despite the high antibiotic concentrations in exudates and tissues, the serum concentration remains very low in local antibiotic treatment when using gentamicin beads, even when high numbers of beads are used (300-600) or when patients have impaired renal function. Toxic side effects do not occur [39]. The beads are placed in as much as possible of the entire infected area, to promote high local antibiotic concentration where needed. When treatment is effective, the wound will be dry within 5-7 days. Prolonged secretion in the presence of beads is a sign of non-healing. After two weeks, the beads are removed. If healing is not yet probable, debridement must be repeated and new beads are again inserted for 2 weeks. So, step by step debridement can be performed in osteomyelitis, searching for the optimal balance between the removal of infected, less vital tissue and the preservation of tissues needed for continuity. The corresponding two-week schedule is an important advantage for the patient as well as the surgeon [38].

Other antibiotics can be admixed into bone cements, such as tobramicin, clindamycin, and vancomycin. However, not all antibiotics are suitable or will diffuse out of the cement. Several other carriers have been studied. Bone grafts and new bone substitutes are especially promising because

they can be used in combination with reconstructive measures. Resorbable carriers have the advantage of having no need for removal; however, the resorption process of the biomaterial may lead to serious wound secretion starting one week postoperatively, and persisting during the process of resorption, which may last for several weeks. In Europe, combinations of aminoglycosides have been used with collagen (Collatamp®, Septocoll®) or plaster of Paris.

Antiseptics have the advantage that there is no fear of bacterial resistance, and perhaps they will increase in importance in the future. The disadvantage can be their relative toxicity for the tissues, and increased secretion. They can be admixed into a solution for instillation (Lavasept®) into the wound or can be packed in a collagen carrier (Taurolin®) [23].

With local antibacterial treatment, the infected tissues can be freed of their bacterial load stepwise, in combination with stepwise excision of avital tissues. When the carriers are not resorbable, they are helpful in maintaining space needed for reconstruction. Resorbable carriers should be reserved for the cases where no reconstruction is needed. Because of their tendency to provoke secretion, they should be used specifically in the deeper tissues, well closed in by several soft tissue layers. The special properties of the biomaterial may render these useful in specific indications. For example, collagen fleece fibres are suitable in soft tissues or small cavities because they become flat and small, shrinking substantially inside a haematoma.

■ Reconstruction

There are two main reasons for reconstruction: loss of vital soft tissues covering the bone, and loss of bone strong enough to restore a functional limb. Cavities have long been seen as an important reason for non-healing in osteomyelitis. Therefore, reducing cavities by saucerisation and filling has always been an important part of the treatment. However, a persisting cavity, for example in the proximal tibia or femur metaphysis, is no reason in itself to fill with bone graft that can be better used elsewhere. The cavity can be filled with beads that may be left behind, or can be left alone without being filled, because it is sterilised by the treatment. Cancellous grafts are used to bridge defects up to 3-5 cm in a diaphysis. In reconstruction after infection, the best results will be obtained with autologous grafts. Most cancellous bone can be harvested from the iliac bone just lateral to the sacroiliac joint, or from the proximal tibial metaphysis (via a small lateral window). Grafts are also used in the case of windows that weaken the diaphyseal structure too much, and in the lower leg to connect the tibia with the fibula (tibia pro fibula). When cancellous bone grafts are used, stability must be provided for a long period, with an external fixator as the safest solution. An interlocking nail is convenient for the patient, but it has the disadvantage of a possible infection along the entire nail. Should this occur, it can be suppressed by antibiotics until consolidation of the graft, and the infection cured afterwards by reaming the medullary canal when the nail is removed. When cancellous bone grafts are used in osteomyelitis treatment, and soft tissues cannot be closed, the graft can be treated open [7, 28].This will, however, result in the loss of the superficial part of the graft, which can be avoided by the use of artificial skin (Epigard®).

Large bone defects can be reconstructed by the use of segment transport. A segment of healthy bone is transported 1 mm a day by an external fixator [26]. Behind the transported segment, new bone is formed with the characteristics of callus. Over several months, this will consolidate into strong and healthy diaphyseal bone. Large defects can thus be bridged but with much effort from the patient as well as the surgeon. Bridging fifteen centimetres takes about one year. Another possibility for overcoming large bone defects is the use of free vascularised bone segments - from the iliac crest or contralateral fibula, for example. This can be combined with attached muscles and skin coverage, depending on the soft tissue defects. Expert microvascular surgery is needed for these reconstructions. Large soft tissue defects are best filled with a muscle flap, pedicled or free.

■ *Systemic antibiotic treatment*

The role of antibiotics, although secondary, may be important. Surgical measures must create a favourable situation for the application of local as well as systemic antibiotics. Those who promote very radical debridement and large radical reconstructions often refrain from systemic antibiotics, because all contaminated tissues are regarded as having been excised. However, this does not seem to be advisable for the average orthopaedic surgeon treating common osteomyelitis. Therefore, in most osteomyelitis cases, the surgical treatment will be supported by antibiotic therapy.

Reliable information about the causative bacteria is decisive for the success of any kind of antibiotic therapy. The method of taking the samples is very important in orthopaedic infections. The best and most reliable information is given by deep tissue samples, which have been cultured in the laboratory for aerobic as well as anaerobic bacteria. In the laboratory, cultures that remain sterile should be further incubated in enrichment broth for about two weeks to avoid false negative reports. To avoid false positive reports (for example, skin contaminants) the material is subdivided into 6 tubes with enrichment broths. Bacteria are considered as clinically relevant if they grow in 3 or more of these cultures [38]. The

help of, and discussion with, a bacteriologist with knowledge of orthopaedic infections and the special laboratory techniques as needed are mandatory for effective antibiotic treatment.

When the only specimens can be taken from a sinus tract, it has to be considered that these cultures show a discrepancy with cultures from deep-seated tissue. The discrepancy rate rises from 18% to 69% when the sinus tract infection was present longer [24], presenting more polybacterial cultures. The only exception is when *St. aureus* is found in the sinus: in that case *St. aureus* is also found in 80% of the deep tissue.

Penicillin-resistant *St. aureus* is the most frequent causative bacteria, and flucloxacillin is then the best choice. The dose is up to 6 times per day 2 gram i.v. in young healthy patients during the hospital stay. In older patients, the maximal dose may be reduced to 6 times per day 1 gram i.v. to avoid renal problems. When the treatment is switched to oral administration, most patients can stand a dose of 4 times per day 500 mg for a very long period, even lifelong, while feeling uncomfortable with 4 times per day 1 gram. Most authors advise a long treatment of 6-12 weeks, although only a single study has supported the effectiveness of a long-term treatment [18]. If a choice has to be made for an antibiotic that can only be administered intravenously, then a Hickmann catheter can be used.

■ *Conclusion*

To summarise, the treatment of chronic osteomyelitis can be performed based upon the following schedule:
1. debridement of the infection in one or (stepwise) several stages;
2. implantation of a local antibiotic carrier for two weeks, with temporary bone stabilisation;
3. permanent stabilisation and reconstruction by bone graft and soft tissue transfer if necessary;
4. 6-12 weeks systemic antibiotic treatment, of which the first 3 weeks i.v.

INFECTED ARTHROPLASTIES

■ *Early postoperative infections*

In this case, as in all early postoperative infections, it is hoped that the infection is limited to the haematoma and tissue necrosis that has developed in the early postoperative days, and has not involved the bone-prosthesis/cement interface. The decision about whether an infection is present in the early postoperative period, and if it necessitates treatment, is one of the most difficult ones to make. It must be decided fully on clinical judgement based mainly on the aspect of the wound, body temperature and laboratory findings. Aspecific infection symptoms must be

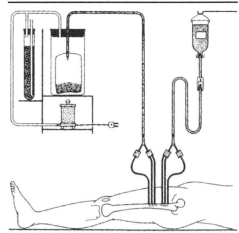

10 *Suction drainage system as used in the past in osteomyelitis: 2 inlet and 2 outlet drains* [36].

distinguished from regular postoperative symptoms. It is difficult to decide if treatment for infection must be started, because this treatment can only be effective if it is aggressive. Giving some oral antibiotic treatment for a few days or weeks is easier to decide, but is harmful because it masks the symptoms of the infection without providing a chance for healing, therefore increasing the delay before effective treatment.

Treatment with systemic antibiotics alone can be a reasonable therapy when only superficial infection is present, with induration and oedema, but without subcutaneous collections of haematoma or pus. When such collections are present or deep infection seems to be present, operative debridement is necessary. Upon operation, a connection between the subcutaneous layers and the deeper tissues of the joint under the fascia must be carefully looked for, because it is almost always found. In that case, the whole field of the primary operation is regarded as infected and must be debrided. Then local treatment may be as follows:

– Suction drainage system: 2 inlet and 2 (larger) outlet drains are used. Lavage with Ringer's solution without additives is used, 3-4 litres per day. The infusion must be performed with low pressure, only gravity forces (*fig 10*). The outlet needs some suction, about 25 cm H_2O. After 7-10 days, the system must be removed. These drainage systems require much attention because the drains clog and leak. After 10 days, gram-negative superinfection becomes very frequent.

– Gentamicin PMMA beads are used in the limited space of the new joint. In a total hip, about 120 beads can be placed, in a knee joint 60 - 90 beads. After 2 weeks they are removed, or the debridement is repeated.

– Gentamicin-containing collagen fleeces can be used in this indication, due to the limited space, the relatively high gentamicin concentration (up to several thousand µg/ml) and the resorbability, which makes reoperation unnecessary.

In cases of early postoperative infection around a prosthesis, treatment with systemic antibiotics is always indicated. Even in the case of operative debridement, it is never sure if the bone/cement and prosthesis/bone interfaces are involved. These have not been reached by the debridement and local antibiotics, so systemic antibiotics must be added. A retained infected prosthesis is outweighed by an aggressive, high-dosed and long term systemic antibiotic treatment. Systemic antibiotics should therefore be given for 3-6 months and intravenously as long as possible. In case of adhesive *St. epidermidis*, clindamycin should be used, or rifampycin, combined with another antibiotic.

Late prosthesis infections

These infections are always deep, and the interface between prosthesis, bone and cement is involved. The treatment is very comparable with the treatment of chronic osteomyelitis, the reconstruction having specific aspects. Treatment with systemic antibiotics alone is only indicated to reduce infection symptoms in patients who cannot be operated. However, when a fistula closes during antibiotic therapy, there is a high risk of severe sepsis when the effectiveness of the therapy diminishes or the therapy is stopped. Deep prosthesis infection can cause life-threatening septicaemia, especially in rheumatoid patients. Operative treatment includes removal of all prosthetic components and all bone cement, including every small distal fragment! In case of non-loosening, this may be a difficult operation requiring much skill and special instruments. Sometimes trochanteric osteotomy and large femoral windows are necessary. Removal of some types of well-fixed, non-cemented prostheses (for example, Lord, Zweymuller) may cause severe bone damage. Hydroxyapatite coatings when used in the proximal part of the femoral stem permit extraction with less difficulty after some forceful hammering, if necessary, after longitudinal osteotomy of only the lateral proximal femoral cortex. When prosthesis and cement are removed, and all granulation tissue and abscess walls have been excised, gentamicin PMMA beads are placed in the entire infected area. Beads are placed deep in the femoral canal with a special introducer. A cortical window is permanently or temporarily closed with sutures or cerclages. A large number of beads are used to achieve a high gentamicin concentration and to avoid the development of resistance. The fascias are tightly closed. Beads are also placed subcutaneously when the subcutis is thick. Drains are placed in the joint to reduce the volume of the haematoma, which can be very large in a Girdlestone hip. If the volume of the haematoma is too large, the concentration of

gentamicin remains correspondingly low. Therefore, it is best to use a deep drain under the fascia, used just as gravity drainage. A suction drain is placed in the subcutis to suction away the haematoma that has permeated through the fascia and to prevent the formation of abscesses subcutaneously. The suprafascial drain is therefore removed later than the deeper one. In selected cases, direct reimplantation of the prosthesis can be performed. This "one-stage revision" is done:

– in aseptic loosening;

– in low grade infections: which often means infections not recognised by improper bacteriological diagnosis. This may explain the high infection rate of some revision series. If local and systemic antibiotic therapy is well applied in low-grade infections, then a one-stage revision could be a reasonable alternative to a two-stage revision. However there is no comparative study at all in the literature;

– if the patient can only stand one operation and the infection is low-grade, with low virulence bacteria;

– in severe infections of prostheses: some centres with a large amount of experience have advocated one-stage revision with individualised antibiotic-cement mixtures. There is a need for special bacteriological diagnostic investigations preoperatively, and a large selection of antibiotics that have to be admixed in bone cement in the form of sterile powder.

In general orthopaedic practice, the best policy seems to be to restrict the indication for one-stage revision to aseptic and questionable infected cases. The risk for reinfection requiring re-revision should be weighed against an extra operation in two-stage revisions and two or more weeks of extra hospital stay. In any event, a one-stage reimplantation should never be done when a patient cannot physically and psychologically stand another revision for a reinfected hip. After 2 weeks the beads are

Table III. – Criteria for healing of an ortho-paedic infection.

no fever
no secretion
no warmth, redness
no induration
no cyclic pain related to secretion or fever
no use of antibiotics
normal ESR, CRP, leucocyte count

removed, and if necessary the whole procedure is repeated once or twice.

Reimplantation

When healing seems appropriate (table III), a decision must be made about reimplantation. Reimplantation must be technically possible, depending on the skills of the surgeon and availability of special revision prostheses, and bone grafting may be necessary. The use of allograft bone for reconstruction may be dangerous in infected cases. Reimplantation must only be considered when healing seems appropriate. However, it is never 100% sure that this is the case, so surgeon and patient have to take a calculated risk. It is better in infected cases not to reimplant, and to create a Girdlestone hip when:

– there is no adequate bone stock and repair is not reasonably possible;

– a severe infection is caused by a virulent bacteria, and the patient can only stand one operation (the debridement).

If healing of the infection is uncertain after a few weeks of therapy, it is better to postpone making the decision of whether reimplantation has to be performed. During 6-12 months, the patient is observed with a temporary Girdlestone situation, and a reimplantation is planned only if healing is more appropriate (normalised soft tissues and ESR), and the patient is still willing to take the risk of relapse (fig 11).

Acknowledgements – Figures 4, 5 and 6 were first published in Walenkamp GH. Traitement de l'air. In : L'infection en chirurgie orthopédique. Paris : Expansion scientifique francaise, 1990 : 14-21

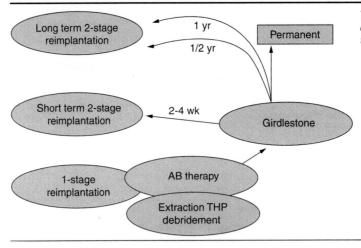

11 *Schedule illustrating the one - and two-stage revision in infected THR.*

References

[1] Bansai VP, Mittal PK, Ashokraj G. Humoral immune responses in osteomyelitis. *Int Orthop* 1992 ; 16 : 297-301

[2] Blomgren G. Hematogenous infection of total joint replacement. An experimental study in the rabbit. *Acta Orthop Scand [suppl]* 1981 ; 187 : 1-64

[3] Cruse PJE. A five-year prospective study of 23, 649 surgical wounds. *Arch Surg* 1973 ; 107 : 206-209

[4] Eiff CH, Von Bettin D, Proctor RA, Rolaufs B, Lindner N, Winkelman W et al. Recovery of small colony variants of *Staphylococcus aureus* following gentamicin bead placement for osteomyelitis. *Clin Infect Dis* 1997 ; 25 : 1250-1251

[5] Elek SD, Conen PE. The virulence of Staphylococcus Pyogenes for man. A study of the problems of wound infection. *Br J Exp Pathol* 1957 ; 38 : 573-586

[6] Elson RA, Jephcott AE, McGechie DB, Verettas D. Bacterial infection and acrylic cement in the rat. *J Bone Joint Surg Br* 1977 ; 59 : 452-457

[7] Enami A, Mjoeberg B, Larsson S. Infected tibial nonunion: good results after open cancellous bone grafting in 37 cases. *Acta Orthop Scand* 1995 ; 66 : 447-451

[8] Espehaug B, Engesaeter LB, Vollset SE, Havelin LI, Langeland N. Antibiotic prophylaxis in total hip arthroplasty. Review of 10,905 primary cemented total hip replacements reported to the Norwegian arthroplasty register,1987 to1995. *J Bone Joint Surg Br* 1997 ; 79 : 590-595

[9] Friedrich B. Biomechanische Stabilität und posttraumatische Osteitis. Experimentelle Untersuchungen zur Aetiologie und ihre Konsequenzen für die Klinik. *Hefte Unfallheilkd* 1975 ; 122 : 1-110

[10] Gastrin B, Lovestad A. Postoperative wound infection: relation to different types of operation and wound contamination categories in orthopaedic surgery. *J Hosp Infect* 1989 ; 13 : 387-394

[11] Gernaat-Van Der, Sluis AJ, Hoogenboom-Verdegaal AM, Edixhoven PH, Spies Van Rooijen NH. Prophylactic mupirocin could reduce orthopedic wound infections; 1,044 patients treated with mupirocin compared with 1,260 historical controls. *Acta Orthop Scand* 1998 ; 69 : 412-414

[12] Gillespie WJ, Walenkamp G. Antibiotic prophylaxis in patients undergoing surgery for proximal femoral and other closed long bone fractures. Cochrane Library, 1998

[13] Gristina AG, Barth E, Webb LX. Microbial adhesion and the pathogenesis of biomaterial centered infections. In : Gustilo RB ed. Orthopaedic infections. Diagnosis and treatment. Philadelphia : WB Saunders, 1989 : 3-25

[14] Gristina AG, Costerton JW, Webb LX. Microbial adhesion, biofilms and the pathophysiology of osteomyelitis. In : d'Ambrosia RD ed. Orthopaedic infections. New Jersey : Slack, 1989 : 49-69

[15] Gristina AG, Naylor PT, Myrvik QN. Molecular mechanisms of muculoskeletal sepsis. In : Esterhai JL ed. Musculoskeletal infection. Park Ridge : American Academy of Orthopaedic Surgeons, 1992 ; 2 : 13-28

[16] Haley RW. Surveillance by objective; A new priority directed approach to the control of nosocomial infections. *Am J Infect Control* 1985 ; 13 : 78-89

[17] Haley RW, Culver DH, White JW, Etal. The efficacy of infection surveillance and control programs in preventing nosocomial infections in US hospitals. *Am J Epidemiol* 1985 ; 121 : 182-205

[18] Hedström SA. The prognosis of chronic staphylococcal osteomyelitis after long-term antibiotic treatment. *Scand J Infect Dis* 1974 ; 6 : 33-38

[19] Josefsson G, Kolmert L. Prophylaxis with systemic antibiotics versus gentamicin bone cement in total hip arthroplasty: a ten year survey of 1688 hips. *Clin Orthop* 1993 ; 292 : 210-214

[20] Klemm KW. Antibiotic bead chains. *Clin Orthop* 1993 ; 295 : 63-76

[21] Lidgren L, Lindberg L. Post-operative wound infections in clean orthopaedic surgery. Review of a 5-year material. *Acta Orthop Scand* 1974 ; 45 : 161-169

[22] Lidwell OM, Lowbury EJ, White W, Blowers R, Stanley SJ, Lowe D. Effect of ultraclean air in operating rooms on deep sepsis in the joint after total hip or knee replacement: a randomised study. *Br Med J* 1982 ; 205 : 10-14

[23] Lob G, Burri C, Mutschler W. Die lokale antibakterielle Therapie mit Taurolin-gel 4% bei akuter und chronischer Osteitis. *Hefte Unfallheilkd* 1983 ; 165 : 216-218

[24] Mackowiak PA, Jone SR, Smith JW. Diagnostic value of sinus tract cultures in chronic osteomyelitis. *JAMA* 1978 ; 239 : 2772-2775

[25] Malchau H, Herberts P. Prognosis of total hip replacement. Revision and re-revision rate in THR: A revision risk study of 148, 359 primary operations. The National Hip Arthroplasty Registry of Sweden, 1998

[26] Morandi M, Zembo MM. The Ilizarov compression-distraction osteosynthesis: a method of treatment for infected pseudarthrosis and segmental bone defects. In : d'Ambrosia RD ed. Orthopaedic infections. New Jersey : Slack, 1989 : 163-190

[27] Norden C, Gillespie WJ, Nade S. Infections in bones and joints. Oxford : Blackwell, 1994

[28] Papineau LJ. L'excision-greffe avec fermeture retardée delibérée dans l'osteomyélite chronique. *Nouv Presse Méd* 1973 ; 2 : 2753

[29] Patzakis MJ, Wilkins J. Factors influencing infection rate in open fracture wounds. *Clin Orthop* 1989 ; 243 : 36-40

[30] Persson U, Persson M, Malchau H. The economics of preventing revisions in total hip replacement. *Acta Orthop Scand* 1999 ; 70 : 163-169

[31] Peters KM, Koberg K, Zwadio-Klarwasser G, Zilkens KW. Immunreaktionen bei der chronischen posttraumatischen osteomyelitis. Eine aktuelle Standortbestimmung. *Z Orthop* 1991 ; 129 : 313-318

[32] Proctor RA, Balwit JM, Vesga O. Variant subpopulations of *Staphylococcus aureus* as cause of persistent and recurrent infections. *Infect Agents Dis* 1994 ; 3 : 302-312

[33] Ritmann WW, Perren SM. Corticale Knochenheilung nach Osteosynthese und Infektion. Biomechanik und Biologie. Berlin : Springer-Verlag, 1974

[34] Schurman DJ, Smith RL. Bacterial biofilm and infected biomaterials. In : Esterhai JL ed. Musculoskeletal infection. Park Ridge : American Academy of Orthopaedic Surgeons, 1992 ; 10 : 133-147

[35] Vasey H,. L'épidémiologie de l'infection post-opératoire. In : L'infection en chirurgie orthopédique. Paris : Expansion scientifique francaise, 1974 : 127-146

[36] Walenkamp GH. A clinical, pharmacokinetic and toxicological study. Katholieke Universiteit Nijmegen, 1983

[37] Walenkamp GH. L'infection en chirurgie orthopédique. In : Traitement de l'air. Paris : Expansion scientifique francaise, 1990 : 14-21

[38] Walenkamp GH. How I do it: Chronic osteomyelitis. *Acta Orthop Scand* 1997 ; 68 : 497-506

[39] Walenkamp GH, Vree TB, Van Rens TH. Gentamicin-PMMA beads. *Clin Orthop* 1986 ; 205 : 171-183

[40] Whyte W. The role of clothing and drapes in the operating room. *J Hosp Infect* 1988 ; 11 (suppl C) : 2-17

[41] Whyte W, Hodgson R, Tinkler J. The importance of airborne bacterial contamination of wounds. *J Hosp Infect* 1982 ; 3 : 123-135

[42] Wymenga AB. Joint sepsis after prophylaxis with one or three doses of cefuroxime in hip and knee replacement surgery. Katholieke Universiteit Nijmegen, 1991

Deep venous thrombosis: prophylaxis and treatment

R Mollan

Abstract. – *Orthopaedic and trauma surgeons require to be informed about deep venous thrombosis (DVT) to protect their patients and themselves. This chapter is a comprehensive statement about DVT prophylaxis and treatment as it applies to orthopaedic surgery at this time. However, much more information is needed about DVT in trauma; internal fixation makes assessment much more amenable to non-invasive detection methods.*

The profession is urged to move away from the concept of the ideal prophylactic agent, and to take general measures that are known to reduce the risk of DVT. Protection against DVT must be tailored to local practice. Methods will depend on the rate of DVT in their patients, the degree of risk in individual patients, what is available in terms of mechanical and chemical agents, and cost. Strategy will be modified with the availability of accurate, non-invasive detection systems.

In each centre, the prophylaxis policy should be determined, protocols written, and arguments documented for future examination. Protocols for treatment of established disease are much more uniform. However, the question of postoperative assessment must be given a higher priority, and especially the protocols for dealing with assessment of possible DVT on re-referral.

Accurate, non-invasive methods of detection are now available, and this service is extremely cost-effective compared to the cost of complications of the disease, or readmission and assessment by invasive means.

© 2000, Editions Scientifiques et Médicales Elsevier SAS. All rights reserved.

Keywords: *deep venous thrombosis, prophylaxis, treatment, orthopaedic surgery, trauma, non-invasive detection, screening, strain gauge plethysmography, venography.*

Is deep venous thrombosis a problem?

The prevalence of deep venous thrombosis (DVT) is high. Without prophylaxis, DVT was historically reported at 40% to 80% in hip and knee arthroplasty. In contemporary practice without prophylactic agents, the rate is reducing somewhat, 32% (16% distal, 16% proximal) after total hip replacement, and 66% (50% distal, 16% proximal) after total knee replacement [6]. Even with chemical prophylaxis, DVT rates are significant: calf thrombosis 15.4% with low molecular weight (LMWT) heparin versus 32.1% in the control; and in proximal thrombosis, 15.4% with LMWT heparin and 17.9% in the control [48]. The prevalence of DVT in trauma is largely unknown, but it is high in proximal femoral fracture, and well recognised in fracture of the lower limb, (67%) [19], spinal fracture with neurological

Raymond Mollan, *Professor, MD FRCS, Consultant Orthopaedic Surgeon, Musgrave Park Hospital, Stockman's Lane, 167 Bangor Road Belfast BT9 7JB, Northern Ireland.*

sequelae, and pelvic fracture. The prevalence of DVT is low in spinal reconstruction surgery [41].

In the past decade, there has been a steady improvement in anaesthetic and surgical techniques, and more rapid mobilisation of patients after surgery. Past practice and observation is not valid for use in comparison with contemporary practice, and as the prevalence of DVT varies with patient selection, management and prophylactic precautions, these variables must be standardised for clinical trials and research.

Clinical examination is of no benefit in asymptomatic disease, and is of poor sensitivity and specificity in symptomatic disease. Therefore, expeditious access to accurate, non-invasive detection techniques is essential. While studies from other centres are a useful guide to prevention, local audit of DVT by screening after common surgical procedures is required to assess the local prevalence and to determine best practice.

The site of DVT is important. Calf vein thrombosis is common, especially after knee arthroplasty and major lower limb trauma. However, it is when the thrombosis extends

to the popliteal vein, 20% in the case of knee replacement surgery, that there is a significant risk of embolisation. Single investigations will not detect a propagating thrombus, and only a non-invasive screening system, or effective anticoagulation will help protect the patient.

Pulmonary embolism is a major cause of death in patients undergoing surgery. It accounts for 10% of hospital deaths, and 0.9% of all admissions [17, 39]. The prevalence of pulmonary embolism is disputed and reported from 0.27% to 10% depending on the method of detection. While micro-emboli can be detected only for a short time following surgery [1], recent studies with iterative lung scans, transthoracic and transoesophageal echocardiography show that 76% to 90% of patients with pulmonary embolism remained asymptomatic after orthopaedic surgery. In a study of 64 replacement joints, 5% developed pulmonary emboli in which venography had demonstrated isolated distal thrombi [20]. This and many other clinical studies which report pulmonary embolism emphasise the caution required in interpretation of more optimistic assertions [33].

Chronic pulmonary embolism leading to pulmonary hypertension within a few years is overlooked. Post phlebitic syndrome (PPS) is a major cause of morbidity and a major financial burden, and careful studies reveal an excess of symptomatic PPS due to DVT following arthroplasty [11, 29]. Recurrent venous thromboembolism is a serious problem. Thirty percent of patients treated with warfarin for 3-6 months after the first episode have a further thromboembolic event within 8 years. These recurrent events carry a poor prognosis: 5-12% are fatal pulmonary emboli, which suggests that oral anticoagulation should be continued for an extended time. These studies contain patients with cancer, but in our ageing population many people undergoing arthroplasty will develop cancer in any event. Interestingly, subsequent surgery, recent trauma and fracture were associated with a decreased risk of a further embolic event [36].

Patients are aware of and anxious about thrombosis, and information is easily accessed through the Internet. DVT is the commonest cause of re-admission to hospital after total hip and knee replacement [40]. Prophylaxis with chemical agents can cause serious wound complications and can be expensive. The orthopaedic surgeon requires to be cognisant of the issues, and take steps to ensure that practice can be explained. A consensus group has highlighted the need for awareness and for the use of prophylaxis in orthopaedic patients [45], but it must be emphasised that prophylaxis does not necessarily imply chemical methods, but applies to the whole range of measures that should be considered to protect the patient. The issues that surround DVT prophylaxis are complicated by the paucity of independent research funds, the methods which have been used to detect the disease and complicating events, and the imbalance between the marketing of chemical and mechanical methods of prevention. Orthopaedic surgeons can be forgiven for finding it difficult to reach a consensus on many aspects [21].

What is known about DVT?

DVT after total hip replacement is resistant to the methods of prevention normally used in other surgical specialities [38], suggesting that the thrombogenic process in orthopaedic patients is different. Knowledge of the natural history since the classical thesis of Virchow in 1859 has only begun to advance with the introduction of safe and more accurate diagnostic screening methods [28]. The relative contribution of Virchow's three classical factors (injury to the vessel wall, hypercoagulability and venous stasis) have been extensively studied experimentally; these have been of limited help clinically. Indeed, in assessing the

efficacy of anticoagulation of agents, the presence of a wound in the clinical situation has often been overlooked. Clinical observations and studies are paramount. While torsion of the femoral vein during dislocation of the hip was thought to be a major factor, improved venography [16] has demonstrated that thrombi are predominantly associated with a venous valve cusp in the thigh or sinus in the calf. These sites would suggest that stasis or turbulence might have a strong aetiological effect. Vascular stasis is a well recognised factor in thrombogenesis in the use of tourniquets, general and spinal anaesthesia, pain and post-operative immobilisation which interfere with the calf muscle pump. Thrombosis has been correlated in terms of site with areas of maximum stasis. Strain-gauge plethysmography confirms the prolonged nature of vascular disturbance after total hip replacement and proximal femoral fractures, continuing long after discharge from hospital [36].

Chemical agents are commonly used to combat hypercoagulability. Changes in blood coagulation and fibrinolytic markers have been studied in total hip replacement, but there is poor correlation between these changes and the development of DVT. Recently the use of thromboelastography, a mechanical method that measures whole blood coagulation, has added valuable information [50].

Detection of DVT

Detection of postoperative DVT, and associated complications, requires objective diagnostic tests, as the clinical diagnosis is highly non-specific. Clinical examination is misleading, and the symptoms and signs can be caused by non-thrombotic disorders. Ascending contrast venography is invasive, painful and technically impossible in some 10% of patients. It requires a radiologist skilled in the high contrast technique and in the interpretation of results. Venography is a "snapshot" in time of what is a dynamic process. It is expensive and is therefore unsuitable for repetition. Indeed, in clinical trails where venography is considered to be the gold standard, once patients report the technique, it becomes very difficult to recruit new patients to the trial. While having no place as a screening test, venography is essential in assessing the degree and site of thrombosis once the diagnosis has been established by other means.

Venous ultrasonography includes B-mode ultrasound, Duplex ultrasonography and Colour flow ultrasonography. These are standard techniques for evaluating patients with symptomatic DVT [4]. They depend however on the quality of the technician [13]. Duplex and Colour flow methods are not usually immediately accessible in orthopaedics, nor are they cost-effective or easily organised screening systems. Doppler

ultrasound can be very accurate in skilled hands, but there is great variability. Both limbs need careful comparison and there is significant inter-observer variability. Doppler is generally not performed alone, but with B-mode or Duplex evaluation. Failure to compress the vein is the most reliable sign of DVT; echogenicity is less reliable. Colour imaging allows rapid identification of blood vessels and enhances accuracy. Ultrasonography is much less sensitive in the detection of asymptomatic DVT, and thus is of limited value in post-operative orthopaedic patients and for screening in audit or clinical trials.

Plethysmography includes the old impedance method, which relies on a sensor which is sensitive to skin blood flow and emotion. It lacks sensitivity, yet has been used widely in the absence of something better [5]. The strain-gauge system was developed to overcome the disadvantages of the impedance method. The strain-gauge as a sensor is much more objective, and the system has been computerised to permit an automatic correlation with a huge database derived from venography tests. This has been shown to be a major advance [27]. We have found non-invasive strain-gauge plethysmography to be accurate for the detection of proximal thrombosis and significant calf thrombosis, with an extremely high negative predictive value.

D-dimer, a whole blood test to detect cross-linked fibrin, a breakdown product in thrombosis, has been evaluated. There is a considerable variation in reported results. Its value is claimed as a negative predictor of DVT, but as D-dimer has a half-life of 6 hours, patients with stabilised thrombus, not undergoing active fibrin deposition, will not give detectable elevations. A positive D-dimer test is not diagnostic of DVT, specificity is very low, and a positive test can indicate sepsis, liver disease, trauma, metastatic cancer, and will be elevated post-operatively from the surgical wound.

What can be done to prevent DVT?

It is impossible to recommend a single, ideal prophylactic agent to protect patients in such a multifactorial disease. Indeed, all methods leave a residual incidence of thromboembolism which needs evaluation and thought. Up to one-third of patients undergoing hip surgery may still develop DVT despite chemical prophylaxis, and these are often asymptomatic. Protection against DVT must be based on an understanding of the natural history of the disease in orthopaedic patients; on reducing the factors that enhance risk; and on audit of the local policy. Indeed, protection might be a better word, as prophylaxis is inextricably linked with chemical agents. Accurate, non-invasive detection techniques, and new methods of assessing venous function and blood coagulability continue to enhance knowledge. In the past, because of inability to properly assess methods to prevent stasis, chemical methods were highlighted because they were easier to assess. Particularly in recent times, these new systems have permitted a direct assessment of physical methods such as early mobilisation, exercise regimens, compression stockings, pneumatic compression, intra-operative calf muscle stimulation and mechanical foot and calf pumps. Chemical agents, such as warfarin, and LMW heparins inhibit procoagulant activity, but carry the risk of bleeding complications, and, in the case of newer agents, delay in wound healing. Warfarin inhibits vitamin K-dependent clotting factors II, VII, IX and X. It also inhibits some naturally occurring anticoagulants such as protein C and S, which can induce a paradoxical hypercoaguable state. This is why, in the treatment of DVT with heparin, warfarin should be overlapped with the heparin for 4-5 days. Warfarin has been popular as a prophylactic agent in the United States [23]. It is safer, but not as efficacious as heparin [35].

Heparin binds to antithrombin III and inhibits thrombin and activated factor X. Intravenous administration of unfractionated heparin requires hospitalisation and sequential laboratory tests to balance the levels and avoid systemic bleeding complications. LMWT heparins are about one-third the molecular weight of standard heparin, 4,000-6,000 Dalton versus 12,000-15,0000 Dalton. LMWT heparin binds to antithrombin III, as does standard heparin, but it will not bind to antithrombin III and thrombin at the same time. The half-life of LMWT heparin is 4-6 hours as opposed to the 30-60 minutes of the standard heparin. The advantages are the increased bioavailability and increased plasma half-life, which give the potential for outpatient treatment and DVT prophylaxis. LMWT heparins are equally efficacious as the standard heparin, and in some cases they have improved on the efficiency of heparin as much as halving rates of DVT. There is a benefit for LMWT heparin over standard heparin shown in meta-analysis, but this seems to hold only for high prevalences of DVT [34]. On the other hand, they carry with them enhanced bleeding levels and wound complications that can prove disastrous in joint replacement.

PROPHYLAXIS WITH LOW MOLECULAR WEIGHT HEPARINS

In high risk patients: Dalteparin sodium, 5,000 IU by subcuticular injection into the abdominal or lateral thigh, one to two hours pre-operatively, then 5,000 IU each evening for five weeks.

In low risk patients: Dalteparin sodium, 2,000 IU by subcuticular injection into the abdominal or lateral thigh, one to two hours pre-operatively, then 2,000 IU each evening for seven to ten days.

The corresponding dose of Tinzaparin is 3500 IU in low risk and 4,500 IU in high risk; and of Enoxaparin the dose is 20 mg in low risk and 40 mg in high risk.

Where bleeding complications are expected, e.g. in knee replacement surgery, the pre-operative and first post-operative doses may be omitted to reduce the risk. In all cases, formularies should be consulted for special warnings, precautions, interactions and side-effects. There is a slight difference in European and North American practice. Whereas in Europe Enoxaparin is approved for pre-operative use (40 mg once daily), in North America it is commenced post-operatively with a dose of 30 mg twice daily. The anticoagulant effect induced by heparins is inhibited by protamine.

Who should receive prophylaxis for DVT?

It is important to repeat that prophylaxis is not simply chemical agents and specific mechanical devices. These are simply adjuncts to a totality of care that should be directed towards protection of the patient. All patients undergoing major orthopaedic surgery should have prophylaxis, either mechanical or chemical, or both. Patients with previous thromboembolism, malignant disease and those over 40 years old are at high risk regardless of the degree of surgery. Patients who are confined to bed would be best with mechanical methods of prophylaxis because of the low risk of their producing complications and the possibility that chemical prophylaxis might prejudice subsequent surgery. All surgical patients should have measures taken in their management to reduce the risk of DVT, even if it is just advice to carry out specific exercise patterns.

What needs to be done?

The choice of prophylaxis must be based on a number of criteria. Historically, regimens have been developed on the basis of high prevalence, and an inability to properly assess mechanical methods. With contemporary populations of patients who have much lower levels of DVT, the bleeding complications and delayed wound healing of chemical methods assume much greater significance, and specific mechanical measures should be the first choice. Intra-operative and post-operative Dextran 70 has not been popular in the past, and indeed has been abandoned in France because of reported occurrences of hypersensitivity reactions. While allergy is still a risk, it does not have the problems of bleeding and we continue to use it routinely, finding it effective in both arthroplasty and fractures of the neck of the femur. The complication of fluid overload should not be an issue with modern post-operative fluid management.

Newer chemical anticoagulation agents should be treated with great caution. They must be subjected to stringent independent clinical trial in a small number of recognised centres of excellence before widespread marketing and distribution. In addition to assessing efficacy of reducing DVT, careful attention must be paid to wound healing and bleeding complications. The dangers experienced in Europe as a result of the plethora of total hip replacements must be a warning in other areas of clinical orthopaedic practice. Specific inhibition of thrombin with hirudin has begun early clinical trial. Previous dose ranging studies produced unwelcome bleeding at high doses, and the effect of this drug on bleeding and wound healing must be carefully evaluated before widespread use. Eriksson et al [9] have shown desirudin, a recombinant hirudin, begun preoperatively, to be more effective than unfractionated heparin. There has been discussion about the choice of the reference drug in the desirudin study.

If DVT levels are high in the incident population, peri-operative management of risk factors, good surgical technique, good analgesia and fluid management, mechanical methods of prophylaxis, early mobilisation, exercise patterns and chemical prophylaxis will give good protection. Bleeding complications of the chemical will be balanced by the high prevalence of the disease. Where DVT levels are low, the cost of chemical prophylaxis and the high rate of bleeding complications become more major determinants of practice, and general measures coupled with the safe mechanical methods can be supplemented by screening with non-invasive systems in the post-operative period [31]. The ability to carry out, in the outpatients department, an accurate, non-invasive test in patients referred back to hospital for assessment would be essential to reduce the high costs of readmission, prevent anxiety in suspicious circumstances, and confidently detect those with DVT. Once a diagnosis of DVT is made, the patient should be admitted, treatment commenced and venography undertaken to assess the site and degree of disease.

In the past, not enough attention was paid to the wide range of techniques which play an important role in reducing the risk. Careful attention to pre-operative assessment, taking steps to correct cardiac, respiratory and other problems prior to surgery seems so basic. Discontinuing oral contraceptives before surgery, reducing anxiety by information and reassurance, the use of spinal anaesthesia [7], maintenance of blood volume, good surgical planning and technique, pain relief following surgery, early postoperative mobilisation with formal exercise programmes [26], foot and leg compression pumps [43] are all important cumulative methods of prevention. All are methods of prophylaxis, and should be documented in protocols.

In Musgrave Park Hospital, Belfast, where the average over the past five years of total hip replacements is 1,064 and total knee replacements is 627 per year, the combination of: the posterior approach to the hip [12]; spinal anaesthesia; regional nerve blocks; intra-operative electronic stimulation of calf muscles [22]; peri-operative Dextran 70; and early mobilisation has reduced the incidence of proximal DVT in total hip replacement to 4%. Now that we are cognisant of the importance of such factors which protect the patient, investigations which do not standardise for these in their protocols must be suspect.

For how long should DVT prophylaxis be given?

DVT after discharge from hospital in patients who did not have thrombosis on discharge is well established. In total hip replacement and fractured neck of femur, the risk period may be as long as six weeks; in knee replacement, the period seems to be much shorter. It is impractical and very costly to continue chemical prophylaxis after discharge from hospital, but mechanical methods, especially in those who are less well motivated or who have problems mobilising should be formalised, and compliance checked regularly. Non-invasive screening may pick up those at risk who exhibit poor venous function, and this deserves more study. Where patients are very immobile after discharge, chemical methods might have a place until the risk period is over. As the suspicion of DVT is the most common reason for readmission, protocols should be instituted to permit rapid and accurate evaluation of the venous system to detect DVT.

DVT IN KNEE SURGERY

Comparison with changes in blood flow after total hip replacement identified different patterns of altered haemodynamics in knee replacement. This suggests that there are different mechanisms of venous stasis and thrombogenesis in hip and knee arthritis, and in subsequent surgery for these conditions. These findings correlate with the importance of stasis as an aetiological factor. The relative lack of adequate trials of prophylaxis in knee replacement surgery makes recommendation difficult.

The prevalence of DVT in total knee replacement in the absence of prophylaxis is 70% to 80%; however the relative prevalence of pulmonary embolism is considerably less than in total hip replacement. Only one-fifth of DVT occurs in the proximal venous segment, and this is as a result of extension from calf vein thrombosis. Bilateral disease occurs in 10% to 15%, with a similar prevalence in the contralateral limb. The use of a tourniquet has both positive and negative effects, which probably cancel out.

Regional and continuous epidural anaesthesia is beneficial [3]. Continuous passive motion offers theoretical advantages which have not been proven.

Chemical prophylaxis is less efficacious than in total hip replacement, and in North America, warfarin is the most popular agent. However, an INR (International Normalised Ratio, which is the recommended method for reporting prothrombin time results for the control of anticoagulation) of over 3, results in bleeding complications of 8% to 10%, and the recommendation is to maintain the INR between 2 and 2.5. Warfarin has decreased the prevalence to 30% to 40%. The use of LMW heparins has been associated with bleeding complications that are more significant in knee surgery [49] and Dextran 70 continues to be our choice. General measures are paramount where chemical agents can cause disaster. Calf and foot compression pumps reduce the prevalence of thrombosis, but flow has been shown to be reduced for only a few days after surgery [25]. The advent of accurate non-invasive systems provides the opportunity for post-operative surveillance, for rapid diagnosis and reassurance for the inevitable 5% to 10% of patients re-referred with warm painful knees. We do not treat calf vein thrombosis [14], but if specific treatment is not given, then careful surveillance is required to detect those which might propagate proximally into the popliteal vein.

Arthroscopy is associated with a low incidence of venous thrombosis 4.2%, but surveillance can yield much higher levels 17.9% [8]. Because meniscectomy, arthrotomy, patellectomy, synovectomy and arthrodesis have rates of 25% to 67%, they should be considered high-risk procedures, particularly in patients over 40 years [44].

Fractures and DVT

In proximal femoral fractures, adjusted-dose warfarin and Dextran 70 have both been shown to be moderately effective, the latter reducing the risk of fatal pulmonary embolism in this group. There is, however, the problem that 10% to 15% will have DVT prior to internal fixation [15], and this should be borne in mind when clinical trials are presented. A meta-analysis of aspirin concluded an approximate 50% reduction in fatal and non-fatal complications in this group, similar to that for subcutaneous heparin. A large trial using 162 mg of aspirin daily for five weeks has commenced and will assess the effects of aspirin on vascular mortality, and both venous and arterial morbidity [37].

PPS has been reported as high as 51% following long bone fracture in the lower limb [2]. In displaced fractures of the pelvis, 33% had DVT detected by venography, and 58% on magnetic resonance venography [32]. However, in general, clinical experience and emerging studies of trauma patients reveal a

low prevalence of DVT and pulmonary embolism which do not justify aggressive prophylaxis [42], but the advent of accurate non-invasive methods of detection will be welcomed. The picture continues to be confused with some centres reporting significant DVT rates, deaths from embolism and poor results from established prophylactic methods [18]. In high risk patients such as those with femoral neck fracture, large bone fracture over 40 years, major pelvic fracture and unstable spinal injuries, chemical prophylaxis with standard heparin, 5,000 International Units (IU) twice daily, mechanical prophylaxis with standardised exercise programmes and compression pumps, and below knee anti-embolism stockings would be advised. The protocol needs to be individually adjusted in multiple trauma patients. In low risk situations, chemical prophylaxis should be omitted and mechanical methods used with early mobilisation a priority.

Treatment of established DVT

In the case of calf vein thrombosis, the danger is propagation to more proximal sites with the increased risk of embolisation. Because of the risk of bleeding and wound complications from full anticoagulation and the low risk of complication if the clot remains confined to the calf, either no chemical treatment or outpatient treatment with warfarin or LMWT heparin can be advised.

It is important that the options be discussed with the patient and informed consent obtained. Where there is the facility for surveillance with accurate, non-invasive detection systems, these should be used to detect failure of treatment and extension into the popliteal vein. If extension of the clot occurs, then admission and full anticoagulation should be commenced. A venogram will confirm the site and extent of the thrombus.

Where the facilities do not exist to screen the patient for extension of the thrombus, some consider that the risk of bleeding into the wound outweighs the risks of extension and subsequent complications. This will be determined by the degree of existing bleeding, which in knee replacement can be considerable. However, as 20%-30% of calf thrombi will extend within 2 weeks of presentation, a consensus of physicians would treat with anticoagulant for 3-6 months. If oral anticoagulation is chosen, then warfarin can be used in this group, stabilising the INR between 2 and 3 for a minimum of three months. Mobilisation with formal exercise patterns and below-knee anti-embolism stockings should also be instituted.

In the case of a proximal thrombosis, the patient should be admitted to hospital and full anticoagulation should be commenced immediately. The site and degree of thrombosis should be determined by contrast venography. If the thrombus extends into the pelvic veins, or is unstable on contrast screening, then serious consideration should be given to inserting a vena caval filter [46]. The decision should be left to those skilled in its use, and in our own centre, thoracic surgeons are not convinced of the benefit [24].

Patients with a proximal DVT should be admitted to hospital and receive an initial bolus of 5,000 IU standard heparin. An intravenous infusion of 30,000 IU standard heparin per day should be erected, and subsequently adjusted to maintain the activated partial thromboplastin time of between 1.5 and 2.5 times normal value. Oral anticoagulation can be commenced on day 2 to 4, and should be continued for a minimum of three months. For a full description of the issues and guidelines, the reader is directed to Guidelines on Oral Anticoagulation: Third edition, British Journal of Haematology, 1998, 101, 374-387. Once oral anticoagulation has been stabilised for two consecutive days, the infusion can be discontinued. Overlap of warfarin on heparin must be for a minimum of 5 days. This inpatient treatment will take a period of 5-10 days.

Alternatively, low molecular weight heparin, enoxaparin 1 mg/kg body weight or 90 IU of anti-factor Xa per kg body weight can be injected subcutaneously twice daily. More prolonged prophylaxis should be discussed with physicians, for those patients who have cancer, protein deficiency or lupus.

Warfarin should be adjusted to hold the INR between 2 and 3. Treatment with LMWT heparin has the advantage of fewer thromboembolic events, improved venographic outcome, improved survival, and fewer bleeding events in general, but not specifically in orthopaedic post-operative patients. LMWT heparin can be discontinued at day 10, or if the INR falls below 2, and these patients can be discharged from hospital earlier and managed as outpatients, provided there are no contraindications such as pulmonary embolism, recurrent thromboembolism, bleeding disorders or peptic ulcer disease. LMWT heparin binds to platelets, and every 2-3 days the platelet count should be measured. If it falls below 100,000, or half the baseline value, the heparin should be discontinued, and haematological advice sought. It should be remembered that protamine does not completely reverse haemorrhagic events due to LMWT heparin.

In all patients with renal impairment, marked obesity and bleeding events, or where the surgeon does not usually treat this complication, the advice of a physician skilled in this area should be sought.

In all cases, patients should be treated with regular exercise patterns and below-knee stockings for two years [36]. Some centres are now advocating external compression therapy to reduce venous volume and increase venous flow velocities.

Ilio-femoral thrombosis produces a high risk of PPS, and in addition to complete anticoagulation, catheter directed thrombolysis should be seriously considered. Thrombotomy is controversial, and rarely used outside a few centres in Europe.

Because most pulmonary emboli are asymptomatic, a chest radiograph on admission and subsequent pulmonary scanning will give an objective assessment of this complication.

Conclusion

Orthopaedic and trauma surgeons require to be informed about DVT to protect their patients and themselves. The profession must move away from the concept of the ideal prophylactic agent, and take many measures which are known to reduce the risk of DVT. Protection against DVT will be tailored to their local practice. Methods will depend on the rate of DVT in their patients, the degree of risk in individual patients, what is available in terms of mechanical and chemical agents, and cost. The methods might be modified with the availability of accurate, non-invasive detection systems. In each centre, the prophylaxis policy should be determined, protocols written, and arguments documented for future examination. Protocols for treatment of established disease are much more uniform; however, the question of postoperative assessment must be given a higher priority, and especially the protocols for dealing with assessment of possible DVT on re-referral. Accurate, non-invasive methods of detection are now available, and this service is extremely cost-effective compared to readmission and assessment by invasive means.

Much more information is needed about DVT in trauma. The advent of accurate, non-invasive detection methods and the widespread use of internal fixation have resulted in the disease being much more amenable to investigation.

I would wish to express my sincere thanks to all those who over many years have toiled with me in Belfast to improve our knowledge of this disease and to help protect our patients.

I would also thank the Green Park Health Care Trust, Belfast, for the time and facilities afforded to me in the preparation of this chapter.

References

[1] Abraham P, Carter D, Millot JR, Leftheriotis G, Pidhorz L, Saumet JL. Prolonged asymptomatic micro-embolism after hip or knee arthroplasty. *J Bone Joint Surg Br* 1997 ; 79 : 269-272

[2] Aitken RJ, Mills C, Immelman EJ. The postphlebitic syndrome following shaft fractures of the leg. A significant late complication. *J Bone Joint Surg Br* 1987 ; 69 : 775-778

[3] Ayers DC, Dennis DA, Johanson NA, Pellegrini VD Jr. Instructional course lectures. Common complications of total knee arthroplasty. *J Bone Joint Surg Am* 1997 ; 79 : 278-311

[4] Benson GJ, Oishi CS, Hanson PB, Colwell CW, Otis SM, Walker RH. Postoperative surveillance for deep venous thrombosis with duplex ultrasonography after total knee arthroplasty. *J Bone Joint Surg Am* 1994 ; 76 : 1649-1657

[5] Brown JG, Ward PE, Wilkinson AJ, Mollan RA. Impedance plethysmography: a screening procedure to detect deep-vein thrombosis. *J Bone Joint Surg Br* 1987 ; 69 : 264

[6] Clarke MT, Gregg PJ, Harper WM, Green PJ. Screening for deep-venous thrombosis after hip and knee replacement without prophylaxis. *J Bone Joint Surg Br* 1997 ; 79 : 787-791

[7] Davis FM, Laurenson VG, Gillespie WJ, Wells JE, Foate J, Newman E. Deep vein thrombosis after total hip replacement. A comparison between spinal and general anaesthesia. *J Bone Joint Surg Br* 1989 ; 71 : 181-185

[8] Demers C, Marcoux S, Ginsberg JS, Laroche F, Cloutier R, Poulin J. Incidence of venographically proved deep vein thrombosis after knee arthroscopy. *Arch Intern Med* 1998 ; 158 : 47-50

[9] Eriksson BI, Ekman S, Lindbratt S, Baur M, Bach D, Torholm C et al. Prevention of thromboembolism with use of recombinant hirudin: results of a double-blind, multicenter trial comparing the efficacy of Desirudin (Revasc) with that of unfractionated heparin in patients having a total hip replacement. *J Bone Joint Surg Am* 1997 ; 79 : 326-333

[10] Fender D, Harper WM, Thompson JR, Gregg PJ. Mortality and fatal pulmonary embolism after primary total hip replacement. Results from a regional hip register. *J Bone Joint Surg Br* 1997 ; 79 : 896-899

[11] Francis CW, Ricotta JJ, Evarts CM, Marder VJ. Long-term clinical observations and venous functional abnormalities after asymptomatic venous thrombosis following total hip and knee arthroplasty. *Clin Orthop* 1988 ; 232 : 271-278

[12] Gallus A, Raman K, Darby T. Venous thrombosis after elective hip replacement: the influence of preventive intermittent calf compression and of surgical techniques. *Br J Surg* 1983 ; 70 : 17-19

[13] Garino JP, Lotke PA, Kitziger KJ, Steinberg ME. Deep venous thrombosis after total joint arthroplasty. The role of compression ultrasonography and the importance of the experience of the technician. *J Bone Joint Surg Am* 1996 ; 78 : 1359-1365

[14] Haas SB, Tribus CB, Insall JN, Becker MW, Windsor RE. The significance of calf thrombi after total knee arthroplasty. *J Bone Joint Surg Am* 1992 ; 74 : 799-802

[15] Hefley WF Jr, Nelson CL, Puskarichmay CI. Effect of delayed admission to the hospital on the preoperative prevalence of deep-vein thrombosis associated with fractures about the hip. *J Bone Joint Surg Am* 1996 ; 78 : 581-583

[16] Kalebo P, Anthmyr BA, Eriksson BI, Zachrisson BE. Phlebographic findings in venous thrombosis following total hip replacement. *Acta Radiol* 1990 ; 31 : 259-263

[17] Karwinski B, Svendsen E. Comparison of clinical and postmortem diagnosis of pulmonary embolism. *J Clin Pathol* 1989 ; 42 : 135-139

[18] Knudson MM, Lewis Fr, Clinton A, Atkinson K, Megerman J. Prevention of venous thromboembolism in trauma patients. *J Trauma* 1994 ; 37 : 480-487

[19] Kudsk KA, Fabian TC, Baum S et al. Silent deep vein thrombosis in immobilised multiple trauma patients. *Am J Surg* 1989 ; 158 : 515-519

[20] Laupacis A, Rorabeck C, Bourne R, Tugwell P, Bullas R, Rankin R et al. The frequency of venous thrombosis in cemented and non-cemented hip arthroplasty. *J Bone Joint Surg Am* 1996 ; 78 : 210-212

[21] Laverick MD,, Croal SA,, Mollan RA. Orthopaedic surgeons and thromboprophylaxis. *Br Med J* 1991 ; 303 : 549-550

[22] Laverick MD, McGivern RC, Crone MD, Mollan RA. Comparison of the effects of electrical calf stimulation and the venous foot pump on venous blood flow in the lower leg. *Phlebology* 1990 ; 5 : 285-290

[23] Lieberman JR, Wollaeger J, Dorey F, Thomas Bj, Kilgus DJ, Grecula MJ et al. The efficacy of prophylaxis with low-dose warfarin for prevention of pulmonary embolism following total hip arthroplasty. *J Bone Joint Surg Am* 1997 ; 79 : 319-325

[24] Martin JR, Marsh JL, Kresowik T. Phlegmasia cerulea dolens: a complication of use of a filter in the vena cava. A case report. *J Bone Joint Surg Am* 1995 ; 77 : 452-454

[25] McNally MA, Bahadur R, Cooke EA, Mollan RA. Venous haemodynamics in both legs after total knee replacement. *J Bone Joint Surg Br* 1997 ; 79 : 633-637

[26] McNally MA, Cooke EA, Mollan RA. The effect of active movement of the foot on venous blood flow after total hip replacement. *J Bone Joint Surg Am* 1997 ; 79 : 1198-1201

[27] McNally MA, Crone MD, Mollan RA. A practical screener for deep venous thrombosis after total hip replacement. *Hip Int* 1996 ; 6 : 140-148

[28] McNally MA, Kernohan WG, Croal Sa, Mollan RA. Deep vein thrombosis in orthopaedic patients. Improving the specificity of diagnosis. *Clin Orthop* 1993 ; 295 : 275-280

[29] McNally MA, McAlinden MG, O'Connell BM, , Mollan RA. Postphlebitic syndrome after hip arthroplasty. *Acta Orthop Scand* 1994 ; 65 : 595-598

[30] McNally MA, Mollan RA. Total hip replacement, lower limb blood flow and venous thrombogenesis. *J Bone Joint Surg Br* 1993 ; 75 : 640-644

[31] McNally MA, Mollan RA, Buxton MJ. Reducing the cost of post-operative deep vein thrombosis. *J Manage Med* 1993 ; 7 : 23-29

[32] Montgomery KD, Potter HG, Helfet DL. Magnetic resonance venography to evaluate the deep venous system of the pelvis in patients who have an acetabular fracture. *J Bone Joint Surg Am* 1995 ; 77 : 1639-1649

[33] Murray DW, Britton AR, Bulstrode CJ. Thromboprophylaxis and death after total hip replacement. *J Bone Joint Surg Br* 1996 ; 78 : 863-870

[34] Nurmohamed MT, Rosendaal FR, Buller HR, Dekker E, Hommes DW, Vandenbroucke JP, et al. Low molecular weight heparin versus standard heparin in general and orthopaedic surgery: A meta-analysis. *Lancet* 1992 ; 340 : 152-156

[35] Patterson BM, Marchand R, Ranawat C. Complications of heparin therapy after total joint arthroplasty. *J Bone Joint Surg Am* 1989 ; 71 : 1130-1134

[36] Prandoni P, Lensing AW, Cogo A, Cuppini S, Villalta S, Carta M et al. The long-term clinical course of acute deep venous thrombosis. *Ann Intern Med* 1996 ; 125 : 1-7

[37] Prentice C. Thromboprophylaxis in elective orthopaedic surgery - what is the purpose? *J Bone Joint Surg Br* 1997 ; 79 : 889-890

[38] Salzman EW, Harris WH. Prevention of venous thromboembolism in orthopaedic patients. *J Bone Joint Surg Am* 1976 ; 58 : 903-913

[39] Sandler DA, Martin JF. Autopsy proven pulmonary embolism in hospital patients: are we detecting enough deep vein thrombosis? *J R Soc Med* 1989 ; 82 : 203-205

[40] Seagroatt V, Tan HS, Goldacre M. Elective total hip replacement: incidence, emergency readmission rate and postoperative mortality. *Br Med J* 1991 ; 303 : 1431-1435

[41] Smith MD, Bressler EL, Lonstein JE, Winter R, Pinto MR, Denis F. Deep venous thrombosis and pulmonary embolism after major reconstructive operations on the spine. a prospective analysis of three hundred and seventeen patients. *J Bone Joint Surg Am* 1994 ; 76 : 980-985

[42] Spain DA, Richardson JD, Polk HC Jr, Bergamini TM, Wilson MA, Miller FB et al. Venous thromboembolism in the high-risk trauma patient: Do risks justify aggressive screening and prophylaxis? *J Trauma* 1997 ; 42 : 463-469

[43] Stranks GJ, Mac Kenzie NA, Grover ML, Fail T. The A-V impulse system reduces deep vein thrombosis and swelling after hemiarthroplasty for hip fracture. *J Bone Joint Surg Br* 1992 ; 74 : 775-778

[44] Stringer MD, Steadman CA, Hedges AR, Thomas EM, Morley TR, Kakkar VV. Deep vein thrombosis after elective knee surgery. An incidence study in 312 patients. *J Bone Joint Surg Br* 1989 ; 71 : 492-497

[45] THRIFT (Thromboembolic Risk Factors Consensus Group). Risk of and prophylaxis for venous thromboembolism in hospital patients. *Br Med J* 1992 ; 305 : 567-574

[46] Vaughn BK, Knezevich S, Lombardi AV Jr, Mallory TH. Use of the Greenfield filter to prevent fatal pulmonary embolism associated with total hip and knee arthroplasty. *J Bone Joint Surg Am* 1989 ; 71 : 1542-1548

[47] Virchow R. Die Cellular Pathologie. In : Ihrer Begrundung auf Physiojlogische undpathologische Gewebelehre. Berlin : Verlag von August Hirschwald, 1859

[48] Warwick D, Bannister GC, Glew D, Mitchelmore A, Thornton M, Peters TJ et al. Perioperative low molecular weight heparin. Is it effective and safe? *J Bone Joint Surg Br* 1995 ; 77 : 715-719

[49] Warwick DJ, Whitehouse S. Symptomatic venous thromboembolism after total knee replacement. *J Bone Joint Surg Br* 1997 ; 79 : 780-786

[50] Wilson SD, Cooke EA, Mc Nally MA, Mollan RA. Coagulation changes after total hip replacement. *J Bone Joint Surg Br* 1996 ; 78 (suppl) : 63

A pragmatic approach to prophylaxis of thromboembolic complications in orthopaedic surgery

P Haentjens
R Lemaire

Abstract. – The efficacy of in-hospital prophylaxis against venous thromboembolic disease after elective total hip arthroplasty is well documented in the literature. Warfarin, low molecular weight heparins, early ambulation, aspirin, and the arteriovenous impulse foot pump system have been accepted as efficacious forms of prophylaxis against deep venous thrombosis after total hip arthroplasty. Consequently, orthopaedic surgeons generally use pharmacological or mechanical methods, or both, as prophylaxis against this complication. By contrast, there has been recent debate in the literature concerning the options for prophylaxis against venous thromboembolic disease after hospital discharge.
The purpose of this paper is to describe the incidence of venous thromboembolic disease in orthopaedic and trauma surgery, and to review the current options of prophylaxis for this complication, both during hospitalisation and after.

Keywords: deep venous thrombosis (DVT), venous thromboembolism, prevention, total hip arthroplasty, total knee arthroplasty, trauma surgery.

Thromboprophylaxis - why?

Prevention of thromboembolic complications is a permanent concern in orthopaedic and trauma surgery. Deep venous thrombosis (DVT) may result in fatal or non-fatal pulmonary embolism (PE); non-fatal PE may result in chronic respiratory deficiency; DVT not complicated by PE may also result in post-thrombotic syndrome (PTS), the incidence of which is often underestimated. A "post-thrombotic syndrome study group" in Amsterdam followed for 5 years a group of patients who had presented a first symptomatic DVT: 47% developed moderate PTS and 24% severe PTS, usually within the first two years [8]. Similarly, Verstraete [46] reported 30% PTS in patients with symptomatic calf vein thrombosis and 50% to 60% in those with symptomatic proximal DVT. The risk may be lower for asymptomatic DVT, but it is certainly not zero.

Over the past twenty years, many studies have been devoted to the occurrence of DVT

Patrick Haentjens, M.D., Ph.D., Professor, Department of Orthopaedics and Traumatology, University Hospital, A.Z.-V.U.B., Brussels, Belgium.
Roger Lemaire, M..D, Professor, Department of Orthopaedic and Trauma Surgery, University Hospital, C.H.U. du Sart-Tilman, Liège, Belgium.

following total hip arthroplasty (THA) and, to a lesser extent, total knee arthroplasty (TKA) and hip fractures. Following THA, the figures range from 40% to 70%, with extension to the popliteal or proximal veins in half of the cases; following TKA, the figures range from 40% to 84%, with 9% to 20% proximal DVT. After fracture of the proximal femur, figures ranging from 43% to 91% have been reported [10, 18]. Although it clearly appears that patients who undergo TKA or THA and those with a fractured hip are exposed to a high risk of DVT, there is no reason to consider the risk of DVT as irrelevant in other categories of orthopaedic or trauma patients. For example, following arthroscopic knee surgery performed on an outpatient basis, Roth [41], using duplex sonography, noted DVT in 8.2% of 122 patients, most of them aged 40 or younger. The incidence was higher in patients who had undergone more than a simple meniscectomy; no DVT was noted in a group of patients receiving low molecular weight (LMW) heparin. DVT may also occur in patients with fracture of the pelvis, or with any other fracture of the lower limb. For a long time, it has been known from retrospective studies that plaster cast immobilisation of the lower limb generates a risk of DVT, not only following major or minor fractures but also following lesions affecting soft tissues only, such as knee or

ankle sprains [4]. Kock et al [28] prospectively studied 241 outpatients with a mean age of 33 years receiving ambulatory treatment with an above-the-knee or below-the-knee plaster cast for minor injuries. They recorded 3.9% DVT in the group without prophylaxis and none in the group receiving LMW heparin. These figures are much lower than those noted after THA, TKA, or hip fracture, but they should not divert attention from the fact that these patients may also develop DVT. Every surgeon who was trained before DVT prophylaxis became widely used can remember at least one patient with a "trivial" injury or operation who either lost his life due to PE or developed chronic venous insufficiency.

What are the indications for prevention? The end point issue

Thus, a large proportion of our patients are definitely at risk from DVT, albeit to a variable degree. Should they all be given prophylaxis? This question has received quite diverging answers. One of the reasons is the choice of the prophylaxis target. Some authors focus on prevention of PE, particularly of fatal PE, and do not seem to be too concerned about DVT itself, particularly asymptomatic DVT. In addition, PTS does not appear to be a widespread concern: this may be explained by the difficulty in diagnosing this complication which develops over several years and may be of varying severity. By contrast, others have decided to prevent any type of venous thrombosis, on the assumption that a demonstrable DVT is a manifestation of a thrombotic condition which has the potential to end up in more severe complications. Judging from the recent literature, these two extreme positions are impossible to reconcile, mainly because the proponents of one particular tendency always criticise the methodology of those clinical trials which have produced results that do not fit with their own attitude. Using death from PE as a clinical end point may appear convenient, but the diagnosis of a fatal PE is by no means easy, especially if it occurs late in an already sick individual. Any error in identifying a single case of fatal PE may offset the conclusions of a study with fatal PE as an end point, as the incidence of fatal PE is, fortunately, very low. It is generally admitted that due to advances in anaesthesia, surgical technique and post-operative rehabilitation, the incidence of fatal PE is now much lower than it was a few decades ago [17, 44]. Murray et al [34] have also argued that the efficacy of thromboprophylaxis should be related to total postoperative mortality, which would introduce a potential bias. Studies with death rate from PE as a clinical end point require very large numbers of patients. They also ignore other clinically relevant events, such as symptomatic DVT and chronic venous insufficiency. Using any clinical event as an end point may be preferable, but the problem of an indisputable definition of these end points remains, as currently used definitions leave ample room for subjectivity. Using surrogate end points such as demonstrable DVT or PE - whether symptomatic or not - one faces the objection that a reduction in surrogate end points may not necessarily lead to a reduction in fatal PE and morbidity from venous thrombosis. Such statements are typical of a present trend towards "evidence-based medicine" where reasoning and logical deduction from established physiopathological data must be supported by empirical data and clinical facts. To those who hold the key to the safe in our European health care systems, this trend has a definite link with cost efficiency concerns, and any information is welcome if it dismisses an investigation or treatment that is considered not cost-efficient. We should therefore be extremely cautious when defining the outcome of DVT prophylaxis measures: not every surgeon would agree that prophylaxis is only justified in preventing fatal PE following major trauma, in patients undergoing THA or TKA, or hip fracture surgery. It has also been suggested that DVT prophylaxis should be limited to those patients who have individual

thrombophilic risk factors [44]. Screening for thrombophilia could therefore be of interest, but would also be time and resource consuming, with a cost efficiency which is, as yet, unknown if such screening were to be applied to all patients undergoing surgical or orthopaedic treatment. Moreover, restricting prophylaxis to patients with a higher risk may appear questionable from the medical, ethical and medico-legal viewpoints.

Which prophylactic agents are available to the clinician? Unravelling the meta-analyses

Next comes the choice of a prophylactic method, with a wide array of available pharmacological or mechanical methods, including aspirin, dextran, fixed low dose unfractioned heparin, adjusted dose unfractioned heparin and dihydroergotamine, LMW heparin, heparinoid, fixed mini-dose and adjusted dose of oral anticoagulant therapy, graduated elastic compression stockings, external pneumatic compression, and foot pulse technology, all of which have been investigated in multiple trials. Most clinical trials, however, have been performed in patients undergoing THA or TKA and the results have been summarised in systematic reviews and meta-analyses.

All reviews found that multiple agents or combinations thereof are effective forms of prophylaxis for DVT after hip arthroplasty, but that none decreases the rate to zero [10, 35, 42]. In addition, there is much overlapping in the 95% confidence intervals for the probability of DVT and especially proximal DVT. Nevertheless, all review papers have published guidelines together with evidence supporting their recommendations.

ORAL ANTICOAGULANTS

The broad conclusion of several recently published papers by North American groups was that routine chemical thromboprophylaxis in THA was justified, and that the treatment most commonly used in North America was low-dose warfarin, rather than unfractioned heparin [42]. In the case of the American Orthopedic Association guidelines, priority is given to outcomes that are major contributors to morbidity in North America (e.g. major bleeding events), but it is acknowledged that other considerations may be as important. The task of assigning relative values to different types of outcome is left to patients and their clinicians.

LOW MOLECULAR WEIGHT (LMW) HEPARINS

In many parts of Europe, oral anticoagulant therapy is now rarely used as a routine prophylaxis and LMW heparins have largely

replaced unfractioned heparin, because they are at least as effective, they cause less heparin-induced thrombocytopenia, and they are more convenient to use [48]. They can be given subcutaneously and laboratory monitoring is unnecessary, except in patients with renal insufficiency and possibly those with a body weight of less than 50 kilograms or more than 80 kilograms [48]. Historically, the demonstration that LMW heparins are safe and effective for the prevention of venous thromboembolism led to the licensing of several of these compounds during the mid 1980s in Europe, but only since 1993 in the United States (enoxaparin Clexane®). The results of several North American studies involving enoxaparin, comparing a once-daily with a twice-daily dosage regimen, led the Food and Drug Administration to approve the twice-daily regimen for the prevention of venous thrombosis after elective hip or knee surgery. In all the North American studies, LMW heparin treatment was started postoperatively, and a twice-daily regimen was included as one of the comparison groups. In three studies, there was a lower incidence of thrombosis with the twice-daily regimen, which was statistically significant in two studies. In European studies, however, once-daily dosing and twice-daily dosing yield similar thrombosis rates, and these are consistently lower than in North America, where postoperative dosing has been the standard. In Europe, treatment with LMW heparin is started pre-operatively, which may explain these differences. Once-daily dosing, which is also more convenient, has therefore become standard practice in Europe [24].

META-ANALYSES

A meta-analysis of 52 trials involving methods to prevent DVT in 10,929 patients who had a THA was published by Freedman et al [16]. They found that, for the control group, the absolute risks were 49% for total (proximal and distal) DVT, 26% for proximal DVT, 22% for distal DVT, 1.2% for symptomatic PE, and, most surprisingly, 0% for fatal PE. LMW heparin and warfarin were the most effective protections against proximal thrombus. The risk of proximal thrombosis was 6.3% in patients treated with warfarin and 7.7% in patients treated with LMW heparin. Aspirin (11.4%), intermittent pneumatic compression (13.3%) and low-dose heparin (19%) were also found to reduce the risk compared to the control groups. Although warfarin and LMW heparin were most effective for the prevention of a proximal thrombus, they were also associated with a risk of clinically important bleeding (1.7% for warfarin and 2.3% for LMW heparin). Only low-dose heparin was associated with a higher rate of bleeding complications (3.5%). The authors also found that warfarin, intermittent pneumatic compression, and LMW heparin were effective for the prevention of a symptomatic PE, but aspirin and low-dose heparin were not effective (0.2% for warfarin, 0.3% for intermittent pneumatic compression, 0.4% for LMW heparin, 1.3% for aspirin, and 1.4% for low-dose heparin). Finally, this meta-analysis found no significant differences between agents regarding the risk of death from PE, or from any other cause. In 1994, Imperiale and Speroff [25] carried out a meta-analysis to determine the efficacy of the accepted methods of prophylaxis of venous thromboembolism, following THA. For the control group, the risks are consistent with what is reported in the previous meta-analysis: 47% for all DVT, 23% for proximal DVT and 4% for PE. Imperiale and Speroff also found that LMW heparin and warfarin were the most effective for prevention of proximal thrombus. Dextran (9%), heparin (14%), and intermittent pneumatic compression (13%) were also found to reduce the risk compared to that in the control groups, but aspirin (16%) was not effective. Despite a good overall agreement between the results of both meta-analyses, several results are not consistent. Imperiale and Speroff [25] concluded that LMW heparin treatment was superior to all other methods for the prevention of proximal and distal thrombi (17%). They also concluded that only LMW heparin and intermittent pneumatic compression were effective for the prevention of a PE (0.7% for LMW heparin and 0.7% for intermittent pneumatic compression). A possible explanation for the differences between the results of both meta-analyses concerns the inclusion of original studies over a broad period of time, or the variety of methods used to diagnose venous thromboembolism. Interestingly, Imperiale and Speroff's [25] paper provides a comprehensive tabular display of the "number needed to treat" (NNT) for those agents which demonstrated a statistically significant treatment efficacy. For this analysis, the NNT is the number of patients undergoing THA who need to be treated with a particular prophylactic method to prevent one outcome event as compared to untreated controls. The NNT to prevent all DVT is 3.2 with LMW heparin, 3.9 with compression stockings, 4.3 with warfarin, 4.5 with heparin, 5.7 with dextran. To prevent proximal DVT only, the NNT is 5.4 with warfarin, 6.3 with LMW heparin, 7.2 with dextran, 10 with compression stockings, 11 with heparin. To prevent PE, the NNT is 49 with LMW heparin, 51 with compression stockings. Such figures may be used as a basis to evaluate the cost-efficiency of different prophylactic measures.

Several preparations of LMW heparins are available. These LMW heparins share a number of properties, but they differ in profile concerning distribution of molecular weight, specific activities (measured as the ratio of anti-factor Xa to anti-factor IIa activity), rates of clearance from plasma, and recommended dosage regimens [48]. Thus, it

may be assumed that not all LMW heparins have similar clinical benefits. Leizorowicz and Haugh [30] performed a meta-analysis on the data from 32 clinical trials, including a total number of 15,863 patients who had been treated with various preparations of LMW heparins following the dosage recommended by the manufacturers. This meta-analysis included the following preparations of LMW heparins for in-hospital prevention against venous thromboembolism: Kabi 2165/dalteparin (Fragmin ®); CY 216/nadroparin (Fraxiparine®); CY 222, PK 10169/enoxaparin (Clexane®/Lovenox®); LHN-1/tinzaparin (Logiparin®/Innohep®); OP 2123/parnaparin (Fluxum®). This meta-analysis showed that nadroparin was superior to all other LMW heparins for the in-hospital prevention of both DVT and PE. Unfortunately, these data are only available in the form of a paper published in the proceedings of a symposium [30]. To the best of our knowledge, there are no other studies directly comparing the in-hospital use of LMW heparin.

WHAT IS THE RISK OF A BLEEDING COMPLICATION?

There is still debate about whether heparin (LMW heparin or unfractionated heparin) is less safe than warfarin in relation to the risk of haemorrhagic complications. The relative safety of LMW heparin as compared to unfractionated heparin in the prophylaxis of postoperative DVT has now been examined by several meta-analyses [1, 18, 31, 36]. All studies came to the same conclusion, namely that there was no significant difference in major bleeding complications between the LMW heparin and the unfractionated heparin groups of patients. In the early 1990s, three studies that compared LMW heparins to low-intensity warfarin (with the dose adjusted to reach an I.N.R. of 2.0 to 3.0), found no difference in the rates of thrombosis or bleeding [21, 24, 39]. A review representing only the North American experience with LMW heparins concludes that the risk of serious bleeding, especially for wound-related bleeding complications, was significantly higher for patients treated with heparin than for those treated with warfarin [11]. By contrast, in the recent meta-analysis performed by Freedman et al [15], only low-dose heparin was associated with a statistically significantly higher risk of major wound-bleeding (2.56%) and total major bleeding (3.46%), compared to the risk with the placebo (0.28%). There was little difference in the rates for both major wound-bleeding and total major bleeding complications between all the other agents, namely, LMW heparin, warfarin, aspirin, low-dose heparin, pneumatic compression, and placebo, as there was overlap in the 95% confidence intervals for the probability of both major wound-bleeding and total major bleeding for all these agents. On the basis of 16 cases of spinal haematoma reported in

the first 44 months since enoxaparin was released for general use in the United States in May 1993 [23], the FDA issued a warning that spinal haematoma can occur as a complication of spinal or epidural anaesthesia in patients receiving LMW heparin as thromboprophylaxis [15]. An important factor contributing to the higher frequency of spinal haematoma in the United States is that higher doses of enoxaparin are given, 30 mg twice daily, as compared with 40 mg once daily in Europe [23]. An audit examining the cause of postoperative bleeding in patients treated with LMW heparins suggests that up to 80% of bleeding episodes are associated with initiation of treatment too soon after surgery [48]. In North America, therefore, it is recommended that the first dose of fractioned heparin should not be given for at least twelve hours after the operation, to reduce the risk of bleeding [15, 42]. In continental Europe, however, there are insufficient data to recommend such a delay: treatment with LMW heparin is started pre-operatively, which may explain why thrombosis rates are consistently lower than those in North America, where postoperative dosing only is the standard [24]. In Europe, the first dose of LMW heparin is given pre-operatively the night before surgery; the second dose is given postoperatively on the evening of the day of surgery. Subsequently, the daily dose of LMW heparin is given using a standard protocol. Several unanswered questions remain with regard to the actual frequency of major bleeding among patients undergoing elective THA. Since a history of clinically significant bleeding increases the risk of subsequent postoperative bleeding, most clinical studies exclude these patients. Consequently, published results of safety may not apply to this patient subgroup, and more importantly, may underestimate the bleeding risk in daily clinical practice. More information is needed to determine the scope of this problem of major wound bleeding with anticoagulant drugs and whether it increases the risk of infection. Indeed, a theoretical risk of infection exists but we found no evidence for it. Moreover, randomised controlled trials are rarely done to study possible harmful exposures. When harmful outcomes are infrequent, investigators must find an alternative to randomised controlled trials or meta-analyses. A cohort study, particularly one in which the information comes from a large administrative database with longer term data, might be more appropriate.

HOW CAN SIDE-EFFECTS BE REDUCED?

Blood loss after elective THA can be effectively reduced by using aprotinin. In a single centre study, our anaesthesiologists found that patients treated with aprotinin had significantly less blood loss and required fewer blood transfusions than patients treated with a placebo [27]. At least two well-designed clinical studies (double-blind, placebo-controlled clinical trials) in patients undergoing THA confirmed substantial and statistically significant reductions in mean postoperative blood loss after perioperative aprotinin therapy, without increasing the risk of subsequent venous thromboembolism. Significant reductions in transfusion requirements were also confirmed [19, 33]. More recently, tranexamic acid has been found to reduce blood loss in patients undergoing TKA [26] and THA [13]. This effect, linked to fibrinolytic inhibition, has been noted in TKR patients following administration of the drug either before or towards the end of operation. In THA patients however, similar blood loss reduction was noted when the drug was administered at induction of anaesthesia [13], but not when it was administered towards the end of operation [5]. Although the possible effect of tranexamic acid on incidence of DVT has not been specifically studied in prospective randomised clinical trials, no significant increase of symptomatic thrombotic events has been reported so far. The drug is currently used in both our departments, following THA and TKA, with a clear reduction in blood loss, transfusion requirements as well as volume and extent of haematomas, thus removing the spectre of the "Fragmin knee" or "Clexane knee" which obviously worries a number of overseas surgeons. Clinical trials have been undertaken to quantitatively evaluate blood loss and haematoma reduction and the possible influence on thromboembolic complications. No interaction is to be expected between LMW heparin and tranexamic acid anyway, as the latter is merely an anti-fibrinolytic agent, and does not interfere with the coagulation process.

DEXTRAN

Dextran is only moderately effective in preventing DVT and has inherent risks such as fluid overload and anaphylactoid reaction, although the latter can be minimised by hapten inhibition [35]. During the early 1980s, the anaesthesiologists in both authors' departments adopted this regimen but discontinued it when, some years later, a fatal anaphylactic shock occurred in one department after dextran re-exposure, and several non-fatal similar events occurred in the other.

ASPIRIN

A meta-analysis published in 1994 by the Antiplatelet Trialists' Collaboration has demonstrated that antiplatelet therapy (mainly aspirin) in elective hip surgery is only moderately effective for protection against DVT, but the observed reduction in the risk of PE is substantial. The effects of aspirin on DVT and PE were documented very recently by the publication of the results of the Pulmonary Embolism Prevention Trial [43] involving 13,356 hip-fracture patients and 4,088 patients undergoing elective hip or knee arthroplasty. The primary end points of mortality and morbidity from PE and DVT were diagnosed on clinical grounds, with confirmation by standard procedures, such as lung scanning, venography and ultrasound. Among all 17,444 randomised patients, the risk of PE or DVT was significantly reduced by 34%. The authors claim that among elective arthroplasty patients, the proportional effects of aspirin were comparable to those among patients with hip fracture. This conclusion is open to question, as symptomatic PE or DVT was confirmed in 23 (1.1%) of the patients assigned aspirin and 28 (1.4%) assigned a placebo. Moreover, the tabulated results among THA patients, clearly show that the number of events was remarkably similar in the aspirin group and control group, suggesting that the effects of aspirin on non-fatal vascular events and deaths in elective arthroplasty patients did not differ significantly. If combined with those of the previous meta-analysis, however, the results of the PEP Trial show that antiplatelet treatment significantly reduces the risk of clinical PE and DVT by at least one-third (6.4% versus 8.8% for controls), and of fatal PE by about one-half (0.8% versus 1.6% for controls). Interestingly, much of the benefit of aspirin emerged after the first postoperative week when most other prophylactic strategies, such as heparin and elastic compression stockings, had been stopped.

MECHANICAL METHODS

Elastic stockings and intermittent pneumatic compression have been accepted as efficacious forms of mechanical prophylaxis against DVT after THA. Salvati et al [42] provide a tabular display of a number of investigations demonstrating that the overall rate of DVT in patients treated with intermittent pneumatic compression sleeves was not significantly different from that in patients treated with warfarin. Nevertheless, tolerance of the device is a problem for some patients [47]. There is, however, no risk of major postoperative bleeding [25]. Recently, Warwick et al [47] conducted a randomised controlled trial and concluded that the foot pump is a suitable alternative to LMW heparin for prophylaxis against thromboembolism after THA, because it produced fewer soft-tissue side effects (bruising of the thigh and oozing of the wound, postoperative drainage, and swelling of the thigh), and there was no difference in prevalence of DVT, as determined by venography on the sixth, seventh, or eighth postoperative day, between the two groups. One patient who used the foot pump had a non-fatal PE. When asked about the acceptability of the device, 11% of the patients said it was uncomfortable, 17% reported sleep disturbance, and 3% stated they had stopped it. Conversely, 8% found it relaxing.

WHAT IS THE ROLE OF ANAESTHESIA?

Many studies have demonstrated that epidural and spinal anaesthesia reduce the risk of postoperative DVT by approximately one-half, irrespective of the type of postoperative anticoagulant prophylaxis. In their review paper, Salvati et al [42] again provide a clear table of the recent results of European multicentre studies, documenting that epidural anaesthesia reduces the risk of DVT in patients who receive heparin, LMW heparin, or hirudin [14]. In addition, epidural anaesthesia also reduces the risk of PE.

WHAT IS THE ROLE OF EARLY MOBILISATION?

Finally, one retrospective study [7] has documented the incidence of DVT with a delayed weight-bearing rehabilitation protocol after THA. Buehler et al [7] previously reported an increased risk of proximal DVT. This experience indicates that the decreased mobility was at least partially responsible for the thromboembolic complications.

For how long should postoperative antithrombotic prophylaxis be continued?

It has been recognised that even the most effective in-hospital prophylaxis is associated with delayed venous thromboembolic events after hospital discharge [3, 45]. Consequently, prophylaxis against venous thromboembolic disease after hospital discharge has received increased attention. In daily clinical practice various approaches have been suggested and are being used. Prophylaxis in hospital and then discharge without additional surveillance or prophylaxis is probably the most common approach [9]. Another option is to screen all patients routinely with ascending venography [40] or duplex ultrasonography [32] before discharge from the hospital, and to treat only those patients with proximal DVT. The efficacy and safety of a routine use of adjusted low-dose warfarin for 12 weeks after surgery, for the prophylaxis of DVT after THA, has been documented by Paiement et al [37] who performed neither phlebography nor sonography regularly. Recently, this issue was further addressed in six randomised controlled trials of patients receiving standard prophylaxis with low molecular weight heparin (enoxaparin, dalteparine, nadroparin, ardeparin) continued for 3 to 6 weeks after hospital discharge [6, 12, 20, 22, 29, 38]. All European investigators used ultrasound or venography as a diagnostic tool. The results confirm both the substantial rate of thrombosis after hospital discharge despite receiving in-hospital prophylaxis with LMW heparin, and the overall reduction in venous thrombosis with prolonged prophylaxis after hospital discharge. On the other hand, one North American trial using clinical end points rather than venography or ultrasonography to determine the effect of extended ardeparin prophylaxis for 6 weeks after discharge, found no significant difference in the overall incidence of symptomatic DVT, PE, or death [22]. Despite several concerns and controversies, the results of our Belgian multicentre trial [20], when combined with those of the other European studies, support a potential benefit for continued low-molecular-weight heparin prophylaxis after hospital discharge, especially when patients are less mobile after surgery. The European studies all showed a relative risk reduction of at least 50% when patients received continued treatment with LMW heparin after hospital discharge.

Conclusion

In conclusion, on the European continent a vast majority of orthopaedic surgeons have clearly opted for systematic chemical DVT prophylaxis. Most surgeons use LMW heparins and frequently continue prophylaxis for several weeks after hospital discharge. The *indications have also been extended to a number of patients undergoing outpatient surgery or presenting bone or soft tissue trauma requiring plaster cast immobilisation. Moreover, LMW heparin is usually started pre-operatively, even in patients who will undergo spinal or epidural anaesthesia, and an increasing number of centres are using tranexamic acid to reduce the risk of bleeding which may be associated with LMW heparin administration. Chemical DVT prophylaxis must, of course, go together with a number of other measures to reduce the risk of venous thromboembolism, e.g. early mobilisation, compression stockings and other mechanical means whenever applicable.*

This policy regarding DVT prophylaxis, which has been adopted on a large scale in continental Europe, may be considered by some as non-scientific and therefore not acceptable, as the ultimate, large-scale prospective randomised clinical trial, which should provide an unbiased and unquestionable answer to our problems, is still awaited. Nevertheless, the issue of the prophylaxis target will always remain a matter of debate: should we strive to prevent all DVT or only proximal DVT; all PE, or only fatal PE? It is fair to leave the decision to the individual surgeon who is in charge of the individual patient, rather than imposing a strategy that would be based on a population health ethic of efficiency, with a predominant concern for cost-efficiency, rather than an individual patient ethic. Surgeons in *continental Europe have apparently adopted a consensual attitude towards DVT prophylaxis, based mainly on LMW heparin administration, early mobilisation and elastic compression stockings. World-wide, however, clinicians do not treat groups of patients uniformly, but consider local circumstances, individual responses and tailor their therapy accordingly. These issues relate to the applicability of clinical data to the local setting, and to what extent evidence from the literature can be applied to routine clinical practice in any jurisdiction. Given that the same data forms the basis for the estimated treatment effect, clinicians may focus on local circumstances, and this may lead to variability in treatment recommendations. For example, clinicians practising in the United States of America may reject low molecular weight heparin therapy as a treatment for patients with total joint replacement, and prefer oral anticoagulant medication instead. Clinicians practising in some parts of the United Kingdom may systematically reject pharmacological prevention, but consider foot pump technology or early screening by strain-gauge plethysmography. Finally, clinicians from Australia, New Zealand, and South Africa, having participated in the PEP Trial, may consider aspirin. Ultimately, the decision of assigning a relative value to different types of outcome is left to patients and their clinicians.*

References ➤

References

[1] Anderson DR, O'Brien BJ, Levine MN, Roberts R, Wells PS, Hirsch J. Efficacy and cost of low-molecular-weight heparin compared with standard heparin for the prevention of deep vein thrombosis after total hip arthroplasty. *Ann Intern Med* 1993 ; 119 : 1105-1112

[2] Antiplatelet Trialists' Collaboration. Collaborative overview of randomized trials of antiplatelet therapy, III, Reduction in venous thrombosis and pulmonary embolism by antiplatelet prophylaxis among surgical and medical patients. *Br Med J* 1994 ; 308 : 235-246

[3] Arcelus JI, Caprini JA, Traverso CI. Venous thromboembolism after hospital discharge. *Semin Thromb Hemost* 1993 ; 19 (suppl 1) : 142-146

[4] Bauer G. Thrombosis following leg injuries. *Acta Chir Scand* 1944 ; 90 : 229

[5] Benoni G, Lethagen S, Nilsson P, Fredin H. Tranexamic acid, given at the end of the operation, does not reduce postoperative blood loss in hip arthroplasty. *Acta Orthop Scand* 2000 ; 71 : 250-254

[6] Bergqvist D, Benoni G, Björgell O, Fredin H, Hedlundh U, Nicolas S et al. Low-molecular-weight heparin (enoxaparin) as prophylaxis against venous thromboembolism after total hip replacement. *N Engl J Med* 1996 ; 335 : 696-700

[7] Beuhler KO, D'Lima DD, Petersilge WJ, Colwell CW Jr, Walker RH. Late deep venous thrombosis and delayed weightbearing after total hip arthroplasty. *Clin Orthop* 1999 : 361 : 123-130

[8] Brandjes DP, Büller HR, Heijboer H, Huisman MV, De Rijk M, Jagt H et al. Randomised trial of effect of compression stockings in patients with symptomatic proximal-vein thrombosis. *Lancet* 1997 ; 349 : 759-762

[9] Bulstrode CJ. Declaration of interest. *Acta Orthop Scand* 1998 ; 69 : 343-344

[10] Clagett GP, Anderson FA, Geerts W, Heit JA, Knudson M, Lieberman JR et al. Prevention of venous thromboembolism. *Chest* 1998 ; 114 (suppl 5) : 531S-560S

[11] Colwell CW Jr, Collis DK, Paulson R, McCutchen JW, Bigler GT, Lutz S et al. Comparison of enoxaparin and warfarin for the prevention of venous thromboembolic disease after total hip arthroplasty. Evaluation during hospitalization and three months after discharge. *J Bone Joint Surg Am* 1999 ; 81 : 932-940

[12] Dahl OE, Andreassen G, Aspelin T, Muller C, Mathiesen P, Nyhus S et al. Prolonged prophylaxis following hip replacement surgery. Results of a double-blind, prospective, randomised, placebo-controlled study with dalteparin. *Thromb Haemost* 1997 ; 77 : 26-31

[13] Duquenne P, Lhoest L, Henkes W, De Sart F. Tranexamic acid reduces postoperative blood losses associated with elective total hip replacement. Proceedings 4th EFORT Meeting, Brussels, 1999 : 113-114

[14] Eriksson BI, Ekman S, Baur M, Lindbratt S, Bach D, Kälebo P, Close P. Regional block anaesthesia versus general anaesthesia. Are different antithrombotic drugs equally effective in patients undergoing hip replacement? Retrospective analysis of 2354 patients undergoing hip replacement receiving either recombinant hirudin, unfractionated heparin or enoxaparin. [abstract]. *Thromb Haemost* 1997 ; (suppl 487)

[15] Food and Drug Administration Public Health Advisory. Reports of epidural or spinal hematomas with the concurrent use of low molecular weight heparin and spinal/epidural anesthesia or spinal puncture. Rockville : United States Department of Health and Human Resources, 15 December 1997

[16] Freedman KB, Brookenthal KR, Fitzgerald RH, Williams S, Lonner JS. A meta-analysis of thromboembolic prophylaxis following elective total hip arthroplasty. *J Bone Joint Surg Am* 2000 ; 82 : 929-938

[17] Gillespie W, Murray D, Gregg PJ, Warwick D. Risks and benefits of prophylaxis against venous thromboembolism in orthopaedic surgery. *J Bone Joint Surg Br* 2000 ; 82 : 475-479

[18] Green D, Hirsh J, Heit J, Prins M, Davidson B, Lensing AW. Low-molecular-weight heparin: a critical analysis of clinical trials. *Pharmacol Rev* 1994 ; 46 : 89-109

[19] Haas S, Fritsche HM, Ritter H, Lechner F, Blümel G. Führt eine perioperative Gabe des plasmainhibitors Aprotinin zu einer Steigerung des postoperativen Thromboserisikos? In : Betzler M, Quintmeier A, Raute M eds. Chirurgisches Forum '91 für experimentelle und klinische Forschung, Berlin : Springer-Verlag, 1991 : 371-374

[20] Haentjens P, on behalf of the Belgian Nadroparin Post-Hospital Discharge in Orthopedics Study Group (NPHDO). Post-hospital discharge prevention of deep vein thrombosis with nadroparin calcium after elective total hip replacement. *Haemostasis* 1998 ; 28 (suppl 2) : 292

[21] Hamulyak K, Lensing AW, Van Der Meer J, Smid WM, VanOoy A, Hoek JA. Subcutaneous low-molecular weight heparin or oral anticoagulants for the prevention of deep-vein thrombosis in elective hip and knee replacement? *Thromb Haemost* 1995 ; 74 : 1428-1431

[22] Heit JA, Elliot CG, Trowbridge AA, Morrey BF, Gent M, Hirsh J. Ardeparin sodium for extended out-of-patient prophylaxis against venous thromboembolism after total hip or knee replacement. A randomized, double-blind, placebo-controlled trial. *Ann Intern Med* 2000 ; 132 : 853-861

[23] Horlocker TT. Low-molecular-weight heparin. Correspondance. *N Engl J Med* 1998 ; 338 : 687-688

[24] Hull R, Raskob G, Pineo G, Rosenbloom D, Evans W, Mallory T et al. A comparison of subcutaneous low-molecular-weight heparin with warfarin sodium for prophylaxis against deep-vein thrombosis after hip or knee implantation. *N Engl J Med* 1993 ; 329 : 1370-1376

[25] Imperiale TF, Speroff T. A meta-analysis of methods to prevent venous thromboembolism following total hip replacement. *JAMA* 1994 ; 271 : 1780-1785

[26] Janssen AJ, Andreica S, Claeys M, D'Haese J, Camu F, Jochmans K. Use of tranexamic acid for an effective blood conservation strategy after total knee arthroplasty. *Br J Anaesth* 1999 ; 83 : 596-601

[27] Janssens M, Joris J, David JL, Lemaire R, Lamy M. High-dose aprotinin reduces blood loss in patients undergoing total hip replacement surgery. *Anesthesiology* 1994 ; 80 : 23-29

[28] Kock HJ, Schmit-Neuerburg KP, Hanke J, Rudofsky G, Hirche H. Thromboprophylaxis with low-molecular-weight heparin in outpatients with plaster-cast immobilisation of the leg. *Lancet* 1995 ; 346 : 459-461

[29] Lassen MR, Borris LC, Anderson BS, Jensen HP, Skejo Bro HP, Andersen G et al. Efficacy and safety of prolonged prophylaxis with a low molecular weight heparin (dalteparin) after total hip arthroplasty - the Danish Prolonged Prophylaxis (DaPP) Study. *Thromb Res* 1998 ; 89 : 281-287

[30] Leizorovicz A, Haugh MC. A meta-analysis of clinical trials of low-molecular-weight heparin in surgical patients. In : Turpie AG, Büller HR eds. Proceedings of the Third International Symposium on Recent Advances in Anti-thrombotic Therapy. Chichester : ADIS International, 1994 : 37-50

[31] Leizorowicz A, Haugh MC, Chapuis FR, Samama MM, Boissel JP. Low-molecular-weight heparin in prevention of perioperative thrombosis. *Br Med J* 1992 ; 305 : 913-920

[32] Maloney WJ, Harris WH, Woolson ST, Schutzer S. The safety of discontinuing prophylaxis for venous thromboembolic disease based on a negative B-mode ultrasound. *Orthop Trans* 1995 ; 95 : 307

[33] Murkin JM, Haig GM, Beer KJ, Cicutti N, McCutchen J, Communale ME et al. Aprotinin decreases exposure to allogeneic blood during primary unilateral total hip replacement. *J Bone Joint Surg Am* 2000 ; 82 : 675-684

[34] Murray DW, Britton AR, Bulstrode CJK. Thromboprophylaxis and death after total hip replacement. *J Bone Joint Surg Br* 1996 ; 78 : 863-870

[35] Nicolaides AN. Consensus statement. Prevention of venous thromboembolism. *Int Angiol* 1997 ; 16 : 3-38

[36] Nurmohamed MT, Rosendaal FR, Büller HR, Dekker E, Hommes DW, Vandenbroucke JP et al. Low-molecular-weight heparin versus standard heparin in general and orthopaedic surgery: a meta-analysis. *Lancet* 1992 ; 340 : 152-156

[37] Paiement GD, Wessinger SJ, Hughes R, Harris WH. Routine use of adjusted low-dose warfarin to prevent venous thromboembolism after total hip replacement. *J Bone Joint Surg Am* 1993 ; 75 : 893-898

[38] Planes A, Vochelle N, Darmon JY, Fagola M, Bellaud M, Huet Y. Risk of deep venous thrombosis after hospital discharge in patients having undergone total hip replacement: double-blind randomised comparison of enoxaparin versus placebo. *Lancet* 1996 ; 348 : 224-228

[39] RD Heparin Arthroplasty Group. RD heparin compared with warfarin for prevention of venous thromboembolic disease following total hip or knee arthroplasty. *J Bone Joint Surg Am* 1994 ; 76 : 1174-1185

[40] Ricotta S, Iorio A, Parise P, Nenci GG, Agnelli G. Post discharge clinically overt venous thromboembolism in orthopaedic surgery patients with negative venography - An overview analysis. *Thromb Haemost* 1996 ; 76 : 887-892

[41] Roth P. Thromboembolieprophylaxe bei ambulant durchgeführten Arthroskopischen Meniskusoperationen. *Orthop Praxis* 1995 ; 31 : 345-348

[42] Salvati EA, Pellegrini VD Jr, Sharrock NE, Lotke PA, Murray DW, Potter H et al. Recent advances in venous thromboembolic prophylaxis during and after total hip replacement. *J Bone Joint Surg Am* 2000 ; 82 : 252-270

[43] The Pulmonary Embolism Prevention (PEP) Trial Collaborative Group. Prevention of pulmonary embolism and deep vein thrombosis with low dose aspirin: pulmonary embolism prevention (PEP) trial. *Lancet* 2000 ; 355 : 1295-1302

[44] Thomas DP. Whither thromboprophylaxis after total hip replacement? *J Bone Joint Surg Br* 2000 ; 82 : 469-472

[45] Trowbridge A, Boese CK, Woodruff B, Brindley HH, Lowry WE, Spiro TE. Incidence of post-hospitalization proximal deep venous thrombosis after total hip arthroplasty. A pilot study. *Clin Orthop* 1994 ; 299 : 203-208

[46] Verstraete M. Prophylaxis of venous thromboembolism. *Br Med J* 1997 ; 314 : 123-125

[47] Warwick D, Harrison J, Glew D, Mitchelmore A, Peters TJ, Donovan J. Comparison of the use of a foot pump with the use of low-molecular-weight heparin for the prevention of deep venous thrombosis after total hip replacement. A prospective, randomized trial. *J Bone Joint Surg Am* 1998 ; 80 : 1158-1166

[48] Weitz JI. Drug therapy: Low-molecular-weight heparins. *N Engl J Med* 1997 ; 337 : 688-698

Blood saving in orthopaedic surgery

HH Mehrkens
W Puhl

Abstract. – Medical reasons and even forensic obligations call for careful and critical management of blood and blood components in orthopaedic surgery; several different measures are suitable to cope effectively with these requirements. The top ranked measure is careful surgical technique, followed by strict indications for transfusing any blood component, accepting a certain degree of normovolaemic anaemia. At the same time, this may contribute to preventing thromboembolic complications. All options of autologous transfusion techniques are highly recommendable and applicable. Starting from normovolaemic haemodilution as a basic principle, acute pre-operative normovolaemic haemodilution (ANH), different kinds of autologous blood predonation (ABD) and mechanical intra-/postoperative wound blood salvaging (MAT) should be combined into a comprehensive programme, always according to the individual circumstances of a specific hospital. Drug-induced blood saving measures - such as administration of rhEPO and antifibrinolytics or induced hypotensive anaesthesia - are of only minor importance. Creating and practising such a comprehensive autologous transfusion programme requires close co-operation and consensus among the participating orthopaedic surgeons, anaesthesiologists and transfusion medicine specialists. Provided adequate efforts are made, nearly all major elective orthopaedic surgery - apart from septic and tumour surgery - can be carried out without allogeneic blood transfusion; this not only has medical advantages, but it can also be worthwhile in economic terms.

Keywords: *blood saving, normovolaemic anaemia, transfusion, autologous transfusion techniques, drugs.*

Introduction

Major orthopaedic surgery often entails blood consuming procedures. Prior to the "AIDS era", in general there was little concern about blood transfusion; however, since the mid-1980s, there has been increasing awareness of transfusion-associated risks among surgeons, anaesthesiologists, and patients as well. The main concern to our population is focused on the risk of HIV-infection, particularly since the spectacular problems of haemophilic patients have come under public discussion. In spite of the fact that blood transfusion today can be used under the highest possible safety quality standards, a residual risk can never be completely excluded.

However, from the medical point of view, AIDS is not in the first rank of potentially transmittable diseases. In Germany, we presently calculate a risk of roughly about 1:

H-Hinrich Mehrkens, Prof. Dr. med., Head of the Department of Anesthesiology and Intensive Care Medicine.
Wolfhart Puhl, Prof. Dr med., Head of the Orthopedic Department, Medical Director of the Rehabilitation Hospital, Ulm Orthopedic and Neurologic Clinic of Ulm University, D-9081 Ulm, Germany.

1 million units of transfused blood. By number, of course, hepatitis is still much more important; the estimated rate has now been lowered to about 1: 20-50000 (HCV, HBV) [13]. Presumably, the most frequent transfusion incidents are still related to incompatibility reactions, mainly due to any kind of clerical error. More recently, a growing matter of concern has been suspected immunosuppression and immunomodulation by homologous blood transfusion [3, 41], but this still has to be definitely assessed in detail.

Nevertheless, with regard to blood transfusion, some other aspects must be considered: first of all, its necessity - the main question is the "acceptable" or "tolerable" haemoglobin concentration (Hb) - and also the limited resources of banked blood. Thus, there are sufficient arguments to justify reducing the use of allogeneic blood.

Blood saving techniques

(table I)

Blood loss caused by surgical procedures may first of all be influenced by the surgeon

Table I. – Blood saving techniques.

1.	Careful surgical technique
2.	Strong indication for blood transfusion/acceptance of limited "normovolaemic anaemia"
3.	Use of autologous blood transfusion techniques
4.	Administration of specific drugs (e.g. Erythropoi-etin, Hemostyptica)

himself; therefore, careful surgical technique is always top ranked in any discussion about blood saving measures.

According to a statement by the American Association of Blood Banks (AABB) in 1983, autologous blood is the safest (and least risky) kind of blood transfusion [1]. However, before any blood transfusion therapy is undertaken, very careful consideration must be given to its indication. There is no question that in former times blood was often used open-handedly and more than was really needed, when the transfusion trigger of the "magic ten" (Hb = 10.0 g/dl) was followed uncritically. Nowadays, there is a world-wide consensus that the transfusion trigger should always be a specific number, depending on the individual clinical status. In general, blood

Table II. – Blood saving by means of autologous transfusion techniques.

1. Acute preoperative normovolaemic haemodilution (ANH)

2. Preoperative donation of autologous blood (ABD)
   a) full blood (aFB)
   b) full blood + separation:
      - packed RBCs (aRBCs)
      - fresh (frozen) plasma (aFFP)
   c) blood components by mechanical apheresis (MCP):
      - packed RBCs (aRBCs)
      - fresh (frozen) plasma (aFFP)

3. Intra- and postoperative wound blood salvaging:
   a) mechanical autotransfusion (MAT) by wash centrifuge processing of packed RBCs (waRBCs)
   b) autotransfusion of unprocessed/unwashed wound blood

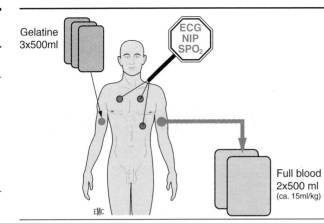

1 *Acute pre-operative normovolaemic haemodilution (ANH).*
Immediately prior to the operation, phlebotomy of about 15m/kg bodyweight is collected into normal blood bags (CPDA-1 stabiliser) and simultaneously replaced by artificial colloid solutions.

transfusion is dispensable with a Hb > 7.5 g/dl under conditions of normovolaemia, normoxia and not substantially impaired coronary function [32, 45]. The primary goal of any blood substitution therapy must be to achieve normovolaemia at all times during perioperative treatment. Adequate volume replacement is therefore necessary and can be ensured, at first, by the administration of artificial colloids such as gelatines or hydroxyethylstarch solutions.

Tolerating a certain status of (normovolaemic) anaemia is a first important (nonsurgical) step in reducing the use of blood transfusions; in other words, haemodilution is the basis of a systematic blood-saving concept. However, the understanding of haemodilution is twofold: one is the general measure (as described above); the second is haemodilution as a specific measure, such as in "acute pre-operative normovolaemic haemodilution" (ANH).

Blood saving by autologous transfusion techniques *(table II)*

ACUTE PRE-OPERATIVE NORMOVOLAEMIC HAEMODILUTION (ANH)

Acute pre-operative normovolaemic haemodilution was introduced into clinical practice by Messmer et al in late 1996/early 1997 [20, 30]. In spite of the fact that its real blood saving effect in terms of volume is rather limited, there are general advantages provided by improved blood fluidity, which is of particular interest in orthopaedic surgery as regards preventing thromboembolism [9, 20].

This specific kind of haemodilution is performed immediately prior to the operation by withdrawing a full blood volume of about 15 ml/kg body weight into a normal CPD-A1-blood bag; the blood should be retransfused within 6 hours as "warm blood", or at least 72 hours as "fresh blood", and is simultaneously replaced by

an isovolaemic artificial colloid solution (e.g. gelatine or hydroxyethylstarch). The technique is easy and not expensive. There is no need for special personnel or equipment apart from a simple hand springbalance (or electronic rocking balance). Nevertheless, some extra time (about 15-20 minutes) must be allowed. Withdrawn units of autologous full blood are retransfused in a reverse order. Currently, pre-operative haemodilution seems to be undergoing a certain "revival" in the U.S.A. [31], whereas it does not appear to be used on a large scale in Europe.

■ *Indication for acute pre-operative normovolaemic haemodilution (ANH)* *(fig 1)*

– expected blood loss > 1000 ml

■ *Contraindications*

– Hb < 11.0 g/dl (= Hct < 0.33),

– unstable coronary heart disease,

– severe aortic stenosis,

– myocardial infarction < 6 months,

– severe pulmonary dysfunction (FEV$_1$ < 1.5 l; paO$_2$ < 65 mmHg),

– hypoproteinaemia 45 g/l,

– acute general infection (leucocytosis, fever > 38.0° C).

PRE-OPERATIVE DONATION OF AUTOLOGOUS BLOOD (ABD)

Since major orthopaedic surgery is mainly elective, the predeposit of autologous blood is highly recommendable and most effective in terms of blood saving. Transfusion of blood components (packed red cells and fresh frozen plasma) is a therapeutic standard nowadays [37], and the same rule should apply to the use of autologous blood. However, in the case of limited needs, full blood (e.g. 1-2 units) is accepted as well, because, on the one hand, no disadvantages have been found [21] and, on the other hand, autologous donation of full blood can be carried out quite easily everywhere, with little cost and effort, to help relieve the banked blood pool.

Because of the limited preservation time (depending on the kind of stabiliser: 35 to 49 days), the predeposit of autologous blood must be completed according to the scheduled date of surgery. There is still some debate on the appropriate way of organising autologous pre-operative blood donation - whether it should be done by the supplying blood bank rather than by the hospital itself, or the anaesthesiology department in particular. There are some striking arguments in favour of the in-hospital option (with the anaesthesiology department being in charge):

– critical observation and monitoring are ensured;

– a minimal rate of rejection (according to Isbister's statement: "fit for operation means fit for donation, too" [17]);

– an optimal course of organisation under the responsibility of only one department;

– the patients gain confidence in the institution and its personnel, who will be in charge of their further treatment;

– increased contact leads to increased motivation of patients and personnel due to a better relationship;

– economic advantages.

Following the German guidelines [37], autologous blood units should always be procured if the likelihood of blood transfusion is calculated to be superior to 10% (subject to the patient's ability and willingness). Pre-operative donation should start about 4 weeks prior to the operation, with intervals of 3 to 4 days between donations, and a final interval of about 7 days before the date of surgery. As a positive side effect, a certain degree of erythropoesis stimulation is quite welcome; moreover, the efficiency of pre-operative blood donation may be supported by intravenous administration of Fe (ca. 200 mg) at every donation [5].

Although it is no longer "state of the art", full blood predeposit is the simplest and least expensive kind of ABD *(fig 2A)*.

Following the given guidelines, full blood from phlebotomy is immediately separated into its components, packed red cells and fresh plasma; the preservation time of the

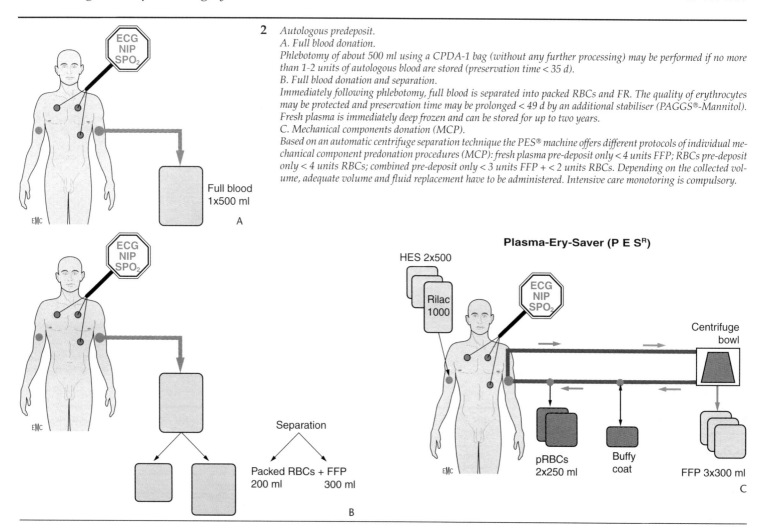

2 *Autologous predeposit.*
A. Full blood donation.
Phlebotomy of about 500 ml using a CPDA-1 bag (without any further processing) may be performed if no more than 1-2 units of autologous blood are stored (preservation time < 35 d).
B. Full blood donation and separation.
Immediately following phlebotomy, full blood is separated into packed RBCs and FR. The quality of erythrocytes may be protected and preservation time may be prolonged < 49 d by an additional stabiliser (PAGGS®-Mannitol). Fresh plasma is immediately deep frozen and can be stored for up to two years.
C. Mechanical components donation (MCP).
Based on an automatic centrifuge separation technique the PES® machine offers different protocols of individual mechanical component predonation procedures (MCP): fresh plasma pre-deposit only < 4 units FFP; RBCs pre-deposit only < 4 units RBCs; combined pre-deposit only < 3 units FFP + < 2 units RBCs. Depending on the collected volume, adequate volume and fluid replacement have to be administered. Intensive care monotoring is compulsory.

red cells may be prolonged up to 49 days by an additional special stabiliser (PAGGS®-Mannitol), while the plasma can be stored deep-frozen for many months [38] *(fig 2B)*.

Pre-operative blood donation can be optimised by using special equipment, such as the mechanical separation system PES® (Haemonetics Comp., Germany). Various protocols [12, 40, 46] are available to meet individual requirements regarding amount and type of blood components to be provided for a specific operation.

For a patient in full medical fitness, a total amount of at least 3 units of plasma (300 ml each), plus 2 units of red cells (250 ml each), can be collected in one session, thus making the procedure most economic and quite cost-effective, too [28] *(fig 2C)*.

■ **Indications for pre-operative autologous blood donation (ABD)**

– major elective surgery (including tumour operations),

– expected blood loss > 1000 ml,

– likelihood of blood transfusion > 10%.

■ **Contraindications**

– anaemia Hb < 11.5 g/dl (= Hct < 0.34),

– unstable coronary heart disease,

– myocardial infarction < 6 months,

– severe aortic stenosis,

– severe pulmonary dysfunction (FEV_1 < 1.5 l; paO_2 < 65 mmHg),

– hypoproteinaemia < 45 g/l (plasmapheresis: < 60 g/l),

– acute general infection (leucocytosis, fever > 38.0 °C).

Intra- and postoperative wound blood salvage

As early as 1868, the German surgeon R.V. Volkmann claimed: "...it is so easy to collect and retransfuse the shed wound blood that one only can wonder at the fact that this procedure has not yet been applied much more often..." [43]. For some time, wound blood recycling was a life-saving emergency treatment for life-threatening haemorrhagic shock, using primitive retransfusion systems which provided only filtering of the shed wound blood. Today, special washing-centrifuge machines are available, which automatically process high quality washed erythrocyte concentrates [11, 33, 34], directly from the intraoperative wound blood or/and from the postoperative drainage blood. Through processing, 60-80% of red cells can be harvested; however, it must be considered that all plasma is eliminated at the same time as all wash solution, tissue

debris and other undesired substances. Therefore, the greater the blood loss, the more need there is for fresh (frozen) plasma, either homologous or autologous if possible [38].

For reasons of cost-effectiveness, the complete mechanical autotransfusion system should only be activated if the collected volume of shed wound blood exceeds 1000 ml (without irrigation fluids), permitting the harvest of about 2 units of red cells. Therefore, in the beginning, a suction line and a (simple) collection reservoir are used, to be completed only later, if it is sure that processing is worth doing [10] *(fig 3)*.

Processed red cells are not for preservation, but must be transfused promptly. Apart from emergencies, in orthopaedic surgery other less complicated recycling systems, which do not use any washing and separating process, are not in general recommended [8, 26, 35]. Recycling of shed wound blood is also contraindicated if bacterial or tumour cell contamination is present; however, salvaged tumour blood may be retransfused after radiation (50 Gy [16]).

INDICATION FOR MECHANICAL AUTOTRANSFUSION (MAT)

– "real" blood loss > 1000 ml.

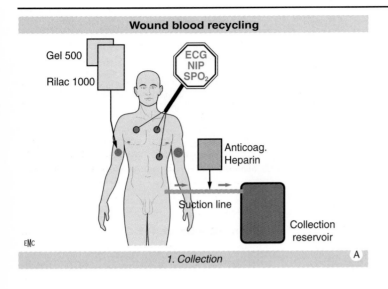

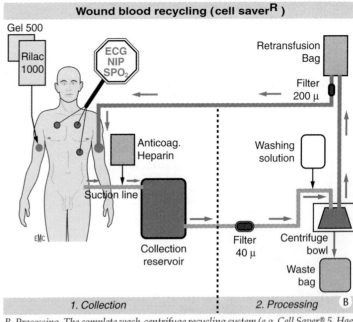

3 *Intra / postoperative wound blood salvaging.*
A. Collection. As a first step of the recycling procedure wound blood is anticoagulated and suctioned from the field into a simple collection reservoir until processing is worth doing (blood loss > 1000 ml).

B. Processing. The complete wash-centrifuge recycling system (e.g. Cell Saver® 5, Haemonetics Comp.) is only started if more than 1 litre of wound blood has been collected. Processed pRBCs are automatically pumped into the retransfusion bag ready for immediate administration to the patient.

Table III. – Hb guideline values.

Hb [g/dl]		Judgement
12.0-17.0	→	Normal
10.0-12.0	→	Optimal
7.5-10.0	→	**Tolerable**
6.0-7.5	→	Critical
< 6.0	→	Alarming

Table IV. – Intervention limits of special laboratory parameters.

Lab-Parameter	% of normal	absolute
Serum protein (PROT)	40	30.0 g/l
Clotting factors (CLOTF)	30	30.0 %
Thrombocytes (THR)	20	30 G l/1

CONTRAINDICATION

– wound blood contaminated by bacteria or tumour cells.

Clinical practice of blood management

The implementation of any blood management programme calls for well-agreed interdisciplinary co-operation between orthopaedic surgeons, anaesthesiologists and transfusion specialists. Basic principles of action should be followed, in accordance with international standards, and modified according to the individual conditions of the specific hospital. In spite of the indubitable improvements in blood bank safety, efforts to reduce allogeneic

Table V. – Scheme of volume and blood substitution therapy (modified after Lundsgaard Hansen) [24].

Blood loss related to tBV	COL	RBCs	FFP	THR	Threshold Value
< 1.0 l = < 20 %	+	-	-	-	
< 2.5 l = < 50 %	+	(+)	-	-	Hb < 7.5 g/dl
< 5.0 l = < 90 %	+	+	(+)	-	Prot < 30.0 g/l
< 7.5 l = < 150 %	(+)	+	+	-	THR < 50 G l/1
> 7.5 l = 150 %	(+)	+	+	+	

Compared to Lundsgaard-Hansen, threshold values of Hb [32] and protein [4] are lowered and human albumine 5% solution has entirely been dispensed with.

blood transfusion as far as possible are still worthwhile. However, successful results can only be achieved through the common involvement of all disciplines in this field.

Within a clinical concept of blood substitution therapy, utmost attention has to be paid to maintenance or restoration of normovolaemia rather than normaemia. This is because the human organism is able to tolerate anaemia much better than hypovolaemia, i.e. if normovolaemia (and additional normoxia) is provided, a considerably reduced Hb will be sufficient to meet oxygen supply requirements. This may be particularly true in orthopaedic surgery due to its high risk of thrombo-embolic complications, which should be effectively lowered by improved rheology [38].

As a result of the ongoing international debate, the following Hb values may be used for guidelines, keeping in mind that the transfusion trigger must always be an individual value based on specific circumstances and clinical signs [6, 38] (table III).

According to a NIH statement in 1989, blood transfusions are normally not necessary with Hb > 7.5 g/dl [31]. The main limiting factor to accepting a certain degree of normovolaemic anaemia is impaired coronary function [45].

Further intervention limits are provided in table IV.

The Bern Component Scheme [24] can serve as a suitable basis for volume and blood substitution therapy (table V).

Relevant blood losses are primarily substituted by artificial colloids (COL, e.g. gelatine or hydroxyethylstarch solutions). Red cells (RBCs) are not transfused unless blood loss exceeds about 50% of estimated total blood volume (tBV) under conditions of normal starting values and normal organ function. Blood loss > tBV requires fresh plasma (FFP) substitution to maintain haemostasis. At the least, platelets (THR) become necessary if blood loss exceeds 1.5 times tBV. 5% human albumin solutions are completely replaced by artificial colloids [42] and should as a rule be eliminated from blood substitution therapy [4].

Mechanical AUTOTRANSFUSION (MAT)
intra-a/o postop wound blood processing
by wash centrifuge technique

Autologous BLOOD PREDONATION
1. Full blood → aFB; 2. Full blood + separation → aRBCs + (LNA)
3. Mechanical Component Predep. → aFFP / aRBCs / aFFP + aRBCs

HAEMODILUTION
a. general: limited normovolaemic anaemia (LNA)
b. specific: acute preop normovolaemic haemodilution (ANH)

4 *Step by step autologous transfusion programme composition. Based on haemodilution as a general principle (= limited normovolaemic anaemia), different autologous techniques can be combined to form a comprehensive programme according to individual circumstances.*

Table VI. – *Average blood loss (BL) of typical major orthopaedic operations (RKU) (Rehabilitationskrankenhaus, Ulm).*

Operation	BL intraop [ml]	BL postop [ml]	BL total [ml]
TKR	350 ± 250	1 100 ± 700	1 450 ± 950
THR	900 ± 500	1 150 ± 450	2 050 ± 950
Revision THR	2 300 ± 1 200	1 400 ± 550	3 700 ± 1 750
Spondylodesis	1 650 ± 1 100	800 ± 650	2 450 ± 1 750
Scoliosis OP	2 800 ± 1 500	900 ± 400	3 700 ± 1 900

Data derived from 1 y surgical activities in the RKU, orthopaedic clinic of Ulm university: estimated blood loss intra- and postoperative (until the next morning after surgery), special attention should be paid to the order of magnitude of postoperative blood loss; indicating the importance of postoperative wound blood salvaging.

Table VII. – *Autologous transfusion techniques related to typical major orthopaedic operations (RKU) (Rehabilitationskrankenhaus, Ulm).*

Operation	ANH	FPPD	MAT	RBCs PD
TKR	+	+ (1x)	+	-
THR	+	+ (2x)	+	-
Revision THR	+	+ (3x)	+	+ (2x)
Spondylodesis	+	+ (2-3x)	+	+ (0-1x)
Scoliosis OP	+	+ (3x)	+	+ (2x)
	acute preop norm vol. haemodilution	fresh plasma predonation	mechan. autotransfusion	red blood cells predonation

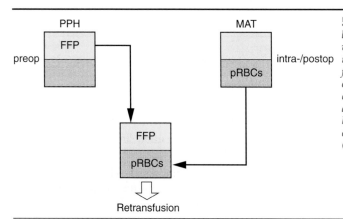

5 *Fresh plasma predeposit combined with intra-/postoperative wound blood processing. Full capacity autologous blood is regenerated for retransfusion by a combination of pre-deposited fresh plasma (FFP) collected by plasmapheresis (PPH) and processed washed, packed RBCs harvested from intra- and postoperative wound blood salvaging (MAT).*

Whatever the strategy of perioperative haemotherapy to be used, ranking the measures to be applied should be considered as follows:

– every effort must be made to avoid blood transfusion; in practice, this means acceptance of normovolaemic anaemia in connection with adequate volume substitution therapy;

– autologous blood components should be made available and must be used whenever and wherever possible;

– use of homologous blood components if inevitable.

USE OF AUTOLOGOUS TRANSFUSION

Next to cardiovascular surgery, orthopaedic surgery is a most suitable field of application. To achieve the aim of using no allogeneic blood, it is necessary to exhaust all available options of autologous transfusion techniques by a comprehensive programme (ATP). This means finding the best way to combine the different measures,

always taking the individual circumstances of a specific hospital into account [25, 38, 39] *(fig 4)*.

The first step in setting up such a programme is an analysis of the amount of blood loss associated with all types of operations; an illustrative survey is given in the table VI.

According to the "regular" blood losses listed in table I, patients at the RKU (Rehabilitationskrankenhaus, Ulm) are prepared and managed using the different autologous transfusion techniques *(table VII)*.

Regardless of operation type, plasma pre-donation, pre-operative haemodilution and mechanical autotransfusion are applied to all patients; red cell pre-donation is reserved for patients expected to undergo a blood loss exceeding approximately 2.5 litres. Putting the main emphasis on plasma pre-donation and mechanical autotransfusion result in independence of the date of surgery, and rather "large-scale" pre-donated units of autologous plasma may also serve for "ideal" volume substitution, particularly in maintaining essential normovolaemia in the postoperative period [25, 38].

In major orthopaedic surgery, a combination of pre-deposited autologous plasma (by plasmapheresis) and intra- and postoperative wound blood processing represents the proper method of "regenerating" a patient's own blood to full capacity. For over 15 years, our practical experience has proven its applicability and effectiveness in compensating moderate surgical blood loss (< ca. 2.5 l) and in entirely avoiding allogeneic blood transfusions *(fig 5)*.

With regard to the individual circumstances of a specific hospital (number of beds, types and numbers of operations, internal/external blood bank), various models of volume and blood substitution therapy are possible:

1. Only full blood (aFB) from pre-operative donation and warm blood (aWB) from pre-operative haemodilution are provided *(table VIII)*.

2. Blood components: red cells (aRBCs) and plasma (aFFP) from pre-operative donation with following separation, warm blood (aWB) from pre-operative haemodilution and washed red cells (awRBCs) from wound blood processing/mechanical autotransfusion are provided *(table IX)*.

3. Blood components: red cells (aRBCs) and plasma (aFFP) from pre-operative mechanical component donation with the PES® system, warm blood (aWB) from pre-operative haemodilution and washed red cells (awRBCs) from wound blood processing are provided *(table X)*.

Table VIII. – Volume and blood substitution therapy - model 1: pre-operative blood donation and pre-operative haemodilution.

Blood loss related to tBV	COL	aWB	aFB	RBCs	FFP	THR	Threshold Value
< 1.0 l = < 20 %	+	-	-	-	-	-	
< 2.5 l = < 50 %	+	+	+	(+)	-	-	Hb < 7.5 g/dl
< 5.0 l = < 90 %	+	+	+	+	(+)	-	Prot < 30.0 g/l
< 7.5 l = < 150 %	(+)	+	+	+	+	-	THR < 50 G 1/l
> 7.5 l = > 150 %	(+)	+	+	+	+	+	
	colloids	autol.	autol.	(homol.)	(homol.)	(homol.)	

Sample autologous transfusion techniques (pre-operative donation → autologous full blood and pre-operative haemodilution → autologous warm blood) may compensate for moderate blood losses < ca. 2 litres: over this amount, homologous blood components are needed.

Cost aspects

Today, medical care is submitted to strong economic pressures. Acting in this field is therefore crucial, even when forensic obligations must be followed on the one hand and limited financial resources considered on the other. The ongoing controversial debate on costs related to autologous versus homologous blood components is not very helpful, as many different local and national conditions have to be considered. However, in Germany, autologous transfusion programmes are used cost-effectively, depending on specific efforts [28, 29, 39]. This is well demonstrated by extensive personal clinical experience showing that an autologous transfusion programme has advantages not only in medical terms, but also in economic terms (See Section "Intra- and postoperative wound blood salvage", and table XI).

Additional administration of specific drugs

Compared to autologous transfusion techniques, administration of specific drugs has only limited importance in the field of blood saving, but some of the following drugs are relevant *(table XII)*.

RECOMBINANT HUMAN ERYTHROPOETIN (RHEPO)

The hormone erythropoetin is known as the most important stimulus of erythropoiesis; it is an established treatment in patients suffering from renal anaemia. Over the past ten years, the administration of rhEPO has been seen to increase the amount of autologous blood that can be collected prior to any blood consuming surgery; its efficacy has been proved in numerous studies. RhEPO administration is not a routine

therapy to facilitate pre-operative blood donation in general, but should be restricted to special patients unable to donate the requested amount of autologous blood units (e.g. for reasons of anaemia). The recommended dosage has not yet been established: current investigations suggest a regimen, with a weekly subcutaneous injection, of about 400 IU/kg for 4 weeks prior to surgery, systematically coupled with supplementary iron therapy [14]. Recently, a more cost-effective regimen has been advocated, rhEPO coupled with pre-operative haemodilution instead of pre-operative blood donation [15].

APROTININ

Aprotinin, a proteinase inhibitor, is well known and routinely used to reduce blood loss in cardiac surgery. However, its exact mechanism of action is still to be clarified. Besides cardiac surgery, there is some evidence of its effectiveness in orthopaedic surgery as well. A significant reduction in allogeneic blood requirements has been demonstrated subsequent to high dose aprotinin (initial bolus of 2x 10^6 KIU immediately prior to surgery followed by an infusion of 5x 10^5 KIU/h until the end of surgery) [7, 18, 44]. In spite of its proven efficacy, aprotinin is not recommended for routine therapy (not even by its supporters [18]) because of some serious reservations, which are particularly focused on the problem of incalculable immunological sensitisation (with possible subsequent severe anaphylactoid reactions) [19]. Aprotinin

Table IX. – Volume and blood substitution therapy - model 2: pre-operative blood donation plus separation and pre-operative haemodilution and wound blood processing/mechanical autotransfusion.

Blood loss related to tBV	COL	aWB	aRBCs	aFFP	awRBCs	RBCs	FFP	THR	Threshold Value
< 1.0 l = < 20 %	+	-	-	-	-	-	-	-	
< 2.5 l = < 50 %	+	+	+	(+)	(+)	-	-	-	Hb < 7.5 g/dl
< 5.0 l = < 90 %	+	+	+	+	+	-	-	-	Prot < 30.0 g/l
< 7.5 l = < 150 %	(+)	+	+	+	+	(+)	-	-	THR < 50 G 1/l
< 7.5 l = < 150 %	(+)	+	+	+	+	+	+	+	
	colloid	autol. warm blood	autol. red blood cells	autol. fresh frozen plasma	autol. washed red blood cells	(homol.) red blood cells	(homol.) fresh froz. Plasma	(hom.) platelets	

Comprehensive autologous transfusion programme with emphasis on pre-operative donation plus separation in connection with pre-operative haemodilution and wound blood processing; autologous blood supply may be sufficient to compensate for blood loss < ca. 5 litres (= 90- 100% of tBV); considerable organisational efforts are necessary, pre-donating carried out in hospital or outside in cooperation with serving blood bank.

Table X. – Volume and blood substitution therapy - model 3: pre-operative mechanical blood component donation and pre-operative haemodilution and wound blood processing/mechanical autotransfusion.

Blood loss related to tBV	COL	aWB	aRBCs	aFFP	awRBCs	RBCs	FFP	THR	Threshold Value
< 1.0 l = 20 %	+	-	-	-	-	-	-	-	
< 2.5 l = 50 %	+	+	-	+	(+)	-	-	-	Hb < 7.5 g/dl
< 5.0 l = 90 %	+	+	+	+	+	-	-	-	Prot < 30.0 g/l
< 7.5 l = 150 %	(+)	+	+	+	+	-	-	-	THR < 50 G 1/l
> 7.5 l = 150 %	(+)	+	+	+	+	(+)	(+)	(+)	

Comprehensive autologous transfusion programme with emphasis on pre-operative mechanical component donation and wound blood processing in connection with pre-operative haemodilution, normally no red cell pre-deposit unless expected blood loss exceeds 2.5 litres; "large-scale" providing of autologous plasma to be used for maintenance of normovolaemia, particularly in the postoperative period as "ideal physiological volume substitute" too. Total blood loss > 7.5 litres may be compensated without allogeneic blood. In hospital, organisation is most efficient; consequent and optimal application provided this programme can even be classified "cost-effective" in spite of increased technical efforts.

Table XI. – Cost comparison autologous vs. homologous blood components (Rehabilitationskrankenhaus, Ulm).

Blood components	Autol. RKU	Homol. German Red Cross
RBCs (200 ml)	EUR 56.50 [1]	--
RBCs (200 ml)	EUR 43.50 [2]	EUR 64.00
wRBCs (MAT/200 ml)	EUR 31.50 [3]	--
FFP (300 ml)	EUR 40.50 [4]	EUR 60.00

[1] 1 unit predonated red blood cells (PES®) including discarding rate 38%
[2] 1 unit predonated red blood cells (PES®) including discarding rate 20%
[3] 1 unit processed washed red blood cells based on 3.7 U/ mechanical autotransfusion application
[4] 1 unit predonated plasma (PES®) including discarding rate 16%
One year data basis (RKU 1997) demonstrating cost-effectiveness of an elaborate autologous transfusion programme which becomes all the more relevant as the perioperative blood loss increases.

Table XII. – Additional drug-induced blood saving means.

Drug	Effect
Erythropoetin (EPO)	Erythropoesis stimulation
Aprotinin	Haemostasis
Desmopressin; Tranexamic acid	Haemostasis
Sodiumnitroprusside; Nitroglycerine	Induced hypotension

should therefore be considered as a possible alternative, when conventional blood saving techniques are inapplicable.

OTHER ANTIFIBRINOLYTIC DRUGS

Following a recent meta-analysis of randomised trials in cardiac surgery, it was concluded that contrary to previous presumptions, desmopressin - a synthetic analogue to vasopressin - does not influence surgical blood loss. However, another fibrinolysis inhibitor, tranexamic acid, decreases the exposure of patients to allogeneic blood transfusion perioperatively [23]. This has also been confirmed in relationship to total knee arthroplasty when tranexamic acid has been given in a total dose of 20-35 mg/kg (administered once prior to the release of the thigh tourniquet, and once or twice postoperatively) without any increase in thrombo-embolic complications [2].

INDUCED HYPOTENSION

In spite of the fact that induced hypotensive anaesthesia is well known for its effect on decreasing intraoperative blood loss and the need for blood transfusions, its use has not become a clinical routine. Reduction of mean arterial blood pressure (MAP) to 50-60 mmHg may be achieved by a variety and combination of certain drugs: at first, short-acting vasodilators (e.g. nitroprusside, nitroglycerine, urapidil, prostaglandin E_1), supplemented by volatile anaesthetics and/or betablockers (e.g. esmolol) to improve effect and prevent side-effects (e.g. tachycardia, rebound hypertension). Careful monitoring takes place and complications are rarely reported in healthy individuals. However, the main concern is for the elderly and those patients with possibly impaired vital organ blood circulation (e.g. myocardium, brain, kidney). Therefore, careful indication, together with consideration of the potential complications, appropriate choice of drugs and invasive monitoring, are essential for the safe practice of induced hypotension [22, 36].

Conclusion

Major orthopaedic surgery is known to be associated with considerable blood loss quite often requiring adequate volume and blood substitution. In contrast to the "pre-AIDS era" a growing awareness of uncritical use of blood transfusions can be noticed among all physicians nowadays, and there is general agreement that blood sparing measures are compulsory. In orthopaedic surgery, in particular, it is possible to carry this out.

In general, two sorts of blood saving are possible:

Reduction of surgical blood loss

– Mainly by careful surgical technique;

– Additionally, by the administration of special drugs, e.g. antifibrinolytics, induced hypotensive anaesthesia.

Reduction of allogeneic blood transfusions

– Primarily, by lowering the transfusion trigger to about 7.5 g/dl Hb (with acceptance of a certain status of normovolaemic anaemia);

– Secondly, by the replacement of allogeneic blood by autologous blood as far as possible, using the given options: pre-operative blood donation, pre-operative haemodilution, wound blood, processing/ mechanical autotransfusion (e.g. implementation of a comprehensive autologous transfusion programme using all techniques in a well combined way);

– In selected patients, additional pharmaceutical stimulation of erythropoesis by administration of rhEPO can be helpful.

Whatever strategy of blood saving is used in detail, normovolaemia has a key position in all therapeutic activities. It has been proven that nearly all major elective orthopaedic surgery can be carried out without any allogeneic blood transfusion. Even in emergencies, septic and tumour surgery, autologous transfusion techniques may be partly used to considerably reduce allogeneic blood requirements. In spite of all medical and even economical advantages, there is some evidence of decreasing enthusiasm in using autologous transfusion techniques. Of course, a continuous process of re-evaluation is necessary to cope with changing requirements, but success in blood saving and reduction of allogeneic blood transfusion will always result from common involvement, and close interdisciplinary co-operation.

References ➤

References

[1] American Association of Blood Banks. Bulletin. Arlington, Virginia, 1983

[2] Benoni G, Fredin H. Fibrinolytc inhibition with tranexamic acid reduces blood loss and blood transfusion after knee arthroplasty: a prospective, randomised, double-blind study of 86 patients. *J Bone Joint Surg Br* 1996 ; 78 : 434-440

[3] Blumberg N. Allogeneic transfusion and infection: economic and clinical implications. *Semin Hematol* 1997 ; 34 (suppl 2) : 34-40

[4] Bormann BV. Volumentherapie in der operativen Medizin. *Krankenhaus Arzt* 1993 ; 66 : 44-51

[5] Bormann BV, Aulich S. Autologe Transfusionsverfahren: Nutzen und Risiko. *Dtsch Ärzteblatt* 1993 ; 90 : 2159-2164

[6] Bormann BV, Friedrich M. Hämodilution. *Klin Anästhesiol Intensivther* 1993 ; 43 : 161-171

[7] Capdevila X, Calvet Y, Biboulet P, Biron C, Rubenovitch J, D´Áthis F. Aprotinin decreases blood loss and homologous transfusions in patients undergoing major orthopedic surgery. *Anesthesiology* 1998 ; 88 : 50-57

[8] Caroli GC, Borghi B, Pappalardo G, Oriani G, Valbonesi M, Ferrari M et al. Consensus Conference Risparmiare sangue: quali ancora i dubbi e i problemi? (Saving blood: which are still the doubts and problems?). *Minerva Anesthesiol* 1994 ; 60 : 285-293

[9] Coburg AJ. Die akute normovolämische Hämodilution in klinischer Anwendung. *Anaesthesiol Wiederbeleb* 1977 ; 104 :

[10] Geiger P, Gelowicz-Maurer M, Mehrkens HH, Wollinsky KH. Maschinelle Auto-transfusion im Baukastenprinzip. *Hämatologie* 1994 ; 3 : 136-139

[11] Geiger P, Matscheko J, Gelowicz-Maurer M, Mehrkens HH, Seifried E. Qualitätssichernde Untersuchungen im Rahmen der maschinellen Autotransfusion mit dem Vacufix-Inline-Filtersystem. *Hämatologie* 1995 ; 4 : 78-83

[12] Geiger P, Ventour W, Gelowicz-Maurer M, Junker K, Mehrkens HH. Erste klinische Erfahrungen mit dem MCSR-3/2p-Gerät zur automatisierten Eigenplasmapherese und buffycoat-armen Erythrozytenspende. *Hämatologie* 1995 ; 5 : 1-5

[13] Glück D, Maurer C, Kubanek B. Studie des Berufsverbands Deutscher Transfusionsmediziner/ Robert-Koch Instituts zur Epidemiologie von HIV- und Hepatitisinfektionen bei Blutspendern. *Beitr Infusionsther Transfusionsmed* 1997 ; 34 : 1-4

[14] Gombotz H. Subcutaneus epoetin alfa as an adjunct to autologous blood donation before elective coronary artery bypass graft surgery. *Semin Hematol* 1996 ; 33 (suppl 2) : 69-72

[15] Goodnough LT, Monk GT. Erythropoetin therapy in the perioperative setting. *Clin Orthop* 1998 ; 357: 82-88

[16] Hansen E, Hofstädter F, Taeger K. Autologe Transfusion bei Tumoroperationen. *Infusionsther Transfusionsmed* 1994 ; 21: 337-347.

[17] Isbister JP. Autotransfusion. An impossible dream? *Anaesth Intensive Care* 1984 ; 12 : 236-240

[18] Janssens M, Joris J, David JL, Lemaire R, Lamy M. High-dose aprotinin reduces blood loss in patients undergoing total hip replacement surgery. *Anesthesiology* 1994 ; 80 : 23-29

[19] Kasper SM, Schmidt J, Rütt J. Is aprotonin worth the risk in total hip replacement. *Anesthesiology* 1994 ; 81 : 517-518

[20] Klövekorn WP, Pichlmaier H, Ott E. Akute präoperative Hämodilution - eine Möglichkeit zur autologen Bluttransfusion. *Chirurg* 1974 ; 45 : 452-458

[21] Kretschmer V, Weippert-Kretschmer M. Eigenblut als Vollblut oder Blutkomponenten. *Beitr Infusionsther* 1993 ; 31 : 209-214

[22] Larsen R, Kleinschmidt S. Die kontrollierte Hypotension. *Anaesthesist* 1995 ; 44 : 291-308

[23] Laupacis A, Fergusson D. Drugs to minimize perioperative blood loss in cardiac surgery: meta-analysis using perioperative blood transfusion as the outcome. The international study of perioperative transfusion (ISPOT) investigators. *Anesth Analg* 1997 ; 85 : 1258-1267

[24] Lundsgaard-Hansen P, Tschirren B. Die Verwendung von Plasmaersatzmitteln und Albumin im Rahmen der Komponententherapie. *Klin Anästhesiol Intensivther* 1980 ; 21 : 120-135.

[25] Mehrkens HH. Autologe Bluttransfusion in der Orthopädie: Effektivität und Grund-sätze der interdisziplinären Zusammenarbeit. *Chir Gastroenterol* 1992 ; 8 : 106-112

[26] Mehrkens HH. Klinischer Einsatz und Kontraindikation der maschinellen autlogen Transfusion. *Beitr Infusionsther* 1993 ; 29 : 146-157

[27] Mehrkens HH. Pre-operative autologous plasmapheresis - 9 years experience in orthopedic surgery. *TBC (France)* 1994 ; 3 : 215-219

[28] Mehrkens HH, Geiger P. Autologous transfusion vshomologous transfusion: cost analysis. [abstract]. *Anästhesiol Intensivmed Notfallmed Schmerzther* 1998 ; 33 (suppl 3) : 373-374

[29] Meierhofer N, Schmied D. Fremdblutsparende Mabnahmen: Kostenvergleich-Eigenblut versus Fremdblut. *Hämatologie* 1994 ; 3 : 22-30

[30] Messmer K, Lewis DH, Sunder-Plassmann L, Klovekorn WP, Mendler N, Holper K. Acute normovolemic hemodilution. *Eur Surg Res* 1972 ; 4 : 55-70

[31] Monk TG, Goodnough LT. Acute normovolemic hemodilution. *Clin Orthop* 1998 ; 357: 74-81

[32] NIH Publication 1989 ; 89-2974a

[33] Orr MD, Gilcher RO. Autotransfusion. Perioperative blood salvage in non heparinized patients. *Crit Care Med* 1976 ; 4 : 103

[34] Paravicini D. Intraoperative Autotransfusion. *Beitr Infusionther Klin Ernahr* 1986 ; 15 : 15-18

[35] Paravicini D. Maschinelle Autotransfusion (MAT). *Klin Anästhesiol Intensivther* 1993 ; 43 : 172-177

[36] Pasch T. Indikationen, Effektivität und Grenzen der kontrollierten Hypotension. *Klin Anästhesiol Intensivther* 1993 ; 43 : 89-95

[37] Richtlinien zur Blutgruppenbestimmung und Bluttransfusion. (Hämotherapie). Aufgestellt vom wissenschaftlichen Beirat der Bundesärztekammer und vom Paul-Ehrlich-Institut. Überarbeitete Fassung 1996. Köln : Deutscher Ärzte-Verlag, 1996

[38] Schleinzer W, Mehrkens HH, Weindler M, Wollinsky K, Pohland H. Klinisches Kon-zept der autologen Transfusion: Hämodilution, maschinelle Autotransfusion, Plasmapherese, Eigenblutspende. *Anästh Intensivmed* 1987 ; 28 : 235-241

[39] Schleinzer W, Singbartl G, Buchholz K. Aufbau, Organisation und Kostenanalyse eines transfusionsmedizinischen Bereichs innerhalb einer Anästhesieabteilung. *Beitr Infusionsther* 1993 ; 29 : 261-287

[40] Taborski U, Müller-Berghaus G. Verfahren zur Herstellung eines resuspendierten Erythrozytenkonzentrats während einer maschinellen Plasmapherese: Geringe Spendehäufigkeit bei gleicher Qualität des Erythrozytenkonzentrats. *Beitr Infusionsther* 1990 ; 26 : 273-276

[41] Tartter PI. Transfusion-Induced Immunosuppression and Perioperative Infections. *Beitr Infusionsther* 1993 ; 31 : 52-63

[42] Vogt N, Bothner U, Georgieff M. Vergleich von Humanalbumin 5 % und 6 % HES 200/0, 5 als ausschliebliche Kolloidkomponente bei groben chirurgischen Eingriffen. *Anästhesiol Intensivmed Notfallmed Schmerzther* 1994 ; 29 : 150-156

[43] Volkmann RV. Drei Fälle von Exartikulation im Hüftgelenk. *Dtsch Klin* 1868 ; 22 : 381-382

[44] Wollinsky KH, Mehrkens HH, Freytag T, Geiger P, Weindler M. Vermindert Aprotinin den intraoperativen Blutverlust? *Anästhesiol Intensivmed Notfallmed Schmerzther* 1991 ; 26 : 208-210

[45] Zander R. Der optimale Bereich der Hämoglobinkonzentration: Physiologie und Klinik. *Chir Gastroenterol* 1992 ; 8 : 119-127

[46] Zeiler TA, Kretschmer V. Automated blood component collection with the MCS 3p cell separator: evaluation of three protocols for buffy-coat poor and white cell-re-duced packed red cells and plasma. *Transfusion* 1997 ; 37 : 791-797

Bone substitutes

J Delecrin
N Passuti
F Gouin
D Heymann

Abstract. – Bone substitutes constitute an alternative to bone grafts. They must be biocompatible, osteoconductive and slowly resorbed, allowing progressive bone formation. Clinical applications must be very precisely defined and validated by comparative studies. The combination of bone substitutes and osteogenic cells or active substances provides osteoinductive properties and a local therapeutic activity.

© 2001, Editions Scientifiques et Médicales Elsevier SAS. All rights reserved.

Keywords: bone substitutes, bioactive ceramics, osteoinduction, clinical applications.

Introduction

Bone grafts are frequently used in bone and joint surgery. However, the complications related to harvesting of autologous bone grafts and the potential infectious and immunological risks (hepatitis, human immunodeficiency virus (HIV), prions, etc.) related to allografts and xenografts have encouraged the search for alternatives to bone grafts. Animal-origin or synthetic bone substitutes must allow direct interactions with biological media to ensure bioactivity. These early exchanges must induce new bone growth in contact with the substitute, resulting in a real chemical bond with the bone. Progressive bone ingrowth of the substitute requires resorption of the substitute and apposition by differentiated bone tissue; biocompatibility is therefore an essential parameter to avoid recycling of substances with cytotoxic effects. Preclinical development (in vitro and in vivo studies) must evaluate these parameters and determine the bone ingrowth kinetics of a substitute as a function of the site and local conditions of use. We will therefore describe the various types of bone substitutes according to their animal, biological, or synthetic origin and define the basic mechanisms of osteoconduction (properties of a material to receive and guide bone ingrowth from the bone tissue in which it is implanted) and the parameters which regulate bone ingrowth of the material. Finally, we will discuss the current possibilities of combinations of bone substitutes and osteogenic cells or active substances designed to make the biomaterial osteoinductive or active on an associated pathological process.

Various types of bone substitutes

This section is confined to a description of the main characteristics of bone substitute materials considered to be bioactive (new bone growth in contact with the material, with establishment of continuity between the material and the bone matrix by means of physicochemical processes). Autografts and allografts, bio-inert materials (integration into bone without interposition of a layer of fibrous tissue), such as dense ceramics (alumina or zirconium oxide), and biotolerated materials (integration into bone with interposition of a layer of fibrous tissue), such as acrylic cement derivatives and metallic bone substitutes, will not be discussed.

SYNTHETIC CALCIUM PHOSPHATE CERAMICS

This category comprises all materials submitted to pressure and heat treatment during formation (sintering). The basic products are synthetic (hydroxyapatite powder [HA], tricalcium phosphate, etc.) and biocompatible. Their osteoconductive properties are determined by their physicochemical characteristics. The mechanical characteristics of most of the products in this category are poor before implantation (at best equal to the resistance to compression of trabecular bone) and improve with subsequent bone ingrowth after implantation [55].

XENOGRAFTS

Xenografts are bone substitutes derived from animals; only bovine products are currently marketed in France. Although bone is a tissue with no detectable risk of infectivity for prion diseases, the immunogenic, viral or bacterial infectious risks, and the risk of transmission of known or unknown non-conventional pathogens justify identification of the geographical origin of the animals and implementation of several steps of treatment. Some products are ceramised. As heat treatment eliminates all organic residues, these substitutes are more closely related to calcium phosphate ceramics, as described in the previous paragraph. Other products are submitted to chemical and heat treatments designed to eliminate cell debris, destroy proteins and lipids, and inactivate viruses and prions. In every case, the three dimensional structure and the mineral phase of bovine bone are preserved, while preservation of the organic protein phase (particularly collagen) depends on the treatment.

"COMPOSITES"

These substitutes combine calcium phosphate granules with a bovine or porcine organic compound. One of the objectives of these combinations (collagen, pig skin gelatine and glycerol) is to improve the ease of use of the product, particularly by

Joël Delecrin, M.D.
Norbert Passuti, M.D.
François Gouin, M.D.
Dominique Heymann, M.D.
Clinique chirurgicale orthopédique, CHU, Hôtel Dieu, place Alexis Ricordeau, 44093 Nantes, France.

All references to this article must include: Delecrin J, Passuti N, Gouin F and Heymann D. Bone substitutes. Editions Scientifiques et Médicales Elsevier SAS (Paris). All rights reserved. Surgical Techniques in Orthopaedics and Traumatology, 55-010-F-10, 2001, 8 p.

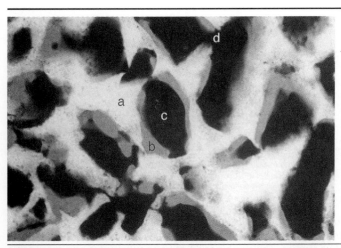

1 *Macroporous calcium phosphate ceramic colonised by newly formed bone in the macropores. a. Ceramic; b. new bone; c. macropore; d. interpore porosity.*

providing a malleable material. However, they are associated with a risk of possible problems of transmission of diseases and antigenic reactions.

IONIC CEMENTS

Ionic cements are malleable products that can potentially be injected. Ionic cements (or hydraulic cements) are composed of a powder, a mixture of basic and acidic calcium phosphate, to which the addition of water triggers hardening, forming a moderately crystallised hydroxyapatite. These cements possess osteoconductive properties, but their mechanical properties are limited and highly dependent on the conditions of preparation of the mixture.

CORAL DERIVATIVES

Coral derivatives are probably the best known and most widely publicised family of bone substitutes. Madrepore coral is a natural product with a mineral composition comprising 99% calcium carbonate. Various physicochemical treatments give rise to products with various chemical compositions (HA or calcium carbonate), various physical characteristics (porosity), and variable organic contents. Many studies [5, 22, 43, 49] have demonstrated the osteoconductive potential of this material when implanted in bone. The reported problems of local tolerance [22, 43] raise the problem of organic residues when the raw material has not been "ceramised".

OTHER PRODUCTS

We will only mention plaster of Paris or calcium sulphate, for which the first human applications were performed in 1892. This compound, with a very low porosity, is absorbed in several weeks (2 to 5 weeks in man) and replaced by bone in the sporadic cases reported in the literature.

In vivo behaviour: osteoconduction (fig 1)

Implantation of a calcium phosphate ceramic is followed by biodegradation of the material, consisting of resorption related to

the solubility of the material (early physicochemical process) combined with degradation related to a cellular process. From the first hours after implantation, some crystals dissolve within the ceramic and are mixed with biological ions and subsequently precipitate (release of calcium and phosphorus ions), resulting in the formation of biological apatite crystals, similar to those of bone [7]. This is followed by calcification of the matrix and mechanical modification of the implants. The chemical nature, structure, and porosity of the material influence the biodegradation process. The cell reaction starts rapidly with a phagocytosis phenomenon involving mononuclear histiocytes. Polynuclear cells (osteoclasts and macrophages) very rapidly contribute to degradation of the ceramic. In parallel with these cellular phenomena, osteoid tissue is formed in contact with the implant. This bone growth is the result of differentiation of mesenchymal cells, peripherally and centripetally. Bone, initially fibrillary, then becomes lamellar. True bone, characterised by osteocytes and mineralised bone matrix, is therefore formed within the implant. This is always a slow process. For example, in the study by Galois et al [20], bone ingrowth in small implants (6 mm wide by 10 mm long) reached a depth of only 1.6 mm to 2.3 mm, 4 months after implantation in bone.

Biodegradation and osteoconduction therefore depend on various factors:

– chemical factors;

– physicochemical factors: porosity and crystal size;

– biological factors: site of implantation and type of bone tissue.

Parameters influencing osteoconduction of calcium phosphate ceramics

The reactivity of the bone substitute with the biological medium depends on its physicochemical and structural

characteristics, as well as the mechanical and biological qualities of the local environment in which it is implanted.

Evaluation of the influence of the various characteristics specific to the material or related to the environment encounters a number of difficulties. These various parameters interact with each other and they have not been exhaustively described in the literature, making it difficult to establish analytical comparisons.

PARAMETERS RELATED TO THE MATERIAL

The most extensively studied of the numerous characteristics of ceramics are the influence of porosity (concerning the structure) and the influence of the calcium phosphate phase (concerning the composition).

■ *Structure*

The porosity of calcium phosphate ceramics can be classified into three types: macroporosity created by the addition of a pore-forming agent during synthesis and which corresponds to a pore diameter greater than several tens of microns (arbitrarily defined as ≥ 100 μm); microporosity, the residual porosity after sintering and with a pore diameter of less than ten microns and the interconnection porosity between macropores when pores of the surface of the material communicate with deeper pores. In this case, the porosity is described as being "open". Each of these three types of porosity can be defined by the mean pore diameter and the percentage volume occupied by the pores compared to total volume of the material.

Optimal macropore size

Several studies [14, 20, 30] have shown that bone ingrowth can occur for pore diameters less than 100 μm, and even for diameters on the order of 40 μm, but this growth is less extensive than that observed with larger pore sizes. The results for pore diameters greater than 100 μm are less homogeneous and sometimes contradictory. The difficulty of interpretation is due to the fact that the other characteristics of the material are either different, or poorly defined, or sometimes unknown, and the results of various studies cannot be compared simply in terms of the macroporosity parameter. Few studies have reported higher bone ingrowth rates for macroporosities less than 200 μm. Frayssinet et al [17], comparing identical calcium phosphate phases and the same porosity percentages, reported high bone contact rates for pore diameters less than 200 μm compared to diameters of 300 to 400 μm and greater than 600 μm. Eggli et al [14] obtained better results with macroporosities of 50 to 100 μm compared to macroporosities of 200 to 400 μm for certain calcium phosphate phases and only for certain time-points, but these results are influenced by the different porosity percentages and interpore porosity between the various materials. A greater number of studies appear to indicate that more abundant bone ingrowth is obtained with pore diameters greater than 500 µm.

Optimal macroporosity percentage

Fewer studies have analysed the influence of macroporosity percentage on the new bone growth rate. Gauthier et al [21] did not note any significant difference between macroporosity percentages of 40% and 50% for ceramics presenting similar microporosity (33%), calcium phosphate phases and pore diameters (300 µm). In contrast, significantly lower results were obtained for the group of ceramics with 30% macroporosity. They also concluded on the predominant influence of pore diameter compared to porosity percentage on bone ingrowth, but these conclusions only apply within the limits of the experimental plan adopted by these authors. Finally, in relation to clinical applications, they considered that, beyond these limits (30% and 50% porosity), a material with 20% macroporosity more closely resembles a dense material. Under these conditions, the possibilities for bone ingrowth intimately depend on the resorbability of the calcium phosphate phase. On the other hand, beyond 60% macroporosity, the mechanical resistance becomes too low to allow easy implantation of the material [3].

Interconnection porosity

The theoretical importance of interconnection porosity is based on the need for passages between surface macropores and deep macropores to allow deep and abundant colonisation of the ceramic. This raises the problem of determination of the optimal diameter to globally promote bone ingrowth [30] and, more specifically, the minimum diameter allowing the passage of osteogenic cells [41].

Microporosity

Microporosity is a residual phenomenon related to the conditions of synthesis. It decreases when the temperature of synthesis increases due to fusion of the constituent particles, which increases the density of the ceramic. These microporosity variations have a decisive influence on dissolution phenomena and therefore osteoconduction, as increased density decreases the degradation process [33, 36, 37]. Trecant et al [55] have demonstrated the decisive role of microporosity in the improvement of the mechanical properties of ceramics after implantation, and attributed this phenomenon to dissolution-reprecipitation processes within the micropores.

Total porosity

Total porosity is defined as the sum of macroporosity, microporosity and interconnection porosity and can be as high as 70 to 80% of the total volume for the ceramics commonly used in clinical practice [24]. This global parameter corresponds to a decisive characteristic in relation to the mechanical [38] and biological properties.

Changing porosity

The variations of porosity after implantation reflect biodegradation of the material with a reduction of microporosity due to microcrystalline repreciptation and an increase of macroporosity and interconnection porosity due to resorption. However, it should be noted that some ceramics without interconnection porosity after synthesis are deeply colonised due to the secondary appearance of connections between pores as a result of resorption. Resorption rates, indissociable from the osteoconductive process, vary with respect to all of the parameters influencing osteoconduction and can therefore only be established for a specified material and for a given site of implantation and at a given time. The multifactorial variations of porosity account for the discordant results reported in the literature for the quantification of resorption within the same calcium phosphate phases. For example, quantification of resorption has revealed low (5.4%) [14] or even undetectable levels for certain HAs, levels of 45% [53], 56% and 71% [14] for certain tricalcium phosphates (TCP), values in the order of 30% for certain biphasic calcium phosphates comprising HA and TCP (BCP) [30].

■ *Composition*

The calcium phosphate ceramics used as bone substitutes differ in terms of a large number of physicochemical characteristics. The calcium phosphate phase, essentially HA or TCP (used alone or in the form of mixtures), is the parameter that has been most extensively studied. Moreover, the influence of certain characteristics is partly based on in vitro studies and extrapolation of the results obtained with calcium phosphate ceramic coatings or with inert materials.

Hydroxyapatite and β-tricalcium phosphate

These two phases are soluble and therefore potentially degradable in vivo, but with different kinetics (cf. infra). As tricalcium phosphate (β-TCP) is clearly more soluble than HA [11, 13, 32, 33, 37], resorption of a ceramic, and therefore its reactivity with the surrounding bone, are all the more rapid and complete when the ceramic contains a higher proportion of β-TCP [17]. This explains the clinical use by some teams of mixtures of β-TCP and HA in ratios of about 50/50 or 40/60 [24] to promote, in the short-term, resorption and therefore substitution by means of TCP, and to maintain, in the longer term, a bioactive substitute in situ by means of HA.

Crystallinity

Ceramics with identical calcium phosphate phases can be differentiated at the crystal scale in terms of crystal size, polycrystalline grain size, quality of grain joints, perfection of crystals and amorphous phases, presence of impurities and possible ionic substitutions. All of these characteristics can influence the reactivity of the ceramic with the biological medium. The potential for degradation of the material therefore increases with decreasing crystal and polycrystalline grain size and with an increasing number of imperfections and amorphous phases, and with certain ionic substitutions [18, 37].

Surface characteristics

The numerous surface characteristics can essentially influence the initial molecular and cellular events, which determine the subsequent cellular reactions in terms of recruitment, adhesion, proliferation and differentiation [4]. Among these various characteristics, the specific surface area, defined by the surface area developed per gram of material, has been shown to have an important influence on in vitro cytotoxicity [17]. Other studies have shown that the surface energy [4] and the chemical nature [2] of the surface can influence the type of proteins that rapidly adhere to the material, and that the crystallinity [26], roughness [35], and chemical nature of the surface also influence the cellular reaction.

■ *Form*

Thickness

Bone ingrowth in a macroporous ceramic, an exclusively osteoconductive material, is centripetal and its deep penetration varies according to the structure and composition of the material, but also according to its thickness. Uchida et al [57] and Shimazaki et al [53] showed, for various types of ceramics and for small implants measuring 2 and 3 mm in diameter, respectively, that bone ingrowth may be limited to the periphery of implants. Eggli et al [14] and Delécrin et al [10] demonstrated significant differences in bone ingrowth for zones situated at a depth of 0.7 mm and 1.6 mm, respectively, compared to the surface of the implant. These findings raise the clinical problem of matching of the material in terms of structure, composition and thickness to a given site of implantation in order to obtain complete bone ingrowth as far as the centre of the material.

Particle size

The bone ingrowth obtained with ceramics injected in the form of granules, varying in size from several tens to several hundreds of microns, essentially varies according to the granule diameter. Determination of the optimal particle size raises the problem of determination of the minimum diameter likely to activate a reactive process, in addition to resorption-substitution, such as a macrophage reaction, which would have harmful effects on bone ingrowth [61].

■ *Parameters related to the environment*

Regardless of its characteristics, incorporation of an osteoconductive bone substitute depends on the biological and mechanical conditions of the site of implantation.

■ *Mechanical factors*

The stability of the recipient site is a necessary and essential condition for integration of autologous bone grafts. This has been extensively documented in clinical studies concerning the contribution of instrumentation to the reduction of the non-union rate and especially applies to synthetic bone substitutes.

The rigidity and constraints exerted at the fracture site influence the formation of bony callus, which in the context of traumatology is reflected by specific choices of the relative rigidity of the fixation material-fracture site. Bone ingrowth inside a ceramic is partly dependent on the same processes of bone repair-formation and, by analogy, would also be influenced by these mechanical conditions of relative rigidity of the implant-recipient site.

■ *Biological factors*

Incorporation of osteoconductive substitutes largely depends on the quality of the bone surrounding the recipient site [9].

– Intrinsic factors: they correspond to the osteogenic capacities of bone tissue, which are determined by the type of bone, cortical or cancellous, the density of bone stem cells in the adjacent bone marrow, the abundance of the local blood supply, and all physiological processes such as ageing, or pathological processes such as osteonecrosis, which influence cellular activity.

– Factors related to the implantation technique: the quality of the bone environment around the bone substitute can also be defined in terms of the degree of contact and the distance between the bone and the biomaterial, and the quality of surgical roughening, essential parameters related to the implantation technique.

CLINICAL APPLICATIONS

The large number of parameters (related to the material and to the environment) affecting osteoconduction and therefore the function of calcium phosphate ceramics makes evaluation of their clinical efficacy a complex enterprise.

Only randomised, controlled studies can help to justify the choice of a particular biomaterial, and must be based on a limited range of indications and sites, with comparison versus a reference method, generally autologous bone graft, and clearly defined criteria for assessment of clinical efficacy.

Several articles, although not meeting all of these methodological criteria and without pretending to be validated or exhaustive, nevertheless contribute to a more precise definition of the clinical applications of calcium phosphate ceramics.

■ *Anterior cervical fusions*

The main biomaterials used in this indication are dense or low porosity HA and TCP ceramics to ensure limited resorption and relatively high mechanical resistance, and bovine bone substitutes. It is difficult to compare the results obtained with these two types of substitute, as no real comparative studies are available and the correlation between clinical and radiological criteria is sometimes discordant: for example, an excellent clinical result may be obtained despite a fractured graft associated with kyphosis.

Discectomy and fusion

There is a tendency, in this indication, not to associate internal fixation, which is questionable as several cases of fracture of biomaterials have been reported in the literature [9]. Recent articles [44, 50, 51] have reported the results obtained with a bovine substitute. The clinical results, based on 40 [44], 89 [50] and 101 cases [51], were satisfactory at short-term follow-up (6 to 9 months), but the radiological results were less satisfactory, with high kyphosis rates of 25% [44] and 50% [51], associated with 47% of fractures and 75% of vertebral collapse according to Motuo Fotso [44]. Senter [52], using dense blocks of HA in a series of 84 cases in the context of a comparative study versus corticocancellous bone grafts (75 cases), reported excellent clinical results associated with only 5% of fractures. Polo [48], based on a limited series (ten cases) using non-resorbable HA associated with plate fixation, reported a similar trend (good clinical results, only one partial fracture and 0% of kyphosis).

Fusion in traumatology and after corporectomy

In these indications where the implant site is unstable, plate fixation is required, as it has a decisive influence. For example, Motuo Fotso [44], who reported kyphosis in 25% of cases after using a bovine substitute without plate fixation for spinal fusion after discectomy, reported 0% of kyphosis when the same type of graft was used in combination with internal fixation.

Malca [42] confirmed this result by reporting no cases of kyphosis with a bovine substitute used for post-traumatic cervical interbody fusions. The preliminary results [9] of an analysis comparing 35 cases grafted with a bovine substitute (mean follow-up: 28 months) with 21 cases grafted with low porosity TCP (mean follow-up: 14 months), showed a marked difference between the two biomaterials, with 25% of complete non-union (no interbody fusions), 25% of partial non-union (only one interbody fusion) and 15% of kyphosis for the bovine substitute, versus only 7% of partial non-union (no complete non-union) and 5% of kyphosis for TCP. The intermediate results therefore appear to be favourable when calcium phosphate ceramics, which remain mechanically fragile despite their low porosity, are protected by plate fixation.

■ *Thoracic fusions*

Biomaterials have essentially been used in the treatment of scoliosis, particularly in posterolateral and posterior sites, which are favourable sites due to their stability, allowing large contact with the recipient bone. Two populations must be distinguished within this indication: children, with "generous" bone growth, and adults in whom the reference technique requires the addition of a supplementary graft to the in situ decortication grafts.

A first article [49], based on 49 cases grafted with coral, reported satisfactory results with a mean follow-up of 1.3 years, but for patients with a mean age of 14 years, which limits the role of the biomaterial in the quality of the fusion. Another randomised, prospective comparative study [9] was based on a population with a mean age of 18 years (Risser ≥ 4, with 30 patients treated by autologous bone graft and 28 patients treated by biphasic ceramic [mixture of HA and TCP]). With a mean follow-up of 4 years, no difference was demonstrated between the two groups in terms of maintenance of correction and back pain. The absence of iliac crest pain in the group grafted with ceramic biomaterial, versus the persistence of a painful donor site in 19% of patients in the other group, with the longest follow-up, constitutes the essential advantage of using a substitute for autologous bone grafts in this indication.

■ *Lumbar fusions*

Lumbar fusions correspond to a wide range of indications and graft sites (interarticular, and/or interbody, and/or intertransverse). The assessment criteria for quality of the fusion are also difficult to define. Under these conditions, the data available in the literature are particularly limited and poorly contributive. A report by the Société d'Orthopédie de l'Ouest [9] emphasised the need for clinical evaluation, especially for the lateral intertransverse site, which is both very frequent and poorly conducive to bone ingrowth, and which may be the only graft site in the case of complete lamino-arthrectomy.

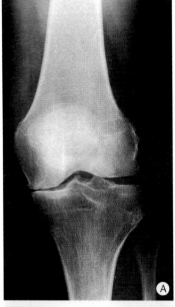
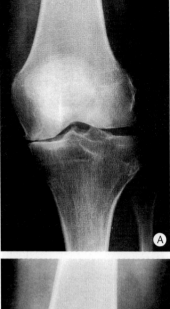
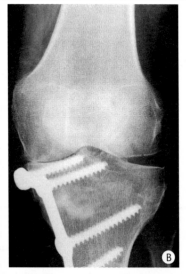
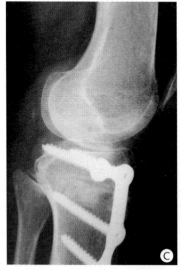
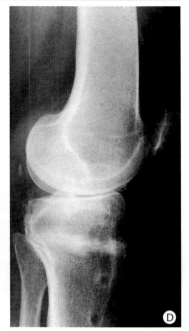
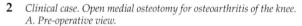
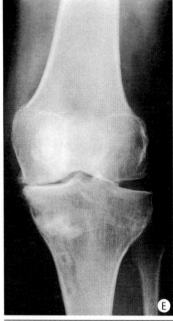

2 *Clinical case. Open medial osteotomy for osteoarthritis of the knee.*
A. Pre-operative view.
B, C. Early post-operative view. Osteosynthesis and filling of the cavity with calcium phosphate ceramic.
D, E. Three years later, complete incorporation of the bone substitute.

■ **Filling of acetabular bone defects during revision of total hip replacement**

In this indication, the bone substitute is used to fill the bone defect, without a primarily mechanical role, which is either ensured by the acetabular implant or palliated by prolonged resting of the hip. Two studies [39, 46] demonstrated that the efficacy of the bone substitute partly depended on local mechanical conditions: site and dimensions of the bone defect and type of acetabular implant.

Oonishi [46] reported 40 cases of massive bone defects in the acetabulum filled by HA granules, with weight-bearing between the tenth and twelfth week. Based on a follow-up of 3 to 9 years, he reported only two cases of radiolucent lines at the bone-substitute interface and two cases of measurable migration of the acetabular implant, requiring surgical revision in one case. Levai [39], in the context of a multicentre study of 100 cases using a bovine bone substitute, reported 14 cases of migration at 2 years of follow-up, and three migrations with clinical failure in a subgroup of 32 cases followed for 5 years. The mechanisms common to these failures and migrations were mechanical or technical: defective reconstruction of the anterior and posterior columns, and incorrect choice of acetabular implant.

■ **Filling of post-traumatic bone defects of the tibial plateau**

Only one randomised, comparative study comparing HA with autologous bone graft has been published in the literature for this indication [6]. On the basis of radiological satisfaction criteria, the authors concluded that HA was just as effective as autologous bone graft, with the methodological reservation that the mean follow-up was different between the ceramic group (34.5 months) and the autologous bone graft group (15.4 months). These results appear consistent with the fact that the proximal tibial epiphysometaphyseal site is a site biologically and mechanically favourable to new bone growth.

■ **Filling of medial epicondylar osteotomies** *(fig 2)*

Filling of medial epicondylar osteotomies by calcium phosphate ceramics is an attractive technique. Leaving to one side the discussion of the tibial osteotomy technique, when the surgeon decides to perform medial epicondylar osteotomy, the disadvantages of the conventional technique (autologous grafts, allografts, cement) and the uncertainties associated with absence of filling theoretically constitute an ideal indication for calcium phosphate ceramics. However, no studies have been published on the subject; the first case was reported in 1995 [24] as part of a more general series, with a good result after more than 2 years. The same team reported 20 cases filled by biphasic macroporous ceramic granules or rods, combined with stable plate fixation, with no cases of delayed consolidation or local complications. A heterogeneous, but large series [43] reported 174 cases with a high reoperation rate (24 out of 174 cases), but usually related to the use of bovine substitutes. The diversity of the implants, the form and the associated fixation prevents any definitive conclusions on the value of these substitutes in this indication.

■ *Filling of cavities after bone tumour curettage*

Several papers have reported good results with ceramics used to fill cavities after bone tumour curettage [22, 27, 28, 54, 56]. One of these studies [27] was randomised and prospective and demonstrated equivalent results for autologous graft and bioactive glass. This indication, with small volumes and bone continuity corresponding to a GESTO type 1 defect [23], is a good indication for ceramics.

Combinations: ceramic-osteogenic cells-active substances

The current fields of investigation into calcium phosphate bone substitutes tend towards improvement of the osteogenic properties of ceramics and the use of ceramics as a drug delivery system.

CERAMIC-OSTEOGENIC CELL COMBINATIONS

Although most calcium phosphate ceramics possess varying degrees of osteoconductive properties, none of them are osteoinductive, which therefore limits their use to the filling of small defects. Various ceramic-osteogenic cell combinations (designed to improve the kinetics of colonisation of ceramics) have been proposed in order to overcome this deficiency *(table I)*. Two conditions are required for the development of this type of material: the cellular component associated with calcium phosphate ceramics must be able to synthesise bone tissue as rapidly as possible, and the synthetic support must be able to receive the cells so that they can grow and retain their functional activities (particularly the presence of macropores).

Two main sources of osteogenic cells can be considered:

– differentiated osteoblasts derived from bone explants: clinical applications are limited by their poor proliferative property and the difficulty of maintaining the phenotype of these cells in vitro;

– bone marrow mesenchymal stem cells, essentially comprising osteoblasts, fibroblasts and adipocytes. These cells possess marked proliferation capacities and an intense osteogenic property (expression of osteocalcin, osteopontin, alkaline phosphatase, vitamin D receptors, capacity

Table I. – Osteogenic cells and active substances combined with calcium phosphate ceramics.

Cells	Active substances
Osteoblastic precursor clones [16]	Bone morphogenetic protein [59, 60]
Polyclonal culture of osteoblastic stem cells [29]	Growth hormone [25]
Total bone marrow cells [47]	Transforming Growth Factor-β1 [40]
Bone marrow mesenchymal cells after subculture [45]	Platelet Derived Growth-Factor [1]
Fraction of bone marrow mononuclear cells	Bisphosphonate [12]
Osteoblasts derived from bone explants	Anticancer drugs [58]
	Antibiotics [62]
	Plasmid DNA coding for parathyroid hormone and BMP-4 [15]

to mineralise an extracellular matrix). They can either be cloned to obtain a clone of osteogenic cells expressing the best possible osteogenic capacities (monoclonal population), or a polyclonal population can be used. The use of bone marrow stem cells also introduces, into the site of implantation, cells involved in the degradation of ceramics, such as osteoclasts, monocytes-macrophages, as well as haematopoietic stem cells.

CERAMIC-ACTIVE SUBSTANCE COMBINATIONS

Drug substances, administered orally or by injection, often have an excessively short half-life and a risk of systemic toxicity in order to achieve the desired local effect. Drug delivery systems (DDS) are being developed in order to overcome these disadvantages. The principle of these DDS is to regularly deliver pharmacologically active substances in situ, for prolonged periods, in sufficient quantities without inducing toxicity.

These techniques require the control of numerous parameters:

– binding of the active substance to the material: this is usually based on a mechanism of adsorption of the active substance onto the material. This binding is reversible, allowing release of the adsorbed molecules;

– delivery of the active substance: the release kinetics required to obtain a local therapeutic effect must be defined, and persistence of the active substance must be controlled after adsorption and release;

– preservation of the biological activity of the adsorbed and released drug;

– absence of any harmful modification of the mechanical and biological properties of the support prior to implantation.

Such combinations have already been considered, using calcium phosphate ceramics as the matrix. These combinations are able to ensure two synergistic actions in situ: a therapeutic action by prolonged release of an active substance and a support activity for bone ingrowth of the ceramic. Recent studies have shown that this type of

delivery system can be used to induce osteoinductive properties in the ceramic (combination with osteogenic proteins), or to treat certain bone diseases (infections, tumours, osteoporosis [1, 12, 16, 25, 29, 40, 45, 47, 58, 59, 60, 62] *(table I)*. More recently, a new concept has been developed by Fang et al [15], in which the calcium phosphate ceramic is considered to be a system for the release of plasmid deoxyribonucleic acid (DNA) coding for osteogenic factors (BMP [bone morphogenetic protein], PTH [parathormone]). This system, implanted in the rat femoral diaphysis, allowed the transfer of mesenchymal stem cells in situ, leading to the growth of a genetically modified cell population able to produce osteogenic proteins.

Conclusion

Bone substitutes constitute an alternative to bone grafts, but an "ideal" biomaterial must be biologically safe, possess mechanical properties similar to those of bone, and, finally, be defined in terms of clinical efficacy. The safety of a bone substitute depends on the quality of its reproducibility, its biocompatibility, and the absence of toxicity of the material. This preclinical evaluation is fundamental and should allow predictive risk analysis prior to implantation. No certification system has yet been developed for these devices, but the regulation concerning their marketing has been in force since June 1998, date of the introduction of European Community (CE) marking.

One of the mechanical problems is that porosity is necessary for osteoconduction, but makes the material less mechanically resistant. Osteoconduction corresponds to the passive property of a material to receive new bone growth, by vascular and cellular invasion from the recipient bone tissue in contact with the material. Osteoconduction is dependent on the pore size and the interconnection between pores. At the present time, osteoconductive materials have relatively poor mechanical properties, requiring very specifc conditions of use.

Clinical evaluation of bone substitutes must be based on comparative studies in man. In practice, randomised, controlled studies can help to define the choice of a biomaterial, but these studies raise certain problems, as the results depend on the type of indication (site, bone structure), the reference used, and the assessment criteria (definition of the efficacy of a bone substitute). Evaluation of the efficacy of a biomaterial is complex as it must be multifactorial. Factors involved in the reproducibility of the results are the volume of the defect to be filled, the patient's age, loading and mechanical constraints, and the condition treated.

Current research is tending to integrate osteoinductive properties into the bone substitute, by combining either osteogenic cells derived from the patient, or active substances which are subsequently released in situ during degradation of the material. These methods, currently under evaluation, should improve bone ingrowth kinetics and accelerate the formation of differentiated bone in large volumes of biomaterial.

The clinical applications of bone substitutes already validated should be submitted to retrospective studies, but especially medical device monitoring in order to identify problems encountered after use of a biomaterial, and to demonstrate any serious incidents (systemic toxicity) or absence of bone ingrowth with mechanical failure.

Nevertheless, bone substitutes now offer treatment options to replace autologous grafts in a variety of indications and clinical situations, under strictly defined conditions of use. The possibility of composites combining osteogenic cells or specific active substances (growth factors, antibiotics, antimitotics) with specifically defined materials will open up extensive fields of application, especially as these active materials will be inserted by minimally invasive surgical techniques.

References

[1] Arm DM, Tencer AF, Bain SD, Celino D. Effect of controlled delivery of platelet derived growth factor from a porous hydroxyapatite implant on bone ingrowth. *Biomaterials* 1996 ; 17 : 703-709

[2] Bleiberg I, Glowacki J, Anklesaria P, Greenberger JS. Origin of stromal cells associated with osteoclast recruitment in s.c. implants of bone particles in chimeric mice. *Exp Hematol* 1992 ; 20 : 957-961

[3] Bouler JM, Trecant M, Delécrin J, Royer J, Passuti N, Daculsi G. Macroporous biphasic calcium phosphate ceramics: influence of five synthesis parameters on compressive strength. *J Biomed Mater Res* 1996 ; 32 : 603-609

[4] Boyan B, Hummert TW, Dean DD, Schwartz Z. Role of material surfaces in regulating bone and cartilage cell response. *Biomaterials* 1996 ; 17 : 137-146

[5] Braye F, Irigaray JL, Jalot E, Oudadesse H, Weber G, Deschamps N et al. Resorption kinetics of osseous substitute: natural coral and synthetic hydroxyapatite. *Biomaterials* 1996 ; 17 : 1345-1350

[6] Bucholz RW, Carlton A, Holmes R. Interporosis hydroxyapatite as a bone graft substitute in tibial plateau fractures. *Clin Orthop* 1989 ; 240 : 53-62

[7] Daculsi G, Legeros RZ, Heughebaert M, Barbieux. Formation of carbonate apatite crystals after implantation of calcium phosphate ceramics. *Calcif Tissue Int* 1990 ; 46 : 20-27

[8] Daculsi G, Passuti N. Effect of the porosiy for osseous substitution of calcium phosphate ceramics. *Biomaterials* 1990 ; 11 : 86-87

[9] Delécrin J. Biomatériaux et arthrodèses vertébrales. *Ann Orthop Ouest* 1998 ; 30 : 162-163

[10] Delécrin J, Aguado E, Nguyen JM, Pyré D, Royer J, Passuti N. Influence of local environment on incorporation of ceramic for lumbar fusion. Comparison of laminar and intertransverse sites in a canine model. *Spine* 1997 ; 22 : 1683-1689

[11] Den Hollander W, Patka P, Klein C, Heidental G. Macroporous calcium phosphate ceramics for bone substitution: a tracer study on biodegradation with 45Ca tracer. *Biomaterials* 1991 ; 12 : 569-573

[12] Denissen H, Van Beek E, Van Den Bos T, Deblieck J, Klein C, Van Den Hoof A. Degradable biphosphonate-alkaline phosphatase complexed hydroxyapatite implants in vitro. *J Bone Miner Res* 1997 ; 12 : 290-297

[13] Ducheyne P, Radin S, King L. The effect of calcium phosphate ceramic composition and structure on in vitro behavior - I-Dissolution. *J Biomed Mater Res* 1993 ; 27 : 25-34

[14] Eggli PS, Müller W, Schenk RK. Porous hydroxyapatite and tricalcium phosphate cylinders with two different pore size ranges implanted in the cancellous bone of rabbits. A comparative histomorphometric and histologic study of bone in growth and implant substitution. *Clin Orthop* 1988 ; 232 : 127-138

[15] Fang J, Zhu YY, Smiley E, Bonadio J, Rouleau JP, Goldstein SA et al. Stimulation of new bone formation by direct transfer of osteogenic plasmid genes. *Proc Natl Acad Sci USA* 1996 ; 93 : 5753-5758

[16] Faucheux C, Bareille R, Rouais F, Amédée J, Lebendörfer A, Dard M. Biocompatibility testing of a bovine hydroxyapatite ceramic material with the use of osteo-progenitor cells isolated from human bone marrow. *J Mater Sci Mater Med* 1994 ; 5 : 635-639

[17] Frayssinet P, Mathon D, Azimus E, Autefave A. Céramiques phosphocalciques : influence de leurs caractéristiques sur leur ostéoconductivité. In : *Actualités en biomatériaux*. Paris : éditions Romillat, 1998 ; vol 4 : 121-125

[18] Frayssinet P, Tourenne F, Rouquet N, Conte P, Delga C, Bonel G. Comparative biological properties of HA plasmasprayed coatings having different crystalinities. *J Mater Sci Mater Med* 1994 ; 5 : 11-17

[19] Frayssinet P, Trouillet JL, Rouquet N, Azimus E, Autefage A. Osseointegration of macroporous calcium phosphate ceramics having a different chemical composition. *Biomaterials* 1993 ; 14 : 423-429

[20] Galois L, Mainard D, Bordji K, Membre H, Marchal L, Foliguet B et al. Céramiques phosphocalciques : influence de la taille des pores sur la réhabitation osseuse de deux céramiques phosphocalciques, l'HA et le bTCP. In : *Actualités en biomatériaux*. Paris : éditions Romillat, 1996 ; vol 3 : 361-380

[21] Gauthier O, Bouler JM, Aguado E, Pilet P, Daculsi G. Macroporous biphasic calcium phosphate ceramics : influence of macropore diameter and macroporosity percentage on bone ingrowth. *Biomaterials* 1998 ; 19 : 133-139

[22] Gouin F. Comblement des cavités osseuses par les biomatériaux. *Ann Orthop Ouest* 1998 ; 30 : 166-169

[23] Gouin F. Évaluation des biomatériaux. Table ronde du GESTO (Ph. Chiron). *Rev Chir Orthop* 1998 ; 84 (suppl 1) : 60-63

[24] Gouin F, Delécrin J, Passuti N, Touchais S, Poirier P, Bainvel JV. Comblement osseux par céramique phosphocalcique biphasée macroporeuse. *Rev Chir Orthop* 1995 ; 81 : 59-65

[25] Guicheux J, Heymann D, Trécant M, Gautier H, Faivre A, Daculsi G. Association of human growth hormone and calcium phosphate by dynamic compaction: in vitro biocompatibility and bioactivity. *J Biomed Mater Res* 1997 ; 36 : 258-264

[26] Hambleton J, Schwartz Z, Khare A, Windeler SW, Luna M, Brooks BP et al. Culture surfaces coated with various implant materials affect chondrocyte growth and metabolism. *J Orthop Res* 1994 ; 12 : 542-552

[27] Heikkila J, Mattila K, alan AJ. Bone healing in benign tumour induced cavities filled with bioactive glass. A randomised prospective clinical study. *3rd EFORT Congress*, Barcelona 24-27 April 1997, Abstract 018

[28] Inoue O, Ibaraki K, Shimabukuro H, Shingaki Y. Packing with high-porosity hydroxyapatite cubes alone for the treatment of simple bone cyst. *Clin Orthop* 1993 ; 293 : 287-292

[29] Jaiswal N, Haynesworth SE, Caplan AI, Bruder SP. Osteogenic differentiation of purified, culture-expanded human mesenchymal stem cells in vitro. *J Cell Biochem* 1997 ; 64 : 295-312

[30] Klawitter JJ, Bagwell JG, Weinstein AM, Sauer BW, Pruitt JR. An evaluation of bone growth into porous high density polyethylene. *J Biomed Mater Res* 1976 ; 10 : 311-321

[31] Klawitter JJ, Hulbert SF. Application of porous ceramics for the attachment of load bearing internal orthopedic applications. In : Journal of biomedical matererials research. Symposium n° 2 (part 1). New York : John Wiley and Sons, 1971 : 161-229

[32] Klein CP, De Groot K, Driessen AA, Van Der Lubbe HB. A comparative study of different b-whitlockite ceramics in rabbit cortical bone with regard to their biodegradation behaviour. *Biomaterials* 1986 ; 7 : 144-146

[33] Klein CP, Driessen AA, De Groot K. Relationship between the degradation behaviour of calcium phosphate ceramics and their physical-chemical characteristics and ultrastructural geometry. *Biomaterials* 1984 ; 5 : 157-160

[34] Kühne JH, Barti R, Frisch B, Hammer C, Jansson V, Zimmer M. Bone formation in coraline hydroxyapatite. Effects of pore size studied in rabbits. *Acta Orthop Scand* 1994 ; 65 : 246-252

[35] Larsson C, Thomsen P, Lausmaa J, Rodahl M, Kasemo B, Ericson LE. Bone response to surface modified titanium implants: studies on electropolished implants with different oxide thicknesses and morphology. *Biomaterials* 1994 ; 15 : 1062-1074

[36] Legeros RZ. Biodegradation and bioresorption of calcium phosphate ceramics. *Clin Mater* 1993 ; 14 : 65-88

[37] Legeros RZ, Parsons JR, Daculsi G, Driessens F, Lee D, Liu ST et al. Significance of the porosity and physical chemistry of calcium phosphate ceramics. Biodegradation - Bioresorption. In : Bioceramics : material characteristics versus in vivo behavior. New York : Academy of sciences, 1988 : 268-271

[38] Le Huec JC, Schaeverbeke T, Clement D, Faber J, Le Rebeller A. The influence of porosity on mechanical resistance of hydroxyapatite ceramics under compressive stress. *Biomaterials* 1995 ; 16 : 113-118

[39] Levai JP, Boisgard S. Acetabular reconstruction in total hip revision using a bone graft substitute. Early clinical and radiographic results. *Clin Orthop* 1996 ; 330 : 108-14

[40] Lind M, Overgaard S, Sob ale K, Nguyen T, Ongpipattanakull B, Bunger C. Transforming growth factor beta 1 enhances bone healing to unloaded tricalcium phosphate coated implants: an experimental study in dogs. *J Orthop Res* 1996 ; 14 : 343-350

[41] Lu JX, Anselme K, Flautre B, Hardouin P, Galur A, Descamps M et al. Évaluation in vitro de la biocompatibilité de deux biocéramiques de porosité identique à base d'hydroxyapatite ou de phosphate tricalcique. In : Actualités en Biomatériaux. Paris : éditions Romillat, 1998 ; vol 4 : 137-146

[42] Malca SA, Rocke PH, Rosset E, Pellet W. Cervical interbody xenograft with plate fixation. *Spine* 1996 ; 21 : 685-690

[43] Meynet JC. Ostéotomie tibiale de valgisation par ouverture interne : place des substituts osseux. *Ann Orthop Ouest* 1998 ; 30 : 171-174

[44] Motuo Fotso MJ, Brunon J, Duthel R. Résultats des xénogreffes intersomatiques cervicales par un substitut osseux. *Rachis* 1993 ; 5 : 241-246

[45] Ohgushi H, Okumura M, Yoshikawa T, Inoue K, Senpuku N, Tamai S et al. Bone formation process in porous calcium carbonate and hydroxyapatite. *J Biomed Mater Res* 1992 ; 26 : 885-995

[46] Oonishi H, Kushitani S, Iwaki H, Sakai K, Ono H. Long term clinical results of using HAP in revision of total hip replacement involving massive bone defects in the acetabulum. *Bioceramics* 1992 ; 8 : 157-162

[47] Petite H, Kacem K, Triffit JT. Adhesion, growth and differentiation of human bone marrow stromal cells on non-porous calcium carbonate and plastic substrata: effects of dexamethasone and 1, 25 dihydroxyvitamin D3. *J Mater Sci Mater Med* 1996 ; 7 : 665-671

[48] Pollo C, De Coexe B, Collard A, Gilliard C. Discectomie cervicale antérieure et fusion intersomatique par greffons d'hydroxyapatite et vis plaque. *Rachis* 1997 ; 9 : 39-46

[49] Pouliquen JC, Noat M, Verneret C, Guillemin G, Patat JL. Le corail substitué à l'apport osseux dans l'arthrodèse vertébrale postérieure chez l'enfant. *Rev Chir Orthop* 1989 ; 75 : 360-369

[50] Rawlinson JN. Morbidity after anterior cervical decompression and fusion. The influence of the donor site on recovery, and the results of a trial of surgibone compared to autologous bone. *Acta Neurochir* 1994 ; 131 : 106-118

[51] Savalainen S, Usenius JP, Hernesniemi J. Iliac crest versus artificial bone grafts in 250 cervical fusions. *Acta Neurochir* 1994 ; 129 : 54-57

[52] Senter HJ, Kortyna R, Kemp WR. Anterior cervical discectomy with hydroxyapatite fusion. *Neurosurgery* 1989 ; 25 : 39-43

[53] Shimazaki K, Mooney V. Comparative study of porous hydroxyapatite and tricalcium phosphate as bone substitute. *J Orthop Res* 1985 ; 3 : 301-310

[54] Taminiau A, Pooley J, Manfrini M, Tigani D, Capanna R. Implant of biphasic ceramic (Tricalcium phosphate/hydroxyapatite) in cystic cavities after bone tumour curettage: Preliminary results. In : Langlais F, Tomeno B eds. Limb salvage-major reconstruction in oncologic and nontumoral conditions. Berlin : Springer-Verlag, 1991 : 193-195

[55] Trecant M, Delécrin J, Nguyen JM, Royer J, Passuti N, Daculsi G. Influence of post-implantation physicochemical changes in a macroporous ceramic on its mechanical strengh. *J Mater Sci Mater Med* 1996 ; 7 : 227-229

[56] Uchida A, Araki N, Shinto Y, Yoshikawa H, Kurisaki E, Ono K. The use of calcium hydroxyapatite ceramic in bone tumour surgery. *J Bone Joint Surg Am* 1990 ; 72 : 298-302

[57] Uchida A, Nade S, McCartney E, Ching W. Bone ingrowth into three different porous ceramics implanted into the tibia of rats and rabbits. *J Orthop Res* 1985 ; 3 : 65-77

[58] Uchida A, Shinto Y, Araki N, Ono K. Slow release of anticancer drugs from porous hydroxyapatite ceramic. *J Orthop Res* 1992 ; 10 : 440-445

[59] Urist MR, Lietze A, Dawson E. β-tri calcium phosphate delivery system for bone morphogenetic protein. *Clin Orthop* 1984 ; 187 : 277-280

[60] Urist MR, Nilsson O, Rasmussen J, Hirota W, Lovell T, Schmalzreid T et al. Bone regeneration under influence of a bone morphogenetic protein (BMP) beta tricalcium phosphate (TCP) composite in skull trephine defects in dogs. *Clin Orthop* 1987 ; 214 : 295-304

[61] Van Der Meulen J, Koerten HK. Inflammatory response and degradation of three types of calcium phosphate ceramic in a non-osseous environment. *J Biomed Mater Res* 1994 ; 28 : 1455-1463

[62] Yamamura K, Iwata H, Yotsuyanagi T. Synthesis of antibiotic-loaded hydroxyapatite beads and in vitro release testing. *J Biomed Mat Res* 1992 ; 26 : 1053-1064

Management of the multiply injured patient

F Walcher
B Maier
I Marzi
W Mutschler

Abstract. – *The overall management of multiply injured patients needs to be adapted to the individual association of injuries and to the systemic situation during intensive care treatment. On the scene resuscitation and rapid but safe transport to an appropriate trauma centre are the first steps of the essential life-saving procedure. Operative treatment in multiply injured patients is carried out in three stages. In the first stage, life-saving operations are performed, such as control of massive intra-abdominal or thoracic bleeding and cerebral decompression. The second urgent stage of the so called "day-one-surgery" includes operative procedures to allow for intensive care therapy, and to prevent subsequent major disabilities. Stabilisation of fractures and debridement of soft-tissue injuries or open fractures are necessary to reduce the systemic inflammatory response during the early period of intensive care, thus reducing the risk of multiple organ failure. Within approximately one week after trauma, "second-look" procedures are carried out to stabilise soft-tissue repair and to optimise infection control. After stabilisation of the overall condition of the patient, the remaining reconstructive procedures are performed in the third stage of operative treatment.*

© 2000, Editions Scientifiques et Médicales Elsevier SAS. All rights reserved.

Keywords: multiply injured patients, polytrauma, fracture stabilisation.

Introduction

The multiply injured patient is defined by the conjunction of injuries to different organ systems, even when isolated lesions would not in themselves be life-threatening. The threat comes from the simultaneous occurrence of injuries, which include orthopaedic trauma, brain injury, and chest and abdominal lesions.

Numerous scoring systems have been developed over recent years to classify individual trauma patients, and to assess the probability of survival. These rating systems have also been used for the clinical decision-making process in managing the individual patient. Overall patient management must take numerous individual factors which influence the planning of the operative procedures into consideration. The principles of therapeutic strategies are recommended as guidelines for the management of multiply injured patients.

Felix Walcher, M.D.,
B Maier, M.D.,
I Marzi, M.D., Ph.D.,
Abteilung fürUnfall-, Hand- und Wiederherstellungschirurgie, Chirurgische Universitätsklinik, 66424 Homburg/Saar, Germany.
Wolf Mutschler, *M.D., Ph.D., Chirurgische Klinik und Poliklinik der Universität, Nußbaumstraße 20, 80336 München, Germany.*

Abbreviations

AIS	Abbreviated Injury Scale
APACHE	Acute Physiology and Chronic Health Evaluation
ARDS	Acute Respiratory Distress Syndrome
CT	Computer Tomography
DPL	Diagnostic Peritoneal Lavage
GCS	Glasgow Coma Scale
ISS	Injury Severity Score
MTOS	Major Trauma Outcome Study
MESS	Mangled Extremity Severity Score
MODS	Multiple Organ Dysfunction Syndrome
MOF	Multiple Organ Failure
PTS	Polytrauma Score
RTS	Revised Trauma Score
SIRS	Systemic Inflammatory Response Syndrome
TRISS	Trauma and Injury Severity Score TS Trauma Score

The multiply injured patient may already have several risk factors prior to injury, e.g. age, respiratory or cardiac diseases, etc. With trauma, major life-threatening cofactors suddenly arise. During prehospital care, the multiply injured patient presents mainly acute haemorrhage, due to severe musculoskeletal injuries or abdominal and pelvic lesions. Within the first hours after admission, prolonged haemorrhagic shock and severe brain damage represent the major life-threatening factors. After the initial operative treatment, with haemorrhage control and stabilisation of major fractures, other risk factors must be taken into account when planning the next steps of therapy. In particular, it has been discussed that delaying surgical procedures for a couple of days after trauma can lead to a kind of "second hit" that can trigger a potential increased systemic inflammatory response syndrome (SIRS). This inflammatory response may also be responsible for increased patient mortality due to the development of a multiple organ dysfunction syndrome (MODS). In particular, acute lung failure may occur [7, 8]. This working hypothesis is based on studies concerning inflammatory response after trauma and helps to plan the operative procedures [49]. After stabilisation of the systemic situation, the time-consuming operative reconstruction procedures may be a cause for the development of further additional systemic inflammation.

With increasing knowledge of the above-mentioned pathophysiology, the present management of the multiply injured patient is divided into three stages of operative therapy. These have to be adapted to the overall situation of the patient [36, 42]. Again, this working hypothesis is based on experimental investigations, clinical findings and surgical practice.

Prehospital care

Improvements in rescue systems have led to a decrease in the immediate mortality rate after trauma. Over the past twenty years, a better understanding of the pathophysiology of haemorrhagic shock and resuscitation, as well as the resulting aggressive management of the multiply injured patient, has led to a decrease in morbidity and less frequent multiple organ failure [21, 48]. Rapid utilisation of helicopter transport may have an impact on patient mortality [29, 51]. The beneficial presence of the emergency physician is also important [59]. Physical examination of the patient on the scene should lead to the first decisions regarding the priorities for life-saving procedures. The neurological status is determined by the Glasgow Coma Scale (GCS) [56]. Basic procedures such as stabilisation of central circulation by volume replacement, intubation and mechanical ventilation, drug administration and compression of external bleeding prior to patient rescue and transportation, must be decided and organised by the emergency physician (usually a trauma surgeon and/or anaesthesiologist). Information about the trauma mechanism is an important addition to clinical examination and diagnostic evaluation, since most of the patients suffer amnesia or are unconscious. The emergency physician or paramedic must, therefore, summarise the mechanisms of trauma and assess the forces that caused the injuries. This information is an essential part of the report to the clinical trauma team in the emergency room.

Haemorrhagic shock results mainly from massive abdominal or thoracic bleeding after traumatic rupture of parenchymal organs or major vessels, and severe injuries to extremities. Well-planned resuscitation is the major therapy leading to decreased morbidity of the multiply injured patient during prehospital care. In cases of thoracic trauma, insertion of chest tubing and controlled ventilation are required prior to transportation. Initial on the scene splinting of fractures is essential; bleeding due to injury to extremities requires temporary external compression. Since control of bleeding due to blunt abdominal or thoracic trauma is not possible on the scene, the priority is immediate transport of the patient to the nearest appropriate trauma centre. In these cases, volume replacement should be limited until the bleeding is controlled in the operating theatre.

The increase of intracerebral pressure in cases of brain damage with intracerebral bleeding increases the mortality rate in the prehospital period. Thus, the immediate transport of patients with serious head injuries to a specialised trauma unit is most important for successful treatment. The overall outcome of patients with traumatic brain injury has been significantly improved by reducing the number of secondary systemic insults [43]. Hypercapnia and hypoxia have been avoided by controlled ventilation with high concentrations of inhaled oxygen.

Emergency room

CLINICAL EVALUATION

The management of the first hour after admission to the shock room of the multiply injured patient should be organised by algorithms providing guidelines for diagnostic and therapeutic procedures. Each member of the trauma team and the consulting medical specialists should constantly bear in mind their role and their part in the team. The decision to undertake diagnostic and operative procedures should be co-ordinated by the trauma surgeon in co-operation with the medical consultants.

Immediately after arrival in the emergency room, the emergency physician must make a short but sufficient report to the trauma team. A precise physical re-examination should be carried out. The trauma surgeon must summarise the overall situation, in particular the present condition of circulation, ventilation and neurological status. Repeated evaluation of possible bleeding is required during resuscitation management, because restoration of the circulation sometimes results in further bleeding.

The prerequisite for successful surgical treatment is the immediate analysis of life-threatening injuries. Life-saving surgical therapy has to be decided within minutes after admission, in particular to control blood loss from thoracic, abdominal, pelvic or external bleeding, and the need for cerebral decompression in cases of increased intracerebral bleeding or contusion.

SCORING SYSTEMS

The development and use of scoring systems became popular in the early seventies. The standard trauma scores, developed and validated in the United States, are used for a variety of reasons [60]: valid classification and severity of injury, triage, clinical decision making and assessment of outcome. Moreover, a uniform validation allows for comparisons between quality of management and operative treatment [12]. Some scoring systems may be used for follow-up evaluations of intensive care patients [62].

Different kinds of scoring systems have been developed. Some are used for grading the severity of trauma patients without estimating the pathophysiological response of the patient (ISS, AIS). It has been demonstrated that they have predictive value for remote complications such as adult respiratory distress syndrome (ARDS) and multiple organ failure (MOF).

The commonly-used description of multiply injured patients is given by the Injury Severity Scale (ISS), which measures the severity of anatomical injury of trauma patients. The ISS developed by Baker [4] is based on the Abbreviated Injury Scale (AIS) presented in 1971. Using the AIS, the severity of injury is graded for non-fatal lesions from 0 (no injury) to 5 (critical) in 5 body areas. Based on these ratings, an ISS was devised by summing the squares of the three highest AIS values obtained for one patient, the maximum being 3x25 = 75. In a large series of trauma evaluations, it was shown that death rates increase in the presence of injuries in a second and third body area. The overall prediction of outcome correlates acceptably to mortality [4]. The ISS correlates well with the Polytrauma Score (PTS), designed in 1985. This score is an anatomical injury severity score, taking the patient's age into consideration [44].

Other scoring systems grade the physiological response to trauma. In 1974, the Glasgow Coma Scale (GSC) was introduced and has proved to be a simple, reliable method for assessing coma and altered levels of consciousness [56]. The GSC has shown a good correlation to the functional outcome of the survivors. Signs of central nervous system activity are a positive predictor of survival. Severe head injury serves as a negative predictor of survival [40]. The Trauma Score (TS) designed by Champion [16] aids rapid assessment and field triage of trauma victims. This scoring system describes the pathophysiological changes caused by the trauma, including respiratory and haemodynamic parameters in combination with the Glasgow Coma Scale.

A third kind of scoring system assesses the severity of trauma in relation to physiological response. The Hospital Trauma Index (HTI) is a modification of the AIS. It contains additional physiological elements of the trauma victim. Both, the ISS and AIS disregard the age of the patient as a major risk factor. Therefore, physiological status on admission (using the trauma score) and anatomical characteristics of trauma (using the ISS) related to age are combined in the TRISS method [16]. The Trauma Score has been replaced by the Revised Trauma Score (RTS) which may have a better predictive value than the TRISS method [13]. The TRISS methodology is used to assess probability of survival of a single patient. By the TRISS method, it is also possible to calculate the expected outcome for a whole group of trauma patients treated at one institution; the reference group of patients is derived from the major trauma outcome study (MOTS) [15]. Thus, as a scoring system, the TRISS method acts as a kind of external quality control to identify potential differences between institutions and to point out areas for improvement.

The Acute Physiology and Chronic Health Evaluation (APACHE II) was created to stratify critical illnessess of patients being admitted to the intensive care unit (ICU) [33]. The rating is based on pathophysiological data, chronic diseases and the age of the individual patient. The score correlates closely to subsequent death due to the acquired illness. Goris et al presented the Multiple Organ Failure Score (MOF) in 1985 [23]. During follow-up, the MOF score is applied daily in the ICU to assess severity of organ dysfunction or failure.

In conclusion, it is important to be aware that no scoring system gives sufficient confidence to predict the outcome of individual patients, but can help in planning and clinical decision-making in the management of a multiply injured patient. It can also contribute to introducing improvements to patient care within an institution, by comparing the quality of management.

Diagnostic evaluation

In addition to the information obtained from the physical examination in the shock room, diagnostic evaluation is carried out if there is no necessity for immediate operative intervention.

THORAX

An X-ray of the chest is the first radiological procedure after admission to the emergency room. Since blunt thoracic trauma often results in a number of intrathoracic injuries and lung contusion, early CT evaluation of the thorax can reveal other severe lesions. In these patients, even after insertion of chest tubing, a unilateral or bilateral pneumothorax can persist which can be missed by X-ray examination [26, 42].

ABDOMEN

The initial diagnostic evaluation of the abdominal cavity is still a matter of debate. We prefer sonography to visualise or exclude free fluid collection within the pleura spaces and/or peritoneal cavity, and in other compartments (pelvis, retroperitoneum, abdominal wall), indicating laceration of parenchymal organs, bowel injury or contusion of soft tissue [47]. It has been shown that sonography provides an accurate and rapid indicator of the need for emergency laparotomy [9]. Sonography re-evaluation of the abdomen and the costodiaphragmatic sinuses is routinely required within one hour after the first ultrasound examination.

To clarify the intra-abdominal situation as revealed by sonography, further evaluation must be performed by computer tomography, if the condition of the patient allows it. Others prefer the initial standardised CT examination which includes head, body and proximal extremities [38], because the precise location of the injury cannot be given with ultrasound technique alone. In respect to the initial abdominal CT diagnosis, the need for I.V. contrast and bowel opacification is still controversial [19, 54]. In cases of pelvic ring fracture, a CT evaluation of the abdomen should also be performed due to the higher incidence of occult abdominal injuries [5]. Basic diagnostic procedures to check the urogenital systems may also be indicated.

The well-known method of diagnostic peritoneal lavage (DPL) has been replaced by sonography and CT [17, 25]. although for many years it was been a reliable diagnostic tool in detecting intra-abdominal lesions.

HEAD AND CEREBRUM

Clinical signs of increased intracerebral oedema, or on the scene anamnestic information of primary unconsciousness, prior to anaesthesia, must lead to further investigation by cranial CT. Repeated evaluation within 24 hours is needed in cases of small asymptomatic epidural hematomas (which are frequently managed nonoperatively), unclear neurological defects or persisting unconsciousness [55].

EXTREMITIES

A conventional X-ray study of the spine and pelvis is required to clarify the need for immediate stabilisation. Additional selected X-ray investigations are performed if the clinical examination reveals fracture signs in the extremities. As a lack of pulse rate and abnormal Doppler ultrasound findings can account for rupture or occlusion of major vessels, an angiography can clarify the situation and justify immediate operative exploration.

Table I. – Three-stage concept for the management of multiply injured patients.

Stage 1	Stage 2	<<<--->>>	Stage 3
Day-One-Surgery			
Life saving operations	stabilisation	intermediate	delayed procedures
haemorrhage control of - abdomen - chest - pelvis - extremities cerebral decompression	musculoskeletal injuries - long bone fractures - open fractures - joint fractures - soft tissue injuries - compartment syndrome - spinal cord injuries - pelvic fractures	second looks	definitive stabilisation of fractures reconstruction of - acetabulum - joint injuries - soft tissue defects - hand and foot fractures - maxillofacial injuries - urological injuries

Table II. – Risk factors for the development of multiple organ failure [50, 52].

parameters	risk factors
age	> 55 years
ISS	> 24
lactate	> 2.5 mmol/L
base excess	> 8 mmol/L
blood transfusion	> 5 units of packed red blood cells

Principles of operative management

Over the last decades, a better understanding of the inflammatory response of multiply injured patients has led to the development of a balanced operative strategy in three stages [57], which is now the widely-accepted treatment (table I) [42]. The surgical therapy has been adapted to the overall situation during intensive care treatment. The surgeon must bear in mind that different risk factors can increase the incidence of MODS [50]. These findings can be interpreted as predictors of outcome (table II) [52]. Different scores and scoring systems have also been developed and they can play a role in the decision-making process for the individual patient.

Within the first hours of admission, haemorrhage control and fracture stabilisation must be completed. This so-called "day one surgery" is followed by a period of stabilisation of the patient. The trauma surgeon must be aware that additional operative treatment during this period can have deleterious effects on the overall condition of the patient ("second hit") and can increase peri-operative mortality due to an overwhelming inflammatory response [41, 49]. This so-called "second hit" reaction has led to the knowledge that long surgical therapy at an inappropriate time can increase peri-operative morbidity. Overall planning of the surgical therapy must also consider the consequences of different operative procedures, followed by additional treatments, for example, temporary initial stabilisation of long bone fractures by external fixators should be substituted by

Table III. – Priorities of life-saving operations.

First priority	Second priority	Third priority
massive bleeding of the thoracic and abdominal cavity rupture of major vessels	increased intracerebral pressure and intracerebral bleeding	haemorrhage caused by - unstable fractures - abdominal trauma - pelvic trauma - other major injuries

definitive osteosynthesis. Haemorrhage control of the abdomen by local tamponade must be followed by a second look operation within a definite time limit.

FIRST OPERATIVE PERIOD

The sequence of initial operative procedures on admission is decided by the leading trauma surgeon. Even within the first period of operative treatment, an order of merit must be established regarding the different operative priorities *(table III)*. Priority of immediate life-saving operations must be given to massive bleeding of intra-abdominal, thoracic organs or major vessels. Most life-threatening bleeding of the abdomen is caused by rupture of the spleen, and less frequently by injuries of the liver, bowel and pancreas. Second priority, but required immediately, is given to decompression of increased intracerebral pressure. If the GCS < 8 points after trauma, intracranial pressure should be continuously determined by a intracranial pressure transducer. The third priority is given to bleeding caused by unstable fractures of the extremities or the pelvic ring. Procedures for haemorrhage control and stabilisation of the pelvic ring by external or internal fixation may be performed in association with urgent laparotomy. Scattered bleeding in the abdomen and the thoracic cavity may be controlled by a local tamponade, so-called "packing".

SECOND OPERATIVE PERIOD

After the initial life saving procedures and completion of the diagnostic procedure, the operative stabilisation of relevant fractures takes place. Some call this stage, "delayed primary surgery" *(table I)* [36]. The procedures performed in "day one surgery" are an essential prerequisite for intensive care treatment. The trauma team, with the medical consultants, must decide the order of priority of the injuries and the possibility of performing simultaneous operative procedures.

Initial stabilisation of musculoskeletal injuries should be the major goal of the second stage of surgical therapy. It is well known that there is an increased morbidity and mortality even in the post-traumatic period of multiply injured patients with unstable fractures of long bones [10]. Early stabilisation of unstable fractures of long bones, as well as spinal and pelvic fractures, is therefore needed for intensive care therapy [37, 39]. Pain, haematoma and

instability of fractures activate the inflammatory response of local and systemic defense systems and may lead to an overwhelming SIRS [49]. This situation of "auto-aggressive inflammation" increases postoperative morbidity due to respiratory failure or sepsis associated with MOF [18]. The influence of pro- and anti-inflammatory mediators in the development of multiple organ dysfunction or failure have been demonstrated in numerous experimental and clinical studies. However, the precise interpretation of data remains difficult, due to varying beneficial and detrimental effects on the overall local and systemic situation of the multiply injured patients [49].

Concerning soft tissue trauma in particular, different operative aspects must be taken into account while planning fracture stabilisation.

Open fractures are mainly stabilised by external fixation, after accurate debridement of the fracture area. During delayed surgical therapy, external fixation should be replaced by other methods of osteosynthesis [2]. However, some studies have recently shown that primary stabilisation of open fractures by intramedullary, unreamed nailing, even in polytraumatised patients, generated no increased morbidity due to infection, instability or failure of implants, as compared to delayed reamed intramedullary nailing [32]. A definitive recommendation on how to stabilise open fractures does not seem possible now.

Severe joint fractures are either reconstructed initially or may be stabilised in the early period of treatment by external fixation after reduction. Depending on the extent of soft tissue defect and bone loss, anatomical reconstruction can be a challenge for the trauma team. However, these time-consuming procedures must be planned during the third stage of operative treatment. In particular, pre-operative diagnostic evaluation by CT scan or conventional tomography is necessary to plan the exact reconstruction procedure. When indicated, surgeons must deal with specialised techniques, including bone grafting and microsurgical tissue transfer.

Within recent decades, studies indicate that fracture stabilisation by extension or cast has been replaced by temporary or definitive osteosynthesis [11, 31]. Soft tissue injury associated with closed fractures is often less obvious and can easily be underestimated compared to open fractures. The method of stabilisation for multiply injured patient differs from that used for patients with an

isolated injury. There is controversy on how to stabilise fractures of long bones in cases of multiply injured patients. Several authors have shown that reaming for intramedullary nailing increases the occurrence of acute respiratory distress syndrome (ARDS), in particular in patients suffering blunt thoracic trauma with lung contusion. It was demonstrated by Pape et al that, in patients with severe chest trauma, there was a higher incidence of postoperative ARDS and mortality when early femoral nailing was done [45]. It has been argued that fat marrow embolisation due to increased intramedullary pressure, or release of vasoconstricting mediators during reaming, favour lung failure in multiply injured patients. In contrast, van Os et al stated that the presence of thoracic trauma should not be regarded as a contraindication for early stabilisation of major fractures by reamed nailing [58]. To reduce the possible iatrogenic trauma of the reaming process, techniques for unreamed intramedullary nailing have been developed. For example, reduced morbidity after initial unreamed antegrade nailing when managing open fractures has been demonstrated [34]. Other minimally invasive techniques have also been presented for definitive initial biological stabilisation of long bones using retrograde nailing [24], bridge plating [61], or indirect plate osteosynthesis [35].

Nevertheless, based on our clinical experience, we continue to recommend external fixation for early stabilisation of long bones in cases of multiply injured patients. The initial procedure is for the day one surgery and is followed by delayed nailing during the third stage of operative management [53].

Debridement of severe soft tissue injury is an essential part of the second stage surgical procedure. Mediators being released by contused and necrotic tissue are significantly reduced by the debridement. This prevents activation of the inflammatory systems. A vital tissue is susceptible to infection and therefore represents a further factor leading to increased systemic inflammatory response. Time-consuming reconstructive procedures by debridement of the resulting tissue defects have to be delayed for a few days until a stable systemic condition is achieved.

Amputation or salvage of a limb may be an essential question immediately after admission of the patient. The Mangled Extremity Severity Score (MESS) can help to decide how to handle amputation on the premises with an adequate team using microsurgical techniques. The MESS takes into account the age of the patient, the duration of ischaemia, additional injuries to other areas of the body and the soft tissue injury of the extremity [30]. It has been shown that reperfusion of ischaemic tissue after a time-consuming replantation may reactivate the systemic inflammatory response and can be hazardous for the overall condition of the multiply injured patient. It has also been demonstrated, by a series of studies, that a MESS above 7 points is an indication for amputation. Initial ranking according to the MESS, after admission of the patient to the shock room, should therefore lead to a definite decision whether to amputate or to salvage the limb.

A similar grading procedure should be applied in cases of severe open fractures (Gustilo IIIc) with ischaemia of the limb [28]. However, isolated injuries of major vessels of the extremities, with resulting short periods of ischaemia, require immediate revascularisation within approximately 6 hours after trauma [3].

The compartment syndrome of extremities, mostly occurring in the lower leg, is a menace to the polytraumatised patient. Increased intracompartmental pressure may have different causes: bleeding within the compartment due to persisting instability of fractures and contusion of soft tissue due to direct trauma or local inflammation after penetration injuries. A fasciotomy must be performed when the difference between diastolic and intracompartmental pressure is below 30 mm Hg. Stabilisation of fractures by external fixation is mostly recommended in cases where a fasciotomy must be performed. However, studies have recently been presented demonstrating good results with intramedullary stabilisation after fasciotomy [22]. Covering the resulting skin defect is performed by temporary synthetic overlay. Closing of skin by mesh-graft transplantation or dynamic suture should be planned during the third stage of surgical management.

Clinical signs of spine injuries with neurological defects have led to the administration of steroids, according to the NASCIS protocol, immediately after admission [14]. When injury to the cervical spine is suspected, adequate on-the-scene stabilisation with a stiff collar must be guaranteed until a definitive diagnostic evaluation can be completed. Unstable spine fractures, irrespective of their localisation, must be stabilised initially within 24 hours after trauma, thus giving the possibility of intensive care treatment. Lumbar spine fractures are mainly stabilised initially by posterior internal fixation, whereas fractures of the cervical and thoracic spine are mostly stabilised by anterior instrumentation.

Evaluation of the abdomen by computer tomography and ultrasound should clarify the need for laparotomy in the case of visceral injuries. Since blunt abdominal trauma is often associated with pelvic fractures and injuries of the urogenital tract, diagnostic evaluation and surgical treatment have to be managed in co-operation and co-ordination with the associated specialists: trauma, visceral and urological surgeons. In cases of complicated pelvic fractures with an unstable pelvic ring or concomitant pelvic soft tissue trauma, mortality rises significantly [46]. Severe pelvic injury is one

Table IV. – Criteria that count for/against the timing of operation procedures in the third period.

FOR	AGAINST
> 5 days after trauma	1 to 4 days after trauma
reduction of MOF-score	persistance/increase of MOF-score
improvement of oxygenation	failure of oxygenation
reduction of capillary leak (flow period)	persistance of capillary leak (tissue oedema)
stabilisation of coagulation	failure of coagulation
reduction of elastase and C-reactive protein	increase of elastase and C-reactive protein
normalisation of lactate	persistance of elevated lactate

of the leading prognostic criteria and requires special attention. Initial stabilisation of the pelvic ring is therefore needed immediately after admission. According to the fracture location, specific types of stabilisation are recommended [46]. Since additional urgent laparotomy is needed in cases of massive bleeding of intra-abdominal organs, stabilisation of the pelvic ring should be performed by internal osteosynthesis, e.g. in cases of unstable open-book fractures with integrity of the posterior part of the pelvic ring, plating of the symphysis can replace external fixation [37]. In these cases, combined packing of the abdominal and pelvic cavity may be advantageous, in particular since "second look" operations are needed in the follow-up. Unstable posterior pelvic ring disruption and vertical shear injuries with severe venous bleeding need initial external fixation. The application of the pelvic clamp provides direct transverse compression over the iliosacral region, thus reducing excessive blood loss by restoration of the intrapelvic space and providing earlier tamponade [20, 27]. The pelvic clamp does not interfere with subsequent laparotomy or necessary diagnostic procedures [20]. If injuries of the posterior pelvic ring (sacroiliac displacement, sacroiliac fracture dislocation or sacrum fractures) are present, computer tomography should be performed [46].

For severe arterial bleeding in the pelvic cavity, it has been reported that haemorrhage control can be performed by angiographic embolisation [1, 6]. However, it is important to be aware that most life-threatening bleeding due to pelvic injuries is caused by lacerations of the pelvic venous plexus, which are inaccessible to the embolisation procedure. Reconstruction of acetabular fractures should be performed during the third stage of operative management. However, dislocation of the hip must be reduced immediately. Prior to the elective operative procedure, detailed information on the fracture morphology should be available by CT evaluation.

Maxillofacial injuries with unstable fractures (Lefort I-III) must be managed simultaneously with other injuries during the second stage of operative treatment. However, massive bleeding from injuries to the nasopharyngeal region can contribute to

haemorrhagic shock and therefore must be stopped by local tamponade in the emergency room, and followed by early operative treatment. Fractures with loss of cerebrospinal fluid have to be temporarily closed because of the possibility of septic complications. Medical specialists who deal with the treatment of severe neurotrauma must therefore take part in the initial surgical treatment of maxillofacial injuries. After a time delay, the definitive time-consuming reconstruction of the maxillofacial fractures can be performed, once swelling of the soft tissue has been reduced.

INTERMEDIATE PERIOD

After the first two stages of operative management, further surgical procedures should be avoided for several days and up to one week. Intensive care therapy should stabilise respiratory function and systemic inflammatory status. Only second look operations should be performed to prevent septic complications due to necrotic tissue and haematoma. Early reconstruction procedures can lead to a so-called "second hit" or cause an "additional injury" that can have a fatal effect on the general status of the multiply injured patient and trigger an overwhelming SIRS. On the other hand, a "missed opportunity" to reconstruct certain injuries can prolong or increase the need for surgical procedures in dealing with tissue repair.

The end of the intermediate phase is determined by different clinical signs and laboratory analyses *(table IV)* [42]. Reduction of the MOF score indicates general stabilisation of the patient. However, isolated organ functions can still be impaired. Decisions concerning the best time for beneficial interventions as well as the timing of the third operative period are still difficult and subjective.

THIRD OPERATIVE PERIOD

The last stage of the operative procedure is reconstructive. Time-consuming elective operations must be arranged with the associated surgical consultants to coordinate operative conditions. It is recommended that different surgical interventions be performed simultaneously if the patient's medical condition allows multiple surgical interventions. However, the whole team must be aware of the possibility of a "second hit" that can again lead to an overwhelming inflammatory response.

A sensitive clinical view together with objective findings and increased knowledge about the pathophysiology are essential prerequisites for the successful management of the multiply injured patient.

References

[1] Agolini S, Shah K, Jaffe J, Newcomb J, Rhodes M, Reed J. Arterial embolization is a rapid and effective technique for controlling pelvic fractures hemorrhage. *J Trauma* 1997 ; 43 : 395-399

[2] Antich-Adrover P, Marti-Garin D, Murias-Alvarez J, Puente-Alfonso C. External fixation and secondary intramedullary nailing of open tibial fractures. *J Bone Joint Surg Br* 1997 ; 79 : 433-436

[3] Austin O, Redmaond H, Burke P, Grace P. Vascular trauma - A review. *J Am Coll Surg* 1995 ; 181 : 91-108

[4] Baker S, O'Neill B, Haddon W. The injury severity score: A method for describing patients with multiple injuries and evaluating emergency care. *J Trauma* 1974 ; 14 : 187-196

[5] Ballard R, Rozycki G, Newman P, Cubillos J, Salone J, Ingram W et al. An algorithm to reduce the incidence of false-negative FAST examination in patients at high risk for occult injury. Focused assessment for the sonographic examination of the trauma patient. *J Am Coll Surg* 1999 ; 189 : 145-150

[6] Bassam B, Cephas G, Ferguson K, Beard L, Young J. A protocol for initial management of unstable pelvic fractures. *Am Surg* 1998 ; 64 : 862-867

[7] Baue A. Multiple organ failure, multiple organ dysfunction syndrome, and the systemic inflammatory response syndrome - where do we stand? *Shock* 1994 ; 2 : 385-397

[8] Bernard GR, Artigas A, Brigham KL, Carlet J, Falke K, Hudson L et al. Report of the American-European consensus conference on ARDS: definitions, mechanisms, relevant outcomes and clinical trial coordination. *Intensive Care Med* 1994 ; 20 : 225-232

[9] Bode P, Edwards M, Kruit M, Van Vugt A. Sonography in a clinical algorithm for early evaluation of 1671 patients with blunt abdominal trauma. *AJR Am J Roentgenol* 1999 ; 172 : 905-911

[10] Bone L, McNamara K, Shine B, Border J. Mortality in multiple trauma patients with fractures. *J Trauma* 1994 ; 37 : 262-264

[11] Bone L, Sucato D, Stegemann P, Rohrbacher B. Displaced isolated fractures of the tibial shaft treated with either a cast or intramedullary nailing. *J Bone Joint Surg Am* 1997 ; 79 : 1336-1341

[12] Bouillon B, Lefering R, Vorweg M, Tiling T, Neugebauer E, Troidl H. Trauma score systems: Cologne validation study. *J Trauma* 1997 ; 42 : 652-658

[13] Boyd C, Tolson M, Copes W. Evaluating trauma care: The TRISS method. Trauma score and injury severity score. *J Trauma* 1987 ; 27 : 370-378

[14] Bracken M, Shepard M, Collins W. A randomized controlled trial of methylprednisolone or naloxone in the treatment of acute spinal cord injury. *N Engl J Med* 1990 ; 322 : 1405-1411

[15] Champion H, Copes W, Sacco W, Lawnick M, Keast S, Bain L et al. The major trauma outcome study: Establishing national norms for trauma care. *J Trauma* 1990 ; 30 : 1356-1365

[16] Champion H, Sacco W, Carnazzo A. Trauma score. *Crit Care Med* 1981 ; 9 : 672

[17] Davis J, Morrison A, Perkins S, Davis F, Ochsner M. Ultrasound: Impact on diagnostic peritoneal lavage, abdominal computed tomography and resident training. *Am Surg* 1999 ; 65 : 555-559

[18] Deitch E. Multiple organ failure. *Ann Surg* 1992 ; 216 : 117-134

[19] Federle M, Peitzman A, Krugh J. Use of oral contrast material in abdominal trauma CT scans: Is it dangerous ? *J Trauma* 1995 ; 38 : 51-53

[20] Ganz R, Krushell R, Jakob R, Kuffer J. The antishock pelvic clamp. *Clin Orthop* 1991 ; 267 : 71-78

[21] Garner A, Rashford S, Lee A, Bartolacci R. Addition of physicians to paramedic helicopter services decreases blunt trauma mortality. *Aust N Z J Surg* 1999 ; 69 : 697-701

[22] Georgiadis G. Tibial shaft fractures complicated by compartment syndrome: Treatment with immediate fasciotomy and locked unreamed nailing. *J Trauma* 1995 ; 38 : 448-452

[23] Goris RJ, Te Boekhorst TP, Nuytinck JK,, Gimbrere JS. Multiple-organ failure. Generalized autodestructive inflammation ? *Arch Surg* 1985 ; 120 : 1109-1115

[24] Gregory P, Dicicco J, Karpik K, Dipasquale T, Herscovici D, Sanders R. Ipsilateral fractures of the femur and tibia: Treatment with retrograde femoral nailing and unreamed tibial nailing. *J Orthop Trauma* 1996 ; 10 : 309-316

[25] Healey M, Simons R, Winchell R, Gosink B, Casola G, Steele J et al. A prospective evaluation of abdominal ultrasound in blunt trauma: Is it useful?. *J Trauma* 1996 ; 40 : 875-883

[26] Heffner J, McDonald J, Barbieri C. Recurrent pneumothoraces in ventilated patients despite ipsilateral chest tubes. *Chest* 1995 ; 108 : 1053-1058

[27] Heini P, Witt J, Ganz R. The pelvic C-clamp for the emergeny treatment of unstable pelvic ring injuries. A report on clinical experience of 30 cases. *Injury* 1996 ; 27 (suppl 1) : A38-A45

[28] Helfet DL, Howey T, Sanders R, Johansen K. Limb salvage versus amputation: preliminary results of the mangled extremity severity score. *Clin Orthop* 1990 ; 256 : 80-86

[29] Jacobs L, Gabram S, Szajnkrycer M, Libby M. Helicopter air medical transport: Ten-year outcomes for trauma patients in a New England program. *Conn Med* 1999 ; 63 : 677-682

[30] Johansen K, Daines M, Howey T, Helfet D, Hansen ST. Objective criteria accurately predict amputation following lower extremity trauma. *J Trauma* 1990 ; 30 : 568-573

[31] Johnson K, Cadambi A, Seibert B. Incidence of adult respiratory distress syndrome in patients with multiple musculoskeletal injuries: Effect of early operative stabilization of fractures. *J Trauma* 1985 ; 25 : 375-383.

[32] Keating J, O Brien P, Blachut P, Meek R, Broekhuyse H. Locking intramedullary nailing with and without reaming for open fractures of the tibial shaft. *J Bone Joint Surg Am* 1997 ; 79 : 334-341

[33] Knaus WA, Draper EA, Wagner DP, Zimmerman JE. APACHE II: A severity of disease classification system. *Crit Care Med* 1985 ; 13 : 818-829

[34] Krettek C, Haas N, Schandelmaier P, Frigg R, Tscherne H. Der unaufgebohrte Tibianagel (UTN) bei Unterschenkelfrakturen mit schwerem Weichteilschaden. *Unfallchirurg* 1991 ; 94 : 579-587

[35] Krettek C, Schandelmaier P, Miclau T, Bertram R, Holmes W, Tscherne H. Transarticular joint reconstruction and indirect plate osteosynthesis for complex distal supracondylar femoral fractures. *Injury* 1997 ; 28 (suppl) : A31-A41

[36] Krettek C, Simon R, Tscherne H. Management priorities in patients with polytrauma. *Langenbecks Arch Chir* 1998 ; 383 : 220-227

[37] Leenen LP, Van Der Werken C, Schoots F, Goris RJ. Internal fixation of open unstable pelvic fractures. *J Trauma* 1993 ; 35 : 220-225

[38] Leidner B, Adiels M, Aspelin P, Gullstrand P, Wallen S. Standardized CT examination of the multitraumatized patient. *Eur Radiol* 1998 ; 8 : 1630-1638

[39] Livingstone DH. Management of the surgical patient with multiple system organ failure. *Am J Surg* 1993 ; 165 (suppl) : 8S-13S

[40] Luk S, Jacobs L, Ciraulo D, Cortes V, Sable A, Cowell V. Outcome assessment of physiologic and clinical predictors of survival in patients after traumatic injury with trauma score less than 5. *J Trauma* 1999 ; 46 : 122-128

[41] Maier B, Frank J, Rose S, Marzi I. Primäre und sekundäre Freisetzung von Interleukin 6 und 8 bei der gestuften Polytraumaversorgung. *Unfallchirurgie* 1999 ; 25 : 100-107

[42] Marzi I, Mutschler W. Operative Strategie in der klinischen Versorgung des Polytraumas. *Zentralbl Chir* 1996 ; 121 : 950-962

[43] Meixensberger J, Roosen K. Clinical and pathophysiological significance of severe neurotrauma in polytraumatized patients. *Langenbecks Arch Chir* 1998 ; 383 : 214-219

[44] Oestern H, Tscherne H, Sturm J, Nerlich M. Klassifizierung durch Verletzungsschwere. *Unfallchirurg* 1985 ; 88 : 465-472

[45] Pape HC, Auf'm'Kolk M, Paffrath T, Regel G, Sturm JA, Tscherne H. Primary intramedullary femur fixation in multiple trauma patients with associated lung contusion--a cause of posttraumatic ARDS? *J Trauma* 1993 ; 34 : 540-547

[46] Pohlemann T, Bosch U, Gänsslen A, Tscherne H. The Hannover experience in management of pelvic fractures. *Clin Orthop* 1994 ; 305 : 69-80

[47] Pohlenz O, Bode P. The trauma emergency room: A concept for handling and imaging the polytrauma patient. *Eur J Radiol* 1996 ; 22 : 2-6

[48] Regel G, Lobenhoffer P, Grotz M, Pape H, Lehmann U, Tscherne H. Treatment results of patients with multiple trauma: An analysis of 3406 cases treated between1972 and1991 at a German level I trauma center. *J Trauma* 1995 ; 38 : 70-78

[49] Rose S, Marzi I. Mediators in polytrauma - Pathophysiological significance and clinical relevance. *Langenbecks Arch Chir* 1998 ; 383 : 199-208

[50] Roumen RM, Redl H, Schlag G, Sandtner W, Koller W, Goris RJ. Scoring systems and blood lactate concentrations in relation to the development of adult respiratory distress syndrome and multiple organ failure in severely traumatized patients. *J Trauma* 1993 ; 35 : 349-355

[51] Sampalis J, Denis R, Frechette P, Brown R, Fleiszer D, Mulder D. Direct transport to tertiary trauma centers versus transfer from lower level facilities: Impact on mortality and morbidity among patients with major trauma. *J Trauma* 1997 ; 43 : 288-295

[52] Sauaia A, Moore F, Moore E, Haenel J, Read R, Lezotte D. Early predictors of postinjury multiple organ failure. *Arch Surg* 1994 ; 129 : 39-45

[53] Scalea T, Boswell S, Scott J, Mitchell K, Kramer M, Pollak A. External fixation as a bridge to intramedullary nailing for patients with multiple injuries with femur fractures: Damage control orthopedics. *J Trauma* 2000 ; 48 : 613-621

[54] Stafford R, McGonigal M, Weigelt J, Johnson T. Oral contrast solution and computer tomography for blunt abdominal trauma: a randomized study. *Arch Surg* 1999 ; 134 : 622-626

[55] Sullivan T, Jarvik J, Cohen W. Follow-up of conservatively managed epidural hematomas: Implication for timing of repeated CT. *AJNR Am J Neuroradiol* 1999 ; 20 : 107-113

[56] Teasdale G, Jennett B. Assessment of coma and impaired consciousness. A practical scale. *Lancet* 1974 ; 1 : 81-84

[57] Tscherne H. Schweregrad und Prioritäten bei Mehrfachverletzungen. *Chirurg* 1987 ; 58 : 631-640

[58] Van Os J, Roumen R, Schoots F, Heystraten F, Goris R. Is early osteosynthesis safe in multiple trauma patients with severe thoracic trauma and pulmonary contusion? *J Trauma* 1994 ; 36 : 495-498

[59] Van Wijngaarden KJ, Lafreniere R, Cunningham R, Joughin E, Yim R. Air ambulance trauma transport: A quality review. *J Trauma* 1996 ; 41 : 26-31

[60] Waydhas C, Nastkolb D. Scores in polytrauma - Do they help? *Langenbecks Arch Chir* 1998 ; 383 : 209-213

[61] Wenda K, Runkel M, Degreif J, Ruding L. Minimally invasive plate fixation in femoral shaft fractures. *Injury* 1997 ; 28 : A13-A19

[62] Wong D, Barrow P, Gomez M, McGuire G. A comparison of the acute physiology and chronic health evaluation (APACHE) II score and the Trauma-Injury Severity Score (TRISS) for outcome assessment in intensive care unit trauma patients. *Crit Care Med* 1996 ; 24 : 1642-1648

Bone autografting techniques

C Delloye

Abstract. – The use of autogenous bone is one of the basic procedures in orthopaedic surgery. Autogenous bone remains, even today, the best bone grafting material. Different techniques of procurement and grafting procedures are reported.

Keywords: bone graft, bone autograft.

Introduction

The use of autogenous bone for managing bone defects has been a time-honoured procedure for a century. Although many bone substitutes are available today, such as bone allografts or synthetic materials, the bone autograft is still considered the gold standard.

The main advantages of a bone autograft over an allograft lie in retaining the properties of a fresh, living bone graft without immunity interference or risk of transferring disease.

These properties are:

– Osteogenic capacity: Most of the osteogenic cells from a bone autograft can survive the transplantation act and form new bone in their new environment.

– Osteoconduction capacity: Like any other substitute with a three-dimensional structure, trabecular or cortical bone can form a framework or scaffolding to support the ingrowth of cells.

– Osteoinductive capacity: This property is mainly dependent on the morphogenetic bone protein synthesised by the surviving osteoblasts.

Types of bone autograft

There are two types of bone autograft: cancellous and cortical bone grafts.

Bone grafts can be transferred free, or with their vascular pedicles.

Christian Delloye, Professor, Faculté de Médecine, Université Catholique de Louvain, Orthopaedic Surgeon, St-Luc University Clinics Brussels, Belgium.

FREE CANCELLOUS BONE

This is the most frequently used grafting material and is usually harvested at the iliac crest. Cancellous bone is richer in osteogenic cells than cortical bone because it offers a comparatively larger surface area for the cells. The cancellous bone from the iliac crest is considered to be the most osteogenic, compared to cancellous bone from other sites. This is presumably due to its persistent red marrow content.

Osteogenic cells from cancellous bone are more likely to survive a surgical transplant than those from cortical bone, for two reasons: The cells are in close proximity to the bone surface from which they can derive their nutrients. A distance of 300 µ from the surface is considered the critical distance beyond which an osteogenic cell would not resist anoxia [6]. In a cancellous bone autograft, the blood supply can be re-established within 2 days after transplantation, whereas for cortical bone, revascularisation takes longer.

FREE CORTICAL BONE

In a living cortical bone autograft, the endosteal side is the most active contributor to osteogenesis [4]. However, compared to cancellous bone, cortical bone is less cellular, hence less osteogenic, but is stronger mechanically. Consequently, compact bone will only be considered for grafting when there is a need for a structural graft. Such an indication is rare and may even be performed by a cortical bone allograft. Compact bone is procured at the medial aspect of the tibial diaphysis, or at the fibula.

VASCULARISED BONE

The rationale for transplanting a vascularised bone is that the bone remains viable if its vessels are immediately re-anastomosed. Cell survival after the surgical trauma is optimal. The healing process is then limited to the repair of the host-graft junction. This is similar in a way to a fracture repair. The main advantage is that revascularisation is immediately achieved and avoids the prolonged process of non-vascularised bone graft incorporation.

Among the disadvantages, the fit of the bone for size and shape may not be appropriate. Common donor sites of vascularised bone include the fibula, ribs and iliac crest.

Temporary preservation of the procured bone

As the freshly procured bone is a living tissue, it is imperative to preserve the viability of the osteoblasts as much as possible. The best method is to keep the bone either exposed to air or covered by a swab moistened with saline solution in a container. However, the bone should not be left immersed in saline. Much of the cellular activity can be preserved up to 3 hours [4].

Soaking cancellous bone chips in an antibiotic solution such as gentamycin, vancomycin, rifampicin, cefalotin (at the respective concentrations of 10, 50, 60 and 100 mg/mL for 10 to 30 minutes at room temperature) will cause adsorption and gradual release of the antibiotic by the bone matrix [5, 13]. Morselised cancellous bone can act as a carrier for prolonged antibiotic delivery.

Regarding the size of free cancellous bone chips, they should neither be too large, to

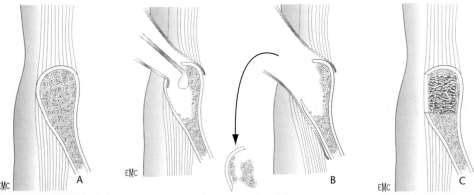

1 *Anterior iliac crest procurement.*
  A. Preoperative aspect.
  B. Cancellous bone procurement (left). Corticocancellous and cancellous bone procurement (right).
  C. Reconstruction of the bone stock with a cancellous bone block allograft.

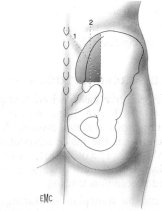

2 *Posterior iliac crest procurement. 1, 2. Recommended incisions.*

ensure nutrient diffusion from the bone surface nor too small, to avoid damage to the cells. The ideal dimension for optimal viability in a spongy bone is considered to be about five millimetres [3].

Preparation of the host bone bed

The host bed must be bleeding and offer raw, cortical or preferably, cancellous bone. No fibrous tissue should be interposed between the graft and host bed.

Techniques of procurement

FREE BONE AUTOGRAFT

■ *Anterior iliac crest*

The patient is placed in a supine position. The iliac tubercle is approached through a skin incision parallel but just inferior to the iliac crest. The tubercle, being the widest part of the crest, contains the largest amount of corticocancellous bone. The incision starts one centimetre behind the anterior superior iliac spine, to avoid injury to the lateral femoral cutaneous nerve. The apex of the crest is incised longitudinally, between the abdominal and gluteus muscles, where the intermuscular plane is relatively avascular. In children, the growing apophysis is split in two, releasing the muscles on either side. The material can either be taken from the inner or the outer aspect of the ilium (*fig 1A*). The corresponding muscles are elevated by subperiosteal dissection over the considered site and retracted. Corticocancellous or cancellous bone is procured with straight and/or curved chisels, curettes and gouges (*fig 1B*).

When particulate cancellous graft is needed, the inner or outer aspect of the cortex is elevated with a chisel, while a gouge or curette procures chips of cancellous bone. Finally, a rongeur may be used to finely cut the cancellous bone into a mouldable putty-like graft. An alternative method for obtaining such material is to use an acetabular reamer that is held against the outer aspect of the ilium. The particulate bone graft material is harvested intermittently. The procedure is stopped once the inner table is reached [10].

When a concave-shaped graft is required, the inner aspect of the ilium is more appropriate for procurement.

When a tricortical graft is considered (e.g., for corrective osteotomies), then a full thickness of the crest should be procured, after both outer and inner aspects have been exposed.

When a dowel is needed in limited quantity, the graft can be taken using a trephine, either percutaneously [9], or through a small incision.

Depending on the quantity of the procured bone, a cancellous bone allograft can be implanted to reshape the defect in case multiple grafting procedures are anticipated, especially in the young (e.g. patient with a tumour) (*fig 1C*). A haemostatic sheet can often be placed on the bleeding area of the donor site. The use of bone wax should be discontinued as it may elicit a foreign body reaction [11].

The aponeurosis is sutured over a wound drainage tube.

■ *Posterior iliac crest*

The largest amount of corticocancellous bone can be procured from this location.

The patient is usually prone but can also be placed in a lateral position with the side to be operated facing upwards. The procurement can be performed separately, or as part of any posterior spine surgery.

The classical incision begins at the posterior superior iliac spine, following the iliac crest for 8 cm anteriorly. Beyond that distance, the clunial nerves cross the iliac crest and their injury can cause a loss of skin innervation. As this procedure crosses the point of pressure over the posterior aspect of the pelvis, it may be complicated by skin necrosis.

Another access is through a more vertical incision, 2 cm lateral to the posterior spine (*fig 2*). This lateral approach has been found to have a lesser incidence of skin complications.

The subcutaneous fat is incised on the line of incision, to expose the gluteus maximus. The gluteal fascia is incised along the crest. The muscle is elevated by subperiosteal dissection. If a large amount of bone is needed, the outer iliac fossa can be exposed as far as the superior border of the greater sciatic notch. The thick portion of bone that forms the notch must be left intact to preserve the stability of the pelvis. The superior gluteal neurovascular bundle should be identified and protected.

If a tricortical bone block is required, the lumbodorsal fascia is dissected free from the inner aspect of the crest. A full thickness segment of the crest can be removed, taking care to preserve the articular surface of the sacroiliac joint.

The bone defect in the crest can be covered by a haemostatic sheet or substituted by a bone allograft in case a recurrent bone graft procurement is anticipated. The aponeurotic plane is sutured over a wound drainage tube.

During spine surgery, the posterior iliac crest can be approached by subcutaneous dissection from the midline to the posterior crest. The dissection can be sharper along the posterior gluteal line, at the tendinous origin of the muscle.

■ *Other sites*

Cancellous bone can be procured from the greater trochanter and the upper tibial metaphysis. Corticocancellous bone can be obtained from a rib during a thoracotomy.

Cortical bone is not often needed, but can be harvested from the medial aspect of the tibial diaphysis or from the fibular diaphysis.

At the tibia, a plate of cortical bone measuring about 30 cm can be taken. To avoid a fatigue fracture, the anterior and posteromedial tibial crests should be excluded from the procurement. No postoperative cast is required and full weight-bearing is allowed immediately.

The middle third of the fibula is also the source of a strong cortical graft.

VASCULARISED AUTOGRAFTS

The transfer of a free vascularised autograft remains one of the best means of reconstructing large skeletal defects. Being living tissue, it has the major advantage of being able to repair itself, and to hypertrophy over a length of time in cases of sustained mechanical loading.

The skin can be transplanted during the same surgery. It can be combined with free bone autografts or massive allografts if necessary.

Common donor sites include the iliac crest, rib, scapula and fibula. A fibula transfer may be preferred when the bony defect to be bridged is over 7 cm. Pre- and peroperative steps include arteriography of both donor and recipient sites, dissection of the vessels at both sites, removal of the bone with a cuff of muscle to protect the nutrient and periosteal blood supply, fixation of the graft, re-anastomosis of one artery and one vein and finally cancellous bone grafting at the bone junction, if necessary. The procurement of the fibula is described briefly.

■ *Free vascularised fibula*

The proximal two thirds of the fibula diaphysis are approached laterally [12]. The distal 10 cm is preferably left intact to avoid any instability problem with the ankle [1]. A tourniquet is used. The plane between the soleus and peroneal muscles is developed. The interosseous membrane is incised close to the fibula. The plane between the peroneal vessels and posterior tibial nerve is dissected including a cuff of the tibialis posterior muscle. The osteotomy is then performed. A cutaneous flap can be transferred in the meantime, if necessary.

Techniques of auto-genous bone grafting

There are numerous techniques for using autogenous bone, whether cortical, cancellous or corticocancellous. It must be emphasised that preparation of the graft bed is extremely important.

RECIPIENT SITE PREPARATION

The recipient site should be bleeding, free from dead tissue or dense fibrotic tissue after a thorough debridement. The site should be stabilised if unstable.

DIAPHYSEAL NON-UNION

Decortication is the usual technique for preparing a cortical bone. The aim is to

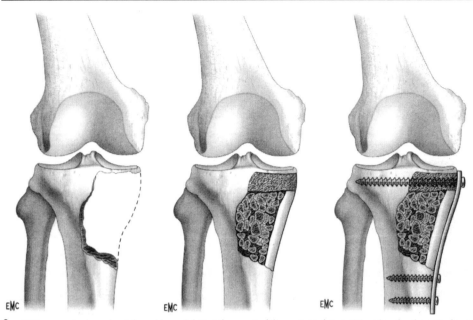

3 *Filling a metaphyseal-epiphyseal bone defect. A fragment of iliac autograft is positioned under the articular cartilage, followed by tibial autograft underneath to serve as support. The rest of the defect is filled with allograft fragments.*

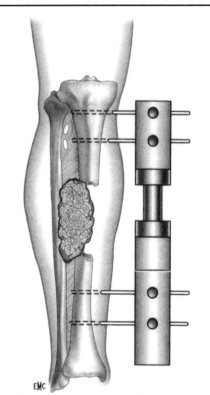

4 *Massive cancellous bone graft placed against the fibula to fill a large loss of tibial bone substance.*

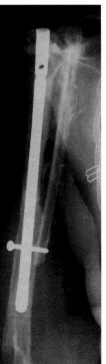

5 *Combined use of an intercalary bone allograft with a vascularised fibula at the shoulder after a tumour resection.*

augment the surface of living bone and hence its osteogenic capacity, by creating several chips of cortical bone that remain vascularised through their periosteum and soft tissues [7].

CORTICAL AND CANCELLOUS BONE AUTOGRAFTING

The bone grafting material can be onlaid or inlaid or both, depending upon the circumstances and the surgeon's choice. Fully autogenous material is only used in

cases requiring a limited amount (eg. a tight non-union), while in other cases, both auto- and allografts will be used (*fig 3*).

In case of a large cortical bone defect, there are many options available: massive cancellous bone grafting (*fig 4*), transfer of a free or vascularised fibula, an intercalary bone allograft or an Ilizarov procedure (*fig 5*). In case of infection, the Ilizarov procedure can be challenged by an autospongious grafting according to Papineau [8], or an intertibiofibular graft.

When there is a cancellous bone loss, the trend is to use allogenous with autogenous bone, or a vascularised bone.

The use of a bone autograft remains imperative in any site where there is no continuous osseous bed to support the graft such as in a lumbar posterolateral arthrodesis, or in a bone block procedure at the hip or shoulder.

Whether the addition of autogenous bone marrow procured by aspiration from the iliac crest is helpful for the "take" of the bone autograft cannot be ascertained by experimental data at present.

Complications

Iliac bone graft harvesting can be a source of complications with an overall rate ranging from 9% to 25% [2]. Osteoporosis and obesity are two major risk factors. The most common complications are protracted pain, haematoma and dysesthesia. Major complications have also been reported such as meralgia paresthetica, injury to the superior gluteal artery and to the sciatic nerve, herniation, pelvic fracture or instability.

A meticulous layered closure of the site and haemostasis are imperative to avoid these complications.

References

[1] Babhulkar SS, Pande K, Babhulkar S. Ankle instability after fibular resection. *J Bone Joint Surg Br* 1995 ; 77 : 258-261

[2] Banwart JC, Asher M, Hassanein S. Iliac crest bone graft harvest donor site morbidity. *Spine* 1995 ; 20 : 1055-1060

[3] Bassett A. Clinical implications of cell function in bone grafting. *Clin Orthop* 1972 ; 87 : 49-52

[4] Gray JC, Elves M. Early osteogenesis in compact bone isografts: a quantitative study of the contributions of the different graft cells. *Calcif Tissue Int* 1979 ; 29 : 225-237

[5] Hernigou P, Glorion C, Girard-Pipau F, Goutallier D. Antibiotic impregnated bone graft, transfer and activity of antibiotics in vitro and in vivo. *J Bone Joint Surg Br* 1991 ; 73 : 185-186

[6] Heslop B, Zeiss I, Nisbet N. Studies on transference of bone. *Br J Exp Pathol* 1960 ; 41 : 269-287

[7] Judet T, Richard L, Arnault O, De Thomasson E, Boury G. Traitement des pseudarthroses de tibia par décortication ostéopériostée de Robert Judet. *Acta Orthop Belg* 1992 ; 58 (suppl I) : 182-186

[8] Papineau L, Alfageme A, Dalcourt JP. Ostéomyélite chronique: excision et greffe de spongieux à l'air libre après mises à plat extensive. *Int Orthop* 1979 ; 3 : 165-176

[9] Saleh M. Bone graft harvesting: a percutaneous technique. *J Bone Joint Surg Br* 1991 ; 73 : 867-868

[10] Stephens H, Feldman B. Simple harvest of particulate autogenous bone graft. *Tech Orthop* 1996 ; 11 : 218-219

[11] Verborgt O, Verellen K, VanThielen F, Deroover M, Verbist L, Borms T. A retroperitoneal tumor as a late complication of the use of bone wax. *Acta Orthop Belg* 2000 ; 66 : (in press)

[12] Weiland A, Moore R, Daniel R. Vascularized autografts. *Clin Orthop* 1983 ; 174 : 87-95

[13] Witsoe E, Persen L, Loseth K, Bergh K. Adsorption and release of antibiotics from morselized cancellous bone. In vitro studies of 8 antibiotics. *Acta Orthop Scand* 1999 ; 70 : 298-304

Bone banking in orthopaedic surgery

C Delloye

Abstract. – *The demand for bone and related allografts has remained high during the past decade and consequently, many bone banks have been established. This chapter reviews tissue and bone banking activity. The purpose of bone banking is to provide surgeons with safe and reliable material. In order to achieve this objective, guidelines must be followed at each step from donor selection to the final supply of the bone. The different approaches for preserving and processing the bones are reviewed and discussed.*

© 2000, Editions Scientifiques et Médicales Elsevier SAS. All rights reserved.

Keywords: bone banking, bone grafts, allografts, sterilisation, disinfection.

Introduction

The basic purpose of bone banking is to provide surgeons with safe and suitable material. In orthopaedic surgery, bone is the most used of human tissues, followed by tendons and cartilage. This primary use of banked bones is related mainly to the spiralling numbers of revision hip arthroplasties, but also to spine, tumour and trauma surgery.

In the United States, about 140,000 bone allografts are used each year. In France, it has been estimated that in 1996, 6,500 femoral heads were implanted, while in the United Kingdom, the figure is about 7,800 [43]. Because the risk of transmission of bacterial or viral disease will never be nil, in Europe there is a trend to favour a more centralised system of tissue banking that would be agreed upon by national authorities.

This chapter reviews the main guidelines for the selection, recovery, processing and preservation of bone and cartilage tissues.

Legislation

There is no European directive concerning human tissues, which so far have not been considered as medical devices. At present, in most European countries there is legislation covering tissue donation, but tissue banking activity itself is legally regulated in only a very few countries (Belgium, France, Scotland, Spain, ...).

The general rule is that where there are no European, national or regional regulations, the European standards of the European Association of Musculoskeletal Transplantation (EAMST)[1] and the European Association of Tissue Banks (EATB)[2] shall be applied.

Donor selection

Selection of a donor presenting minimal risk of transmitting disease to a recipient is one of the major responsibilities of the tissue bank. In the past, bone allografts have transmitted hepatitis B and C, HIV-1 and tuberculosis [51]. HIV and other retroviruses have also been shown to be transmitted through cartilage and tendons [10, 44]. Tissue implantation in orthopaedic surgery is never urgent and is only part of an elective surgical procedure. To reduce the risk, tissue banks perform donor screening. This is carried out using a battery of questions about the life style and medical history of the donor, as well as a series of biological assays. To exclude donors who are risks for disease transmission, several updated guidelines have been published, amongst which those issued by EAMST and EATB.

THE MAIN CRITERIA FOR EXCLUSION OF DONORS ARE:

– Presence or suspicion of any dementia or any central nervous disease such as Alzheimer's or Creutzfeldt-Jakob diseases;

– Risk factors for HIV, B or C hepatitis;

– History of chronic hepatitis or presence of an active hepatitis;

– History of extractive pituitary hormone treatment;

– History, suspicion or presence of HIV or HTLV infection;

– Presence or history of malignant disease (basal cell carcinoma of the skin excluded);

– Presence of connective tissue disease (lupus, rheumatoid arthritis, ...) or chronic steroid use;

– Presence or evidence of infection or prior irradiation at the site of donation;

– Unknown cause of death (without autopsy).

BIOLOGICAL SCREENING

Any donor of tissue will be screened by laboratory assays, including the following tests *(table I)*:

Minimum serological tests:

– Hepatitis B surface antigen (HBs-ag);

– Hepatitis B core antibody (HBc-ab);

– Hepatitis C virus antibodies (HCV);

– HIV1-2 antibodies;

– Syphilis.

Christian Delloye, M.D., Professor, Université Catholique de Louvain, Faculty of Medicine; Orthopaedic Surgeon, St-Luc University Clinics, Avenue E. Mounier, 5388, B-1200 Brussels, Belgium.

[1] EAMST : 53, avenue Mounier, B-1200 Brussels, Belgium

[2] EATB : 10, Roesslestrasse, D-13125 Berlin, Germany

All references to this article must include: Delloye C. Bone banking in orthopaedic surgery. Editions Scientifiques et Médicales Elsevier SAS (Paris). All rights reserved. Surgical Techniques in Orthopaedics and Traumatology, 55-020-E-10, 2000, 6 p.

Table I. – Procedure for femoral head banking.

- Check your patient for selection criteria.

- Obtain oral and preferably witten consent for bone donation.

- Minimal laboratory tests include:

  HIV1-2 antibody assay

  Hepatitis B surface antigen

  Hepatitis B core antibody

  Hepatitis C antibody

  Syphilis (RPR or FTA)

  Anaerobic/aerobic synovial culture

  Rhesus factor

  [liver enzymes]

- Place the head in quarantine and store at - 80 °C or liquid nitrogen.

- Retest your patient at 6 months postoperatively for hepatitis C and HIV (antibody).

- Accurate and reliable record keeping of the bone must be obtained.

OPTIONAL ADDITIONAL BLOOD TESTING

– Polymerase chain reaction (PCR) for HIV and hepatitis viruses. When a quarantine is not possible, a negative PCR for HIV and hepatitis C might be accepted if properly performed by an experienced laboratory;

– HTLV antibody (a legal requirement in France);

– Alanine aminotransferase (ALT) for a living donor (a legal requirement in France). This last recommendation has been established for the detection of patients with liver disease and possible viral hepatitis;

– Rhesus factor, as it is known [33, 34] that a femoral head from a Rhesus positive donor is able to sensitise a Rhesus negative recipient. Consequently, Rhesus matching is necessary for a Rhesus negative female patient with child-bearing potential;

– HLA histocompatibility group matching does not appear necessary to achieve a successful allograft. Although it is known that a bone allograft may elicit an immune response, its significance has not been demonstrated so far [28, 49].

Tissue retrieval

The type of retrieved tissues varies according to circumstances. Femoral heads will be harvested when the donor has undergone a hip arthroplasty, whereas larger bones will be recovered from an organ donor. Table II lists the various kinds of bone allografts.

Permission for tissue retrieval should be obtained according to the national law or regulation. If there is no applicable regulation, informed consent should be obtained from the living donor, or from the next of kin in the case of an organ donor.

Table II. – The various types of bone allografts.

Source	Bone	Procedure
Living donor	Femoral head	Quarantine
Organ donor	Massive bone, tendons	Quarantine via the testing of organ recipients
Deceased donor	Bone	Premortem blood sample required (without haemolysis)
		No quarantine possible
		Validated tissue processing necessary

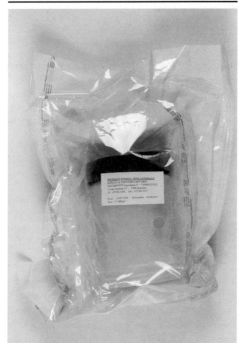

1 *Final aspect of a ready-for-use double container for sterile storage of a femoral head.*

FEMORAL HEADS

Table *I* lists the different steps involved in femoral head banking. The bone is procured as part of the hip arthroplasty and should be examined for quality. Ideally, an X-ray of the femoral head should be kept by the bank for quality assessment. A biopsy to detect occult disease would affect the graft as a whole, and its representativity is questionable. After bacteriologic assay, the bone is immediately placed in a sterile container (*fig 1*).

LONG BONES

In contrast with the femoral head, the procurement of bones and tendons from an organ donor may represent a challenge for the procurement team. In our experience, the procurement team should be conducted by an orthopaedic surgeon and composed of three to four team-mates. We believe that a surgeon is preferable to evaluate the cartilage of a knee or to decide if a meniscus is appropriate for grafting purposes. Whether the recovered tissues should be made ready in their final aspect at the time of procurement or after separate additional processing is a question of logistics. If there is no secondary sterilisation, we prefer on-site final preparation of the tissue at the time of procurement to avoid further handling

and possible contamination. The body is reconstructed with metallic or plastic prostheses that can reshape the skeleton.

Bacteriologic assessment

FEMORAL HEADS

The sensitivity and the negative predictive value of swab cultures have been demonstrated to be low (respectively 39 and 13%) compared to the culture of the whole specimen [55]. Consequently, culturing a representative piece of the bone is more reliable than swabbing. Another approach is the washing of the specimen followed by the culture of an aliquot of water [4, 24]. Any contamination will lead to exclusion of the head unless there is a final sterilisation. However, any positive culture with a pathogenic microorganism such as *staphylococcus aureus, streptococci* from the beta-hemolytic group, *clostridium, pseudomonas* and *enterobacteriae* will cause the exclusion of the specimen.

LONG BONES

Bacteriological screening of the explants by means of swab culturing is not sensitive enough, as this technique can only detect heavily contaminated bone. Culturing samples of soft tissues around the bone or samples of bones is a better method to evaluate the potential contamination of the retrieved bones. The sample should be representative of the tissue. Even more sensitive is the technique of washing the explant to be screened. Each piece is washed with 0.5 or 1 litre of saline from which an aliquot is taken for culture. This last technique is more demanding [24].

The use of antibiotics is controversial. Veen [54] could not show a significant effect of a bacitracin-polymyxin solution when the graft was only rinsed rather than soaked. In the past, we have observed a significant decrease of contaminated specimens when we added an antiseptic to the cryoprotective solution. As soon as a bone is explanted and swabbed, it is important to immediately immerse it in the solution containing the antiseptic for at least one hour [16]. Since 1995, we have been using rifampicin at a dose of 1.2 g/l of saline, because this gram-positive antibiotic has a residual action after the bone has been frozen and thawed. Our contamination rate is now about 4% of explanted bone. If a bone is positive for non-pathogenic contaminants, it is accepted that irradiation in the range of 15 to 25 kGy, depending on the initial bioburden, be performed to obtain a sterile bone segment [27]. The relevance of blood culture at the time of procurement remains controversial because of the high level of laboratory contamination [42].

In conclusion, swabbing the bone, when performed alone, is not sensitive enough and should be discouraged. Culturing a piece from the bone segment or an aliquot from specimen washing is more sensitive. Using duplicate samples will increase the sensitivity and also permit recognition of laboratory contamination.

Microbiological safety

RISKS OF VIRUS TRANSMISSION

The risks of virus transmission through an allograft are not nil; at least four recipients from a non-processed bone have been contaminated by the HIV virus [47, 48] and four others by the hepatitis C virus [12]. The risk is associated with a seronegative window during which a virus-contaminated donor can transmit the virus while his serum still remains negative for antibodies. In 1989, the mean time to seroconvert was 42 days from the time of exposure to the HIV virus [31]. Recent improvement of the sensitivity of anti-HIV assays has resulted in a significant shortening of this pre-seroconversion window period. The risk with the third generation assay is, however, differently appreciated. When the screening is performed with antibody assays alone, Busch et al [9] evaluated this window period to be 22 days, while Lelie et al [38] estimated it as being 37 days. Assuming that there is a tenfold higher incidence of HIV infections amongst tissue donors than amongst blood donors, Lelie [38] estimated the risk of a "window donation" for a tissue to be 6 per one million transplants (one per 166,000 tissues). Concerning hepatitis C, assuming a window period of 14 weeks and an incidence of 61 per tissue donors, the risk for a hepatitis C-contaminated tissue would be one per 6,100 tissue donations.

The risk of a window donation can be lowered by additional safety measures.

USE OF AMPLIFICATION TESTS

The polymerase chain reaction (PCR) is an in vitro amplification of the viral genome that has been intercalated into the patient's DNA. Because the selection and amplification of the target DNA is independent of antibody response, an infecting virus can be detected before seroconversion. This assay is very sensitive and specific. The HIV-DNA polymerase chain reaction is able to shorten the average window period to 16 days from the day of exposure. The residual risk of an infectious tissue would be reduced to 1 in 230,000

donations. The HIV p24 antigen testing will provide the same reduction as the HIV-DNA PCR regarding the window period. The European standards recommend the use of PCR or p24 antigen testing for HIV, and of PCR for hepatitis C, when tissues cannot be kept in quarantine.

QUARANTINE

Quarantine is a waiting period after which the tissue donor is retested if he is living, or in the case of a deceased organ donor, the recipient of organs is tested. This measure is the safest, the least expensive and the most sensitive in tracking hepatitis C and HIV viruses. Therefore, quarantine of tissue should be performed whenever possible.

In case of a living donor, European guidelines recommend a six month quarantine period. This interval remains the same as before, despite the increased sensitivity of HIV antibody assays, because of the longer latency for the hepatitis C virus. In the case of a deceased organ donor, the six month quarantine can be reduced to three months, as a contaminated vascularised organ should expose the recipient to a much earlier viral load [47].

INACTIVATION PROCESSING

Application of a chemical or physical agent can potentially inactivate a contaminated tissue. However, the effectiveness of decontamination should be demonstrated by validated methods before being accepted on a routine basis. The most common decontamination treatments will be reviewed in a later section.

Tissue preservation

DEEP-FREEZING

Deep-freezing is the most convenient and widespread method of tissue preservation. Water contained in the tissue is converted into ice and is therefore no longer available for further chemical reaction.

PRESERVATION TEMPERATURE

The minimal temperature at which the bone must be frozen is -28°C as determined by Bassett [5]. At that temperature, the eutectic point for bone, both the solute and the solvent will completely crystallise. At all temperatures between the freezing point and the eutectic point, there exists a mixture of ice, liquid water and solute.

As a rule, the objective of any storage unit is to reach and maintain a temperature below that point. In practical terms, -40°C is the minimal requirement. There are two usual temperatures: -80°C and -196°C (liquid nitrogen). From a theoretical point of view, maintenance in liquid nitrogen is ideal, as there is no further crystal growth and all

biochemical reactions are suppressed. However, storage in liquid nitrogen requires a high investment to ensure a constant coolant level. This is why most tissue banks use mechanical deep-freezers with a -80°C capacity. At that temperature, persisting biochemical activity has not been demonstrated [21], nor has any detrimental influence on the tissue been reported. Several arguments support this view:

– Comparison of radiographs of large bone segments that have been frozen for years does not show evident densitometric or morphological differences;

– There is no significant correlation between the duration of the storage period and the occurrence of an allograft complication such as a fracture [17].

– There is a rapid extinction of the collagenase activity in bone after freezing storage at -80°C [21].

From the mechanical and immunological points of view, there are no differences for bone between the temperatures of -80° and -196°C [28, 45]. Consequently, any tissue that will be mechanically loaded should preferably be stored frozen rather than freeze-dried.

■ *Duration of storage period*

The European standards limit to 5 years the storage validity for tissue stored below -40°C. Although there is no scientific data to document this, it was felt that the condition of the packaging would have suffered from handling after 5 years of preservation, and also that screening techniques might have improved after such a period, with the availability of more sensitive tests, as reported by Conrad et al [12]. Suppose that you receive a massive bone allograft which has been stored for 9 years. Is the package still in good condition? What about the fact that it was screened using only the second generation antibody assay available at that time for HIV and HCV?

■ *Cartilage protection*

As the chondrocyte is the only cartilage component able to synthesise the matrix of a tissue with no regenerating capacity, cell cryoprotection appears mandatory.

Dimethylsulfoxide (DMSO) is the main agent used to protect the cell from freezing injury [52]. However, the diffusion of the molecule through the various layers of the cartilage remains questionable, as well as its efficacy. Chondrocyte survival is evaluated to be about 20-30% of the population, but the required minimal percentage of surviving cells for satisfactory joint function is not known. The cooling speed of the tissue is also unknown. In a mechanical -80°C freezer, it takes about 5 hours for the deeper parts of the tissue to attain -80°C [18]. To thaw the tissue, the fastest speed is recommended to preserve the highest cell viability. Usually, the frozen tissue is

Table III. – How to measure easily the residual moisture in a freeze-dried or dehydrated tissue.

- At the end of dehydration or freeze-drying, carefully weigh the tissue on an analytical balance.

- Place the sample in an oven at 100 °C for 24 hours.

- Place the sample in the oven again for an additional 24 hours until the tissue reaches a constant weight.

The weight difference is represented by the water still contained in the freeze-dried tissue and must not represent more than 5% of the final weight.

immersed in 37°C heated saline containing antibiotics. A large bone allograft such as a humerus will need 20 minutes at 37°C to reach 20°C. Clinically, there is no apparent superiority of cryoprotected cartilage compared to frozen cartilage without protection [1]. Morphologically, DMSO-treated cartilage displays the same cellular injury pattern as non-protected cartilage, while the cartilage matrix does not appear to suffer from freezing [50].

FREEZE-DRYING

■ *Characteristics of a cycle*

This preservation technique is less widespread because the required material is more sophisticated and expensive. The freeze-drying technique is an application of the triple point of water that allows it to pass directly from the frozen state to the vapour state without melting or denaturation. The sublimation of ice requires freezing and vacuum conditions. First, the wet product is frozen. Then, the frozen sample is exposed to a vacuum for sublimation. The net result will be a dry matter containing less than 5% of residual moisture *(table III)*. As dried material, a freeze-dried bone must be protected from moisture in the air and is therefore packaged under vacuum or in an inert gas *(fig 2)*. The container is either a glass jar or a double plastic envelope. A freeze-dried bone can be stored for 5 years according to the European guidelines. The speed of the freeze-drying procedure depends upon the difference of the vapour pressure of ice between the sublimation chamber and the condenser that traps the water vapour from the sample. A typical cycle for cancellous bone will take approximately 72 hours. Lyophilisation of tissues is usually performed without cryoprotection and consequently, there is no cell survival in a freeze-dried tissue.

■ *Other properties of freeze-dried tissues*

A freeze-dried tissue loses its ability to elicit a humoral immune response, and this loss is greater than after freezing [28].

A freeze-dried bone can be sterilised by ethylene oxide and irradiation. The sequence

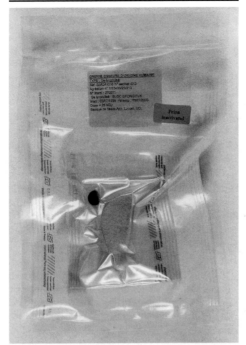

2 *Final aspect of a processed and freeze-dried bone wrapped in a double plastic envelope. The vacuum allows immediate verification of the packaging seal.*

in which sterilisation and freeze-drying should take place remains a matter of debate. Harmful by-products can be generated by the interaction of sterilant and water, such as the appearance of ethylene glycol and free radicals [32]. Mechanically, the strength of a freeze-dried material remains decreased unless it is rehydrated with full recovery after 24 hours [7]. After 30 minutes of rehydration, a freeze-dried cancellous bone has a loss of 20% in ultimate compressive strength and stiffness compared to a fresh bone [14]. Freeze-drying and irradiation, as of a dose of 30 kGy, add their negative effects to the mechanical resistance [39, 53]. When combined, the cancellous bone has a loss of 40% in ultimate compressive strength compared to frozen bone, whereas stiffness is decreased by 20 %. Consequently, freeze-dried bone should not be implanted in a mechanically-loaded area unless it is protected by hardware, for instance in acetabular revision where such material can be used with a supporting ring.

DEHYDRATION

Water is removed from the tissue by a chemical agent such as acetone or ether. This procedure is most often carried out at room temperature. Dehydration is completed when the tissue has less than 5% residual humidity.

Decontamination

This is an additional procedure allowing to decrease the potential bacterial or viral contaminants to the lowest possible level.

However, a decontaminated tissue is not considered to be a sterile tissue unless the decontaminating method has been proved to be truly sterilising (see "Sterilisation").

CHEMICAL AGENTS

The use of antiseptics or antibiotics is often recommended in practice. We advocate their use during the harvesting and thawing phases of the graft [18]. The harvested bone is first swabbed with a sample of adjacent soft tissue to assess a potential initial contamination. The bone is then immersed for 60 to 90 minutes in an antibiotic solution such as rifampicin at a dose of 1.2 g/L. It has been shown experimentally that an antibiotic such as vancomycin can be released from the bone graft for three weeks [29]. Another class of chemical agent is represented by solvent-detergents such as chloroform, ethanol, acetone and ether. These agents are able to inactivate coated viruses such as HIV and hepatitis B and C [25]. However, penetration into the core of the tissue might take longer depending on the nature of the tissue [2], the thickness of the sample and the quantity of fat bone marrow. Hydrogen peroxide has long been used as a bleaching agent and is also effective against viruses and bacteria due to its capacity to form free radicals. For prion disease, contamination through a musculoskeletal tissue has not yet been demonstrated. However, should this occur, one of the two chemical treatments recognised as effective by the World Health Organisation [56] should be applied: sodium hydroxide 1 mol for 1 hour at 20°C or sodium hypochlorite (2% chlorine available) for 1 hour at 20°C. Whether musculoskeletal tissues will mechanically resist such treatment is not known.

PHYSICAL TREATMENT

Irradiation and heat are the two most common physical treatment agents, and will be discussed below. Water jet lavage is another method that may effectively decontaminate a tissue with one decimal reduction of contamination [4]. Another optional treatment is the use of supercritical CO_2 at high pressure (280 bars) and at 50°C for in-depth bone delipidation [23]. The main advantage of this approach is the power of penetration which is not limited by the size of the tissue.

Sterilisation

The basic aim in sterilising musculoskeletal tissue is to reduce the probability of finding a viable microorganism on the sterilised tissue to one in a million [15]. To achieve this goal, it is first necessary to consider the bioburden of the tissue before it is sterilised. In addition, the processing of the tissue should be controlled and standardised to keep the bioburden as low as possible. The effectiveness of the sterilising method will depend on the initial bioburden, the sensitivity of the microorganism to the sterilising agent and the duration of exposure. It should be emphasised that the use of sterilisation in tissue banking does not replace the screening of the donor.

IRRADIATION

The two main sources of irradiation are gamma rays from a cobalt 60 source and accelerated electrons generated by an accelerator. Gamma rays have an excellent penetration capacity. To the contrary, electrons as charged particles cannot penetrate deeply.

In most European countries, the usual and legal dose to sterilise tissue is 25 kGy. One gray (Gy) is equal to 100 rads. Although this dose is appropriate for bacteria, it appears not to be sufficiently effective for the HIV virus [13, 26, 30]. The radiosensitivity of the hepatitis viruses is also not known, but recent clinical data suggest that hepatitis C-contaminated tissues did not transmit the virus after irradiation [12]. Prions are highly resistant to radiation [19, 27]. The mechanical resistance of fresh-frozen irradiated cortical bones is decreased by about 20% in flexion as of a dose of 30 kGy, and in compression, as of a dose of 60 kGy [39, 41]. In contrast, fresh-frozen cancellous bone is not affected by irradiation at 25 kGy when tested in compression [3]. However, when the bone is freeze-dried and irradiated, a negative effect is observed as of a 30 kGy dose [7, 14, 39, 53].

ETHYLENE OXIDE

This alkylating gas was used for a long time, but has now been discontinued in most countries because the by-products it generated produced an inflammatory reaction [32]. Nevertheless, because ethylene oxide is able to penetrate a cortical bone to sterilise musculoskeletal tissue, it is still used in some European countries [35, 46].

HEAT

Autoclaving is another method of sterilisation [11, 20]. However, according to the European standards (EN 554, 555), exposure at 121°C must be reached and maintained for 15 minutes. Unpublished data from our laboratory has indicated that the bone at the centre of whole femoral heads never reaches 121°C during conventional autoclaving at 121°C. Similar observations have been made for long bones [6]. Below the temperature of 121°C, only disinfection can be obtained; spores will resist at lower temperatures. Viral decontamination may be proposed at 80°C for HIV virus [36], but this heat processing remains questionable for hepatitis C in large femoral heads with a diameter greater than 56 mm, because of the limited heat conductivity of bone. Another aspect of viral inactivation is the inability to demonstrate a very high decimal reduction of a process in one single step due to the limited virus load that can be spiked in the sample. As high bioburdens have been reported for hepatitis viruses, no conclusions can be drawn about the effectiveness of the process [35]. Prions are heat resistant and inactivation requires at least autoclaving at 134°C for 30 minutes [8, 19].

Distribution

The bank is responsible for the supply of the tissue, which must be transported in an appropriate container or package that will mechanically protect the tissue. For long distances, an isotherm container with enough dry ice to maintain the required temperature must be provided.

Record keeping

Records should accurately identify all the information pertaining to the donor and all the steps in tissue processing, if any. Release of the tissue should be documented, including the name of the recipient and date of use. All data concerning the donor, his family and the recipients must be treated as confidential. Record keeping should also be organised in such a manner that tissue tracking is possible in any circumstances.

Conclusions

Tissue banking requires multi-step organisation with constant vigilance at each step, from donor selection through the final supply to the surgeon. These efforts are not easy and require dedication to high standards. The final aim is to provide safe and appropriate grafting material. Whether or not he is involved in running a bone bank, the surgeon must co-operate with the tissue bank, by participating in the six month blood testing in the case of femoral heads or by verifying the suitability of the graft he will implant.

References ➤

References

[1] Alho A, Karaharju O, Korkala O, Laasonen E. Hemijoint allografts in the treatment of low grade malignant and aggressive bone tumours about the knee. Int Orthop 1987; 11 : 35-41

[2] Anastasescou M, Cornu O, Banse X, König J, Hassoun A, Delloye CH. Ethanol treatment of tendon allografts: a potential HIV inactivating procedure. Int Orthop 1998; 22 : 252-254

[3] Anderson M, Keyak J, Skinner H. Compressive mechanical properties of human cancellous bone after gamma irradiation. J Bone Joint Surg Am 1992; 74 : 747-752

[4] Anglen J, Apostoles P, Christensen G, Gainor B, Lane J. Removal of surface bacteria by irrigation. J Orthop Res 1996; 14 : 251-254

[5] Bassett C. Clinical implications of cell function in bone grafting. Clin Orthop 1972; 87 : 49-59

[6] Böhm P, Stihler J. Intraosseous temperature during autoclaving. J Bone Joint Surg Br 1995; 77 : 649-653

[7] Bright R, Burchardt H. The biomechanical properties of preserved bone grafts. In : Friedlaender G, Mankin H, Sell K eds. Osteochondral allografts. Boston : Little Brown, 1983 : 241-247

[8] Brown P, Gibbs C, Amya H, Kingsbury D, Rohmer R, Sulima M, Gajdusek D. Chemical desinfection of Creutzfeldt-Jakob disease virus. N Engl J Med 1982; 306 : 1279-1282

[9] Busch MP, Lee LL, Satten GA, Henrard DR, Farzadegan H, Nelson KE et al. Time course of detection of viral and serological markers preceding human immunodeficiency virus type 1 seroconversion: implications for screening of blood and tissue donors. Transfusion 1995; 35 : 91-96

[10] Campbell D, Oakeshott R. HIV infection of human cartilage. J Bone Joint Surg Br 1996; 78 : 22-25

[11] Chiron PH, Gaudy E, Utheza G, Moatti N, Didier J, Izopet J et al. Stérilisation des allogreffes osseuses par la chaleur. Rev Chir Orthop 1993; 79 : 248

[12] Conrad EU, Gretch DR, Obermeyer KR, Moogk MS, Sayers M, Wilson JJ et al. Transmission of the hepatitis C virus by tissue transplantation. J Bone Joint Surg Am 1995; 77 : 214-224

[13] Conway H, Tomford W, Mankin HJ, Hirsch MS, Schooley RT. Radiosensitivity of HIV-1. Potential application to sterilization of bone allografts. AIDS 1991; 5 : 608-609

[14] Cornu O, Banse X, Docquier PL, Luyck S, Delloye C. Effect of freeze-drying and gamma irradiation on the mechanical properties of human cancellous bone. J Orthop Res 2000; 18 : 426-431

[15] Darbord JC, Laizier J. A theoretical basis for choosing the dose in radiation sterilization of medical supplies. Int J Pharma 1987; 37 : 1-10

[16] Delloye C. Current situation and future of tissue banking in orthopaedics. In : Gallinaro P, Duparc J ed. European instructional course lectures. Paris : Masson, 1993 : 161-172

[17] Delloye C, Cornu O, De Nayer P, Vincent A. Complications des allogreffes osseuses massives. Analyse de 145 allogreffes consécutives. Rev Chir Orthop 1996; 82 (suppl 1) : 209-210

[18] Delloye C, De Halleux J, Cornu O, Wegmann E, Buccafusca GC, Gigi J. Organizational and investigational aspects of bone banking in Belgium. Acta Orthop Belg 1991; 57 (suppl 2) : 27-34

[19] Dormont D. Creutzfeldt-Jakob disease and transplantation: facts and fables. Transplant Proc 1996; 28 : 2931-2933

[20] Duparc J, Massin P, Bocquet L, Benfrech E, Cavagna R. Autogreffes tumorales autoclavées. À propos de 12 cas dont 6 tumeurs à haut grade de malignité. Rev Chir Orthop 1993; 79 : 261-271

[21] Ehrlich M, Lorenz J, Tomford W, Mankin H. Collagenase activity in banked bone. Trans orthop Res Soc 1983; 8 : 78

[22] European Association of MusculoSkeletal Transplantation (EAMST) and European Association of Tissue Banks (EATB). Common standards for musculoskeletal tissue banking. Vienna, 1997

[23] Fagès J, Marty A, Delga C, Condoret JS, Combes D, Frayssinet P. Use of supercritical CO_2 for bone delipidation. Biomaterials 1994; 15 : 650-656

[24] Farrington M, Matthews I, Foreman J, Richardson K, Caffrey E. Microbiological monitoring of bone grafts: two years' experience at a tissue bank. J Hosp Infect 1998; 38 : 261-271

[25] Feinstone S, Mihalik K, Kamimura T, Alter H, London W, Purcell R. Inactivation of hepatitis B virus and non-A, non-B hepatitis by chloroform. Infect Immun 1983; 41 : 816-821

[26] Fideler B, Vangness T, Moore T, Li Z, Rasheed S. Effects of gamma irradiation on the human immunodeficiency virus. A study in frozen human bone-patellar ligament-bone grafts obtained from infected cadavera. J Bone Joint Surg Am 1994; 76 : 1032-1035

[27] Forsell J. Irradiation of musculoskeletal tissues. In : Tomford W ed. Musculoskeletal tissue banking. New York : Raven Press, 1993 : 149-180

[28] Friedlaender G, Strong D, Sell K. Studies on the antigenicity of bone. I. Freeze-dried and deep-frozen bone allografts in rabbits. J Bone Joint Surg Am 1976; 58 : 854-858

[29] Hernigou P, Glorion C, Girard-Pipau F, Deriot H, Goutallier D. Libération in vitro et in vivo des antibiotiques à partir des greffes osseuses. Rev Chir Orthop 1992; 78 (suppl 1) : 217

[30] Hernigou P, Marce D, Juliéron A, Marinello G, Dormont D. Stérilisation osseuse par irradiation et virus VIH. Rev Chir Orthop 1993; 79 : 445-451

[31] Horsburgh C, Ou C, Jason J. Duration of human immunodeficiency virus infection before detection of antibody. Lancet 1989; 2 : 637-640

[32] Jackson D, Windler G, Simon T. Intraarticular reaction associated with the use of freeze-dried, ethylene oxide-sterilized bone-patella tendon-bone allografts in the reconstruction of the anterior cruciate ligament. Am J Sports Med 1990; 18 : 1-10

[33] Jensen T. Rhesus immunization after bone allografting. A case report. Acta Orthop Scand 1987; 58 : 584

[34] Johnson CA, Brown BA, Lasky LC. Rh immunization caused by osseous allograft. N Engl J Med 1985; 312 : 121-122

[35] Kearney J. Sterilization of human tissue implants. Tissue Cell Rep 1997; 4 : 33-36

[36] Knaepler H, VonGarrel T, Seipp HM, Ascherl R. Experimental studies of thermal disinfection and sterilization of allogenic bone transplants and their effects on biological viability. Unfallchirurg 1992; 95 : 477-484

[37] LeHuec JC. Study of the thermic effect on bone at 60 degrees C as applied to bone allograft. Chirurgie 1992; 118 : 397-404

[38] Lelie PN, Zaaijer HL, Cuypers HT. Risk of virus transmission by tissue, blood and plasma products. Transplant Proc 1996; 28 : 2939

[39] Loty B. Allogreffes osseuses: aspects fondamentaux et techniques de conservation en 1992. In : Duparc J ed. Conférences d'enseignement 1992. Paris : Expansion scientifique française, 1992 : 211-237

[40] Loty B. Personal communication. 1997

[41] Loty B, Courpied J, Tomeno B, Postel M, Forest M, Abelanet R. Radiation sterilized bone allografts. Int Orthop 1990; 14 : 237-242

[42] Martinez OV, Malinin TI, Valla PH, Flores A. Postmortem bacteriology of cadaver tissue donors: an evaluation of blood cultures as an index of tissue sterility. Diagn Microbiol Infect Dis 1985; 3 : 193-200

[43] Michaud R, Drabu K. Bone allograft banking in the United Kingdom. J Bone Joint Surg Br 1994; 76 : 350-351

[44] Nemzek J, Arnoczky S, Swenson C. Retroviral transmission by the transplantation of connective-tissue allografts. An experimental study. J Bone Joint Surg Am 1994; 76 : 1036-1041

[45] Pelker R, Friedlaender G, Markham T, Panjabi M, Moen C. Effects of freezing and freeze-drying on the biomechanical properties of rat bone. J Orthop Res 1984; 1 : 405-411

[46] Prolo D, Pedrotti P, White D. Ethylene oxide sterilization of bone dura mater, and fascia lata for human transplantation. Neurosurgery 1980; 6 : 529-539

[47] Simonds R. HIV transmission by organ and tissue transplantation. AIDS 1993; 7 (suppl 2) : S35-S38

[48] Simonds R, Holmberg S, Hurwitz R, Coleman TR, Bottenfield S, Conley LJ et al. Transmission of human immunodeficiency virus type 1 from a seronegative organ and tissue donor. N Engl J Med 1992; 326 : 726-732

[49] Stevenson S, Horowitz M. The response to bone allografts. J Bone Joint Surg Am 1992; 74 : 939-950

[50] Tavakol K, Miller R, Bazett-Jones DP, Hwang W, McGann L, Schachar N. Ultrastructural changes of articular cartilage chondrocytes associated with freeze-thawing. J Orthop Res 1993; 11 : 1-9

[51] Tomford W. Transmission of disease through transplantation of musculoskeletal allografts. J Bone Joint Surg Am 1995; 77 : 1742-1754

[52] Tomford W, Fredericks GR, Mankin HJ. Studies on cryopreservation of articular cartilage chondrocytes. J Bone Joint Surg Am 1984; 66 : 253-259

[53] Triantafyllou N, Sotiropoulos E, Triantafyllou J. The mechanical properties of lyophilized and irradiated bone grafts. Acta Orthop Belg 1975; 41 : 35-44

[54] Veen R. Bone allografts. A study into bacterial contamination, sensitivity of cultures, decontamination and contribution to postoperative infection. [thesis], State University of Leiden. 1994 : 1-128

[55] Veen R, Bloem R, Petit P. Sensitivity and negative predictive value of subcultures in musculoskeletal alllograft procurement. Clin Orthop 1994; 300 : 259-263

[56] World Health Organization. Report of a WHO consultation on public health issues related to animal and human spongiform encephalopathies. WHO/CDS/VPH/92. 104, 1992

Acute compartment syndrome

AC Masquelet

Abstract. – Acute compartment syndrome is characterised by abnormal pressure inside a compartment, resulting in ischaemia of muscles and nerves.

All compartments may be involved but the most frequent localisations are in the distal extremities: the forearm and the hand in the upper limb, and the leg and the foot in the lower limb.

Acute compartment syndrome should be considered an urgent vascular problem. Clinical manifestations are linked to ischaemia of the muscles and nerves, but are not specific. Therefore, repeated pressure measurements are very helpful in deciding whether to carry out surgical decompression, which consists of a complete fasciotomy of the compartment.

The possibility of a compartment syndrome should always be considered, especially in uncommon localisations and in cases of delayed syndromes.

Keywords: compartment syndromes, acute compartment syndrome, ischaemia, fasciotomies.

Introduction

Acute compartment syndrome results from increased pressure in a muscle compartment which is limited by a tight osseofascial envelope. The viability of the functional tissues, particularly the nerves and muscles, can be compromised if diagnosis and treatment are not performed early.

Mechanism and aetiologies

The three main mechanisms that elevate pressure are: increased volume within the compartment, compartment constriction and external compression.

INCREASED VOLUME WITHIN THE COMPARTMENT

Any cause which produces swelling and bleeding inside the compartment can obviously precipitate an acute syndrome. The principal causes are fractures, arterial occlusion and intra-compartmental injection of fluids. Physical exercise may initiate a recurrent form of compartment syndrome due to muscle swelling [10, 11, 14].

COMPARTMENT CONSTRICTION AND EXTERNAL COMPRESSION

These reduce the volume of the compartment and can induce local swelling of the soft tissue, resulting in increased pressure. The main causes are closure of a fascial defect, circumferential deep burns (especially electrical burns), or prolonged compression of the limbs whatever the precise aetiology. The increasing pressure always results from bleeding and oedema or both. Up to a critical pressure value, which may vary in time and intensity, the tissue lesions are reversible, which justifies early surgical decompression. Beyond this critical pressure value, the lesions are irreversible, resulting in retractile fibrous transformation of the muscles and nerve paralysis.

Localisations of compartment syndromes

A compartment is a non-extensible space limited by bone, septa and fascia. Fascia usually designates a circumferential fibrous membrane, while a septum inserts on a segment of bone. Septa divide a large volume into several compartments. As compartments are well-defined at the distal extremities, compartment syndrome especially involves the leg, the foot, the forearm and the hand. Nonetheless, a compartment syndrome may occur anywhere at the level of the limbs, including the girdles. In fact, compartment syndrome of the shoulder, arm, pelvic girdle and thigh are not uncommon.

In the leg, the foot or the hand, the acute syndrome may involve one or several compartments. Sometimes an isolated muscle may be affected by high pressure even if it is not enclosed in a true compartment, for example, the pronator quadratus. This muscle is covered by a very thin membrane which inserts on the radius and on the ulna, and slow bleeding from a non-displaced fracture of the radius is likely to produce an acute increase in pressure in the muscle and to compromise its viability [15].

Clinical manifestations

The main components of a compartment are muscles and nerves. Clinical manifestations are linked to ischaemia of these tissues: spontaneous pain, pain on palpation, paraesthesia and paresis are the main indicators of an acute syndrome.

Determining which nerve is affected by ischaemia allows identification of the compartment involved.

Alain-Charles Masquelet, M.D., Professor, Service d'orthopédie et traumatologie, hôpital Avicenne, 125, route de Stalingrad, 93009 Bobigny cedex, France.

All references to this article must include: Masquelet AC. Acute compartment syndrome. Editions Scientifiques et Médicales Elsevier SAS (Paris). All rights reserved. Surgical Techniques in Orthopaedics and Traumatology, 55-030-A-10, 2002, 6 p.

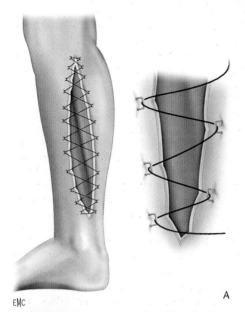

A

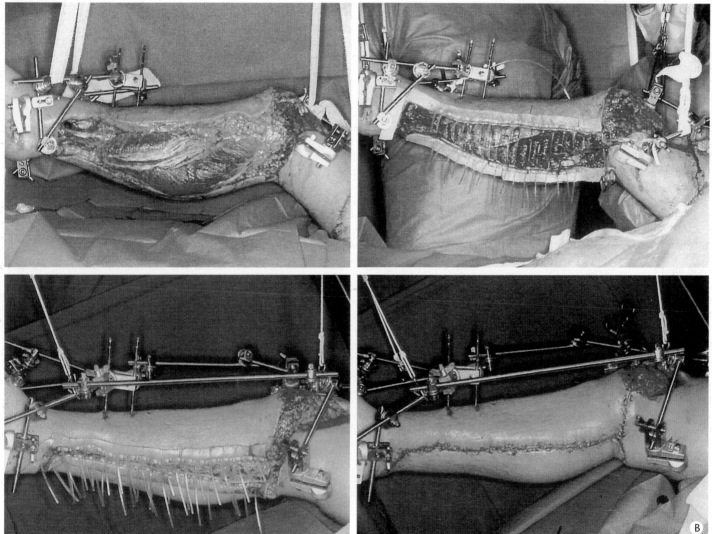

Stretch tests are not specific, but are very sensitive and reflect the muscle lesions.

The value of the interstitial pressure inside the compartment is the most objective datum. Pressure measurement is now facilitated by a quick pressure monitor set. This is recognised as very helpful in deciding whether to perform surgical decompression, but the precise level of pressure at which surgery is indicated remains controversial. To eliminate individual variations, it seems better to assess the difference between the diastolic pressure and the compartment pressure. If the difference is higher than 30 mm Hg, surgery is indicated. This consists of a fasciotomy which widely opens the compartment and decreases the pressure [9].

Principles of surgical procedures

In the acute phase of a compartment syndrome, there is no place for delayed surgery. Even if there is some doubt about the interpretation of the clinical signs and the intramuscular pressure value, it is always better to perform a prophylactic fasciotomy than to leave a true compartment syndrome untreated.

When surgery is indicated, it should be performed in emergency; acute compartment syndrome should always be considered an urgent vascular problem.

Treatment of the late diagnosed compartment syndrome is controversial [5, 6, 13]. Some authors [13] advocate fasciotomy to excise necrotic muscle areas so as to reduce the final functional prejudice. Others advise against operation [5, 6], to avoid infection of necrotic muscle. Moreover, in some localisations such as the anterior compartment of the leg, it may be preferable to preserve the fibrous tissue in order to obtain a tenodesis effect which may avoid a palliative transfer. All cases of compartment syndrome which are seen very late (after 24 to 36 hours) should be thoroughly assessed on an individual basis.

From a surgical point of view, fasciotomy should involve the entire compartment. A partial fasciotomy is inefficient and leads to a muscle hernia which increases muscle swelling.

To perform a complete fasciotomy, we recommend a large skin incision over the entire fasciotomy. A partial skin incision may risk injury to superficial nerves and veins, and subcutaneous fasciotomy may cause muscle injury.

The main nerves which pass through tunnels should be released (for example, the median nerve at the carpal tunnel and the tibialis posterior nerve at the tarsal tunnel).

Obviously, the fasciotomy should not be closed. The skin incision can be closed secondarily using the "shoe lace" technique [3] (fig 1A) or a progressive skin extending procedure (fig 1B) to avoid skin grafting, which entails a functional prejudice. On the other hand, a skin incision over released nerves should be closed primarily.

Surgical treatment according to localisation

COMPARTMENT SYNDROME OF THE FOREARM

■ *Anatomy* (fig 2)

The forearm comprises three compartments: anterior, posterior and lateral.

The anterior compartment includes the flexors of the wrist, the superficial and the

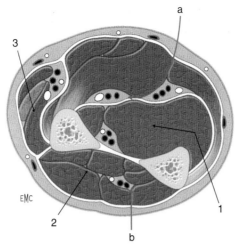

2   *The three compartments of the forearm. 1. Flexor anterior compartment; 2. dorsal extensor compartment; 3. "mobile wad" (radial compartment). a. approach for release of the flexor compartment between the finger flexors and the flexor carpi ulnaris. Retraction of these muscles allows epimysiotomy of the deep flexors (arrow); b. approach for release of the dorsal compartment.*

deep flexors of the fingers, the pronator teres and the quadratus. The course of the ulnar and median nerves is in the anterior compartment. Acute compartment syndrome initiates paresis of finger flexion, pain on passive extension of the fingers and sensory disturbances in the areas innervated by the median and ulnar nerves.

The posterior compartment includes the common extensor of the fingers, the extensors of the index and fifth fingers, the extensor carpi ulnaris, the abductor and extensor pollicis longus, and the extensor pollicis brevis.

The lateral compartment, the so-called "mobile wad", comprises the brachioradialis and the extensors of the carpus.

The boundary between the mobile wad and the posterior compartment is located between the extensor carpi radialis brevis and the extensor digitor communis muscles.

■ *Fasciotomy* (fig 3)

A very long lazy-S skin incision is made over the anterior aspect of the forearm from

the antecubital fossa to the palm of the hand (fig 3A). At the level of the wrist, the incision should remain on the ulnar aspect of the palmaris longus tendon to avoid injury to the sensitive thenar branch of the median nerve. Taking care not to injure the superficial sensitive nerves, the fascia is incised, including the flexor retinaculum to release the median nerve at the wrist.

As advocated by Eaton and Green [4], an epimysiotomy of the deep muscles is performed. The epimysiotomy involves the flexor digitorum profondis, flexor pollicis longus and quadratus pronator. For an early fasciotomy, it is possible to make a skin incision only over the muscle bodies of the forearm without exposing the tendons at the lower third at the forearm. Incision of the palm is always mandatory, but will be closed primarily.

Fasciotomies of the posterior and lateral compartments are necessary when the forearm has sustained compression on both aspects (alcohol and drug abuse, crush syndrome, etc.). The skin incision is gently curved over the posterior aspect of the extensor carpi radialis brevis (fig 3B). Undermining the subcutaneous tissue gives access to the posterior and lateral compartments. The fasciotomy goes from the lateral epicondyle to the dorsal aspect of the distal forearm. Decompression of the dorsal compartment usually ensures decompression of the "mobile wad".

■ *Postoperative course*

The skin incision in the palm is closed and a progressive skin extending procedure is initiated to ensure primary delayed closure of other incisions. A non-constrictive dressing is applied and a splint maintains the elbow at a right angle and the wrist in slight extension. Active motion of the fingers is started the day after the fasciotomy. Elevation of the upper extremity above the level of the heart is recommended to promote venous drainage. Elevation of a non-decompressed limb should be avoided, because it decreases tissue perfusion and exacerbates ischaemia.

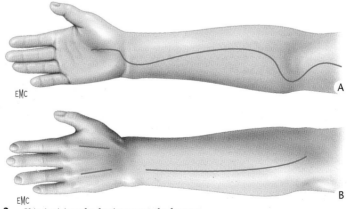

3   *Skin incisions for fasciotomy at the forearm.*
   A. Volar incision.
   B. Dorsal and lateral incisions.

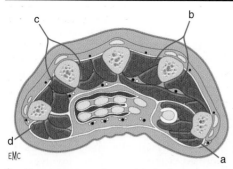

4 *Compartment syndrome of the hand: anatomy and incisions for fasciotomies. a. Radial incision to decompress the thenar muscle; b. dorsal incision over the second metacarpal giving access to the first and second spaces; c. dorsal incision over the fourth metacarpal giving access to the third and fourth spaces; d. ulnar incision to decompress the hypothenar muscles.*

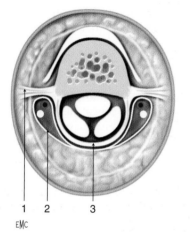

5 *Fasciae and compartments of the fingers. 1. Cleland's ligament; 2. Grayson's ligament; 3. flexor tendon sheath (volar pulleys).*

ACUTE COMPARTMENT SYNDROME OF THE HAND AND DIGITS

■ *Anatomy* (fig 4, 5)

The hand includes several compartments, each of which may be involved in acute compartment syndrome [1, 2, 7, 14] (*fig 4*). The interosseous muscles are divided into four compartments separated by the metacarpal bones. The compartment of the first interosseous muscle is separated from the adductor pollicis by a strong and deep fascia. The thenar compartment comprises the abductor pollicis brevis, flexor pollicis brevis, opponens and adductor pollicis muscles. The hypothenar compartment comprises the abductor, flexor and opponens of the fifth finger.

A crush syndrome usually involves all the compartments. However, some aetiologies such as unconsciousness may implicate only the first web [1, 2] with an acute syndrome limited to the first interosseous muscle and the deep muscles of the thenar compartment. Thus, precise assessment of all compartments should be carried out by clinical examination and by measuring intracompartmental pressure.

Although it is not a true muscular compartment, a finger can be involved in an acute compartment syndrome. A cross-section through a finger (*fig 5*) shows that the subcutaneous tissue is compartmentalised by fascia and volar skin which is not extensible. Excessive swelling or high pressure injections may also cause compression of the neurovascular bundle, resulting in severe disturbances of nerve and vascular supplies.

■ *Fasciotomy at the hand* (fig 4, 6)

Fasciotomy of all interosseous compartments can be performed by two separate dorsal skin incisions. The first is made on the radial side of the second metacarpal bone and gives access to the first and second interosseous compartments. The second incision is made over the fourth metacarpal.

When the first web is involved, we recommend three dorsal incisions. The first is made over the dorsal aspect of the first web and allows a fasciotomy of the first interosseous and adductor pollicis muscles. The second is made over the third metacarpal bone and gives access to the second and third intermetacarpal spaces. The third incision is made over the fourth intermetacarpal space (*fig 6A*).

Fasciotomy of the thenar compartment is performed through a skin incision over the bulky mass of the abductor pollicis brevis muscle.

Fasciotomy of the hypothenar compartment is performed through a skin incision over the ulnar side of the palm. The mobility of the skin allows release of the two adjacent compartments. Fasciotomy of the interosseous muscles is performed, taking care not to damage the extensor tendons (*fig 6B*).

An acute compartment syndrome of the first web space involves the first interosseous compartment and the deep thenar compartment. Release of the two compartments can be performed using a single skin incision on the dorsal aspect of the first web (*fig 7A, B*).

■ *Fasciotomy of the fingers* (fig 8)

Decompression of a finger is achieved by a midaxial incision carried out on the non-dominant side of the finger: the ulnar side for the index, long and ring fingers, and the radial side for the thumb and the little finger. The skin incision joins the axis of motion of the metacarpophalangeal, proximal interphalangeal and distal interphalangeal joints. All vertical bands of connective tissue are released, including the transverse retinacular ligament, Cleland's ligament and Grayson's ligament. The deep dissection is performed volar to the flexor

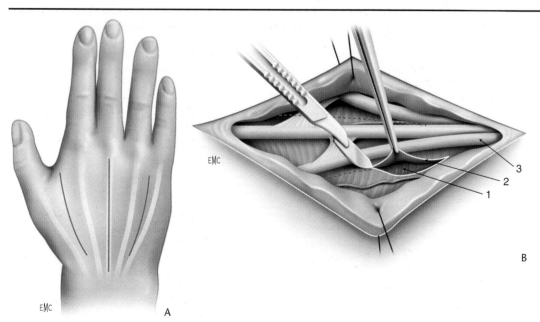

6 *A. Incisions at the dorsum of the hand. When the first web space is also involved, it is preferable to perform three dorsal incisions. The first is designed on the dorsum of the first web. The second is placed exactly over the third metacarpal bone, which provides access to the second and third dorsal interosseous muscles. The third incision is centred on the fourth intermetacarpal space.*
B. Fasciotomy. 1. Interosseous muscle; 2. fascia, incised; 3. extensor tendon.

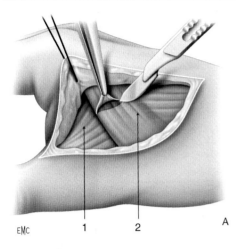

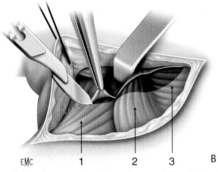

7 *Isolated compartment syndrome of the first web space. Incision of the deep fascia allows decompression of the thenar compartment. Nonetheless, if the pressure remains very high in the thenar muscles, a second appropriate radial skin incision may be mandatory to decompress the abductor pollicis brevis.*

A. The skin incision is centred on the dorsum of the first web space. The first dorsal interosseous muscle is exposed and fasciotomy of the superficial head of the muscle is performed. 1. Adductor pollicis muscle; 2. first dorsal interosseous muscle (superficial head).

B. The distal edge of the superficial head is retracted to expose the adductor pollicis muscle. The fascia that covers the muscle is largely incised to release the pressure inside the compartment of the adductor pollicis muscle. 1. Adductor pollicis muscle; 2. first dorsal interosseous muscle (superficial head); 3. first dorsal interosseous muscle (deep head).

tendons so as to cut all the bands opposite the skin incision. To do so, the two vascular bundles are retracted volarly.

ACUTE COMPARTMENT SYNDROME OF THE FOOT

The foot is frequently a site of traumatic injuries: fractures, dislocations and crush

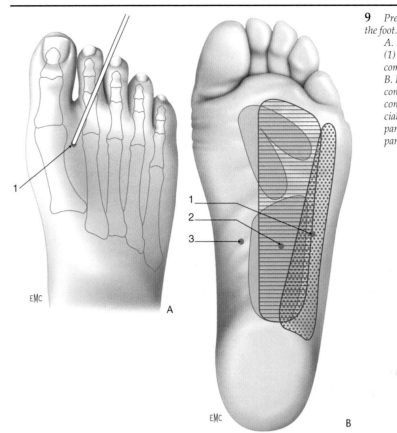

9 *Pressure measurement at the foot.*
A. Pressure measurement (1) in the first interosseous compartment.
B. Pressure in the plantar compartments. 1. Lateral compartment; 2. superficial and deep middle compartments; 3. medial compartment.

syndrome can initiate a compartment syndrome involving one or several compartments [8, 10, 12, 19]. A compartment syndrome in the medial and plantar compartments is not uncommon in the case of an isolated fracture of the calcaneum [8].

■ *Anatomy*

The foot comprises nine compartments separated by very strong and thick fasciae [12]. The medial compartment includes the abductor hallucis and the flexor hallucis brevis muscles. The lateral compartment comprises the abductor and the flexor brevis digiti minimi. The adductor hallucis muscle has its own compartment.

The dorsal and plantar interosseous muscles are contained in four compartments. The superficial middle compartment includes the lumbrical muscles and the flexor digitorum

brevis muscle. The deep middle compartment comprises the quadratus plantaris muscle.

It should be emphasised that the medial, lateral and superficial middle compartments occupy the entire length of the foot.

The compartment of the adductor hallucis and interosseous muscles is limited to the forefoot. The deep middle compartment is limited to the hindfoot.

For pressure measurements at the foot, the existence of several compartments makes it necessary to carry out several measurements in different areas (fig 9A, B).

■ *Fasciotomy*

Fasciotomy of the four compartments of the interosseous muscles is performed by two separate skin incisions which give access to all interosseous compartments (fig 10).

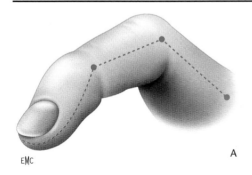

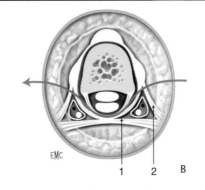

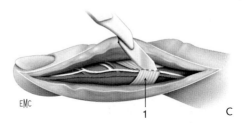

8 *Decompression of the finger.*
A. Skin incision.
B. Cross section showing route of deep dissection. 1. Grayson's ligament; 2. Cleland's ligament.
C. Division of transverse retinacular ligament (1).

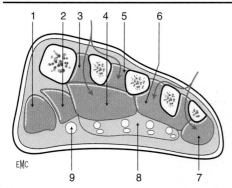

10 *Fasciotomies of the dorsal interosseous compartments at the foot. Two skin incisions are needed. 1. Abductor hallucis: 2. extensor hallucis brevis; 3. first dorsal interosseous; 4. adductor hallucis; 5. second dorsal interosseous; 6. third-fourth dorsal interosseous; 7. lateral compartment; 8. superficial middle compartment; 9. tendon of flexor hallucis longus.*

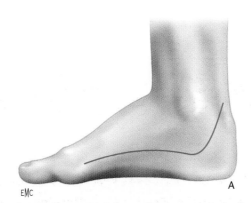

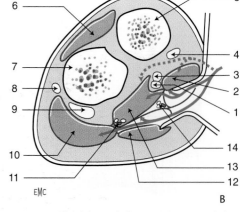

11 *A. Skin incision (Henry's approach).*
B. Medial approach to decompress the four plantar compartments. The abductor hallucis can be retracted plantarly (dotted lines) or dorsally (continuous lines). 1. Flexor digitorum communis tendon; 2. medial compartment; 3. flexor hallucis longus tendon; 4. tibialis posterior tendon; 5. head of the talus; 6. flexor digitorum brevis; 7. anterior tuberosity of the calcaneus; 8. peroneus brevis tendon: 9. peroneus longus tendon; 10. lateral compartment; 11. lateral plantar neurovascular bundle; 12. superficial middle compartment; 13. deep middle compartment; 14. medial plantar neurovascular bundle.

When the plantar compartments are involved, the extensive approach of Henry is suitable for decompression of all plantar compartments *(fig 11A, B)*.

Other localisations

Acute compartment syndrome of the leg is described in the chapter "Fasciotomy for compartment syndrome of the lower leg" and will not be discussed here.

Other localisations of acute compartment syndrome are less frequent. Compartment syndrome may occur at the thigh *(fig 12)*[16, 17], the arm, the deltoid muscle, and the gluteus and psoas muscles.

The pressure elevation is usually caused by increased volume within the compartment resulting from fracture or soft tissue trauma. External compression may occur during unconsciousness or be caused by a crush syndrome.

A particular situation is haematoma in the compartment of the psoas muscle provoked by anticoagulant treatment [18]. The thigh is in flexion, extension is very painful, and compression of the femoral nerve may lead to paralysis of the quadriceps. Early incision of the fascia covering the psoas iliac muscle allows restitutio in integrum.

Since pressure measurement is difficult due to the deep localisation of the muscle, diagnosis may be facilitated by MRI.

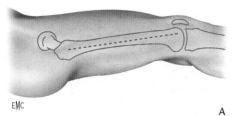

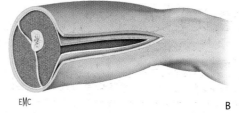

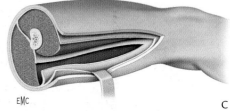

12 *Compartment syndrome of the thigh. Two compartments, anterior and posterior, may be involved.*
A. A single lateral incision is sufficient.

B. Incision of fascia lata decompresses the anterior compartment.

C. The vastus lateralis is released to allow exposure and incision of the septum which decompresses the posterior compartment.

References

[1] Abdul-Wamid AK. First dorsal interosseous compartment syndrome. *J Hand Surg Br* 1987 ; 12 : 269-272

[2] Apoil A, Karren CH, Augereau B, Pupin P. Pathogénie du syndrome de Volkmann de la première commissure de la main et déductions thérapeutiques. *Ann Chir Main* 1982 ; 1 : 210-213

[3] Berman SS, Schilling JD, McIntyre KE, Hunter GC, Bernhard VM. Shoelace technique for delayed primary closure of fasciotomies. *Am J Surg* 1994 ; 167 : 435-436

[4] Eaton RG, Green WT. Epimysiotomy and fasciotomy in the treatment of Volkmann's ischemic contracture. *Orthop Clin North Am* 1972 ; 3 : 175-186

[5] Finkelstein JA, Hunter GA, Hu RW. Lower limb compartment syndrome; course after delayed fasciotomy. *J Trauma* 1996 ; 40 : 342-344

[6] Godinger JJ, Huc DE, Bat JM, Lecestre P, Lortat-Jacob A, Aubert JD et al. Syndrome ischémique post-traumtique des loges de la jambe. *Rev Chir Orthop* 1979 ; 65 : 221-229

[7] Halpern AA, Greene R, Nichols T, Burton DS. Compartment syndrome of the interosseous muscles. Early recognition and treatment. *Clin Orthop* 1979 ; 140 : 23-25

[8] Manoli A, Weber TG. Fasciotomy of the foot: an anatomical study with reference to release of the calcaneal compartment. *Foot Ankle* 1990 ; 10 : 267-275

[9] McQueen MM. Compartment syndromes. In : Court-Brown CM, McQueen MM, Quaba AA eds. Management of open fractures. London : Martin Dunitz, 1996

[10] Muller GP, Masquelet AC. Syndrome de loge d'effort du pied. *Rev Chir Orthop* 1995 ; 81 : 549-552

[11] Phillips JH, Mac Kinnon SE, Murray JF, McMurtry RY. Exercise-induced chronic compartment syndrome of the first interosseous muscle of the hand: a case report. *J Hand Surg Am* 1986 ; 11 : 124-127

[12] Pisan M, Klaue K. Compartment syndrome of the foot. *Eur J Foot Ankle Surg* 1994 ; 1 : 29-36

[13] Shaw CJ, Spencer JD. Late management of compartment syndromes. *Injury* 1995 ; 26 : 633-635

[14] Styf J, Forssblad P, Lindborg G. Chronic compartment syndrome in the first dorsal interosseous muscle. *J Hand Surg Am* 1987 ; 12 : 757-762

[15] Summerfield SL, Folberg CR, Weiss AP. Compartment syndrome of the pronator quadratus: a case report. *J Hand Surg Am* 1997 ; 22 : 266-268

[16] Tarlow SD, Achterman CA, Hayhurst J, Ovadia DN. Acute compartment syndrome in the thigh complicating fracture of the femur. A report of three cases. *J Bone Joint Surg Am* 1986 ; 68 : 1439-1446

[17] Viegas SF, Rimoldi R, Scarborough M, Ballantyne GM. Acute compartment syndrome in the thigh: a case report and a review of the literature. *Clin Orthop* 1988 ; 234 : 232-234

[18] Wells J, Templeton J. Femoral neuropathy associated with anticoagulant therapy. *Clin Orthop* 1977 ; 124 : 155-160

[19] Ziu I, Mosheiff R, Zeligowski A, Lilbergal M, Lowe J, Segal D. Crush injuries of the foot with compartment syndrome: immediate one-stage management. *Foot Ankle* 1989 ; 9 : 185-189

Internal fixation of fractures

C Sommer
T Rüedi

Abstract. – *The goal of modern fracture treatment must be to obtain an optimal outcome with the patient's return to full activity as soon as possible. Today, internal stabilisation is indicated in numerous long bone fractures and most displaced articular fractures of major joints in the adult, whereas external fixation remains the best choice for initial stabilisation of fractures with severe soft tissue injuries and in polytraumatised patients. Two main principles of internal fixation of fractures are defined: 1) stabilisation by interfragmentary compression with screws and/or plates, providing absolute stability leading to direct bone healing. This remains the best way of fixing fractures with a simple pattern as well as metaphyseal and articular fractures. 2) Splinting of a fracture by nailing or bridging plate provides a less rigid (elastic) fixation and the fracture usually unites by indirect bone healing with callus formation. Nailing is the standard treatment for diaphyseal fractures not involving the metaphyseal region of the long tubular bones (femur, tibia, humerus). The choice of reaming or not reaming is still controversial and may be a question of personal preference. New developments in nailing techniques with special interlocking mechanisms have enlarged the spectrum of indications for nailing in the proximal or distal end of the femur. The bridging plate technique is ideal in comminuted fractures of long bones involving the proximal or distal metaphyses. It can be performed using a minimally-invasive technique by percutaneous approach, but reduction by closed manoeuvres remains a major problem.*

Keywords: fractures, internal fixation, bone healing, bridging plate, nailing, minimally-invasive plate.

Introduction

TREATMENT GOALS

The overall aim must be to obtain an optimal functional outcome with return to full activity of the injured limb and patient as soon as possible. To achieve this, we strive not only for rapid fracture healing in an anatomical position, but also for a complete functional restoration of the adjacent joints and soft tissues.

Non-operative treatment with traction or plaster cast requires prolonged immobilisation of the fractured limb and adjacent joints, which almost always leads to muscular atrophy and joint stiffness as well as presenting other risks such as thromboembolism. Furthermore, it is limited to certain types of fractures in which angulation, rotation and shortening can be controlled.

Operative fracture stabilisation should therefore allow for functional aftercare with partial or full weight-bearing within days after the accident.

INDICATIONS FOR OPERATIVE FIXATION OF FRACTURES

A fracture should be treated operatively when conservative treatment is not feasible or is expected to lead to an unsatisfactory result. This is the case in most displaced articular fractures of major joints and numerous long bone fractures in the adult. Open fractures are considered an absolute indication for surgery as well as fractures in the multiply-injured patient. Fractures that cannot be reduced or adequately immobilised by conservative means should also profit from an operative approach.

INTERNAL VERSUS EXTERNAL FRACTURE FIXATION

External fixation is the best choice for initial stabilisation of fractures with severe open or closed soft tissue injuries and as emergency provisional treatment, especially for long bone fractures in severely polytraumatised

patients with an Injury Severity Score (ISS) > 40 [46]. Alternatively, the new solid intramedullary nails that are introduced without reaming offer the possibility of primary internal stabilisation of shaft fractures of the long bones, even in Gustilo grade II or III open fractures. The classical "open reduction and internal fixation" (ORIF) with plates and screws is still the domain of most articular fractures where anatomical reduction and rigid fixation are required. Combined procedures (limited internal plus external fixation) are becoming more and more popular in joint fractures with severe soft tissue injuries (tibial pilon, tibial plateau, distal radius). In our view, this technique should be reserved for relatively simple joint fractures (with soft tissue injury), where the reduction can be achieved by indirect percutaneous manoeuvres. In complex articular fractures, mostly combined with impacted fragments, an open approach is mandatory for adequate reduction and bone grafting.

STABLE VERSUS "LESS RIGID" INTERNAL FIXATION

Anatomical reconstruction with stable

Christoph Sommer, M.D., Consultant in Traumatology. Department of Surgery, Leitender Arzt Chirurgie, Chirurgische Klinik Kantonsspital, 7000 Chur, Switzerland.
Thomas Rüedi, M.D., President AD International.
AD Zentrum, Clavadelerstrasse, CH-7270 Davos-Platz, Switzerland.

All references to this article must include: Sommer C and Rüedi T. Internal fixation of fractures. Editions Scientifiques et Médicales Elsevier SAS (Paris). All rights reserved. Surgical Techniques in Orthopaedics and Traumatology, 55-030-B-10, 2001, 10 p.

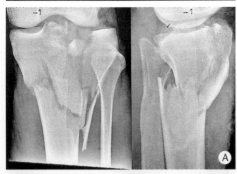

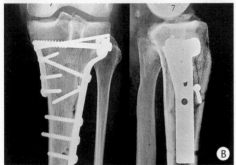

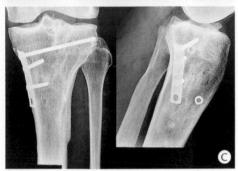

1   Compression principle: buttress plate, anti-glide plate and lag screw for complete articular fracture. A 35-year-old female ski-racer sustained a massive shearing injury with a bicondylar tibia-plateau fracture (A). First the medial plateau was indirectly reduced and fixed by a posteromedial anti-glide plate; the impressed articular fragment in the lateral plateau was elevated and supported by a bicorticocancellous bone block and cancellous bone graft. The final stabilisation of the lateral plateau was achieved by a T-plate in buttress function (B). Healing situation after 3 years with minimal signs of medial osteoarthritis (C).

fixation by interfragmentary compression remains the best way to fix simple as well as metaphyseal and articular fractures. Depending on the location and soft tissue conditions, a classical open approach or the semi-open tunnelling technique may be used. In most articular fractures, an open approach is mandatory for anatomical reduction of impacted joint fragments and bone grafting of metaphyseal defects (*fig 1, 2*).

In more complex shaft fractures of the long bones, anatomical reduction of all fragments is no longer required. Axial and rotational alignment is all that is aimed for, while the most effective fixation appears to be splinting with a locked intramedullary device (*fig 3*). Long, percutaneously introduced plates acting as a "bridge" have also been proposed.

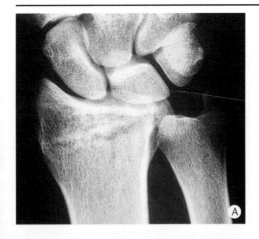

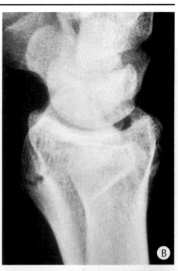

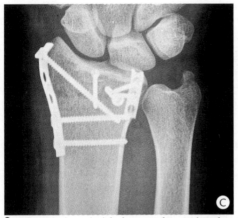

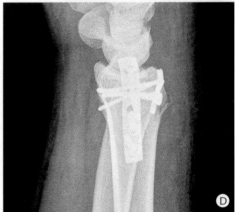

2   Compression principle: buttress plate, spring plate and lag screw for complete articular fracture. A 30-year-old worker fell from 2 metres on his dorsally flexed hand. Unstable, complete intra-articular distal radius fracture with metaphyseal impaction (A, B). Postoperative radiographs after open reduction, bone grafting and stabilisation with a 2.7 plate on the radial pillar with a buttress function; an interfragmentary lag screw for fixation of the Lister tubercle and a 2.0 plate on the dorsoulnar fragment acting as a spring plate (C, D).

Pathophysiology of fracture healing

Fractured bone heals in two different ways: by callus formation (indirect healing) or, provided the fragments are rigidly fixed, without visible callus (direct healing). Both indirect and direct healing require undisturbed vascularity and a certain degree of mechanical stability.

INDIRECT FRACTURE HEALING

The natural process of callus formation starts immediately after the bone is broken, first by forming granulation tissue around and between the fragments. As this tissue matures to fibrous tissue and fibrocartilage, bone formation progresses through a series of different steps to mature cortical bone (*fig 3, 4*).

DIRECT FRACTURE HEALING

Under conditions of rigid fixation, direct osteone remodelling across the fracture line can occur with little or no external callus. Provided there is intimate apposition of the fragment, this healing process is called

"contact healing" (*fig 1, 5*). If, however, there is a gap of less than 1 mm, this is filled with vessels and mesenchymal cells which rapidly transform into bone and this is subsequently integrated into the overall healing process ("gap healing"). However, if interfragmental gaping greater than 1 mm exists under conditions of rigid stability, direct bone healing is disturbed and delayed healing occurs [7].

STRAIN THEORY

Strain is defined as the deformation ratio of a material under given stress. In a simple fracture, the complete deformation induced by motion occurs at one bone-to-bone interface. If the deformation of the repair tissue exceeds the tolerated elongation of the tissue, cellular disruption occurs and tissue differentiation comes to a halt leading to delayed or non-union. In a multifragmentary fracture, the same amount of motion is divided into multiple smaller deformations in each fracture gap which is still tolerated by the repair tissue [31]. This explains why multifragmentary fractures can heal under marked instability while simple fractures do not tolerate even micromotion. As we know that limited micromotion induces callus

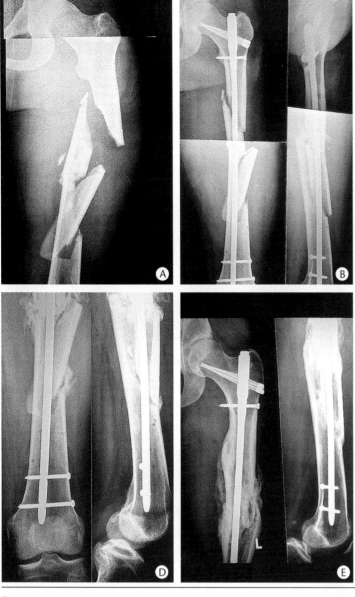

3 *Internal splinting principle: locked un-reamed nail for comminuted shaft fracture. A 28-year-old man was involved in a high-speed car accident and sustained a closed comminuted femoral shaft fracture (A). The fracture was internally splinted by a statically locked unreamed nail (UFN with spiral-blade inter-locking) (B). The fracture healing started immediately by indirect bone healing with marked callus formation well demonstrated on the radiographs after 5 weeks (C, D). After 3 months the fracture had united completely with an on-going remodelling process (E).*

formation [13] and that too much motion leads to delayed or even non-union, the bone implant construct must be adapted to the type of fracture. A simple fracture needs more stability (even absolute, rigid stability with gaps below 1 mm in cases of plate fixation) than a comminuted fracture, where a fixation with relative stability (intramedullary nail or bridging plate) is required.

Biomechanical and biological aspects of different internal fixation principles

There are two main principles for fracture stabilisation: fixation by compression or by splinting. Each of these can be achieved by different implants and applications.

COMPRESSION

Compression of bone fragments is a main factor of stabilisation in a fracture fixation. Furthermore, if adequately performed, it enhances direct bone healing as mentioned above. Compression produces preloading, keeping the compressed surfaces in close contact as long as the compression forces remain larger than the opposite-acting forces. Compression also generates friction between the compressed fragments, increasing the stability of the fixation. It therefore greatly diminishes the forces borne by an internal fixation because the load transfer occurs directly from fragment to fragment. Several biomechanical principles producing compression have been developed for use in different bones and in fracture situations.

■ Lag screw (and protection plate)

Compression by insertion of a lag screw is the simplest way of achieving absolute stability. In articular metaphyseal fragments, a lag screw should be inserted perpendicular to the fracture plane and in the middle of the fragments (*fig 6A*). Respecting these two principles produces an evenly distributed compression over the entire fracture surface and high friction. On the other hand, in axially loaded tubular bones, the optimal inclination of a lag screw bisects the perpendicular to the fracture line and the perpendicular to the long axis of the bone (*fig 6B*).

Lag screw fixation can be used on its own for small bone fragments with one or more screws (i.e. medial malleolus), or in long spiroid shaft fractures of small tubular bones (metacarpals, metatarsals, fibula). In diaphyseal fractures of the long bones (tibia, femur, humerus), lag screw fixation alone is not considered safe enough for axial loading. It should therefore be combined with a so-called neutralisation (or protection) plate, enhancing the stability of the bone implant construct (*fig 5, 6C*).

Lag screws can also be helpful for the reduction manoeuvres in indirect reduction techniques (i.e. minimally-invasive, percutaneous fixation techniques): Insertion of a lag screw in a right angle across a remaining fracture gap allows the still displaced fragment on the opposite side to be pulled towards the nearer fragment and can therefore help reduce the fracture through an indirect reduction technique.

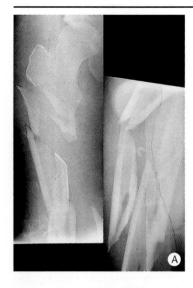
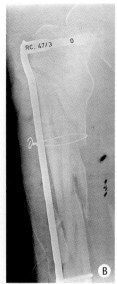
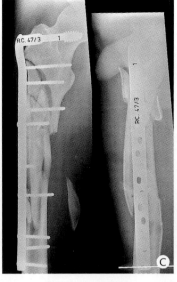
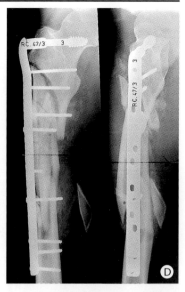

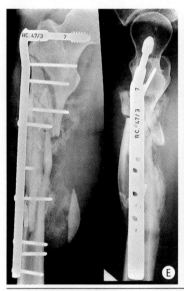
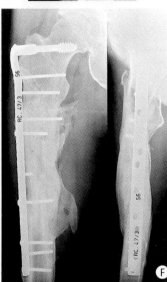

4 *Internal splinting principle: bridging plate for comminuted shaft fracture. A 32-year-old man after a car accident with a comminuted femoral shaft fracture with compartment syndrome (A). Indirect reduction over the plate (dynamic condylar plate) with a tension device and temporary cerclage wire was performed (B) before the definitive stabilisation was achieved by a bridging plate technique (C). Rapid callus formation demonstrated the indirect bone healing after 3 weeks (D) and 7 weeks (E). The radiograph after 1 year (F) showed a complete bone union. Even massively displaced fragments (mid-shaft, medial side) healed.*

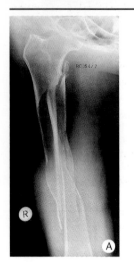
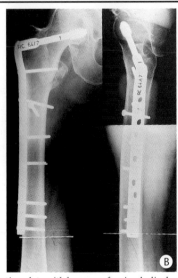
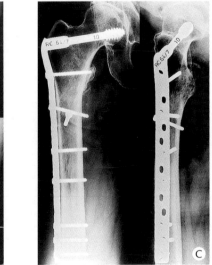
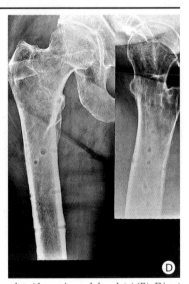

5 *Compression principle: protection plate with lag screw for simple diaphyseal fracture. A 75-year-old man who fell in his room. Long torsional subtrochanteric femur fracture extending to the distal shaft (A). Traditional open reduction and internal fixation (ORIF) by lag screw and protection plate (dynamic condylar plate) (B). Direct fracture healing without visible callus after 10 weeks (C) and 2 years (D).*

■ *Compression plate*

Depending on their function, plates can be applied to the fractured bone according to different mechanical principles. The most frequent application concerns the already mentioned neutralisation plate, protecting the stability of lag screw fixation. Axial compression by a plate can be produced in three different ways: 1) applying a tension device; 2) compression by prebending the plate *(fig 7A, B)*; 3) eccentric screw placement (dynamic compression plate (DCP) *(fig 7C)*. Furthermore a lag screw across the fracture line, placed separately or

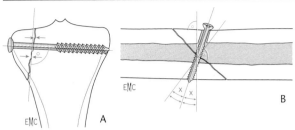

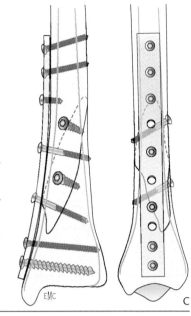

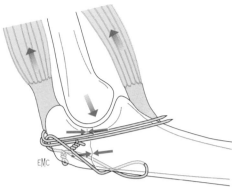

6 *Lag screws and protection plate. The best inclination for lag screws depends on the type of bone and the site of the fracture.*
A. In epimetaphyseal articular fragments, the optimal direction of the lag screw is perpendicular to the main fracture line.
B. In axially loaded tubular bones, the screw bisects the perpendicular to the fracture line and the perpendicular to the long axis of the bone.
C. In diaphyseal fractures of large long bones (i.e. spiroid fracture of the distal tibia), lag screw fixation alone is not stable enough and has to be combined with a neutralisation (or protection) plate.

8 *Tension band principle. In an eccentric loaded bone (typical examples are olecranon or patella), the implant is placed on the traction side. Under loading, the implant converts the tensile forces on this side into compression forces on the opposite side. The two Kirschner wires must be placed close to the articular surface and ideally cross the fracture line in a perpendicular direction. The figure-of-eight wire loop must be well tightened, otherwise the tensile forces will create a gap on the dorsal part of the fracture.*

through a plate hole, may considerably add to compression and stability *(fig 7D, E)*.

■ *Tension band principle*

The tension band principle provides a variant of absolute stability under dynamic conditions. It works only in an eccentrically loaded bone. The implant is applied to the tension or convex side of the bone thereby transforming the tensile forces into compression forces, provided the opposite cortex is well apposed. Typical examples are transverse fractures of the patella or olecranon, where the fixation is achieved by Kirschner-wires and wire-loops *(fig 8)*. The femur is another example of an eccentrically loaded bone where a plate placed on the lateral (or tension) side will exceptionally have a tension band function.

■ *Buttress plate*

In the metaphyseal area most fractures are caused by shearing with articular impaction. As lag screw fixation alone does not provide

enough stability, additional support is required with plates buttressing the reconstructed fracture *(fig 1, 2, 9)*. These plates are specially designed to meet anatomical and biomechanical requirements.

■ *Anti-glide plate*

A plate preventing axial glide of a fracture fragment and shortening is called an anti-glide plate. This principle of fixation was first described for simple distal fibula fractures, where a short 1/3 tubular plate is placed posterolaterally, directly on the proximal end of the spike of the distal fibular fragment [47]. The same method of fixation is helpful in other similar fracture situations with a tendency to axial shortening by gliding, i.e. the posteromedial fracture-dislocation of the tibial plateau (Moore type I) *(fig 1)* [28], shearing fractures of the medial malleolus *(fig 10)* or volar displaced distal radius fractures (Smith fracture).

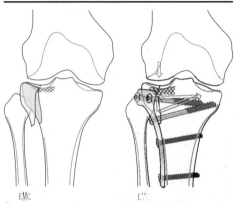

9 *Buttress plate. In metaphyseal split fractures, lag screw fixation alone may be insufficient. Different anatomical preformed plates are available. In this example, the axial forces induced by the femoral condyle are neutralised by a well contoured and tightly fixed L-plate in buttress function.*

■ *Spring hook plate*

The principle of the so-called spring hook plate was first described in the treatment of acetabular fractures [29]. Small posterior wall

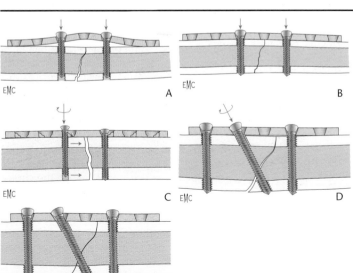

7 *Compression plate principles. Interfragmentary compression of the fracture plane by the use of a plate can be achieved in different ways which are very often combined.*
A, B. Prebending of the plate. In a transverse fracture a sharp bend of about 5° in the middle of the plate is contoured. When fixing the plate to the bone by two screws placed on each side and close to the fracture, the ends of the plate are pushed close to the long bone creating compression forces in the fracture gap opposite the position of the plate.
C. Principle of the dynamic compression plate (DCP). Eccentric placement of a specially designed screw with a spherical head in the oval plate hole leads to a horizontal movement of the screw and the bone fragment (in which the screw is inserted) and creates an adaptation of the fracture fragments with compression within the fracture gap.
D, E. A lag screw placed through a plate hole induces an interfragmentary compression and considerably adds to the stability of the construct.

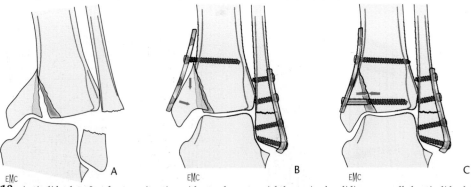

10 *Anti-glide plate. In a fracture situation with a tendency to axial shortening by gliding, a so-called anti-glide plate is very useful. In this example with a shearing fracture of the medial malleolus combined with a avulsion fracture of the distal fibula (type A), a 4 hole 1/3 tubular plate is positioned on the still displaced medial fracture and fixed by a screw just above the proximal end of the distal fragment (A). By tightening the screw, the fracture is indirectly reduced and held in an anatomical position (B). An additional lag screw close to the articular surface enhances the stability and prevents secondary rotational displacement (C).*

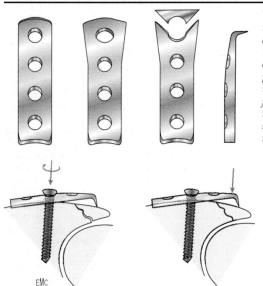

11 *Spring hook plate. In small posterior wall fragments of the acetabulum, one or two spring hook plates are an excellent method of fixation. One end of a 4 hole 1/3 tubular plate is flattened and the end hole is cut out. The two sharp-end spikes are bent at 90° and the plate should be slightly prebent. The plate is placed with the two spikes at the periarticular end of the small fragment and fixed with one or two screws in the intact posterior wall. Care must be taken not to place the sharp hooks over the border of the fragment, to prevent iatrogenic damage of the labrum and/or femoral head.*

fragments, not amenable to lag screw fixation, can be held in place by prepared small 1/3 tubular plates (*fig 11*). The same principle can be used for similar situations in other joint fractures, i.e. for small dorsal fragments in the distal radius (1/4 tubular plate or 2.0 mm mini-plate) (*fig 2*).

INTERNAL SPLINTING

Splinting consists of fixing the fractured bone with a more or less stiff device providing relative (not absolute) stability. Splinted fractures usually unite by indirect bone healing with callus formation (*fig 3, 4*). Splinting can be achieved by various operative techniques: external fixation or intramedullary nails, rods or plates. The effectiveness of a splint depends on the stiffness of the implant and on the interface between bone and implant.

■ *Nailing*

Intramedullary nails offer several biomechanical advantages in fracture fixation. Mechanically, they usually provide correct axial alignment given by the medullary canal and they allow, if desired,

axial gliding. This gliding permits restabilisation by readaptation of the fracture fragments in case of a gap or bone resorption at the fracture surfaces. The biological advantages of intramedullary nails, well known from clinical experience, mostly concern the soft tissue cover of the bone (vascularity) which remains "untouched". The surgical approach to the bone is away from the fracture and the reduction of the main fragments is mainly achieved in a closed way by indirect manoeuvres (manually, reduction over the partially inserted nail, distractor, traction table, etc.). This prevents further damage to the already injured and partly devascularised fragments of the fracture zone.

On the other hand, such closed reduction techniques rely entirely on clinical judgement or measurements (comparing length and rotation to the opposite side) or on indirect visual signs using the fluoroscope. This explains the higher rate of malunion, especially malrotation, of nailed shaft fractures compared to conventional compression plate fixation [3, 34].

Recent developments in nailing techniques have widened the range of indications for

femur fractures: special interlocking mechanisms into the femoral neck (sliding neck screws, spiral blades (*fig 4*), neck screws with the "miss-a-nail technique", etc.) allow internal fixation of nearly all extra-articular proximal femoral fractures with a medullary nail device. On the other hand, there are also several types of nails which are inserted in a retrograde way, mostly for extra- but also intra-articular fractures of the distal femur [14, 15, 39]. There may be some concern about iatrogenic damage of the knee joint due to the transarticular insertion of the nail, although in current studies dealing with this topic, no relevant functional problems are reported. Furthermore, it seems to be an excellent technique especially for older patients with osteoporotic bone and extra-articular distal femur fractures [27].

Reamed nailing

Reaming of the medullary canal permits the insertion of thicker nails with a larger zone of contact with the bone. This increases stiffness but also rotational stability due to friction between implant and bone. While originally very large nails (up to 18 mm) were advocated which required extensive reaming, the present tendency is to smaller diameter nails and less reaming ("reamed to fit"). To obtain fixation, interlocking may become mandatory to prevent telescoping and ensure rotational stability. Reaming also produces bone graft slurry which is considered by some to induce new bone formation [5].

Disadvantages of the reaming procedure may concern the disruption of the medullary blood supply and the obliteration of the vascular canals [24, 36, 41, 43] leading to some necrosis of the diaphyseal cortex. Reaming also creates heat and thinning of the cortical bone depending on the sharpness, design and size of the reamers used. These facts do not seem to be of major clinical significance considering the reported healing rates of 98%-99% in femur fractures treated with reamed nailing [4, 22]. Reports that femoral reaming increases intramedullary pressures, releasing mediators enhancing pulmonary embolisation, are however a serious concern [1, 6, 33]. A higher incidence of pulmonary complications, some of them fatal, has been shown when intramedullary nailing with reaming was performed in severe polytrauma patients with initial pulmonary dysfunction [33].

Unreamed nailing

In addition to the above mentioned disadvantages of reamed nailing, there are other factors which might favour the choice of an unreamed nail: operating time is shorter and intraoperative blood loss decreases [45]. There seems to be evidence that the infection rate in fractures with severe soft tissue injuries is lower when solid unreamed titanium nails are used compared to reamed tubular nails. This was shown in animal experiments [30] and encouraged the initial use of unreamed nails, even in fractures with severe soft tissue damage [16, 20, 40, 42].

Today, the choice of reamed or non-reamed nailing of the long bones is still controversial. Some propose the reamed procedure [8, 9, 22], while others advise unreamed nailing, reporting similar results compared to published data on fractures treated with reamed nails [21, 35]. However, recent prospective randomised studies and meta-analyses quite clearly show that the reaming technique for femoral as well as tibial fractures must still be considered as the gold standard for closed and Gustilo grade I to IIIA open fractures: healing time is shorter and the complication rate (especially the infection rate) is similar to that of unreamed treated fractures [11, 21, 45].

■ ***Bridging plate***

A bridging plate is a non-gliding splint providing only relative stability. The term "bridging" was first used in the German literature ("überbrückende Osteosyn-these") [17]. Bridging is achieved by spanning a fragmented segment of a long bone maintaining axial and rotational alignment as well as correct length without attempting anatomical reduction of the fragments (*fig 12*). Considering the strain theory, larger gaps between the fragments are preferred. This technique is ideal in comminuted fractures of long bones not suitable for traditional nails: fractures involving the proximal or distal metaphyses, or additional injuries prohibiting nailing (severe polytrauma, acetabular fracture, etc.). Compared to traditional compression plate fixation in comminuted fractures of, for example, the subtrochanteric region, bridging plate fixation leads to a more rapid bony union even without a bone graft, and decreases the rate of non-unions and infections (*fig 4*) [2, 12, 17, 18, 23, 38, 44].

Minimally-invasive percutaneous plate osteosynthesis (MIPPO)

Similar concepts of "biological" plate fixation may be achieved by minimally-invasive percutaneous approaches to the bone: the so-called MIPPO (*fig 13*). A cadaveric arterial injection study in the femur has indicated that this MIPPO technique is superior in maintaining arterial femoral vascularity and perfusion when compared to conventional open lateral plate application [10]. Clinical studies using this technique in comminuted fractures of the articular or juxta-articular region of the femur and tibia have reported excellent results with rapid union and low rates of infection and non-union [19, 26, 38, 48, 49]. One of the most significant clinical problems of this technique is the achievement and control of adequate reduction. The correct

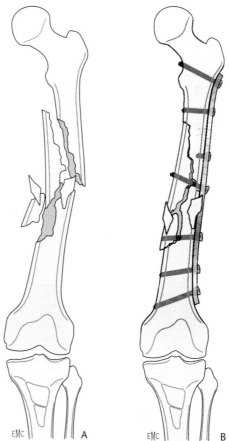

12 *Bridge plating of comminuted diaphyseal fractures.*
A. In special situations, bridge plating of a comminuted femoral shaft fracture may be the best solution for definitive fixation (patient with severe head and/or lung injury, where intramedullary nailing is contraindicated).
B. The main proximal and distal fragments are spanned by a long plate, which is fixed proximally and distally by two or three cortical screws. It is important that the comminuted fracture zone not be touched, thus preserving the remaining vascular supply. Length, axis in both planes, and rotation must be correct. It might be advisable to indirectly reduce and fix large intermediate fragments on the medial side by additional lag screws.

reduction must include length, axis and rotation of the two main (proximal and distal) shaft fragments. Several tools and tricks to ease these difficulties have been developed and published [25, 26].

Indications for different types of internal fixation

Table I attempts to give an overview of the possible indications for the different fixation methods for long bone fractures (femur and tibia). This table is meant to be a "cook book" for standard fracture situations with no, or minor, soft tissue compromise. Each fracture has its own personality and many additional factors (age, compliance and coexisting diseases/injuries of the patient, bone quality, soft tissue condition) must be taken into consideration before choosing the treatment option.

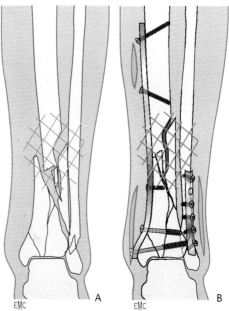

13 *Minimally-invasive percutaneous plate osteosynthesis (MIPPO).*
A. In fractures with severe closed (or Gustilo grade I-IIIA open) soft tissue injuries, the MIPPO technique is a new and promising method of fixation, especially for long bone fractures not suitable for intramedullary nailing.
B. After reduction of the main proximal and distal fragments (including correct length, axis in both planes and rotation), which can be achieved by a temporary external fixator, distractor or traction table, a precontoured long plate is inserted through a short incision and slid along the bone towards the other end. The plate is fixed on both sides by two or three cortical screws, depending on the quality of the bone. Large intermediate fragments might be fixed by lag screws placed separately or through the plate. The main problem of this technique is the achievement and holding of the correct reduction, which must be controlled several times throughout the entire procedure.

Postoperative care for the different types of fracture fixations

GENERAL ASPECTS

Correct postoperative management is essential to improve the functional outcome and to avoid complications. The goals of fracture treatment must be a rapid fracture healing in an anatomical position, combined with complete functional restoration of the joints and soft tissues. This is best achieved by early motion of the involved joints and muscles. The aim should therefore be for a fracture stability which allows motion in all fractures with internal fixation. Several factors can interfere with this aim: the quality of the fractured bone; the localisation and type of fracture; the conditions of the soft tissue and the compliance of the patient. In complex fracture patterns, in extensive soft tissue injuries and in cases of severe osteoporosis, it may therefore be advisable to immobilise the involved joint in an

Table I. – Proposals for indications of fixation principles for standard long bone fractures.

Bone*	Segment*		Fixation principle		Implants (examples)
			Simple fractures**	Complex fractures**	
Femur	Head		Lag screw(s)		3.5, 2.7
	Neck		Lag screws (2-3)		6.5 cancellous 7.0 cannulated
	Trochanteric		Compression/splinting by neck screw + side plate (i.e. DHS)	Bridging plate (young patient) Intramedullary nail	95° CBP, DCS, PFN, Gamma-nail, IMHS
	Shaft	1st fifth (subtroch.)	Compression plate Intramedullary nail	Bridging plate Intramedullary nail (2nd-3rd generation)	95° CBP, DCS, long PFN or long Gamma-nail, Recon. Nail
		2nd-4th fifth	Intramedullary nail (A3-type: dyna. locked)	Intramedullary nail (statically locked)	Reamed or unreamed nails
		5th fifth (+ distal)	Compression plate +/- lag screw(s)	Bridging plate Retrograde nail	DCS, CBP, LISS, Reconstruct. Nail, DFN

	Distal		Lag screws	B-type: Buttress plate
				    +/- Lag screw(s)
				C-type: Bridging plate
				    +/- Lag screw(s)
				    Retrograde nail
					4.5 distal femur buttress plate, CBP, DCP, LISS, Reconstruct. Nail, DFN

Tibia	Proximal		Lag screw(s)
			+/- bone grafting
				B-type: Buttress plate
				    +/- Lag screw(s)
				    +/- bone grafting
				C-type: Bridging plate(s)
				    Anti-glide plate
				    Hybrid fixator
					4.5 L-, T-plate
					
					4.5 DCP, LISS, 4.5 1/2 tub. plate

	Shaft	1st fifth	Compression plate(s) +/- lag screw(s)	Bridging plate (lateral) External fixator	4.5 DCP, LISS
		2nd-4th fifth	Intramedullary nail (A3-type: dyna. locked)	Intramedullary nail (statically locked)	Reamed or unreamed nails
		5th fifth (+ distal)	Compression plate +/- lag screw(s)	Bridging plate External fixator	4.5 DCP, LISS

	Distal		Lag screw(s)
			+/- bone grafting
				B-type: Buttress plate
				    +/- Lag screw(s)
				    +/- bone grafting
					3.5 cloverleaf plate

				C-type: Buttress plate(s)
				    +/- Lag screw(s)
				    +/- bone grafting
				    Hybrid fixator
					2 x 3.5 1/3 tubular plate (double-plate technique)

* Bone and segment are related to the comprehensive classification of fractures [32].
** Simple fractures are defined as A1-3 type (simple spiral, oblique and transverse) and B1-type (spiral, wedge) fractures of the shaft and B1/B2 type (partial articular split/pure impression) fractures of the metaphyseal region.
** Complex fractures are defined as B2/B3 type (bending/fragmented wedge and C type (complete articular) fractures of the metaphyseal region.
Abbreviations: CBP=95° condylar blade plate; DHS=Dynamic hip screw; DCS=Dynamic condylar screw; IMHS=Intramedullary hip screw; LISS=Less invasive stabilisation system; DFN=Distal femur nail; PFN=Proximal femur nail.

articular fracture (or, very seldom, the two neighbouring joints in a diaphyseal fracture). This decision has to be made before or during the operation with regard to achieved stability, soft tissue conditions and the mental state of the patient. The decision for the type of immobilisation (splint, plaster cast, brace, external fixator, etc.) and the required time (2 to x weeks) must be chosen on an individual basis and cannot follow general rules.

ACTIVITY AND WEIGHT-BEARING

It is widely accepted that after the operation the injured limb is elevated above heart level to prevent wound healing problems due to further swelling. Mobilisation of the involved joints usually starts on the first postoperative day under the care of the physical therapist. Active assisted motion may be combined with intermediate continuous passive motion (CPM), especially for fractures of the lower extremity (hip, femur, knee). Medical prophylaxis against thromboembolism is widely used and

recommended, at least during hospitalisation.

In fractures of the upper limb, ambulation is immediately started, whereas in treated fractures of the lower limb (especially below the knee level), bedrest for three to five days is recommended. The level of weight-bearing depends mainly on the localisation and type of fracture as well on the principle and stability of internal fixation *(table II)*. It ranges from immediate full weight-bearing after reamed nailing of a transverse diaphyseal fracture to toe-touch partial weight-bearing (10-15 kg) for most articular fractures and complex diaphyseal fractures treated with unreamed nailing or a bridging plate. In special situations (i.e. complex tibial pilon, tarsal or midfoot fractures), a removable patellar-tendon-bearing (PTB) walking caliper may be adapted after the swelling has completely subsided (after 2-3 weeks), to be used for 2-3 months [37]. This caliper prevents axial and bending forces to the fractured zone, but enables important early motion of the affected joint.

CLINICAL AND X-RAY MONITORING

Recommendations for the patient *(table II)* must be related to the individual healing process which is evaluated clinically and radiologically on a regular basis (4-6 week intervals). On each follow-up examination, the treating physician/surgeon has to be aware of possible warning signs of ongoing or new instability of the fracture fixation: increased redness and swelling, local tenderness and persistent pain are signs which will dictate a reduction in weight-bearing and range of motion.

Radiographic evaluation must be according to the principle of internal fixation. In fixations by compression (lag screws, compression plate, tension band fixation, etc.), direct bone healing without callus formation is ideally expected. The appearance of "irritation" callus indicates an instability of the fracture of variable degrees. If this radiological warning sign is combined with implant loosening, a modification of the treatment regime is strongly recommended: complete rest or re-operation (re-stabilisation +/- bone graft). For indirect

Table II. – Proposals for weight-bearing and follow-up X-ray examination of fractures after internal fixation.

Fracture Site	Fracture Type (A1-C3*)	Principle of Internal Fixation	Weight Bearing (= WB)		Union Time (weeks)	Follow-up X-ray Examinations (weeks)
			Postop. (kg)	Time for full WB (postop. weeks)		
Diaphyseal	Transverse (A3)	Reamed nail	Full	Immediate	10-16	6/12/24
		Unreamed nail	Full	Immediate	10-16	6/12/24
	Oblique (A2) Spiroid (A1) Wedge (B)	Reamed nail	Full, if good contact between nail and inner cortex	Immediate, if good contact between nail and inner cortex	12-18	6/12/24
		Unreamed nail	10-15	6-12, consider dyna-misation	12-18	6/12/24
	Complex (C)	Reamed or unreamed nail, Bridging plate	10-15	8-16	16-24	6/12/18/24
Femur head, neck	Simple, no comminu-tion	Lag screws +/- side plate	10-15	6-10	6-10	6/12
	With comminution	Lag scres +/- side plate	10-15	10-14	12-16	6/12/18
Femur trochanteric	Simple	Compression/splinting by neck screw + side plate	Full	Immediate	6-10	6/12
	Complex	2nd-3rd gen. nail	Full	Immediate	12-16	6/12/18
		Compression/splinting by neck screw + side plate	10-15	8-16	12-20	6/12/18/24
Articular knee	Simple	Lag screws +/- buttress plate	10-15	6-10	6-10	6/12
	Complex	Buttress plate/s	10-15	12-20	12-20	6/12/18/24
		DFN, LISS	10-15	6-10 (?)	12-20	6/12/18
Tibial pilon	Simple, no impression nor impaction	Lag screws +/- buttress plate	10-15	8-12	6-10	6/12
	Complex, with bone graft	Buttress plate/s	10-15 (PTB-walking caliper?)	12-24	12-24	6/12/18/24
Tarsal		Lag screws +/- plate	10-15 (PTB-walking caliper?)	12-16	12-18	6/12/18
Midfoot	Simple	K-wires, screws	10-15	4	6	6
	Complex with lux-ation	Transarticular screw fix., plate	10-15 (PTB-walking caliper?)	12, after implant removal	8-12	6/12

* Bone, segment and fracture type are related to the comprehensive classification of fractures [32]. This advice is for recent fractures with no or minor soft tissue injury, good bone quality, adequate patient compliance and an uncomplicated healing process.

bone healing (nailing, bridging plate, etc.), the appearance and ripening of the callus formation must be carefully observed. In cases with no disturbance of the vascularity of the fracture fragments, the first callus appears after 3-4 weeks, maturing to a sharply delimited fixation callus of homogenous structure within 4-5 months *(fig 3, 4)*.

In positive clinical and radiological findings, weight-bearing is gradually increased with full weight-bearing allowed after 4-16 weeks, according to the type and site of fracture and the method of fixation used *(table II)*. Fracture treatment is completed when the patient regains full working and sports capacity.

References ➤

References

[1] Barre J, Lepuse C, Segal P. Embolies et chirurgie fémorale intra-médullaire. *Rev Chir Orthop Réparatrice Appar Mot* 1997 ; 83 : 9-21

[2] Baumgaertel F, Buhl M, Rahn BA. Fracture healing in biological plate osteosynthesis. *Injury* 1998 ; 29 : C3-C6

[3] Bonnevialle P, Andrieu S, Bellumore Y, Challe JJ, Rongieres M, Mansat M. Troubles torsionnels et inégalités de longueurs après enclouage à foyer fermé pour fracture diaphysaire fémorale et tibiale. Évaluation par scanner de 189 fractures. *Rev Chir Orthop Réparatrice Appar Mot* 1998 ; 84 : 397-410

[4] Brumback RJ, Uwagie-Ero S, Lakatos RP, Poka A, Bathon GH, Burgess AR. Intramedullary nailing of femoral shaft fractures. Part II. Fracture healing with static interlocking fixation. *J Bone Joint Surg Am* 1988 ; 70 : 1453-1462

[5] Chapman M. Closed intramedullary bone-grafting and nailing of segmental defects of the femur. A report of three cases. *J Bone Joint Surg Am* 1980 ; 62 : 1004-1008

[6] Christie J, Robinson CM, Pell A. Transcardiac echocardiography during invasive intramedullary procedures. *J Bone Joint Surg Br* 1995 ; 77 : 450-455

[7] Cornell CN, Lane JM. Newest factors in fracture healing. *Clin Orthop* 1992 ; 277 : 297-311

[8] Court-Brown CM, Christie J, McQueen MM. Closed intramedullary tibial nailing. Its use in closed and type I open fractures. *J Bone Joint Surg Br* 1990 ; 72 : 605-611

[9] Court-Brown CM, Will E, Christie J, McQueen MM. Reamed or unreamed nailing for closed tibial fractures. A prospective study in Tscherne C1 fractures. *J Bone Joint Surg Br* 1996 ; 78 : 580-583

[10] Farouk O, Krettek C, Miclau T, Schandelmaier P, Guy P, Tscherne H. Minimally invasive plate osteosynthesis and vascularity: preliminary results of a cadaver injection study. *Injury* 1997 ; 28 : 7-12

[11] Finkemeier CG, Schmidt AH, Kyle RF, Templeman DC, Varecka TF. A prospective, randomized study of intramedullary nails inserted with and without reaming for the treatment of open and closed fractures of the tibial shaft. *J Orthop Trauma* 2000 ; 14 : 187-193

[12] Gerber C, Mast JW, Ganz R. Biological internal fixation of fractures. *Arch Orthop Trauma Surg* 1990 ; 109 : 295-303

[13] Goodship AE, Kenwright J. The influence of induced micromovement upon the healing of experimental tibial fractures. *J Bone Joint Surg Br* 1985 ; 67 : 650-655

[14] Grass R, Zwipp H. Minimal-invasive Methode zur Behandlung supra-diacondylärer Femurfrakturen. *Zentralbl Chir* 1998 ; 123 : 1247-1251.

[15] Gregory P, Dicicco J, Karpik K, Dipasquale T, Herscovici D, Sanders R. Ipsilateral fractures of the femur and tibia: treatment with retrograde femoral nailing and unreamed tibial nailing. *J Orthop Trauma* 1996 ; 10 : 309-316

[16] Greitbauer M, Heinz T, Gaebler C, Stoik W, Vecsei V. Unreamed nailing of tibial fractures with the solid tibial nail. *Clin Orthop* 1998 ; 350 : 105-114

[17] Heitemeyer U, Hierholzer G, Terhorst J. Der Stellenwert der überbrückenden Plattenosteosynthese bei Mehrfragmentbruchschädigungen des Femur im klinischen Vergleich. *Unfallchirug* 1986 ; 89 : 533-538

[18] Heitemeyer U, Kemper F, Hierholzer G, Haines J. Severely comminuted femoral shaft fractures: treatment by bridging-plate osteosynthesis. *Arch Orthop Trauma Surg* 1987 ; 106 : 327-330

[19] Helfet DL, Shonnard PY, Levine D, Borrelli J. Minimally invasive plate osteosynthesis of distal fractures of the tibia. *Injury* 1997 ; 28 : 42-48

[20] Henley MB, Chapman JR, Agel J, Harvey EJ, Whorton AM, Swiontkowski MF. Treatment of type II, IIIA, and IIIB open fractures of the tibial shaft: A prospective comparison of unreamed interlocking intramedullary nails and half-pin external fixators. *J Orthop Trauma* 1998 ; 12 : 1-7

[21] Herscovici D, Ricci WM, McAndrews P, Dipasquale T, Sanders R. Treatment of femoral shaft fracture using unreamed interlocked nails. *J Orthop Trauma* 2000 ; 14 : 10-14

[22] Kempf I, Grosse A, Taglang G, Bernhard L, Moui Y. L'enclouage centro-médullaire avec verrouillage des fractures récentes du fémur et du tibia. Étude statistique à propos de 835 cas. *Chirurgie* 1991 ; 117 : 478-487

[23] Kinast C, Bolhofner BR, Mast JW, Ganz R. Subtrochanteric fractures of the femur. Results of treatment with the 95° condylar blade-plate. *Clin Orthop* 1989 ; 238 : 122-130

[24] Klein MP, Rahn BA, Frigg R, Kessler S, Perren SM. Reaming versus non-reaming in medullary nailing: interference with cortical circulation of the canine tibia. *Arch Orthop Trauma Surg* 1990 ; 109 : 314-316

[25] Krettek C, Miclau T, Grün O, Schandelmaier P, Tscherne H. Intraoperative control of axes, rotation and length in femoral and tibial fractures. *Injury* 1998 ; 29 : 29-39

[26] Krettek C, Schandelmaier P, Miclau T, Tscherne H. Minimally invasive percutaneous plate osteosynthesis (MIPPO) using the DCS in proximal and distal femoral fractures. *Injury* 1997 ; 28 : 20-30

[27] Kumar A, Jasani V, Butt MS. Management of distal femoral fractures in elderly patients using retrograde titanium supracondylar nails. *Injury* 2000 ; 31 : 169-173

[28] Lobenhoffer P, Gerich T, Bertram T, Lattermann C, Pohlemann T, Tscherne H. Spezielle posteromediale und posterolaterale Zugänge zur Versorgung von Tibiakopffrakturen. *Unfallchirurg* 1997 ; 100 : 957-967

[29] Mast J, Jakob R, Ganz R. Planning and reduction technique in fracture surgery. New York : Springer-Verlag, 1989

[30] Melcher GA, Claudi B, Schlegel U, Perren SM, Printzen G, Munzinger J. Influence of type of medullary nail on the development of local infection. An experimental study of solid and slotted nails in rabbits. *J Bone Joint Surg Br* 1994 ; 76 : 955-959

[31] Müller ME, Allgöwer M, Schneider R, Willenegger H. Manual of internal fixation. Berlin : Springer-Verlag, 1991

[32] Müller ME, Nazarian S, Koch P, Schatzker J. The comprehensive classification of fractures of long bones. New York : Springer-Verlag, 1990

[33] Pape HC, Regel G, Dwenger A, Krumm K, Schweitzer G, Krettek C et al. Influences of different methods of intramedullary femoral nailing on lung function in patients with multiple trauma. *J Trauma* 1993 ; 35 : 709-716

[34] Pröbstel M, Richter FJ, Börner M. Ist die routinemässige postoperative CT-Messung nach Marknagelung von Ober- und Unterschenkelfrakturen indiziert? *Trauma Berufskrankh* 1999 ; 1 : 152-157

[35] Reynders PA, Broos PL. Healing of closed femoral shaft fractures treated with the AO unreamed femoral nail. A comparative study with the AO reamed femoral nail. *Injury* 2000 ; 31 : 367-371

[36] Rhinelander FW. Tibial blood supply in relation to fracture healing. *Clin Orthop* 1974 ; 105 : 34-81

[37] Rüedi T, Allgöwer M. Fractures of the lower end of the tibia into the ankle-joint. *Injury* 1969 ; 1 : 92-99

[38] Rüedi TP, Sommer C, Leutenegger A. New techniques in indirect reduction of long bone fractures. *Clin Orthop* 1998 ; 347 : 27-34

[39] Sanders R, Koval KJ, Dipasquale T, Helfet DL, Frankle M. Retrograde reamed femoral nailing. *J Orthop Trauma* 1993 ; 7 : 293-302

[40] Schandelmaier P, Krettek C, Rudolf J, Tscherne H. Outcome of tibial shaft fractures with severe soft tissue injury treated by unreamed nailing versus external fixation. *J Trauma* 1995 ; 39 : 707-711

[41] Schemitsch EH, Kowalski MJ, Swiontkowski MF, Sanft D. Cortical bone blood flow in reamed and unreamed locked intramedullary nailing: a fractured tibia model in sheep. *J Orthop Trauma* 1994 ; 8 : 373-382

[42] Shepherd LE, Costigan WM, Gardocki RJ, Ghiassi AD, Patzakis MJ, Stevanovic MV. Local free muscle flaps and unreamed interlocked nails for open tibial fractures. *Clin Orthop* 1998 ; 350 : 90-96

[43] Sitter T, Wilson J, Browner B. The effect of reamed versus unreamed nailing on intramedullary blood supply on cortical viability. *J Orthop Trauma* 1990 ; 4 : 232

[44] Sturmer KM. Die elastische Plattenosteosynthese, ihre Biomechanik, Indikation und Technik im Vergleich zur rigiden Osteosynthese. *Unfallchirurg* 1996 ; 99 : 816-829

[45] Tornetta P 3rd, Tiburzi D. Reamed versus nonreamed anterograde femoral nailing. *J Orthop Trauma* 2000 ; 14 : 15-19

[46] Trentz OL. Polytrauma: Pathophysiology, priorities and management. In : Rüedi, TP, Murphy WM eds. AO principles of fracture management. Stuttgart : Thieme-Verlag, 2000 : 661-674

[47] Weber BG. Die Verletzungen des oberen Sprunggelenkes. Bern : Huber-Verlag, 1966

[48] Weller S, Hontzsch D, Frigg R. Die epiperiostale, perkutane Plattenosteosynthese. Eine minimal-invasive Technik unter dem Aspekt der "biologischen Osteosynthese". *Unfallchirurg* 1998 ; 101 : 115-121

[49] Wenda K, Runkel M, Degreif J, Rudig L. Minimally invasive plate fixation in femoral shaft fractures. *Injury* 1997 ; 28 : 13-19

Circular external fixation for fractures

MA Catagni
F Guerreschi
R Cattaneo

Abstract. – The circular external fixator has many applications in fracture management, due to its ease of application, decreased risk of infection, and ability to accommodate soft tissue injuries. It has immense versatility, allowing the frame to be customised to manage any fracture pattern. In addition, there is no need for later operations for hardware removal. Based on our experience, we recommend the Ilizarov fixator for open fractures, war injuries, multilevel fractures, high energy fractures with soft tissue injury, nonunions with and without infection, and fractures with bone loss.

Keywords: external fixation, fractures, circular external fixator, Ilizarov method, open fractures, nonunion fractures, war injuries, infected fractures.

Introduction

Since taking his first steps on earth, man has been plagued with traumatic bone injuries. The first recorded methods of treatment were rest and wooden fragments fixed to the broken limb with flexible reeds. This was perhaps the first use of "external fixation" and is a method still used in China for fracture fixation.

The development in 1952 by Gavrijl Abramovich Ilizarov of a circular external fixator which completely encompasses the limb is thought to be the ideal design for fracture fixation. Originally composed of 32 parts, the Ilizarov device has since been modified by those using it, and new parts have been developed to improve the original design. The constant evolution of the technique, while maintaining the core concepts, attests to the validity of Ilizarov's original idea.

Unfortunately, most surgeons have little training in the use of external fixation, making them reluctant to utilise these methods. Regardless of the method chosen for fixation, three conditions are necessary for the successful treatment of fractures: 1) reduction of the fracture fragments, 2)

MA Catagni, M.D., Chief of the Orthopaedic Department and Ilizarov Unit.
Francesco Guerreschi, M.D., Staff of the Orthopaedic Department.
Roberto Cattaneo, M.D., Honorary Chief of the Orthopaedic Department.
Lecco Hospital, 22053 Lecco, Italy.

stability of the reduction, and 3) vascularisation of the fracture fragments. Our experience has shown that external fixators are particularly useful in cases involving open fractures, war injuries, multilevel fractures, high energy fractures with soft tissue injury, fractures in ischaemic limbs, nonunions with and without infection, and fractures with bone loss [1-11].

Vehicular and industrial accidents often involve high energy fractures associated with extensive bone loss and soft tissue injury. If there is minimal skin injury and bone loss, an external fixator of the surgeon's preference may be applied. If intervention by a plastic surgeon is necessary, it is advisable to initially apply a monoaxial external fixator which will allow ease of tissue transfer and skin grafting. After the soft tissue injuries have been addressed, a more complex fixator such as the circular external fixator may be applied. With minimal skin injury but extensive bone loss or comminution, a circular fixator is advantageous. The surgeon may perform bifocal or trifocal internal transport to address bone loss, and he may customise the frame according to the degree of comminution [1, 3, 5, 8, 10].

War injuries are the most challenging injuries with severe soft tissue damage, bone loss, and often infection. Fixators in this setting must be very simple, versatile and easy to apply [9, 11].

Indications

Based on our experience at Lecco Hospital, internal fixation or external fixation with a monolateral fixator are generally the preferred methods of treatment for humeral and femoral fractures. Both methods are well-tolerated by the patient and provide adequate stability. A circular external fixator is recommended for humeral and femoral fractures with accompanying bone loss. Likewise, in forearm fractures, the indications for an Ilizarov device are limited to fractures with significant bone loss, open fractures, and severely comminuted fractures that can not be reduced or sufficiently stabilised with a monolateral fixator [1-11].

In contrast, the indications for an Ilizarov device in the treatment of tibial fractures are wide ranging. They include acute fractures both open and closed, intra-articular fractures, fractures with bone loss, non-unions with or without infection and malalignment corrections.

Technique

HUMERAL FRACTURES

■ *Fractures of the humerus with bone loss* (fig 1A)

The standard frame consists of a proximal arch, an intermediate ring and a distal block consisting of a full ring and a 5/8 ring

All references to this article must include: Catagni MA, Guerreschi F and Cattaneo R. Circular external fixation for fractures. Editions Scientifiques et Médicales Elsevier SAS (Paris). All rights reserved, Surgical Techniques in Orthopaedics and Traumatology, 55-030-C-10, 2000, 6 p.

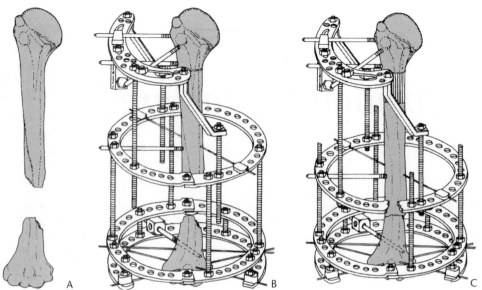

1 A. Humeral fracture with bone loss.
  B. Pre-assembled frame and configuration of positioning pins and wires. Note the proximal osteotomy for distraction osteogenesis.
  C. Final result after achieving union in the docking site and restoring limb length.

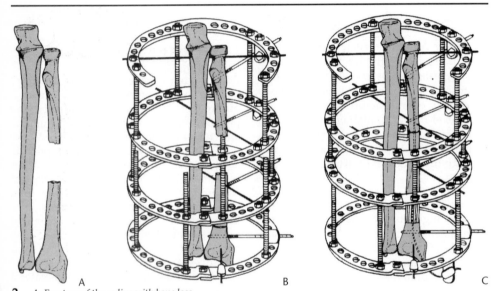

2 A. Fracture of the radius with bone loss.
  B. Pre-assembled frame showing position of pins and wires. Note the distal radius osteotomy for distraction osteogenesis.
  C. Final result.

(fig 1B). The distal block is fixed to the distal humerus with a reference wire at the level of the epicondyles. The wire is directed from posterolateral to anteromedial and is perpendicular to the long axis of the bone. A half-pin is inserted into the proximal humeral epiphysis from posterolateral to anteromedial, perpendicular to the long axis of the bone. The pin is then attached to the proximal arch. These steps centralise the frame on the humerus. Two additional half-pins are inserted in the proximal humerus. Additional wires and half pins are inserted in the arch, rings, and 5/8 ring. Care is taken to avoid damaging the neurovascular structures in this area. A corticotomy is performed at the level of the metaphysis of the longer segment. The fracture level is compressed while the osteotomy is distracted until normal humeral length is

restored *(fig 1C)*. If the nonunion site is opened, it is important to resect the infected and/or sclerotic bone fragments to allow for good surface contact between bone ends.

FOREARM FRACTURES

■ **Fractures of the forearm with bone loss**

Severe fractures of the radius and ulna occasionally result from violent trauma. Function of the extremity can be severely compromised. Before undertaking any reconstructive procedures, one must evaluate the eventual function of the limb expected after treatment. If there is significant neurovascular injury, a primary amputation may need to be considered. If the bone loss is less then 3-4 cm and equal

in both the radius and ulna, which may occur after resection, it is best to apply the monofocal compression technique to both bones. This shortening will not decrease the overall function of the limb. When the bone loss affects one bone more than the other, a frame may be applied for bone transport.

■ **Fractures of the radius with bone loss** *(fig 2A)*

This frame is composed of a proximal 5/8 ring and an additional three full rings. The 5/8 ring is fixed to the proximal radius with one wire directed from anterolateral to posteromedial and a half-pin perpendicular to this wire. The distal ring holds a wire directed from anteromedial to posterolateral and one half-pin posteromedial to anterolateral. On the proximal intermediate transport ring, one inserts a wire from anterolateral to posteromedial and a half-pin perpendicular to this wire. The distal intermediate ring is affixed to the radius in the usual technique, but reinforced with a half-pin inserted from lateral to medial and attached to the ring 1 cm proximal with a ring extension. A corticotomy is performed in the distal part of the radius and bone transport is initiated one week postoperatively at a rate of 0.25 mm three times a day *(fig 2B)*. If good bone regeneratation is evident after a couple of weeks, the bone transport rate can be increased to 0.25 mm four times a day. If the bone loss is the result of resection of necrotic bone, an intramedullary guide wire may be inserted to help maintain proper alignment *(fig 2C)*. If the bone appears hypoplastic at the end of the transport, the fracture should be opened and a bone graft applied.

■ **Fracture of the ulna with bone loss**

The pre-assembled frame is composed of a proximal 5/8 ring and three full rings distally. Two wires or one wire and a half-pin are applied to transfix the ulna to the distal ring. Two wires and a half-pin are applied proximally to secure the ulna to the proximal 5/8 ring. On the distal intermediate ring, one inserts a wire directed anteromedial to posterolateral, with a half-pin inserted posteromedial to anterolateral. On the transporting ring, one directs a wire and a half-pin in the same manner as that in the distal intermediate ring. The corticotomy, timing, rate of transport, and use of a guide wire are the same as for the radius.

FEMORAL FRACTURES

■ **General considerations**

The standard assembly for treating femoral fractures includes incorporating a full ring distally and an arch proximally at the subtrochanteric level. One or two intermediate rings or arches will be incorporated into the fixator, depending on the type and level of the fracture. Fixation distally includes a transverse wire and two half-pins, one inserted from posteromedial to anterolateral and the other from posterolateral to anteromedial. Proximal fixation is achieved by attaching two half-pins to the arch, one from posterolateral to anteromedial and the other from anterolateral to posteromedial. At the intermediate ring or rings, olive wires have been used traditionally to reduce and hold the fracture fragments. Unfortunately, olive wires are not well-tolerated for the duration of treatment. Therefore, half-pins should be applied to the intermediate rings, trying to stay posterior to the iliotibial band so that knee motion is not hindered. The olive wires can then be removed. Frame construction, wire and half-pin placement will be presented for proximal, diaphyseal and distal fractures of the femur. Pre-assembly of the frame is recommended to reduce operating time. Basic configurations can be used and modified as necessary. For fractures in the upper third of the femur, two arches and two rings are recommended. In middle and distal third fractures, one arch and three rings are used.

■ *Fractures of the femur with bone loss* (fig 3A)

In the case of a fracture of the femur with bone loss, with or without shortening, the goal is to restore normal limb length. The pre-assembled frame is to be constructed using two arches proximally connected with hexagonal sockets and then attached to a ring. The distal block will consist of two rings. The proximal arch will be at a level between the greater and lesser trochanter, the intermediate ring approximately 3 cm proximal to the area of bone loss, and the proximal ring of the distal block about 3 cm distal to the fracture. A distal reference wire is inserted in the usual manner. Rotational alignment and fracture reduction are then achieved. Next, a half-pin is inserted at the proximal arch from posterolateral to anteromedial, making sure to stay perpendicular to the proximal segment of the femur. Half-pins and wires are inserted respecting the anatomy of this region. A corticotomy is performed in the subtrochanteric area, and after a five to ten day latency period, distraction can begin with a rhythm of 0.5 to 1 mm per day; the rate therefore will be 0.25 mm two or four times a day depending on the biological response of the regenerate (fig 3B). Bone transport is continued until the defect is corrected. In some cases, it is better to shorten the deficient bone at the fracture site in order to achieve bony contact in a more rapid manner. At the time of docking, the irregular bone ends are resected to increase bone surface contact and ease of compression. If the docking site is not infected, bone graft may be applied. The

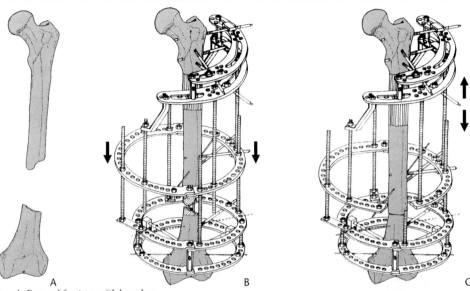

3   *A. Femoral fracture with bone loss.*
       B. Pre-assembled frame fixation and proximal osteotomy for transport.
       C. Final result achieving union and correcting limb length discrepancy.

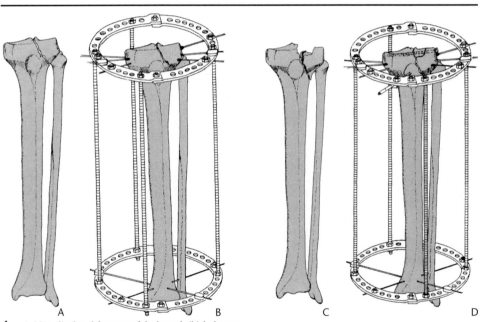

4   *A. Non-displaced fracture of the lateral tibial plateau.*
       B. Fracture reduction with olive wires and application of a two-level Ilizarov frame.
       C. Displaced fracture of the lateral tibial plateau.
       D. Fracture reduction with olive wires and application of a two-level Ilizarov frame.

frame must be left in place until both the regenerate and the docking site have healed (fig 3C).

TIBIAL FRACTURES

■ *Proximal non-displaced intra-articular fractures* (fig 4A)

The preassembled frame consists of two rings, one proximal and one distal. On the proximal ring, two olive wires are inserted from posterolateral to anteromedial and anterolateral to posteromedial, respectively, at an angle of 30 degrees to each other. Another olive wire is inserted from medial to lateral. This causes the fragment to be reduced, allowing interfragmentary

compression. Distally, two wires are inserted, one transversely through the fibula and the other from anterolateral to posteromedial (fig 4B).

Partial weight-bearing is prohibited for at least 45 days. With percutaneous fixation with wires, there is less risk of infection and the fixator can be removed without general anaesthesia.

■ *Proximal displaced intra-articular fractures* (fig 4C)

When there is a compressed fragment, it is necessary to restore joint surface alignment. Open reduction is performed to realign the fragments with olive wires and cannulated screws. A similar apparatus as previously described is applied for reduction of the

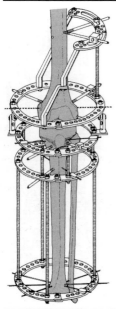

5 *Proximal complex fracture of the tibial metaphysis and epiphysis treated with an Ilizarov frame extended on the femur.*

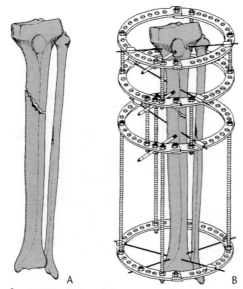

6 A. *Tibia diaphyseal fracture.*
B. *Alignment in the frontal plane with wires and Ilizarov frame.*

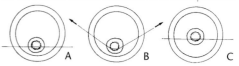

7 A. *Transverse insertion of a wire in a fracture bone segment to reduce a displacement on the lateral plane.*
B. *Fixation of the wire in the desired position on the ring to align the fragment.*
C. *Tensioning of the wire and achieving desired position of the bone fragment.*

fracture. The number of the wires and the position of the olive wires depends on the type of fracture *(fig 4D)*. Range of motion begins immediately, but partial weight-bearing is delayed 45 days.

■ *Proximal complex fractures*

In an open fracture where the fracture involves the joint and the metaphysis, a three-ringed frame will be applied. Fixation of the proximal fracture is as previously described. If the fracture is displaced, it is openly reduced and fixated with olive wires and cannulated screws. The frame is then applied, with transverse olive wires proximally, and a wire through the tibia and fibula distally, perpendicular to the tibial axis. After the wires are tensioned, radiographs are taken. Further reduction of the metaphyseal fracture may be achieved with a wire attached to the intermediate ring. After fracture reduction has been achieved, the frame is further stabilised with a wire at the distal ring from anterolateral to posteromedial and a half-pin on the intermediate ring, perpendicular to the inserted wire.

Partial weight-bearing is delayed 45 days. In special cases, when the fracture is extremely complex and unstable, the frame can be extended onto the distal femur with two levels of fixation *(fig 5)*. The femoral and tibial frame are connected with hinges in line with the centre of rotation of the knee. It is possible to apply distraction at the knee joint in order to avoid compression and displacement of the fracture.

■ *Proximal metaphyseal fractures*

The pre-assembled frame consists of 3 rings: one proximal at the level of the fibular head, the second 2 cm distal to the fracture, and the third 2-3 cm proximal to the ankle joint. To centralise the frame, a transverse proximal wire is inserted perpendicular to the long axis of the tibia. A second wire is

inserted distally through the tibia, perpendicular to its axis. After the frame is centralised, the fracture is reduced with a wire attached to the intermediate ring. The frame is strengthened with another wire on the distal ring (from anterolateral to posteromedial) and two half-pins on the proximal ring (one from anteromedial to posterolateral, and the second from anterolateral to posteromedial). A half-pin is also inserted on the intermediate ring from anteromedial to posterolateral. This configuration provides enough stability to allow partial weight-bearing a few days after surgery. Full weight-bearing occurs in approximately 20 days.

■ *Simple (transverse) diaphyseal fractures* *(fig 6A)*

In this case, the frame consists of four rings, the proximal ring at the fibular head and the distal ring 2-3 cm proximal to the ankle joint. The two intermediate rings lie 3 cm proximal and distal to the fracture. Two reference wires are inserted, one proximal to the fibular head in the tibia transversely, and one distally through the tibia and fibula. After the wires are attached to the rings and tension is applied, check the alignment of the tibial crest and compare rotation to the contralateral foot. Reduction is checked with a radiograph. Olive wires placed transversely on the intermediate rings allow for reduction of the fracture in the frontal plane *(fig 6B)*. If in the lateral plane a recurvatum exists, it is possible to move the wires on the intermediate rings until the fragments are aligned *(fig 7 A, B, C)*.

After fracture reduction, the frame can be strengthened by inserting additional wires or half-pins. Traditionally, four more wires are inserted so that there are two at each level. This fixation is indicated for the younger patient, while in adults half-pins are introduced at the 3 proximal rings

perpendicular to the wires at these levels. Adequate fixation is obtained distally by two crossed wires angled 90 degrees to one another and affixed to the distal ring.

In the open fracture, reduction is achieved through the wound and can be maintained with clamps. It is important to keep the size of the incision to a minimum and to not devitalise the fracture fragments. A similar frame configuration is applied without the need for olive wires.

■ *Diaphyseal fractures with a third (butterfly) fragment*

The frame is built with four rings and the application is similar to previously described, except for the position of the olive wires. Two are applied from the same side. The third is applied opposite to the first two catching the fragment and fixed with a post. It is not necessary to apply tension to the third wire.

In the case of open fractures, reduction can be performed through the wound, and maintained by applying two wires or screws through the fragments. The frame with the crossed configuration of wires and half-pins is then applied without the need for olive wires. The wires or screws can be removed at the completion of fixation.

■ *Diaphyseal fractures at two levels (segmental)* *(fig 8A)*

The pre-assembled frame must contain 5 rings: 2 sets of 2 rings at the level of the proximal and distal fragments, and a ring in between. A reference wire is placed proximally and distally in a transverse manner through the tibia and fibula, perpendicular to their long axes. Tension is applied, being careful to maintain the correct position of the foot with respect to the knee. Then, by means of the insertion of olive wires, reduction in the frontal and sagittal planes can be achieved. Three or four olive wires are usually sufficient to achieve reduction. Additional wires can be inserted for better stabilisation of the fracture fragments, if necessary. At each ring, there should be at least two wires.

In open fractures, reduction can be achieved and temporarily maintained by clamps or

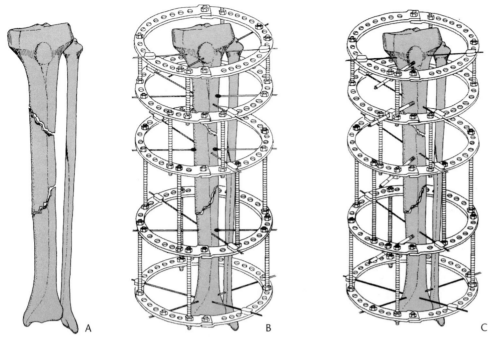

8 *A. Segmental fracture of the tibia.*
B. Reduction of the fracture and external fixation with an Ilizarov frame including 5 rings.
C. Reduction and fixation with a hybrid frame.

wires while applying the required crossed configuration of wires and half-pins *(fig 8B, C)*.

■ *Diaphyseal fractures with bone loss* *(fig 9A)*

The frame consists of five rings: one block of two rings at the level of the proximal metaphysis, one ring above and one ring below the bone gap, the last ring on the distal metaphysis.

The proximal and distal rings are applied in the usual manner with two reference wires,

and the frame is strengthened with additional wires and half-pins *(fig 9B)*. A corticotomy is performed in the region of the metaphysis of the longer segment *(fig 9C)*. Bone is transported at a rate of 0.75 mm per day. Once the bone ends are approximated, the chances of union are improved by performing a resection or remodelling of the bone ends to improve bone surface contact *(fig 9D)*. A fibular osteotomy to remove a small section of bone is necessary to allow for acute shortening of the tibia to achieve bone contact. To

eliminate any overall shortening, lengthening can be continued until normal limb length has been restored. It is also possible to use autogenous cancellous bone graft to increase the likelihood of union *(fig 9E)*.

■ *Pilon fractures* *(fig 10A)*

In pilon fractures resulting from axial loading of the lower leg, it is imperative to restore the articular surface of the distal tibia. A preconstructed frame consists of a block of two rings for the tibia and an intermediate ring connected to a foot frame with threaded rods *(fig 10B)*. The proximal block is fixated to the tibia. The distal ring of the proximal block is placed 3-4 cm proximal to the level of the fracture. The foot frame is fixated with two wires in the heel and two wires in the forefoot *(fig 10C)*. Distraction is performed between the tibia block and the foot frame, causing a kind of ligamentotaxis. The fracture is openly reduced, and the fragments stabilised with olive wires or screws *(fig 11A)*. After wound closure, the intermediate ring and wires are applied at the level of the fracture for further stabilisation. Distraction is maintained between the foot and tibia, preventing stress at the ankle joint surface. Distraction is discontinued after one month *(fig 11B)* and the connecting rods are replaced with hinges, allowing ankle joint range of motion. After another 15 days, the foot frame is removed, and the patient is allowed progressive weight-bearing.

Acknowledgements – This article was edited by Laura L. Meyers, M.D., Ilizarov Fellow, Lecco Hospital, Italy.

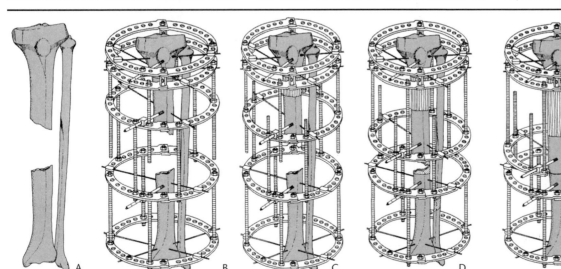

9 *A. Fracture of the tibia with bone loss without shortening.*
B. Application of the Ilizarov frame with 5 levels of fixation.
C. Osteotomy of the proximal metaphysis for proximal - distal bone transport.
D. Before the docking, open debridement of the bone ends.
E. Final result.

Figures 10, 11 and References ➤

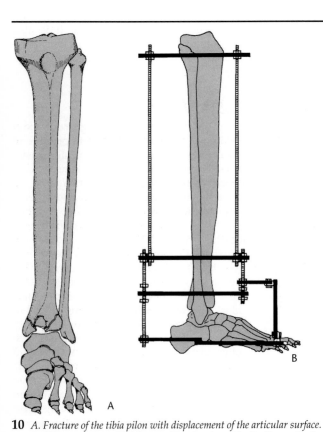

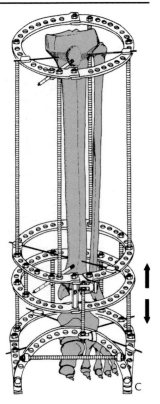

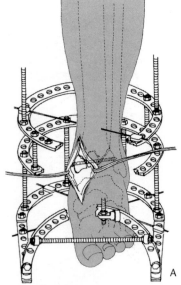

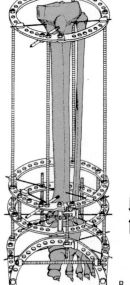

10 *A. Fracture of the tibia pilon with displacement of the articular surface.*
B. Ilizarov pre-assembled frame with extension of the fixation on the foot. The fixation is performed on the proximal block and on the foot.
C. Distraction between the foot and the leg, producing a ligamentotaxis on the ankle joint, helpful for articular surface reduction.

11 *A. Open reduction and fixation with screws and K-wires on the distal ring. Distraction is maintained between foot and leg for at least one month.*
B. Final result with releasing tension on the ankle joint after 30 days (see arrows).

References

[1] ASAMI Group. Operative principles of Ilizarov - fracture treatment, nonunion, osteomyelitis, lengthening, deformity correction. Baltimore : Williams and Wilkins, 1991

[2] Bianchi-Maiocchi A. L'osteosintesi transossea secondo G. A. Ilizarov. Aspetti sperimentali, teorici e clinici. Milano : Medi-Surgical Video, 1985

[3] Bianchi-Maiocchi A, Cattaneo R, Villa A, Catagni MA. Il metodo di Ilizarov nella fissazione esterna delle fratture recenti di Gamba. *Ortop Traumatol* 1983 ; III (n° 3-4) 643-648

[4] Catagni MA, Carvalho G. Tratamento da fratura tibial em pilão com fixador externo Circular de Ilizarov. *Rev Brasil Ortop* 1996 ; 31 : 643-648

[5] Catagni MA, Malzev V, Kirienko A. Advances in Ilizarov apparatus assembly - Fracture treatment, pseudoarthroses lengthening, deformity correction. Milano : Medicalplastic, 1994

[6] Catagni MA, Mendlick M. Femoral fractures. *Tech Orthop* 1996 ; 11 : 160-173

[7] Cattaneo R, Catagni MA, Guerreschi F. Application of the Ilizarov method in the humerus. *Hand Clin* 1993 ; 9 : 729-739

[8] Cattaneo R, Catagni MA, Johnson EE. The treatment of infected nonunions and segmental defect of the tibia by the method of Ilizarov. *Clin Orthop* 1992 ; 280 : 143-152

[9] Cattaneo R, Villa A, Catagni MA, Tentori L. Il metodo di Ilizarov in traumatologia. Medicina militare, atti congresso internazionale di medicina militare, Roma, 24-26 Settembre1986 : 277-280

[10] Ilizarov GA. Transosseous osteosynthesis: theoretical and clinical aspects of the regeneration and growth of tissue. Berlin : Springer-Verlag, 1992

[11] Picariello A, Catagni MA. Fissatore circolare di pronto impiego. Atti Congresso OTODI, Sabaudia, Italy, 1998

Flexible intramedullary devices for fractures in children

JP Metaizeau

Abstract. – The treatment of fractures in children is essentially conservative since young bone heals rapidly and growth remodels many malunions. The techniques of internal fixation developed for the adult skeleton present many disadvantages in children. The surgical approach evacuates the fracture haematoma, damages the periosteum, increases local devascularisation and encourages infection and secondary overgrowth. Fixation which is too rigid encourages cortical union, but it also inhibits the formation of a periosteal callus which is of prime importance in the child. Stable intramedullary pinning carried out with two pre-bent pins allows the stabilisation of nearly all diaphyseal and metaphyseal fractures, while perfectly respecting the healing process and unique biomechanical properties of young bone. The pinning is performed without opening the fracture site, preserving the haematoma and the periosteum, the role of which is essential for bone consolidation. The elasticity of the pins allows slight compression and distraction movements which are particularly favourable for consolidation. The child is discharged from the hospital after a few days. Cast immobilisation is not necessary. The child recovers function rapidly and absence from school is minimised. Complications are infrequent and rarely severe.

Keywords: fractures in children, humeral fractures in children, forearm fractures in children, tibial fractures in children, radial neck fractures in children, internal fixation, flexible intramedullary fixation, long bones.

Introduction

There are a number of differences between fractures in adults and fractures in children. In adults, untreated fractures will lead to nonunion. In children, fractures will consolidate without treatment – in the worse case, with malunion. Our goal is therefore to direct the healing process without disturbing it.

The treatment of fractures in children is essentially conservative since young bone heals rapidly and growth will remodel many malunions. In addition, the techniques developed for the adult skeleton have adverse effects in children and their disadvantages still outweigh their advantages. However, conservative treatment does not always give perfect results; some injuries are liable to sequelae which are not corrected by growth.

It must be noted that children with polytrauma, severe brain injuries, osteogenesis imperfecta, neurological problems, and adolescents near the end of

Jean-Paul Metaizeau, Chief of Department, Paediatric Orthopaedic Surgery, Hôpital Belle-Isle, 57000 Metz, France.

growth cannot always be treated conservatively and may require surgery.

Biomechanical aspects

HEALING OF THE GROWING BONE

The healing process for fractures in children does not pass exactly through the same stages as in the adult [6, 9]. The fracture haematoma contains several ingredients which encourage consolidation: cellular factors such as fibroblasts and chondroblasts, humoural factors such as the morphogenic protein for bone.

The child's very active periosteum plays an essential role by forming an early and very strong primary callus [2]. As of the second week, the new bone envelopes and rapidly immobilises the fracture site, whatever the position of the bone ends. Consolidation is not prevented by a lack of contact between the two fragments, overlapping or displacement. On the other hand, if the fracture site is opened, evacuation of the haematoma and local devascularisation decrease periosteal activity and delay the healing process.

As shown by Firica [1] and McKibbin [5], the conservation of some motions at the fracture

site encourages periosteal osteogenesis. However, some of the possible movements at the fracture site do not encourage consolidation. Movements perpendicular to the bone trabeculae cause shearing in the callus and should be prevented. On the contrary, forces of compression and distraction parallel to the trabeculae stimulate consolidation.

In addition, when placed under axial forces, the bony trabeculae reorientate and thicken along the line of forces, whereas those which are not stressed disappear. The resulting remodelling of bone progressively corrects most of the moderate malunions which often result after conservative treatment, even when well carried out.

The risk of joint stiffness following plaster cast immobilisation is practically non-existent, except in the case of epiphyseal fractures. Everything favours the success of conservative treatment, all the more so as the child is younger.

Rigid internal fixation inhibits the physiological mechanisms of healing. A fixation which is too rigid will encourage a cortical union which appears late and remains weak, but inhibits the formation of

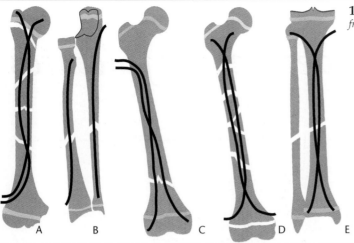

1 *Pinning of the different fractures of long bones.*
A. Humerus shaft fracture.
B. Forearm fracture.
C. Femoral fracture, distal part of the shaft.
D. Femoral shaft fracture.
E. Tibial fracture.

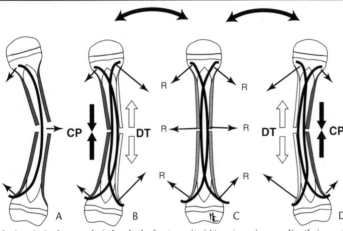

2 *The elastic device. A single curved pin bends the fracture site (A), or two pins equalise their recoil forces (C). If an external force tends to bend the device (B, D), the curve of one of the pins moves close to its original form and its recoil force ("R") diminishes. The other pin will lose its equilibrium, developing an increasing recoil force which opposes the deformation. When the adverse force stops, the fixation returns to its position of equilibrium. In the concavity of the deformation, there appears a compression force ("CP"). In the convexity of the deformation, there appears a distraction force ("DT").*

the periosteal callus which is of prime importance in the child; this callus appears quickly and is strong.

The surgical approach evacuates the fracture haematoma, damages the periosteum, increases local devascularisation, encourages infection and secondary overgrowth of the bone.

In young bone responding to axial stresses, the rigidity of a plate produces a rapid thinning of cortices, adding the risk of recurrent fractures to the other disadvantages.

Finally, the removal of implants requires a second stay in hospital, anaesthesia and an operative risk.

The long scar adds a cosmetic disadvantage which is unacceptable if it can be avoided.

INTRAMEDULLARY NAILING

Open nailing should be prohibited since it does not preserve the main advantage of nailing which is to avoid opening the fracture.

Reaming in children often produces excessive cortical thinning; it also seems to increase the risk of secondary overgrowth.

Femoral nailing also has some specific risks: femoral head necrosis, fracture or narrowing of the neck, coxa valga.

Stable elastic intramedullary pinning (SEIMP)

SEIMP is carried out with two pre-bent pins. It provides effective fixation for nearly all diaphyseal and metaphyseal fractures (fig 1), while perfectly respecting the healing process and the unique biomechanical properties of young bone. This technique presents many advantages and few disadvantages, but it is not meant to supplant conservative treatment. Its aim is only to allow correct treatment of fractures which cannot be treated conservatively without adding iatrogenic complications.

BIOMECHANICAL ASPECTS

When a pre-bent pin is introduced into the medullary canal of the bone (fig 2), it tends to regain its original shape in order to fit the narrow canal, giving three point fixation.

Each of these three points presses on the bone. The two extremities of the pin press on metaphyseal cancellous bone; the apex of the curve presses the inner aspect of the cortex.

A single straight pin does not provide enough contact with the bone and affords no stability in any direction. A single pre-bent pin will induce a deformation (fig 2A), while two pins will equalise their forces and will keep the bone straight (fig 2C).

The principal feature of this type of osteosynthesis is its elasticity (fig 2B, D). If the pin is deformed, it resists by developing a force which opposes the deformation. This returns the pin to its original form on removal of the deforming force. The same applies when a fracture is internally fixed.

In the frontal plane, if a force tends to bend the fixation, one of the pins will approach its position of equilibrium and its recoil force will decrease. The other pin will lose its equilibrium, developing an increasing recoil force which opposes the deformation.

When the adverse force stops, the fixation returns to its position of equilibrium.

In the sagittal plane, the two pins appear to be straight. A flexion or extension force induces a curve which did not exist initially. A recoil force appears in the pins and tends to bring the bone to its position of equilibrium as soon as the deforming force stops.

This also holds for rotation. If one of two fragments is rotated with respect to the other, the two pins are twisted around their long axis, which generates on the cancellous bone a recoil force opposing the deformation. On removal of the deforming force, the fixation returns to equilibrium. The extremity of each pin must be fixed deep in the metaphyseal cancellous bone to achieve this effect. Short pins will slip on the inner aspect of the cortex without twisting, so that no recoil force is generated and displacement of the fragments will occur.

Transverse displacement brings the apex of the curved pins together, but because they tend to keep away from one another, when the deforming force stops, the two pins recover their original shape and reduce the translation.

Axial forces tend to produce telescoping, which has two components: one is perpendicular, the other is parallel to the axis of the bone. The first component is a transverse displacement which discourages consolidation because it is perpendicular to the bone trabeculae and disrupts the bony bridges. The presence of the pins in the medullary canal prevents this displacement. Only the second component remains: this is perpendicular to the fracture line and encourages the consolidation (fig 3).

Overall, in fractures stabilised by pinning, the forces parallel to the fracture line are suppressed, whereas those perpendicular to the fracture, which encourage consolidation, are preserved.

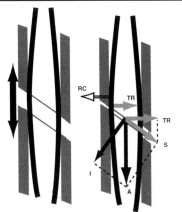

3 *The pins suppress the transverse displacements which cause shearing of the callus, but preserve axial forces parallel to the bone trabeculae. TR: transverse displacements; RC: Recoil. Axial forces are divided into "S" (sliding force suppressed by the pins) and "I" (impaction force preserved).*

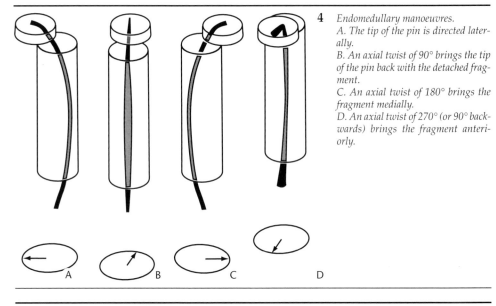

4 *Endomedullary manoeuvres.*
A. The tip of the pin is directed laterally.
B. An axial twist of 90° brings the tip of the pin back with the detached fragment.
C. An axial twist of 180° brings the fragment medially.
D. An axial twist of 270° (or 90° backwards) brings the fragment anteriorly.

Muscle tone, limb movements and weight-bearing result in successive oscillations on either side of the equilibrium. Each point in the fracture site is therefore placed under alternating forces of compression and distraction, which for McKibbin [5] and Firica [1] are particularly favourable for consolidation.

From a dynamic point of view, each movement produces compression on the concave side and distraction on the convexity (fig 2B, D).

Intramedullary pinning is therefore a method of internal fixation particularly well adapted to the conditions found in young bone for fracture healing.

This method encourages consolidation while preserving, in as far as possible, the physiological healing mechanisms in the child (preservation of the periosteum and the fracture haematoma, and the stimulation of periosteal osteogenesis by conservation of some mobility at the fracture site).

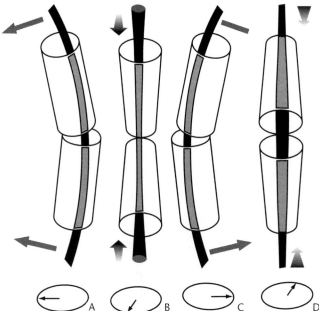

5 *Endomedullary manoeuvres.*
A. The curve of the pin induces a valgus deformity.
B. An axial twist of 90° orients the convexity backwards and produces a recurvatum deformity.
C. After an axial twist of 180°, the convexity faces laterally, and the pin induces a varus deformity.
D. After a twist of 270°, the convexity faces anteriorly, producing a flexum deformity.

Technique

The equipment is very simple, consisting of elastic steel pins, a T handle and a hammer. It is also possible to use titanium pins, but as they are more flexible, for a similar diameter their recoil force is lower. This requires the use of thicker pins than with stainless steel, which is not always possible; the child's medullary canal is frequently very narrow.

Through a short skin incision, a hole is drilled in the metaphysis furthest from the fracture. The diameter of the pin should be close to a third of the diameter of the medullary canal as measured on X-rays. The pin is bent to acquire the shape of a half circle, and its tip is bent more sharply. It is introduced into the bone through a cortical hole and pushed towards the fracture.

If the extremity is not exactly opposite the second fragment, it can easily be rotated from the other end so as to direct it towards the second fragment.

The first pin must not be entered into the cancellous bone of the metaphysis until the second one has been introduced. When both pins are at the same level, if the reduction is not correct, it can be improved by external manipulations. Both pins are then pushed into the cancellous bone. In this way, the two pins are placed so that their forces are balanced.

CORRECTION OF BONE DEFORMATION BY ENDOMEDULLARY MANOEUVRES

Using SEIMP, it is possible to correct the displacement of the bone fragments.

Introducing the pin into the second fragment is possible even if only partial reduction has been achieved. During progression of the first pin, its curve presses on the cortex of the second fragment, progressively reducing part of the displacement. It is then possible to manipulate the fracture via the pin.

If the extremity of the pin does not enter the second fragment by more than one centimetre, rotation of the pin modifies the position of its extremity, so that it moves the second fragment medially, forwards, laterally and backwards (fig 4). If the extremity of the pin is at a distance from the fracture, a twist changes the direction of its curve and the direction of its recoil force, producing valgus, flexion, varus or extension of the fracture (fig 5).

At the end of the operation, the axis of the bone is controlled under image intensification. If an angulation persists, it can be corrected by rotation of the pin, the curve of which is parallel to the deformation (fig 6). Then, the end of the pin is bent at a right angle and cut 0.5 to 1 cm beneath the skin.

The reduction of the displacement is not always perfect, but it is sufficient in a child whose growth will correct slight residual deformity.

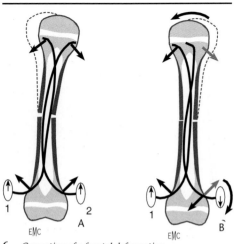

6 *Correction of a frontal deformation.*
A. At the end of the operation, there remains an angulation in the frontal plane.
B. The second pin, where concavity is parallel to the deformation, is twisted 180°. Its recoil force is inverted and opposes the deformation, correcting the angulation.

PARTICULARITIES ACCORDING TO THE FRACTURE SITE

■ *Humeral fractures* (fig 1)

To avoid damaging the ulnar nerve, inserting a pin medially is not recommended. For proximal metaphyseal and diaphyseal fractures, the incision is made just 1 cm proximal to the lateral condyle. The two pins are introduced into the lateral aspect of the humerus and then directed so that their extremities diverge in the proximal metaphysis.

■ *Forearm fractures* [3] (fig 1B, 7)

Only one pin is introduced in each bone. The incision for inserting the radial pin is located on the lateral side of the distal metaphysis, 1 cm proximal to the growth plate. The incision for the ulnar pin is located on the lateral aspect of the proximal metaphysis, 1 or 2 cm distal to the olecranon growth plate.

■ *Femoral fractures*

Fractures of the femoral neck cannot be treated by SEIMP. For subtrochanteric fractures or midshaft fractures, the pins are introduced through each side of the distal metaphysis, 1 or 2 cm proximal to the growth plate (fig 1C, D, 8). For supracondylar fractures and distal shaft fractures, the two pins are introduced through the lateral aspect of the subtrochanteric area. After crossing the fracture site, their extremities are oriented so as to diverge in the distal fragment, and they are pushed through the growth plate into the condyles when the fracture is very distal. There is no risk of creating an epiphysiodesis when introducing two pins into a growth plate, but the manoeuvre must not be repeated several times.

■ *Tibial fractures* (fig 1E)

Indications for SEIMP are rare, as orthopaedic treatment is usually easy.

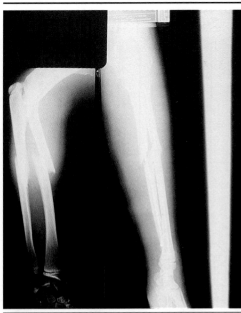

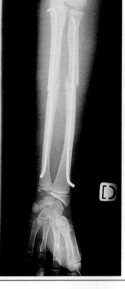

7 *Pinning of forearm fractures.*

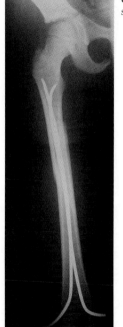

8 *Pinning of a femoral shaft fracture.*

However, when a fracture cannot be stabilised by conservative treatment, SEIMP can achieve a good result. Usually, two pins are introduced through each side of the proximal metaphysis and are pushed downwards.

■ *Radial neck fractures* (fig 9)

This type of fracture can be treated exclusively by endomedullary manoeuvres. A pin 2 to 2.5 mm in diameter is bent, and its extremity is bent more sharply. It is introduced through the lateral border of the distal metaphysis of the radius, 1 cm proximal to the growth plate. The extremity of the pin is directed laterally to the position where the tilt of the head is maximal. The

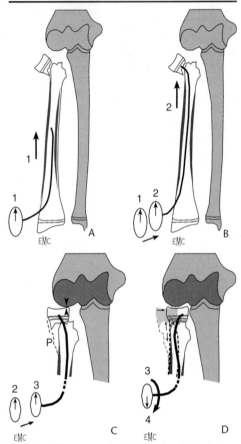

9 *The different steps in pinning of radial neck fractures.*

pin is pushed upwards with a hammer until its extremity reaches the fracture site. Then, the extremity elevates the radial head and brings it back to a horizontal position. At that point, the lateral shift persists; it is corrected by twisting the pin to direct its extremity inwards.

Postoperative care

The child is discharged from hospital after a few days (2 days for fractures of the humerus, forearm or tibia; 5 to 7 days for

Table I. – Complications after 1,582 fractures treated by SEIMP [7].

	Femur	Tibia	Humerus	Forearm
No. of cases	678	181	391	332
%	43%	11%	25%	21%
Reoperation	5.6%	4%	1.4%	5.6%
Skin problems	4.7%	2%	1.4%	2.5%
Axis correction	0.6%	0.5%		0.6%
Infection*	0.3%	0.5%		0.6%
Nonunion		1%		1%
Sequelae	1 case			1 case

* necessitating removal of material.

femoral shaft fractures). The construct is stable and cast immobilisation is not necessary. Functional recovery is rapid and absence from school is minimal.

Complications

The rate of complications is very low, as demonstrated by a study made by several members of the GEOP (a French group of paediatric orthopaedists), on a series of 1,582 fractures treated by SEIMP [7] (table I).

Only two cases (one femoral and one forearm fracture) had sequelae after a severe infection. The main problems were pain over the cut end of the pins or skin breaks requiring that the material be shortened. After femoral fractures, temporary stiffness of the knee is frequent, but resolves after removal of the material. Most complications seen did not necessitate further surgery. However, in about 4% of the children, a new operation was necessary to shorten the pins or to correct the axis.

Conclusion

Stable elastic intramedullary pinning presents many biomechanical advantages for the treatment of fractures in children. It is performed percutaneously, thus preserving the periosteum and haematoma that are essential for bone healing; the risk of infection is very low. The flexibility of the construct allows a slight mobility at the fracture site which encourages consolidation.

The reduction of the displacement is not always perfect, but is sufficient in a child as growth will correct slight residual deformity. Fractures treated with this method heal very quickly with a very low rate of complications.

References

[1] Firica A. L'ostéosynthèse stable élastique. *Rev Chir Orthop* 1981 ; 67 (suppl 2) : 82-92

[2] Jacobsen S. Periosteum: its relation to pediatric fractures. *J Pediatr Orthop (B)* 1996 ; 6 : 84-90

[3] Lascombes P, Prevot J, Ligier JN, Metaizeau JP, Poncelet T. Elastic stable intramedullary nailing in forearm shaft fractures in children: 85 cases. *J Pediatr Orthop* 1990 ; 10 : 167-171

[4] Ligier JN, Metaizeau JP, Prevot J, Lascombes P. Elastic stable intramedullary nailing in children. *J Bone Joint Surg Br* 1988 ; 70 : 74-77

[5] McKibbin B. The biology of fracture healing in long bones. *J Bone Joint Surg Br* 1978 ; 60 : 150-162

[6] Metaizeau JP. Ostéosynthèse chez l'enfant. Montpellier : Sauramps Médical, 1998

[7] Metaizeau JP. Les complications de l'embrochage centromédullaire. Conférence d'enseignement présentée au Congrès de la SFCP, San Sébasia, 1999

[8] Parsch K. Modern trends in internal fixation of femoral fractures in children: A critical review. *J Pediatr Orthop (B)* 1997 ; 6 : 117-125

[9] Teot L. L'enclouage centro-médullaire élastique stable chez l'enfant. In : Cahiers d'enseignement de la SOFCOT. Paris : Expansion Scientifique Française, 1987: 71-90

Comprehensive classification system (CCS) for long bone fractures

ME Müller
J Schatzker
S Nazarian

Abstract. – The Comprehensive Classification System (CCS) is not a classification but a classification system. It is based on the concept that each segment of the skeleton contains triads of fractures, its Types, Groups and Subgroups. The format of the CCS is the hierarchical arrangement of the triads, and the fractures they contain, in ascending order of severity according to their morphological complexity, the energy required to produce them, and their prognosis. The diagnosis of a fracture is given by its exact location and morphology. An alpha-numeric system of coding has been designed to facilitate computer entry and retrieval. Intra- and interpersonal errors in classifying fractures result from a lack of information. Our binary system of questions serves as a check-list when classifying fractures. If a question cannot be answered, it means that further details must be obtained, either through further imaging or at surgery, before the fracture can be classified. Our classification system is based on a careful study of over 100,000 fully documented cases and has been recently validated by Orozco who carefully analysed the X-rays of 54,280 surgically treated fractures, and has provided X-ray illustrations for all Types, Groups and Subgroups as well as a statistical analysis of their incidence.

Keywords: long bone fractures, classification, alpha-numeric system.

"A classification is useful only if it considers the severity of the bone lesion and serves as a basis for treatment and for evaluation of the results."

Maurice E Müller, 1988

History of the CCS

The development of the Comprehensive Classification of Fractures began in 1958. The first important step was the development, for each patient, of the X-ray card [3] on which we fixed a microcopy of the pre-operative X-ray, the postoperative X-ray and those taken at 4 and 12 months after surgery. This allowed us to compile, carefully and completely, 100,000 documented cases over the next 30 years. This enormous collection of data served as the basis for the development of our system for classifying fractures.

In the first edition of the AO Manual [3], published in 1969, we demonstrated the

Maurice E Müller, M.D., Professor.
Joseph Schatzker, M.D., B.Sc, FRCS(C).
Serge Nazarian, M.D., Professor.
Fondation Maurice E Müller, Murtenstrasse 35, P.O.Box 8354, CH-3001 Bern, Switzerland.

division of a long bone into three distinct segments. In the second edition of the AO Manual [4], published in 1970, we demonstrated our concept of the hierarchical organisation of fractures into 3 types, according to their severity, with each type being further subdivided into three groups. We used the fractures of the distal femur for illustration. In 1980, we published in German [2] and, in 1981 in French [5], a detailed description of the whole concept of our classification system. These publications demonstrate the first application of our classification system to the three segments of the femur, and how the fractures of each segment were organised into types, groups and subgroups *(fig 1)*. The definitive publications dealing with our classification system appeared in 1987, in French, as "Classification AO des fractures" [6] and then, more extensively in English in 1990, as the "Comprehensive Classification of Fractures of Long Bones" [7]. In these publications, we demonstrated how our system of classification was applied to all long bones of the skeleton. In addition, these two publications contain the first description of the qualifications for the subgroups. In 1996 we published in our pamphlets [8] on classification of fractures, the binary system of questions. In it, we demonstrated how

the use of appropriate binary questions made mistakes in the classification of a fracture almost impossible. The development of the binary system of questions was stimulated by the publication of Burstein [1] who was critical of the intra- and interpersonal errors when classifying fractures. Finally, the remarkable Atlas of Orozco [9] provides clinical validation of our classification system. Orozco and his colleagues analysed 54,280 fractures treated with internal fixation between 1979 and 1987. This enabled them to demonstrate, with X-rays, the existence of all the fractures of all segments including subgroups, and to provide the reader with a statistical analysis of their incidence.

Principles of the Comprehensive Classification System (CCS)

The CCS is designed in such a way that it can be used to identify and classify all fractures of all long bones in a logical, useful, easy to understand and easy to use manner. It is user friendly. It considers the severity of the bone lesion and therefore is useful as a basis for treatment, and in

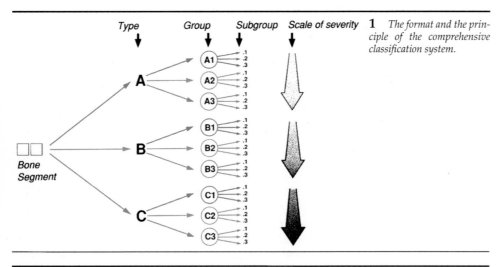

1   *The format and the principle of the comprehensive classification system.*

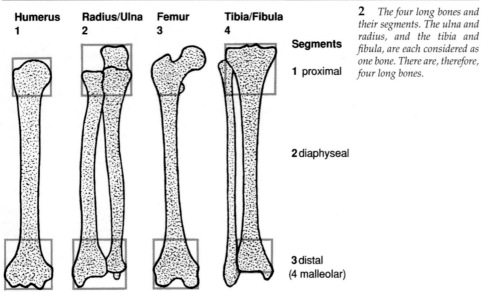

2   *The four long bones and their segments. The ulna and radius, and the tibia and fibula, are each considered as one bone. There are, therefore, four long bones.*

Diagnosis

Location		Morphology		
Bone	**Segment**	**Type**	**Group**	**Subgroup**
1 2 3 4	1 2 3 (4)	A B C	1 2 3	.1 .2 .3
4 Long Bones	3 (4) Segments	3 Types	9 Groups	27 Subgroups

3   *Alpha-numeric coding of the diagnosis for fractures of long bones.*

evaluating its outcome. It is also very useful for teaching and learning about fractures.

The unifying principle of the CCS (*fig 1*) is the division of all bone fractures into triads of fractures which are arranged in ascending order of severity. All long bones are divided into three accurately defined segments (*fig 2*). Each segment in turn has three precisely defined fracture Types which can be further subdivided into three Groups, and each group into three Subgroups. Qualifications of the Subgroups are used, where necessary, for greater definition of these subgroups.

ALPHA-NUMERIC CODE

To facilitate computer entry and retrieval we have designed an alpha-numeric system (*fig 3*) for denoting a fracture. Each bone of the skeleton or group of bones has been given a number. This number, combined with the number of the segment: 1 for proximal, 2 for diaphyseal, and 3 for distal, define the exact location of the fracture. The location combined with the notation of morphology define the diagnosis. Thus 33-C is a Type C fracture of the distal femur. The diagnosis becomes more and more precise as one continues to subdivide the Type into

Groups and then into Subgroups. C1, C2, and C3 are the three Groups of Type C. The ascending order of the numbers reflects the hierarchical organisation of the Groups according to the severity of the lesion which is reflected in its morphological complexity, the energy required to produce it, and the accompanying soft tissue lesion. Thus C2 and C3 are high energy lesions of the distal femur with their accompanying poor prognosis.

GLOSSARY

With the passage of time, the precise meaning of such terms as comminuted or butterfly has become completely corrupted and almost meaningless. To provide accurate terminology for our classification system, we have designed a glossary of terms. In this glossary, each word has such a precise meaning that it is possible to describe a fracture very accurately without the need of an accompanying diagram or X-ray.

– **essence:** That which makes a thing what it is. Most significant part of a thing's nature. A concentrated extract.

– **severity:** A term used to denote morphological complexity, the difficulties of treatment and the prognosis of a fracture.

TERMS FOR DIAPHYSEAL FRACTURES

All fractures of the diaphysis are either simple or multifragmentary.

– **simple:** A term used to characterise a single circumferential disruption of the diaphysis. Simple fractures are spiral, oblique or transverse.

– **multifragmentary**: A term used to characterise any fracture with one or more completely separated intermediate fragment(s). It includes wedge and complex fractures.

– **wedge:** A fracture with one or more intermediate fragment(s) in which, after reduction, there is some contact between the main fragments. The spiral or bending wedge may be intact or fragmented.

– **complex:** A fracture with one or more intermediate fragment(s) in which, after reduction, there is no contact between the main proximal and distal fragments. The complex fractures are spiral, segmental or irregular.

The term **comminuted** is imprecise and should not be used.

TERMS FOR END SEGMENT FRACTURES

Fractures of the end segments are either extra-articular or articular.

extra-articular fractures: These do not involve the articular surface, although they may be intra-capsular. They include apophyseal, metaphyseal and impacted fractures.

– **apophyseal fractures** are usually extra-articular avulsions of the insertions of some ligaments (always A1 fractures).

– **metaphyseal fractures** are either simple or multifragmentary (wedge or complex-their definition corresponds to that for diaphyseal segments).

– **impacted fractures** are stable fractures of the metaphysis or epiphysis in which the fragments are driven one into the other.

articular fractures involve the articular surface. They include partial and complete articular fractures.

partial articular fractures involve only part of the articular surface, while the rest of that surface remains attached to the diaphysis. The fractured joint surface can present different shapes:

– **pure split**: A fracture, resulting from a shearing force, in which the direction of the split is usually longitudinal.

– **pure depression**: An articular fracture in which there is pure depression of the articular surface without a split. The depression may be central or peripheral.

– **split depression**: A combination of a split and a depression, in which the joint fragments are usually separated.

– **multifragmentary depression**: A fracture in which part of the joint is depressed and the fragments are completely separated.

complete articular fractures: The articular surface is disrupted and completely separated from the diaphysis. The severity of these fractures depends on whether the articular surface shows a simple or a multifragmentary rupture or whether the metaphyseal component shows a simple or a multifragmentary (wedge or complex) fracture.

ESSENCE

The essence of a fracture determines its fracture Type, Group, or Subgroup. These are quite different in fractures of the diaphyses and those of the end segments. In fractures of the diaphysis *(fig 4)*, Type A is simple, Types B and C are multifragmentary fractures which are arranged not only in ascending order of morphological complexity, but also in ascending order of energy required to produce them. This arrangement also reflects the accompanying degree of soft tissue trauma. In the end segments, Type A are extra-articular fractures, Type B and C are articular fractures. Their hierarchical arrangement once again reflects not only the morphological complexity but also the energy required to produce them and the soft tissue trauma. Type B are partial articular fractures and Type C are complete articular fractures. For further details please see the accompanying schematic representations *(fig 5)*. The severity of the lesion can be seen by its colour. Green

Diaphyseal fractures

The 3 fracture Types and the 9 fracture Groups of the 4 diaphyseal segments are identical.

Essence: All diaphyseal fractures are divided into 3 Types according to the <u>contact between the two main fragments after reduction</u>: **A** contact > 90 % = simple fracture, **B** some contact = wedge fracture, **C** no contact = complex fracture

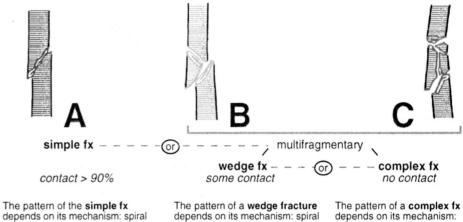

simple fx – – – – (or) – – – – – – multifragmentary

contact > 90%   wedge fx – – – (or) – – – complex fx
some contact   *no contact*

The pattern of the **simple fx** depends on its mechanism: spiral fracture, the result of torsion, oblique or transverse fractures, the result of bending

The pattern of a **wedge fracture** depends on its mechanism: spiral wedge, the result of torsion; bending wedge, the result of bending, fragmented wedge, the result of torsion or bending

The pattern of a **complex fx** depends on its mechanism: spiral complex fx are the result of torsion; segmental and irregular complex fx are usually the result of bending forces

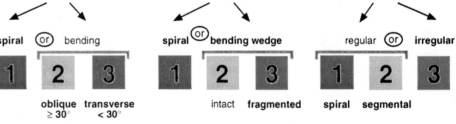

spiral (or) bending | spiral (or) bending wedge | regular (or) irregular

1 **2** **3** | **1** **2** **3** | **1** **2** **3**

oblique transverse
≥ 30° < 30° | intact fragmented | spiral segmental

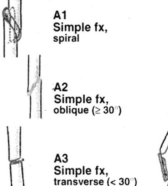

A1
Simple fx,
spiral

A2
Simple fx,
oblique (≥ 30°)

A3
Simple fx,
transverse (< 30°)

B1
Wedge fx,
spiral wedge

B2
Wedge fx,
bending wedge

B3
Wedge fx,
fragmented wedge

C1

Complex fx,

C2
Complex fx,
segmental

C3
Complex fx,
irregular

4   *Diaphyseal fractures.*

reflects a relatively benign low energy lesion with a generally good prognosis. Red reflects a high energy lesion with a serious prognosis.

BINARY SYSTEM OF QUESTIONS

Critics of classification systems [1] have maintained that classification systems are useless because of the high degree of intra- and inter-observer error. We feel that errors mostly result from lack of information. We have therefore designed a set of binary questions which is used as a checklist when classifying a fracture. Please note that the

questions differ when classifying a diaphyseal or an end segment. The first step in the classification of a fracture is the exact definition of its location. If a definite answer cannot be given to the set binary question then classification is not possible until further details become available, either through further imaging or, occasionally, as a result of information obtained at surgery.

■ ***Questions for a diaphyseal fracture*** *(fig 6A, B)*

Step 1. Defines the Type (A, B, C): Is the fracture simple (Type A) or multifragmentary (Type B or C)? If the fracture is

End segment fractures

The 3 fracture Types of 6 of the 8 end segments are identical.
(The 2 exceptions are the proximal segments of humerus and femur)

The fracture Groups of the end segments are different.
Example: 13- Distal humerus

Essence: The fractures of the distal segment of the humerus are divided into 3 Types:
A extra-articular, **B** partial articular, and **C** complete articular

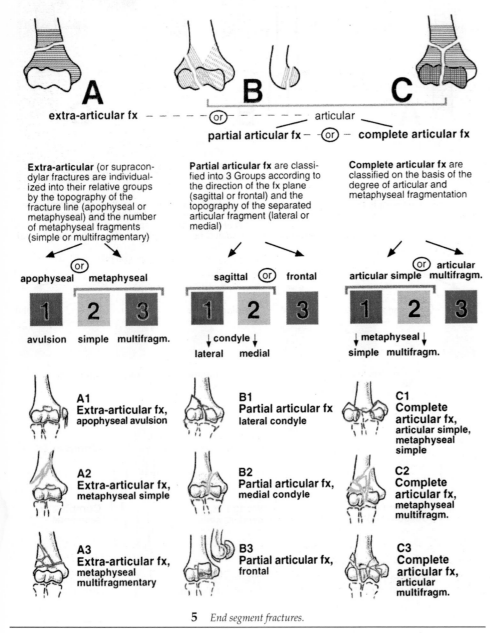

Extra-articular (or supracondylar fractures are individualized into their relative groups by the topography of the fracture line (apophyseal or metaphyseal) and the number of metaphyseal fragments (simple or multifragmentary)

Partial articular fx are classified into 3 Groups according to the direction of the fx plane (sagittal or frontal) and the topography of the separated articular fragment (lateral or medial)

Complete articular fx are classified on the basis of the degree of articular and metaphyseal fragmentation

A1
Extra-articular fx,
apophyseal avulsion

A2
Extra-articular fx,
metaphyseal simple

A3
Extra-articular fx,
metaphyseal
multifragmentary

B1
Partial articular fx
lateral condyle

B2
Partial articular fx,
medial condyle

B3
Partial articular fx,
frontal

C1
Complete
articular fx,
articular simple,
metaphyseal
simple

C2
Complete
articular fx,
metaphyseal
multifragm.

C3
Complete
articular fx,
articular
multifragm.

5   *End segment fractures.*

multifragmentary, it is a wedge fracture (Type B) where, after reduction, there is some contact between the fragments, or it is complex (Type C) where, after reduction, there is no contact between the main fragments.

Step 2. Defines the Group (1, 2, 3) (example for Type C): Is the complex fracture regular (C1 or C2) or is it irregular (Group C3)? If the complex fracture is regular, is it a spiral fracture (Group C1) or is it a segmental fracture (Group C2)?

Step 3. Which is the correct Subgroup?

Step 4. Which is the correct Qualification of the Subgroup?

■ *Questions for an end segment fracture* (fig 6C, D)

Step 1. Defines the Type (A, B, C): Is the fracture extra-articular (Type A) or articular (Type B or C)?

If the fracture is articular, is it partially articular (Type B) where the fracture involves only part of the articular surface, while the rest of that surface remains attached to the diaphysis? Or is it a complex articular fracture (Type C), where the articular surface is disrupted and completely separated from the diaphysis?

Step 2. Defines the Group (1, 2, 3) (example in a partial articular fracture of the distal humerus = Type B): Is the fracture sagittal (B1 or B2) or frontal (Group B3)? If it is sagittal, is it lateral (Group B1) or medial (Group B2)?

Step 3. Which is the correct Subgroup?

Step 4. Which is the correct Qualification of the Subgroup?

IMPORTANCE OF THE COMPREHENSIVE CLASSIFICATION OF FRACTURES

Classification of fractures is important for doctors, insurance companies and for politicians. The surgeon uses a classification to accurately identify the fracture to be treated, with all its specific problems. The insurance company, responsible for the payment, uses the classification to accurately assess what it is paying for, as well as to predict the potential cost of the disability. As governments assume a greater and greater responsibility for the provision of health care, politicians use the classification of fractures to study the incidence of specific injuries, their distribution and their association with employment or recreational activities, as well as to evaluate the effectiveness and outcome of treatment, and its impact on potential disability.

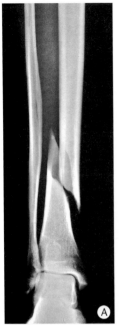
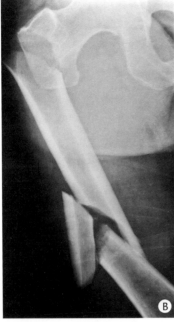
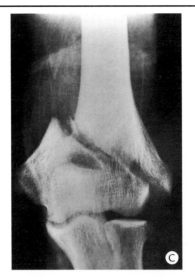
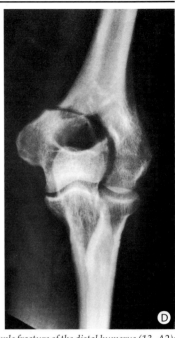

6 *The binary system of questions:*

A. How to proceed in a simple diaphyseal fracture of the tibia (42-A1):
1) Is the fracture **simple (A)** *or multifragmentary (B or C)?*
Type A = simple
2) If the fracture is simple, then is it **spiral (1)** *or bending (2 or 3)?*
Group A1 = simple, spiral fracture
3) If it is spiral, then you have 3 choices according to the location
Subgroup 3 = distal third
Diagnosis: Tibia/fibula diaphysis, simple spiral fracture, distal third
Alpha-numeric code: 42–A1.3

B. How to proceed in a complex diaphyseal fracture of the femur (32–C2):
1a) Is the fracture simple (A) or **multifragmentary (B or C)?**
1b) If it is multifragmentary, is it a wedge fracture (B) or a **complex** *fracture (C)?*
Type C = complex
2a) If the fracture is complex, then is it **regular (1 or 2)** *or irregular (3)?*
2b) If it is regular, is it spiral (1) or **segmental (2)?**
Group C2 = complex, regular, segmental fracture
3) If it is segmental, then you have 3 choices according to the number of fragments
Subgroup 2 = with an additional wedge fragment
4) To indicate the exact location of the segmental fracture and of the wedge, you have to look at the Qualifications of C3.2
+ Q2.4 = proximal diaphysiometaphyseal, wedge distal
Diagnosis: Femur diaphysis, complex, regular, segmental fracture proximal, diaphysiometaphyseal with an additional distal wedge fragment
Alpha-numeric code: 32–C2.2+Q2.4

C. How to proceed in an extra-articular simple fracture of the distal humerus (13–A2):
1) Is the fracture **extra-articular** *(A) or articular (B or C)?*
Type A = extra-articular
2a) If the fracture is extra-articular, then is it apophyseal (1 or 2) or **metaphyseal** *(2 or 3)?*
2b) If it is metaphyseal, is it **simple** *(2) or multifragmentary (3)?*
Group A2 = extra-articular, metaphyseal, simple
3) If it is metaphyseal, simple, then you have 3 choices according to the direction of the fracture line
Subgroup 2 = oblique downwards and outwards
Diagnosis: Extra-articular fracture, metaphyseal, simple, oblique downwards and outwards
Alpha-numeric code: 13–A2.2

D. How to proceed in a partial articular fracture of the distal humerus (13–B2):
1a) Is the fracture extra-articular (A) or **articular (B or C)?**
1b) If it is articular, is it **partial articular (B)** *or complete articular (C)?*
Type B = partial articular
2a) If the fracture is partial articular, then is it **sagittal (1 or 2)** *or frontal (3)?*
2b) If it is sagittal, is it lateral (1) or the **medial condyle (2)?**
Group B2 = partial articular, sagittal, medial condyle fracture
3) If it is a sagittal, medial condyle fracture, then you have 3 choices according to the transtrochlear location
Subgroup 2 = transtrochlear simple, through the groove
Diagnosis: Partial articular fracture, sagittal, medial condyle, transtrochlear simple through the groove
Alpha-numeric code: 13–B2.2

References

[1] Burstein AH. Fracture classification systems. Do they work and are they useful ? *J Bone Joint Surg Am* 1993 ; 75 : 1743-1744

[2] Müller ME. Klassifikation und internationale AO-Dokumentation der Femurfrakturen. *Unfallheilkunde* 1980 ; 83 : 251-259

[3] Müller ME, Allgöwer M, Schneider R, Willenegger H. Manual of internal fixation. Berlin : Springer-Verlag, 1970

[4] Müller ME, Allgöwer M, Schneider R, Willenegger H. Manual of internal fixation. Berlin : Springer-Verlag, 1979

[5] Müller ME, Nazarian S. Classification et documentation AO des fractures du fémur. *Rev Chir Orthop* 1981 ; 67 : 297-309

[6] Müller ME, Nazarian S, Koch P. Classification AO des fractures. Tome I. Les os longs. Berlin : Springer-Verlag, 1987

[7] Müller ME, Nazarian S, Koch P, Schatzker J. The comprehensive classification of fractures of long bones. Heidelberg : Springer-Verlag, 1990

[8] Müller ME, Nazarian S, Schatzker J. CCF comprehensive classification of fractures. Pamphlets I and II. Bern : ME Müller Foundation, 1996

[9] Orozco R, Sales JM, Videla M. Atlas of internal fixation. Fractures of long bones. Heidelberg : Springer-Verlag, 1999

[10] Orthopaedic trauma association, committee for coding and classification. Fracture and dislocation compendium. *J Orthop Trauma* 1996 ; 10 (suppl 1) : 1-155

Fractures with arterial lesions

AE Beris
PN Soucacos

Abstract. – Fractures with arterial lesions run a high risk of leading to muscle necrosis, partial or complete amputation with loss of an extremity and/or its function. It is of paramount importance that the surgeon recognise the implications of the potential or actual vascular injury in order to maximise management of the outcome. Although open fractures run the greatest risk of being combined with an arterial injury, closed fractures may also be associated with a significant vascular lesion.

An important factor in the prognosis of fractures with arterial lesions is ischaemia time. Rapid and proper patient transport with a subsequent decrease in warm ischaemia time are critical factors in decreasing the rate of amputation following severe trauma to the extremities.

On admission, a detailed clinical evaluation should be carried out. When there is clear evidence of arterial injury, the surgeon should not delay treatment by performing arteriography. The principles in the management of acute vascular injuries involve haemorrhage control, timely correction of the ischaemia and careful prevention of potential complications.

Debridement is a critical factor for obtaining good results, particularly for open fractures. The "4 Cs" are a helpful rule of thumb for the surgeon during debridement: Contractility, Colour, Consistency and Capacity to bleed.

In most IIIC fractures, external fixation is recommended as initial treatment. After 2 to 3 weeks, it can be changed to intermedullary nailing or plates and screws. The surgical sequence varies according to the time of cold or warm ischaemia involved. If close to the end of the permitted ischaemia time, the surgeon should proceed directly to revascularisation.

Early wound coverage by local flaps or vascularised tissue transfer minimises infection rate and hospital stay and promotes early bone union.

© 2001, Editions Scientifiques et Médicales Elsevier SAS. All rights reserved.

Keywords: fractures, arteries, open fractures, ischaemia, thrombosis, aneurysm, repair.

Introduction

The potential for serious vascular injury in fractures and dislocations is related to the site and mechanism of skeletal injury. The vasculature of the extremities is vulnerable to trauma in fractures of the skeleton, primarily because of the proximity of the vessels to the bones, their fixed placement around the joints, and their superficial position. Thus, vascular injury should be anticipated with fractures and/or dislocations in vulnerable anatomical areas, such as the knee, elbow and shoulder. Fractures with arterial lesions run a high risk of leading to muscle necrosis, partial or complete amputation with loss of the extremity and/or its function.

Alexandros E Beris, M.D.
Panayiotis N Soucacos, M.D., FACS.
Department of Orthopaedic Surgery, University of Ioannina, School of Medicine, Ioannina 451 10, Greece.

It is of paramount importance that the surgeon recognise the implications of the potential or actual vascular injury to maximise management of the outcome. Survival or not of a limb with combined bony and vascular damage is closely related to the severity of the injury and the timely diagnosis and treatment of the vascular trauma. The focus should not only be on treating the skeletal injury, but primarily on diagnosing and treating the vascular lesion, as well as identifying any damage to nerves, muscles and tendons. To avoid detrimental sequelae, it is better for the surgeon to presume a fracture is complicated with vascular or nerve injury until it be proven otherwise.

Open fractures with arterial lesions

Open fractures may be complicated by arterial lesions. Gustilo and Anderson [11] provided a prognostic classification system for open fractures based predominately on wound size.

– Type I open fractures have a puncture wound with injury to the skin (1 cm or less) from the inside out.

– Type II fractures have a larger skin trauma (> 1 cm) and moderate soft tissue injury.

– Open Type III fractures are the result of a high energy impact, such as those produced in shotgun injuries, traffic accidents and farm accidents, among others. They have a skin defect greater than 10 cm, a comminuted fracture with bone loss, extensive soft tissue and possible vascular injury and are associated with the worst prognosis.

Type III open fractures can be categorised into three subgroups [12]:

– Type IIIA fractures have adequate soft tissue coverage despite the extensive soft tissue injury (local flaps are adequate).

– Type IIIB and particularly Type IIIC open fractures of both the upper and lower extremities are extremely severe injuries that frequently result in limb amputation. High energy impact in Type IIIB fractures results in extensive bony comminution or segmental bone loss, pronounced soft tissue injury, including extensive skin loss, tendon and nerve damage, and muscular and periosteal stripping from the bone.

– Type IIIC fractures are characterised by severe circulatory compromise of the extremity related to complete ischaemia secondary to trauma of the major vessels [21].

The severity of Type IIIB and Type IIIC fractures is emphasised by the high amputation rate. Type IIIB fractures are associated with a rate of amputation of about 16%, while the amputation rate of Type IIIC fractures is as high as 60% to 100% [19, 22]. In type IIIB and IIIC fractures, wound coverage may necessitate the use of vascularised or pedicled fasciocutaneous flaps, or muscle graft.

The aim in treatment today is not just to salvage the limb, but to produce a functional, painless extremity with protective sensation.

Closed fractures with arterial lesions

Although vascular damage occurring in conjunction with fracture-dislocations of the lower extremity is uncommon [5], various vascular injuries can occur from fracture-dislocations, including compression, puncture, laceration and transection. Closed fractures can produce an arterial lesion due to direct injury from the fracture ends. Comminuted fractures may cause arterial lesions by insertion of a bone spike in the artery at the moment of fracture or later during transportation, or during uncontrolled movements or spasms as in drunken states or epileptic seizures. The surgeon should remember that Doppler signals and palpable pulses do not necessarily exclude vascular injury, and that missed diagnosis runs the risk of subsequent amputation, even in closed fractures.

Prognosis

An important factor in the prognosis of fractures with arterial lesions is ischaemia time; the outcome is time dependent. In general, the time limit for warm ischaemia in parts with bulky muscles is about 6 hours [13]. This can be extended up to 12 hours when the part is transported under conditions of cold ischaemia. In cases of trauma to parts with little or no muscle, such as the hand, fingers or foot, the time limit for warm ischaemia can be extended to almost 12 hours, and to 24 hours or more for cold ischaemia.

Rapid and proper patient transport, with a subsequent decrease in warm ischaemia time, are critical factors in decreasing the rate of amputation following severe trauma to the extremities. For transport, a completely amputated part is wrapped in wet gauzes, enclosed in two plastic bags and immersed in a mixture of water and ice (three-parts water to one-part ice). For patients who have fractures with arterial damage and ischaemia of the peripheral part, the limb should be repositioned and immobilised with a posterior splint. A plastic bag containing the water and ice mixture can then be placed around the ischaemic part only.

Time limits refer to real ischaemia time: that is, the time from the accident (and not the time the patient arrives at the hospital) to the time of revascularisation. It is of paramount importance to give exact instructions for the cold ischaemia measures to be taken by those transporting the patient. The importance of cold ischaemia should not be underestimated and should be kept in mind throughout time-consuming procedures, including radiographic examination and other clinical tests and even in the operating theatre.

PROGNOSTIC SCORING SYSTEMS

With growing experience in managing fractures with vascular lesions, surgeons now realise that prognosis is closely dependent on injury to the vessels, nerves, muscle and bone deep in the wound, rather than surface characteristics. Thus, decisions regarding salvageability and outcome cannot accurately be made until the first debridement is complete.

Orthopaedic surgeons are occasionally confronted with extremities that are so mangled that salvage is questionable. Attempts have been made to establish criteria that surgeons can use to determine which severely injured limbs should be salvaged and which should undergo primary amputation.

Several variables play a decisive role in determining the outcome and success of preserving a limb, particularly for open fractures. These include the extent and severity of vascular injury, bone and soft tissue damage, type and duration of limb ischaemia, the patient's age, time elapsed since the initial injury and surgery and the presence of concomitant organ injuries [21]. To help the surgeon determine which limbs should be salvaged and which should be amputated first, several scales using a variety of criteria have been proposed for assessing the severity of the injury. These include the mangled extremity syndrome (MES) [8], the mangled extremity severity score (MESS) [13], and NISSSA (Nerve, ischaemia, soft tissue injury, skeletal injury, shock and age) [18].

MESS takes into account various important parameters for assessing survival of an injured lower limb including age, ischaemia time, local conditions and shock. The sum of these parameters is used to direct the surgeon toward either salvage procedures or amputation. A MESS of 7 to 12 points is a strong indication that the surgeon should proceed to primary amputation. In general, the MESS scoring system holds promise as being a good, objective scoring system for predicting poor outcome and justifying amputation *(table I)*. Lange [16] proposed absolute and relative indications which, in conjunction with the MESS system, provide a helpful guide to determine when to amputate in serious open IIIC tibial fractures. According to Lange, absolute indications for primary amputation include anatomically complete disruption of the posterior tibial nerve in adults and crush injuries with warm ischaemia greater than 6 hours. Relative indications include serious polytrauma, severe ipsilateral foot trauma and anticipated protracted problems in obtaining soft tissue coverage.

The MESS system refers to the lower extremity and Lange [16] to the open IIIC tibial fracture. For the upper extremity the tendency is more toward salvage.

Clinical signs and assessment of arterial injury

On admission, all patients should be examined thoroughly with measures taken to stabilise their general condition. They should be given tetanus prophylaxis and started on antibiotics, as needed, after cultures have been obtained. A broad spectrum cephalosporin is usually sufficient for low impact injuries, while an aminoglycoside (gentamicin) is added for more severe wounds. In severe crush injuries or those with vascular compromise, particularly when there is a high risk of contamination, such as in farm injuries, penicillin G should be administered. A detailed clinical evaluation for colour, temperature, pulsation mobility, sensation and wound condition should be carried out. Culture of the wound, radiographic analysis and Doppler control should be routinely performed. The severity of an arterial injury depends on the extent of vessel damage, collateral circulation and the presence of shock. Every fracture must be checked for additional injury to vessels or nerves. Careful neurovascular examination is imperative in the treatment of open fractures or shotgun injuries. The surgeon must be aware that the absence of haemorrhage or severe signs of ischaemia do not necessarily preclude serious vascular injury. Pulsatile bleeding is a clear sign of arterial injury, as is a large or expanding haematoma. Differences in the colour of the extremities, such as a pale colour of the injured limb, must alert the surgeon to establish a diagnosis rapidly.

Table I. – Mangled Extremity Severity Score. (Reproduced by permission from Helfet CK, Howey T, Sanders R, et al. Limb salvage versus amputation: Preliminary results of the mangled extremity severity score. Clin Othop 1990; 256: 80-86).

Type	Characteristics	Injuries	Points
Skeletal/soft-tissue Group			
1	Low energy	Stab wounds, simple closed fractures, small-calibre gunshot wounds	1
2	Medium energy	Open or multiple-level fractures, dislocations, moderate crush injuries	2
3	High energy	Shotgun blast (close range) high-velocity gunshot wounds	3
4	Massive crush	Logging, railroad, oil rig accidents	4
Shock Group			
1	Normotensive haemodynamics	BP stable in field and in OR	0
2	Transiently hypotensive	BP unstable in field but responsive to intravenous fluids	1
3		Systolic BP less than 90 mm Hg in field and responsive to intravenous fluid only in OR	2
Ischaemia Group			
1	None	A pulsatile limb without signs of ischaemia	0*
2	Mild	Diminished pulses without signs of ischaemia	1*
3	Moderate	No pulse by Doppler, sluggish capillary refill paraesthesia, diminished motor activity	2*
4	Advanced	Pulseless, cool, paralysed and numb without capillary refill	3*
Age Group			
1	< 30 years		0
2	> 30 < 50 years		1
3	> 50 years		2

* Points x 2 of ischaemic time exceeding six hours.
OR: operating room;
BP: blood pressure

The pulse should be equal in both extremities. A diminished or absent pulse strongly suggests partial or complete obstruction of normal blood flow. When clinical examination indicates an absent or diminished pulse, a thorough evaluation of the circulation in the extremity should be performed. This can be easily done with a portable Doppler device, a powerful tool for the rapid assessment of arterial injury in trauma patients. The detection of an arterial signal suggests limb viability. However, it is important to bear in mind that the arterial signal confirms distal patency, and does not exclude proximal vascular injury [1]. In addition, the Doppler device is valuable when pulse palpation is obscured by haemorrhage or oedema.

Johansen [15] described the importance of measuring the ankle-brachial systolic pressure ratio where the normal ankle-brachial systolic pressure ratio is > 0.95. A difference of less than 20 mm Hg (ratio < 0.9) between the extremities is indicative of vascular injury. Overall, the ankle-brachial systolic pressure index for detecting arterial injury is a fast and useful tool, with a specificity of 97% and an overall accuracy of 95% [15]. Duplex ultrasonography can also reliably detect injury to arteries or veins, the presence of arteriovenous fistulas and pseudo-aneurysms. Care must be taken to distinguish between arterial and venous flow. This can be done by differentiating between the magnitude of the signal produced by an artery compared to a vein (the signal is greater for arteries), with subtle changes in the positioning of the probe. The Allen test should also be applied for fractures below the elbow (bifurcation) in order to assess whether the lesion is on the ulnar or radial artery. The Allen test is performed by the patient forming a tight fist. The surgeon then applies pressure and occludes both the ulnar and radial arteries. The patient opens his hand and the surgeon then releases one artery and observes the blood return to the hand; the procedure is repeated for the other artery. If on releasing the artery, the hand does not fill with blood quickly, then there is vascular damage to that artery.

In some cases the limb may be in a position where the bony ends of the fracture site are pressing against the vessel, resulting in a pulseless extremity. The surgeon should proceed with gentle reduction and immobilisation of the fracture and then reassess the circulation of the limb. If there is no return of the pulse, the surgeon should proceed to the operating room without delay.

When there is clear evidence of arterial injury and the site and mechanism of injury have been established, the surgeon should not delay treatment by performing arteriography. Angiography is recommended for patients with complete ischaemia when the limb is without pulsation, or in patients with incomplete ischaemia and when Doppler control suggests major arterial compromise. In a few select cases arteriography can be used to identify occult injury in patients with an abnormal physical examination or when the anatomical localisation of the injury is ambiguous.

Indications for arteriography include:

– multilevel trauma where the exact site cannot be determined;

– knee dislocation or tibial plateau fracture associated with diminished or absent pulse;

– leg or forearm injury with equivocal arterial injury;

– patients with pre-existing arterial disease who have an ischaemic limb;

– suspected arteriovenous fistulas [1].

Displaced fractures of the distal femur and proximal tibia, particularly knee dislocations, have a high risk of concomitant vascular injury and poor collateral circulation to support the distal limb. Angiography is highly recommended for these injuries [5]. An absolute contraindication to arteriography is a history of allergic reactions to contrast media.

For unstable patients, arteriography is best performed in the operating room by a direct needle injection into an arterial segment proximal to the injury site. In injuries of the lower limb when a pulse cannot be clearly detected, the surgeon should expose the proximal superficial femoral artery and clamp it to produce occlusion during the injection of 30 ml of contrast. When patients are stable, they should be evaluated in the arteriography suite. Arterial damage is indicated by an arrest of contrast media, irregular vessel shape, abnormal luminal or venous filling or the expansion of a false aneurysm.

Initial treatment

After the initial evaluation of the patient and assessment of other injuries, the wound is dressed using a sterile technique, the limb is splinted and the patient is taken to the operating room. The extremity is cleaned and a final evaluation is made. During preparations, haemorrhage can be controlled by direct pressure on the arterial wound or proximal vascular structures. Care must be taken if tourniquets are used, as they may increase distal ischaemia. In general, tourniquets are rarely required. Surgeons should also avoid clamping of deep bleeding vessels; it is ineffective and may injure adjacent nerves, increase vascular injury and ultimately compromise subsequent repair. Surgical exploration is indicated with expanding haematomas, which are suggestive of continuing arterial haemorrhage. If delayed, shock, nerve compression, compartment syndrome, or false aneurysm formation may ensue.

If the initial examination suggests obstruction of blood flow as indicated by a diminished or absent pulse, the initial treatment should focus on correction of hypotension and shock. The persistence of ischaemia after management of shock indicates arterial obstruction. As the obstruction of blood flow is caused by some form of arterial interruption, the surgeon should proceed with reduction of any fracture-dislocation which may be the causative factor for extrinsic arterial obstruction or entrapment.

An abnormally harsh, intermittent and oscillatory Doppler signal (bruit) is indicative of an abnormal arteriovenous connection. The early manifestations may include distal ischaemia, arterial thrombosis, false aneurysm and limb oedema and the surgeon is advised to proceed with immediate exploration and vascular repair. This may be delayed if the limb is viable and treatment of other injuries is more pressing.

Blunt injury revascularisation following prolonged ischaemia or deep venous thrombosis often produces a diffuse swelling of the injured extremity. Oedema may also compress the vascular system and soft tissues and further augment ischaemia. It is important to keep in mind that compartment syndrome can also develop in open fractures [2]. In these cases, compartmental pressure should be measured to assess the need for fasciotomy, where incision of the muscle fascia decompresses the affected muscle compartment. A catheter should be inserted into the muscle compartment to determine pressure. Normal compartment pressure is less than 10 mm Hg. Fasciotomy is indicated with compartmental hypertension greater than 40 mm Hg. Fasciotomy is performed with a wide incision across the overlying skin and fascia. A lateral approach is preferred over the leg where all four muscle compartments may have to be decompressed. The surgeon must always be aware of compartment syndrome; particularly in the sedated or unconscious patient, compartment pressure measurements are critical [8]. The criteria for

fasciotomy in vulnerable areas (forearm, tibia and foot) vary according to the method used for measuring compartment pressure. With the older method of continuous infusion monitoring, fasciotomy is recommended when tissue pressure rises above 45 mm Hg. If a self-contained needle manometer is used, fasciotomy should be performed when the compartment pressure rises to within 10 to 30 mm Hg of the patient's diastolic pressure. When uncertain, it is better to perform an unnecessary fasciotomy than not to do one that is needed.

Treatment

The principles in the management of fractures with acute vascular injuries involve haemorrhage control, timely correction of the ischaemia and treatment of fractures and soft tissue injury. Often the treatment can be performed by two orthopaedic teams: a bone team and a vascular team. The bone group debrides the wound and fixes the bone, while the vascular group prepares the contralateral upper or lower limb for a vascular graft. A shunt can temporarily restore blood flow while fixation of the bone takes place. In general, bone fixation is essential because it stabilises the bone and allows for the fine manipulations necessary to perform micro-anastomosis. In addition, further damage to repaired arteries and veins by the gross movements often needed in bone fixation can be avoided by microvascular repair after external fixation of the bone.

DEBRIDEMENT

Debridement is a critical factor for obtaining good results, particularly for open fractures. Surgical enlargement of the wound for an accurate assessment of damage should be done by extensile incisions. This preserves skin viability as well as allowing bone stabilisation later. Before extending the incisions, however, the surgeon needs to carefully consider later wound coverage, so that debridement can be performed through incisions which can be utilised for future pedicle or fasciocutaneous flap advancement in severe open injuries [4].

After adequate exposure has been achieved, the wound is irrigated liberally (6-10 litres) with Ringer's lactate using a pulsed lavage system. Ringer's lactate may be combined with antibiotics. The surgeon should begin debriding wound edges and then proceed to deeper tissues until all necrotic tissue is excised with care taken not to harm intact neurovascular structures. The "4 Cs" are a helpful rule of thumb for the surgeon during debridement: Contractility, Colour, Consistency and Capacity to bleed [10]. Muscle tissue which fails to contract when pinched is pale, disintegrates to the touch and fails to bleed should it be excised.

Skeletal injury should also be assessed and the bone cleaned. Free cortical and grossly contaminated fragments need to be removed, while those with adequate soft tissue attached should be kept. For severe open tibial fractures, the availability of viable soft tissues for bony coverage dictates the extent of additional bone debridement [4]. Finally, it must be stressed that meticulous wound care is essential for the successful management of open fractures, regardless of the type of skeletal fixation ultimately used.

SKELETAL REPAIR

Stabilisation of the skeleton right after debridement improves venous return and local revascularisation, as well as preventing additional soft tissue damage from excessive motion. Stable fixation minimises pain and allows easier surgical access, as well as patient mobilisation. However, it is important for the surgeon to keep in mind that surgical sequence can vary according to ischaemia time. If close to the end of the permitted ischaemia time, the surgeon should proceed directly to revascularisation, either by vascular repair or shunting techniques.

The selection of the skeletal fixation (locked intramedullary nails, plates and screws or external fixation) depends on the location and extent of the wound and the preference of the surgeon. Low velocity injuries can usually be managed as closed fractures, while several factors should be considered in the skeletal fixation of high velocity injuries. The vascularisation of the bone is one such consideration.

Types I, II, IIIA should be managed as closed fractures with the method preferred by the surgeon. Types IIIB and IIIC are better treated with an appropriate external fixator that allows stabilisation and easy access to the wound. Good results have been obtained by the primary use of intramedullary nails but this remains to be proved (Singer RW, Kellan JF. Open tibial diaphyseal fractures: results of an unreamed locked intramedullary nailing. Clin Orthop 1995; 315: 114-119). For tibial fractures, external fixators are the only definitive method of treatment because they do not interfere with the mobilisation of joints and muscle. After an initial use of the external fixator (2-3 weeks) and if the soft tissue envelope permits, the method of fixation is changed to either intramedullary nails for almost all bones, or plate and screws for femur, humerus, radius and ulna.

However, in the presence of extensive soft tissue injury (e.g. Type IIIB), bones such as the femur or humerus should also be managed initially with an external fixator. The wound and joints can be stabilised with minimal soft tissue compromise in open or degloved fracture-dislocations using internal fixation with lag screws and external fixation away from the wound.

Fixation techniques for open fractures of the femur are more dependent on anatomical

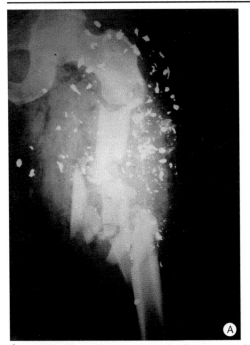 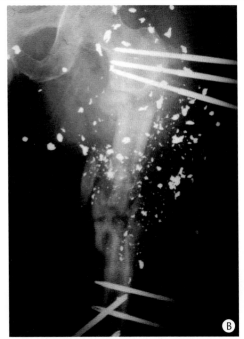 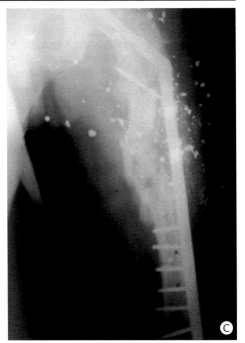

1   A. This 55 year old male sustained a shotgun wound in his left femur with a IIIC
comminuted fracture and laceration of the femoral artery.
B. After his resuscitation, the femur was stabilised with an external fixation device and the femoral artery was grafted with a 6 cm saphenous vein graft.

C. After 3 months, the external fixator was changed to a long angled nail plate as a
bridging plate. Six months later (9 months after the injury), he could walk with full
weight-bearing and with knee flexion of 0-130°.

location than on the type of wound in Type
I, II, IIIA fractures. Intertrochanteric and
subtrochanteric fractures can be effectively
managed with a sliding hip screw or, for the
latter, second or third generation
intramedullary nails can also be used. A
reamed, interlocked intramedullary nail is
appropriate for femoral shaft or distal
fractures without an increase in infection [3].
Type IIIB and IIIC fractures should be
managed initially with external fixation.

In contrast to the femur, fixation of the tibia
is problematic. Because of the poor soft
tissue coverage and vascular supply, plates
and screws and reamed intramedullary nails
are associated with an unacceptably high
rate of infection and should not be applied.
Initial bony stabilisation of the tibia should
be achieved with external fixation. Although
the bone is stabilised without risking further
injury to the blood supply, external fixation
is associated with non-union, malunion, pin
loosening and pin tract infection [20].
Although axial control is difficult, recent
studies indicate that unreamed, interlocked,
intramedullary nails permit excellent bony
alignment, union and low to minimal
infection rates for tibial fractures types I, II,
IIIA and in some cases IIIB [8]. However, in
Singer's (1985) report on intramedullary
nails for IIIA and IIIB tibial fractures, there
was 12% infection and 20% compartment
syndrome. Type IIIC fractures of the tibia
require initial external fixation *(fig 1)*.

VASCULAR REPAIR

The surgical sequence varies according to
the time of cold or warm ischaemia
involved. If close to the end of the permitted
ischaemia time, the surgeon should proceed

directly to revascularisation [17]. This can be
achieved either by vascular repair or
shunting techniques. If the ischaemia time
has been prolonged, the surgeon may opt to
restore perfusion promptly with a temporary
intraluminal shunt, before proceeding to
more time-consuming vascular repair [14].
Although vascular repair should be done
first when no arterial flow is detected by
Doppler ultrasound testing and particularly
if a neurological deficit secondary to
ischaemia is present, bony stabilisation may
need to precede vascular repair. This may
be the case when the bony skeleton is very
unstable, the joints are dislocated, or when
subsequent skeletal manipulations run the
risk of disrupting any arterial reconstruction.
In cases where skeletal repair should
precede vascular repair, shunting techniques
become an invaluable tool. A intraluminal
shunt can be used to secure adequate blood
flow to the limb temporarily.

The aim of vascular repair is to restore a
normal blood flow by securing and
maintaining arterial and venous patency.
Collateral vessels in the forearm and leg
often provide normal perfusion when an
isolated artery is occluded. In these cases,
reconstruction may not be required. On the
other hand, when the extremity is ischaemic,
both arterial continuity and venous outflow
must be restored to avoid early thrombosis,
limb loss or chronic functional ischaemia.

Once the extremity is prepped, adequate
exposure should be achieved to permit
control of vessels proximal and distal to the
wound site. A longitudinal incision over the
vessel is preferred, as it allows extension in
both directions to control bleeding. Only the
popliteal artery should be exposed, using a

medial transverse incision to allow proximal
and distal extension as required.

Until vascular control can be achieved, the
surgeon should not attempt to remove
penetrating objects. Frequently, manual
compression of the brachial artery against
the humerus or of the femoral artery at the
inguinal ligament is sufficient to control
bleeding and allow exposure of a more
distal arterial injury. Ligation of the
collateral vessels should be kept to a
minimum and superficial veins should be
preserved for possible use as vascular grafts.

Surgical treatment of the vascular injury
depends on the mechanism and type of
injury (laceration, transection or blunt
injury). A laceration injury to a vessel is
caused by the impact and penetration of a
object, such as a bullet, glass or bone and is
defined as a tear in the vessel wall. The
presence of an intact vessel wall prevents
retraction and closure of the wound and
leads to persistent bleeding. Debridement of
the vessel wall followed by primary suture
or end-to-end anastomosis is usually
sufficient to manage a simple laceration. If a
small segment of the vessel is resected
(about 1 cm), proximal and distal
mobilisation (about 6 cm) is usually
sufficient to permit primary anastomosis.
Anticoagulation with systemic heparin is
recommended. If this cannot be done
because of other injuries or shock, then
diluted heparin (100 U/ml) should be
instilled in both proximal and distal vessels.

A transection injury is defined as a complete
laceration. Retraction and spasm of the
arterial ends and formation of a temporary
thrombus prevents the persistent bleeding
seen with a simple laceration injury. Delayed

bleeding may be observed in these injuries, due to spasm relaxation or dislodgement of the thrombus. A blunt injury may result in partial or complete transection of the intima, without medial or adventitial disruption, leading ultimately to progressive obstruction and thrombosis. Sometimes, complete obstruction may not occur for hours or days after injury. Characteristic of a contused vessel is the bluish discoloration.

The principles of microsurgery should always by kept in mind: anastomosis on normal vessel edges under normal tension with a perfect technique. When arterial injury is extensive, bridging the defect with a vein graft is the treatment of choice.

The great saphenous vein of the uninjured leg is preferred for venous grafts. When not available, the lesser saphenous, cephalic or basilic veins are also appropriate. These will avoid compromise of venous return in the injured extremity. The use of vein grafts is a time-consuming procedure; it doubles the surgical time for vascular anastomosis. However, it does offer the benefit of performing vessel anastomosis without tension and on healthy intima.

Once arterial repair has been achieved, it is usually advised to postpone venous repair for 10-15 minutes. This allows the blood flow to revascularise the muscles without introducing any residual metabolic waste into circulation. The anaesthesiologist must be made aware if this occurs, in order to replace any additional blood loss.

Upon completion of vessel repair, the reperfused muscles are evaluated. All devitalised tissues are surgically debrided and fasciotomies should be performed at this moment. This is because even if all the compartments are open, there is still an opportunity for compartment syndrome to occur in IIIC open fractures [2].

Arteriovenous fistulas should be repaired by interrupting the fistula tract and then restoring continuity of the artery and vein. This can frequently be achieved by local debridement and direct suture, although the surgical technique depends on the extent of injury.

Once vascular repair is complete, evaluation should take place while still in the operating room. Evaluation of arterial repair consists of performing the patency test and inspecting for adequate distal perfusion of the tissues. It is recommended that the surgeon administer dextran or heparin during and immediately after the procedure to help maintain patency. The vessel and the site of vascular repair should be covered with viable tissue (skin or muscle).

COVERAGE AND POSTOPERATIVE MANAGEMENT

Skin should be just reapproximated but never under tension. In doing so, the surgeon needs to take into consideration not only the condition at the end of the operation, but also the oedema that follows after an extensive procedure. Temporary coverage can be obtained with sterile dressing sponges soaked in normal saline placed over the wound. However, since this can lead to wound dessication, a synthetic biological dressing is preferred. Biological dressings (e.g. Epiguard®) are applied like skin grafts and then are covered with sterile dressing to prevent drying.

Post-operative management should include antibiotics, particularly for open injuries. A second generation cephalosporin plus aminoglycosides for 5 days are adequate. These may be continued subsequently, according to culture and antibiotic sensitivity tests.

Patients who have experienced work-related accidents, such as farmyard injuries, or who have severely contaminated open wounds should also be given penicillin. Patients with open IIIB or IIIC fractures should be brought into the operating room every second to third day for wound inspection and debridement until no necrotic tissue remains. After subsequent debridements to ensure that the zone of injury is clean, closure of the soft tissue wound should take place. Ideally, this should be done within 5 to 7 days, and can be achieved by delayed primary closure, split thickness skin grafting, local flaps or vascularised free tissue transfer as determined by the final defect size and composition. This aggressive approach has changed the prognosis of open fractures by diminishing the postoperative infection rate, the number of additional operations, the hospital stay and the time needed for union [7].

Bone grafting and other secondary reconstruction procedures are recommended 4 to 8 weeks after wound closure. In cases of bone defects, these can be covered by conventional techniques (spongiosa) if less than 5 cm, or by either bone transport or free vascularised bone transplantation (mainly free fibula) for longer defects.

Finally, the early re-establishment of a physiological wound barrier is essential for preventing dessication and contamination of open wounds [4]. In this regard, the surgeon should keep in mind that debridement alone, no matter how adequate, is not always sufficient in preventing infection of open wounds.

References

[1] Bandyk DF. Vascular injury associated with extremity trauma. *Clin Orthop* 1995; 318: 117-124

[2] Blick S, Brumback R, Poka A, Burgess A. Compartment syndrome in open tibial fractures. *J Bone Joint Surg Am* 1986; 68: 1348-1353

[3] Chapman MW. The role of intramedullary fixation in open fractures. *Clin Orthop* 1986; 212: 26-42

[4] Cole JD, Ansel LJ, Schwartzberg R. A sequential protocol for management of severe open tibial fractures. *Clin Orthop* 1995; 315: 84-103

[5] Cone JB. Vascular injury associated with fractures - Dislocations of the lower extremity. *Clin Orthop* 1989; 243: 30-35

[6] Dennis JW, Jagger C, Butcher JL et al. Reassessing the role of arteriograms in the management of posterior knee dislocations. *J Trauma* 1993; 35: 692-697

[7] Godina M. Early microsurgical reconstruction of complex trauma of the extremities. *Plast Reconstr Surg* 1986; 78: 285

[8] Gregory P, Sanders R. The management of severe fractures of the lower extremities. *Clin Orthop* 1995; 318: 95-105

[9] Gregory RT, Gould RJ, Peclet M et al. The mangled extremity syndrome (MES): A severity grading system for multi-system injury of the extremity. *J Trauma* 1985; 25: 1147-1150

[10] Gustilo RB. Management of open fractures and their complications. Philadelphia: WB Saunders, 1982

[11] Gustilo RB, Anderson JT. Prevention of infection in the treatment of one thousand and twenty-five open fractures of long bones. *J Bone Joint Sur Am* 1976; 58: 453-458

[12] Gustilo RB, Mendoza RM, Williams DN. Problems in the management of Type III (severe) open fractures: A new classification of Type III open fractures. *J Trauma* 1984; 24: 742-746

[13] Helfet CK, Howey T, Sanders R et al. Limb salvage versus amputation: Preliminary results of the mangled extremity severity score. *Clin Orthop* 1990; 256: 80-86

[14] Johansen K, Bandyk DF, Thiele BL, Hansen ST. Use of temporary intraluminal shunt: Resolution of a management dilemma in complex vascular injuries. *J Trauma* 1982; 22: 395-398

[15] Johansen K, Lynch K, Paun M, Copass M. Non-invasive vascular tests reliably exclude occult arterial trauma in injured extremities. *J Trauma* 1991; 31: 515-522

[16] Lange RH. Limb reconstruction versus amputation decision making in massive lower extremity trauma. *Clin Orthop* 1989; 243: 92-99

[17] Lemaire R. Traitement des lésions ostéo-articulaires associées à des lésions vasculaires traumatiques. *Acta Chir Belg* 1982; 5: 449-456

[18] McNamara MG, Heckman JD, Corley FG. Severe open fractures of the lower extremity: A retrospective evaluation of the mangled extremity severity score (MESS). *J Orthop Trauma* 1994; 8: 81-87

[19] Ritchie AJ, Small JO, Hart NB et al. Type III tibial fractures in the elderly: Results of 23 fractures in 20 patients. *Injury* 1991; 22: 267-270

[20] Rommens P, Gielen J, Broos P, Gruwez J. Intrinsic problems with the external fixation device of Hoffmann-Vidal-Adrey: A critical evaluation of 11 patients with complex tibial shaft fractures. *J Trauma* 1989; 29: 630-638

[21] Soucacos PN, Beris AE, Xenakis TA, Malizos KN, Vekris MD. Open type IIIB and IIIC fractures treated by an orthopaedic microsurgical team. *Clin Orthop* 1995; 314: 59-66

[22] Zehntner MK, Petropoulos P, Burch H. Factors determing the outcome in fractures of the extremities associated with arterial injuries. *J Orthop Trauma* 1991; 5: 29-33

Management of nonunions: an overview

R Lemaire

Abstract. – This chapter reviews the basic methods (with their indications and contraindications) which may be applied to the treatment of nonunions: internal fixation, external fixation, including the various modalities of compression/distraction osteogenesis possible with annular or unilateral fixators. Combined internal and external fixation is also described. The various techniques of bone grafting are mentioned, whether performed as isolated procedures or combined with internal or external fixation. The indications and results of vascularised bone or composite osteo(myo)cutaneous grafts are presented. The issue of soft tissue coverage is also addressed with reference to local or free flaps. The chapter ends with reflections on the general treatment strategy, whereby a selection may be made between totally different techniques; these techniques must fit into a global strategy that always leaves alternative treatments possible in case of failure. Such factors as the burden of the treatment to the patient, donor site morbidity, and the potential of each technique for minor and major complications, must always be taken into consideration. The treatment must be tailored to the individual case to address all components of the problem. Finally, a survey is presented of available adjunctive non-surgical means to enhance bone healing, such as electrical stimulation, ultrasound, extracorporeal shock waves, bone marrow injection and osteogenic factors.

Keywords: fracture nonunion, pseudarthrosis, internal fixation, external fixation, bone graft, distraction osteogenesis, nonsurgical treatment.

Definition of nonunion

There is no universally accepted definition of nonunion of a fracture. It is known from clinical experience that every given type of fracture tends to unite within a certain time period. If a fracture fails to unite within the time usually required for similar fractures to heal, it will typically be called a delayed union.

What will shift it into the nonunion category is the essentially empirical conviction on the part of the surgeon that it can no longer spontaneously proceed to healing. This conviction is sometimes founded upon evidence, as in the case of a fracture with a large bone defect. On other occasions, there may be no clear-cut indication that healing might not eventually occur, but the surgeon feels he should do something to accelerate a healing process which is at best quantitatively deficient and often appears halted. Many authors have attempted to define nonunion in terms of a specific

Roger Lemaire, M.D., Professor and Chairman, Department of Orthopaedic and Trauma Surgery, University Hospital, Liège (Belgium), Centre Hospitalier Universitaire du Sart-Tilman, 4000 Liège, Belgium.

time after the injury when union has not been achieved: their endpoints vary from fifteen weeks to twelve or more months from injury. In addition to this time requirement, all authors require that the reparative process be stopped completely, which makes spontaneous healing most unlikely.

In some cases with persistent motion at the nonunion site, a synovial-like cavity with fluid will form as a new joint. This will be called a synovial pseudarthrosis, a term which in the English-speaking world is used specifically to designate this precise form of nonunion, whereas the term "pseudarthrosis" is commonly used in several European languages to designate any type of nonunion, whether mobile or not.

Diagnosis of nonunion

In the presurgical era, healing of a fracture was typically assessed based upon the degree of mobility that could be elicited between the bone fragments upon manipulation; a trained surgeon is able to detect angular displacements as low as 2 to 3 degrees [64]. This rarely applies now, as a large number of fractures are treated primarily by internal fixation. The diagnosis of nonunion is now based essentially on analysis of radiographs. The persistence of a radiolucent gap between bone fragments is a clear indication of absence of bony healing. This may be evident on plain AP or lateral films, but the diagnosis may be more difficult if the fracture line is not simple and linear; additional oblique views may be necessary. More elaborate imaging may be required, such as tomograms, CT or MR imaging including 3-D reconstruction, although the presence of stainless steel fixation hardware may significantly interfere with interpretation. Besides, such additional imaging is rarely of great help and optimal use of conventional X-ray imaging remains the usual diagnostic tool.

Other evaluation tools have been investigated, such as medullary phlebography – which of course would not be applicable after medullary nailing, ultrasound transmission, scintigraphy, etc. They are rarely used in clinical practice. In the case of a diaphyseal fracture treated by external fixation, strain gauges on the device may be used to assess the evolution of the rigidity of the system over time: patterns corresponding to normal union, delayed union and nonunion have been defined [16]. Union can be predicted in fractures where bending stiffness reaches 7 Nm per degree and can be considered to have been achieved when it reaches 15 Nm [59]. In clinical practice, such measurements will only be possible in a limited number of cases.

General principles of treatment

The goals of treatment must be well-defined before going into technical considerations. Restoration of function is the ultimate goal, and this most often implies healing of the fracture. The latter is however not a goal in itself, but a requisite for functional recovery. In cases where a long, aggressive and problematical treatment appears necessary to achieve healing of an ununited fracture, such treatment is justified only if a reasonable functional result can be anticipated. If this appears unlikely, due to the condition of the soft tissues, joint stiffness, muscular atrophy or degenerescence from compartment syndrome, or associated neurological problems, a conservative approach (orthosis) may be justified or even, in selected cases, elective amputation.

It is classically stated that three factors are necessary for successful union: firm fixation, good apposition of the fragments and an environment that will promote osteogenesis. This certainly applies to the classical treatment of nonunion, but success has been obtained using other methods of treatment in cases where these conditions were not met, as will be discussed below.

When confronted with an ununited fracture, the first step should be thorough evaluation of the factors which have contributed to this evolution, in order to define the "personality" of the specific nonunion one is to treat. The factors that resulted in nonunion may be related to the initial traumatic injury, to the patient and/or to the treatment.

A first and essential distinction is between nonunions which have always been and still are aseptic and those which are infected or have a history of infection, even if the latter is apparently cleared. Such a distinction may rely on history, physical examination, biology, scintigraphy including indium-labeled leukocyte scintigraphy, aspiration, etc.

Among aseptic nonunions, the treatment will differ depending on the diaphyseal or metaphyseal site of the lesion. A further distinction must be made between nonunions without bone loss and those with bone loss; the latter may result from a bone defect, from shortening or from both. In each subgroup, some ununited fractures are well-aligned while others are malaligned. A final

1 *Schematic drawing of various types of nonunions:*
A. Hypertrophic nonunion.
B. Atrophic nonunion.
C. Nonunion with bone loss without shortening.
D. Nonunion with bone loss and shortening.

and important distinction must be made between atrophic and hypertrophic nonunions [42, 91] *(fig 1)*.

The condition of the soft tissues must be considered in treatment planning. Scar tissues may be fragile and at risk for necrosis; the condition of the soft tissues may restrict the possibilities for surgical approach and for the choice of treatment; deep scarring may interfere with bone transport or with bone realignment.

The vascular status of the limb must be taken into consideration. When in doubt, an arteriogram should be obtained, as some vascular abnormalities may restrict the choice of surgical treatments. Any associated nerve injury must be treated on its own, which may interfere with planning of the treatment of the nonunion.

An algorithm is thus followed, which brings every specific nonunion into one subcategory with specific treatment requirements. In some cases, longitudinal or rotational alignment must be restored; in others, shortening must be corrected; in others, just improving mechanical stability will suffice, while others will require some form of stimulation of osteogenesis. Infected nonunions must first be cleared of their

infection, unless it appears more appropriate to strive for bone healing first and to treat the residual infection secondarily; such a sequence would however not apply to the majority of cases.

In cases where the condition of the soft tissues is a limiting factor, skin grafting, pedicled skin or muscle flaps or free myocutaneous flaps may be necessary before any surgical action on the nonunion.

Treatment methods

Historically, the treatment of ununited fractures has for a long time relied essentially on bone grafting followed by prolonged plaster cast immobilisation. This was already a major improvement over pseudarthrosis resection as advocated in the 19th century. Various methods of bone grafting were used such as onlay or inlay grafts, sliding grafts, etc. Bone grafting is still frequently used, but it is now usually associated with internal or external fixation.

INTERNAL FIXATION

Depending on the type and location of the nonunion, plating or medullary nailing may be selected. Both have advantages and disadvantages: plating requires opening the nonunion site, which entails some damage to the soft tissues, and it carries with it a risk of secondary infection. Nailing can be performed percutaneously in a number of cases; it has a smaller risk of infection but, should an infection be present, there is a risk that it may spread over the entire length of the medullary cavity. Plate fixation was made popular some twenty year ago by the AO-ASIF, but has now been largely superseded by medullary nailing except for very proximal or distal nonunions.

■ Plate fixation

Plate fixation may be used with or without cancellous bone grafting and, wherever possible using compression. The value of compression to secure healing of a nonunion was demonstrated by Danis [23] whose work initiated the AO-ASIF philosophy. The role of compression was however controversial: it is now generally agreed that compression in itself has no specific beneficial effect on bone healing but is associated with improved stability of the fracture or nonunion site. Besides, it has been demonstrated that the compression force applied at operation steadily decreases in a matter of weeks. According to the AO-ASIF principles [91], the nonunion is to be approached by decortication, shingling or petalling and the damage to soft tissues and periosteum must be kept minimal. The fibrous tissue interposed between the bone ends must not be excised, as it will ossify when the nonunion is rigidly immobilised. Cancellous bone grafting is not necessary

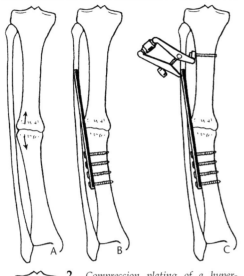

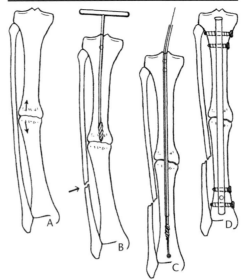

2 *Compression plating of a hypertrophic nonunion of the tibial diaphysis with moderate varus deformity (A). The plate is fixed to the distal fragment (B); the tensioning device is then fixed to the proximal fragment (C) and tension is applied; following correction of the varus deformity, the plate is fixed to the proximal fragment (D), with marked compression on the lateral portion of the nonunion. This may require osteotomy of the fibula if it has healed with marked varus deformity.*

3 *Intramedullary nailing after reaming in a hypertrophic nonunion of the tibial diaphysis with varus deformity (A). The IM guiding rod will often be stopped at the nonunion, and access to the medullary cavity of the distal fragment will require using a hand driven sharp reamer (B). The rod is then driven to the distal epiphysis and flexible reamers are used (C). The nail is inserted (D). Interlocking screws can be dispensed with in numerous cases, as the remnants of the fibrous nonunion provide rotational stability. Osteotomy of the fibula may be necessary to make alignment possible.*

unless the bone ends are sclerotic or when a defect is present or is created by realignment or correction of shortening. In such cases, compression plating is not possible and a neutralisation plate is used. Angular deformity may be corrected by applying a plate under tension on the convex side of the bone (*fig 2*).

Good results have been obtained by plating of nonunions [69], but its indications have clearly declined now, as other techniques have been developed which address more difficult situations than plating. The latter retains some indications in metaphyseal nonunions. Although it has been applied with success in cases with infected nonunion, particularly at the femur, other methods now available are usually considered more appropriate in such cases.

When performing plate fixation even in a good indication, one may face technical problems: it often proves impossible to perform a real decortication as the periosteum may be thin and poorly adherent to bone; the quality of bone may prove insufficient to achieve good fixation with most of the screws. In this case, the classical advice is to use longer screws with nuts, but despite this, screws will sometimes pull out from osteoporotic bone. In such a situation, it is probably best to shift to another technique. If this is not possible, filling the medullary cavity with polymethylmethacrylate will improve screw fixation, but is likely to make subsequent surgery more difficult.

■ *Medullary nailing*

Typical indications for nailing are well aligned nonunions and malaligned nonunions which may be realigned by manipulation; in such cases, nailing is best performed percutaneously, which minimises damage to the soft tissues as well as the risk of infection (*fig 3*).

Reaming and nailing temporarily disturb the blood supply to the endosteum but have been shown to elicit a periosteal vascular reaction which stimulates bone formation [49]. The reaming debris have been said to act as a bone graft, but this is unlikely when percutaneously nailing nonunions without excising the fibrous tissue interposed between the bone ends. In simple cases without bone loss, non-interlocking nails may be adequate, as there is no risk of shortening and rotational stability is provided by what is left of the fibrous union. We have had a 95% success rate using unlocked nails in a series of 102 tibial nonunions [55]; additional plaster cast immobilisation was however necessary in 36%, precisely in those cases that would now be treated by interlocked nailing [50].

It may prove impossible to stick to a percutaneous technique for several reasons: either the correction of a malalignment requires direct action on the bone fragments or sclerosis of the bone ends makes it impossible to pass the guide wire across the nonunion. When nailing has required an open technique, it is probably best to perform cancellous bone grafting to compensate for the damage inflicted to both endosteal and periosteal blood supply. Bone grafting may also be considered in cases with significant bone loss, although it may be better to perform it secondarily if nailing has been done percutaneously.

The idea still largely prevails that compression is a necessary mechanical stimulus to obtain union. Based on this concept, dynamic locking appears preferable [44], either primarily or by secondary removal of the screws at one end of the nail. Success has however been achieved with static locking [3], which cannot be dispensed with in cases with potential rotational or longitudinal instability. Weight-bearing after static interlocked nailing of a femoral or tibial fracture or nonunion is not logical, as no beneficial effect from compression can be obtained, and there is a risk of fracture of one or several locking screws. The risk is reduced if dynamisation is performed 6 to 8 weeks later, but there seems to be a current trend to do without secondary dynamisation. Despite some optimistic reports, it is clear that most surgeons have seen screw fractures under such circumstances. This may pose serious problems when a further surgical action is required, particularly for proximal femoral screws, whether transverse or oblique. Fibulectomy has classically been regarded as necessary in association with nailing of a tibial nonunion. It has been our experience, and other teams' as well [3], that partial fibulectomy is rarely necessary. Isolated osteotomy or segmental resection of the fibula, with subsequent weight bearing in a cast, has also been a classical treatment for tibial nonunion [25], but this treatment mostly applied to well-aligned nonunions following conservative treatment; its indications are exceptional in the nonunions that we now have to treat.

Nailing after plating poses no specific problems, except for the preliminary removal of broken screws, which may be tedious and requires simple albeit specific equipment. Nailing after external fixation poses no technical problem but carries a risk of infection [65]. The risk is proportional to the length of time the pins or wires have been left in place. When nailing is contemplated in such a case, the fixator should be removed first, and the nonunion should be immobilised in a cast for a few weeks or months, depending on the individual case, until it appears safe to perform the nailing. In cases where there was obvious pin tract infection, it may be safe to reconsider the indication for nailing or to take vigorous action, including curettage of the pin tracts, possibly combined with reaming of the medullary cavity and evacuation of all debris, the nailing itself being deferred to a further step.

■ Screw fixation

Simple screw fixation has no place in the management of diaphyseal nonunions; screw fixation combined with a neutralisation plate may be used on rare occasions in nonunion of a long spiral fracture.

Screw fixation finds more indications in the treatment of nonunions of small carpal or tarsal bones, either isolated or associated with cancellous bone grafting.

EXTERNAL FIXATION

■ Fixation

Although unilateral external fixation has been used extensively by certain groups, it has traditionally been reserved for difficult cases in which the local conditions appeared to contraindicate plating or nailing. A variety of constructs have been advocated to increase stability (*fig 4*), including double frames using transfixing threaded pins [89], but interest for such constructs soon faded after the introduction of Ilizarov's annular fixator in the western orthopaedic community [19, 40, 60, 71]. It allowed more versatile applications; it made use of thin smooth wires instead of large threaded pins; given a good knowledge of cross-sectional anatomy, the risk to damage muscles or important soft tissue structures was reduced. This came together with Ilizarov's principles on compression-distraction osteogenesis, which will be discussed below. This initiated a renewed interest in external fixation, as well as the design of improved unilateral fixators, which now permit a similar range of applications owing to their increased rigidity [4, 5, 24].

■ Distraction osteogenesis; Ilizarov's methods

Ilizarov designed a modular system for external fixation using thin wires, and he also developed original methods to achieve healing of nonunion by applying compression, distraction, segmental compression-distraction or distraction-compression or transport osteosynthesis which make it possible to address virtually every possible clinical situation, even in the presence of deformity, shortening, bone defects and infection [19, 40, 60, 71].

Compression osteosynthesis can be applied to hypertrophic, stiff nonunions without bone loss; it only requires two levels of fixation, with compression at a rate of 0.5 mm per day for 2 to 4 weeks. Any pre-existing deformity is corrected gradually, following fibulotomy at the leg, before compression is applied.

Distraction osteosynthesis can be used to treat stiff hypertrophic nonunion with dense fibrous tissue between the bone ends; deformity is corrected gradually, lengthening is achieved if necessary, following

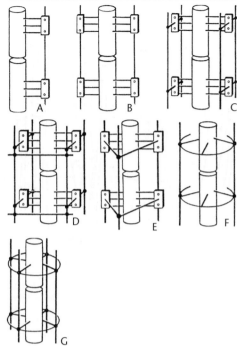

4 *Schematic drawings of various constructs which may be used for external fixation of a fractured or un-united long bone. A. Hemi-frame; B. frame; C. double frame; D. quadrangular triple frame; E. triangular triple frame; F. semicircular construct; G. circular construct. (Reprinted with permission from Huten D., Duparc J. Techniques d'ostéosynthèse des fractures diaphysaires de jambe chez l'adulte. Editions Techniques. Encycl. Méd. Chir. (Paris-France), Techniques chirurgicales, Orthopédie-Traumatologie, 44870, 1992, 18 p.).*

fibulotomy at the leg, by distraction exerted on the interposed fibrous tissue.

Monofocal compression-distraction lengthening osteosynthesis may be used to correct shortening and/or deformity in a stiff nonunion with vascular bone: the bone ends are first put under compression, followed by progressive distraction until the desired correction is achieved.

Sequential monofocal distraction-compression osteosynthesis at the nonunion site can be used to treat nonunion – either atrophic or hypertrophic – with significant instability. Distraction is applied first, which disrupts the interposed tissue and frequently results in some bone regeneration; compression is then applied, which stimulates healing of the nonunion from this bone regenerate.

Distraction osteosynthesis following proximal or distal corticotomy can be used to fill large bone defects without the use of bone grafting. The bone segment produced by the corticotomy is transported gradually across the bone defect until it docks against the other fragment; the nonunion site is then put under compression (*fig 5*). If shortening must also be corrected, distraction is then applied to the corticotomy for lengthening. In order to save time in cases where the bone defect is particularly large, a second corticotomy may be performed either at the other metaphysis or in the transported segment, and distraction is applied to a proximal or distal corticotomy until the

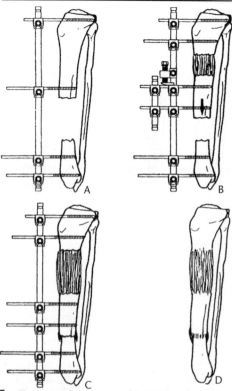

5 *Treatment of a nonunion of the tibial diaphysis with bone loss by segmental bone transport using a unilateral external fixator. (Reprinted with permission from: L. Kinzl, Operative treatment of bone defects in traumatology. EFORT Instructional Course Lecture. 1999, 3, p. 133-143).*
A. Primary stabilisation with two proximal and two distal pins.
B. Two pins added for bone transport following proximal osteotomy; distraction has been applied to the osteotomy.
C. The transported segment has docked against the distal fragment; the docking site has been put under compression.
D. Final result.

required lengthening has been achieved; the corticotomy lengthening serves as a stimulus to the healing of the nonunion.

End-to-end compression can be applied if the nonunion site is fairly perpendicular to the axis of compression; otherwise, surgical reshaping of the fragments through a limited exposure may be necessary, or transverse or oblique compression must be applied using olive wires. At the leg, associated osteotomy of the fibula is necessary when significant malalignment must be corrected or when lengthening must be achieved.

Nonunions with a small or medium-sized bone defect may also be treated by acute or progressive shortening to bring the bone ends into contact, followed by lengthening at a corticotomy in a healthy metaphysis (*fig 6*). Saleh and Rees [80] have made a comparative study of this "compression distraction" technique and the bone transport technique; they found that the former technique required less time and less additional operative procedures than the bone transport technique. The precise limits of acute shortening and bone transport remain unknown and may vary between individual cases.

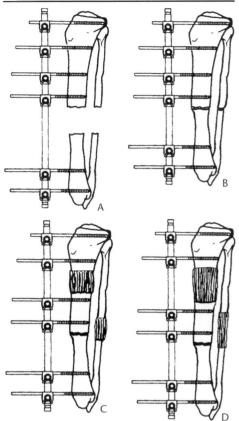

6 *Treatment of a nonunion of the tibial diaphysis with moderate bone loss and shortening by acute or progressive shortening followed by lengthening in a proximal osteotomy or corticotomy. Osteotomy or partial resection of the fibula may be necessary if the fibula is likely to interfere with compression and/ or lengthening.*

A. A unilateral fixator is applied with 2 proximal and 2 distal pins and 2 more pins in the distal part of the proximal fragment.

B. The fragments are brought into contact in one step or in a progressive fashion, depending on the surrounding soft tissues. Compression is applied to the nonunion.

C. A proximal osteotomy is performed and progressive lengthening is undertaken.

D. After restoration of length.

As regards infected nonunions, cases have been noted in which infection spontaneously cleared as healing of a nonunion was achieved through compression; nonunion with sequestrated bone will however require excision of the dead bone and filling in of the resulting defect by bone transport.

When a bone defect is associated with a soft tissue defect, filling the bone defect by bone transport may be associated with soft tissue transport: the latter may be encouraged by using horizontal wires mounted on a transport ring; soft tissue coverage may thus be obtained in some cases without complicated specific operations. When soft tissue transport is not desired, it may be minimised by using longitudinal distraction wires.

Several authors believe that the soft tissue recruitment into the wound from a distant corticotomy site is inadequate in cases with infected nonunion or a high-grade open fracture. Lowenberg et al. (1996) favor a combined approach with early flap coverage, followed by Ilizarov reconstruction as a delayed procedure.

Such a combined approach has not been used extensively, and Ring et al [77] believe this may be one of the reasons why several retrospective studies comparing cancellous bone grafting with Ilizarov type treatment have shown comparable results or only a slight advantage in favour of Ilizarov's methods [22, 34, 61, 72].

Judicious use of the various possibilities offered by the Ilizarov technique may help to solve a variety of difficult problems of nonunions, particularly at the tibia. Compliance with the usual conditions required for the success of Ilizarov's technique is considered essential. Fixation of the fragments should be stable, transsection of the bone should be made by corticotomy rather than osteotomy, the corticotomy should preferably be metaphyseal, there should be no initial gap between bone ends. Distraction should be started only after a 7 to 14 day latency period and should be gradual: 1 mm per day, preferably 0.25 mm four times each day. Regarding corticotomy, which was initially presented as an essential requisite for success, it does not really appear to be essential, as it has been shown both clinically and experimentally that complete osteotomy is just as effective [15, 85]. Effective distraction osteogenesis over an intramedullary nail following reaming of the medullary cavity appears as a further evidence [14, 75, 83].

The Ilizarov technique provides solutions for virtually every nonunion a surgeon may be confronted with; it is however used on a limited scale by many surgeons for several reasons. One reason is its technical difficulty, which can be overcome through training and experience; another reason is the length of time during which the fixator must be left in place, which interferes with a number of activities and may be psychologically disturbing, not to mention minor but frequent tolerance problems with the wires. It does however have significant advantages such as the possibility to bear full weight all through the treatment. It is better tolerated at the leg than at the thigh, even if incomplete rings are used at the thigh; semicircular rings are preferred at the humerus for the same reason [52].

COMBINED INTERNAL AND EXTERNAL FIXATION

This combination may be considered when femoral or tibial lengthening is necessary in the treatment of a nonunion with shortening. The use of an unlocked nail will help to control alignment, but will not allow for removal of the external fixation before the consolidation of bone is complete. This is made possible by using interlocking nails, with the proximal locking screws inserted at the time of nailing and the distal screws once the desired lengthening has been achieved. This makes it possible to reduce the time in a frame to a fraction of the time that would be required if only external fixation were used.

The combination of internal and unilateral external fixation for bone lengthening was proposed nearly fifty years ago [11] and was subsequently applied to the correction of large bone defects [14, 75]. It appears to offer several advantages over external fixation on its own: the risk of malalignment and of fracture of the bone regenerate is reduced, the time in frame is dramatically shortened; in the case of femoral lengthening, the method allows for earlier rehabilitation and more rapid resumption of knee movement. Clinical experience has shown that reaming and nailing do not compromise the quality of the bone regenerate or the consolidation. As pin tract infection is to be anticipated, it is recommended to avoid contact between the pins of the external fixator and the intramedullary nail. Such a combination may be considered in any case in which treatment includes lengthening by distraction osteogenesis, either in the nonunion site or in a secondary corticotomy or osteotomy; the benefit will be all the more substantial as the required amount of lengthening is important. The method may also be of interest for segmental bone transport without lengthening *(fig 7)*.

BONE GRAFTING

■ *Non-vascularised bone grafts*

Bone grafting as an isolated procedure

Bone autografting has been for many years the basic technique used to treat ununited fractures. Numerous techniques have been described. Massive cortical grafts were used initially, as they were considered to provide both mechanical stabilisation and an osteogenic stimulus. In fact, massive cortical grafts are poorly osteoinductive and they are mechanically fragile, so that with both inlay and onlay graft techniques, prolonged immobilisation in a plaster cast was necessary. Onlay grafts were performed either by placing long, thin iliac grafts around the nonunion which had been approached by decortication [74] or by fixing a massive cortical autograft to both fragments with screws [17, 38] *(fig 8)*. Dual onlay grafts were used to treat nonunions in osteoporotic bone, with both grafts fixed with the same set of screws in such a way as to grip the fragments like a vice [12].

Massive sliding grafts were used to bridge limited bone defects [32] *(fig 9B)*; the technique was applied to nonunions of the femur and tibia. This however resulted in a potentially dangerous bone fragilisation which precluded early rehabilitation; besides, if it failed, the resulting situation was difficult to control. Whole fibular transplants have been used as avascular struts to bridge defects in the forearm bones: they are stronger than tibial grafts of similar

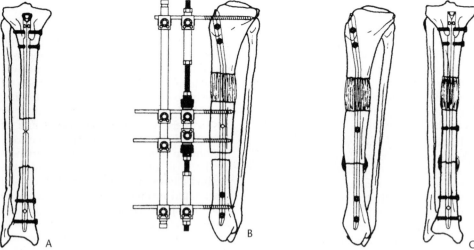

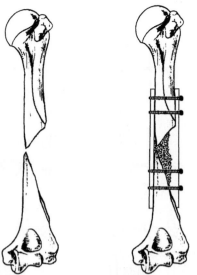

7 *Schematic drawing of bone segment transport to bridge a large defect in the tibial diaphysis using a unilateral external fixator and an IM nail. (Reprinted from L. Kinzl. Operative treatment of bone defects in traumatology. EFORT Instructional Course Lecture. 1999, 3, p. 133-143, with permission).*
A. The nail is inserted and is locked by proximal and distal screws.
B. A proximal osteotomy is performed after the fixator has been fixed proximally, distally and to the segment to be transported; distraction is started in the osteotomy.
C. After the transported segment has docked against the distal fragment, the docking site is put under compression, the nail is locked to the transported segment and the fixator is removed.

8 *Dual onlay graft in a nonunion of the humeral diaphysis with bone loss. Two corticocancellous grafts, procured from the proximal metaphysis of a tibia, are affixed to the bone by the same set of lag screws and hold the fragments like a vice. Autologous cancellous bone chips are packed inbetween the fragments and grafts.*

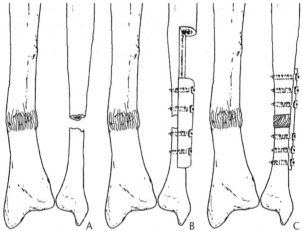

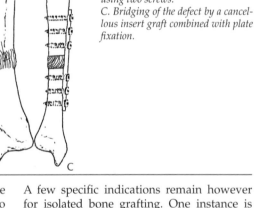

9 *A. Nonunion of the distal ulna with bone defect.*
B. Bridging of the defect by a sliding graft which is fixed to each fragment using two screws.
C. Bridging of the defect by a cancellous insert graft combined with plate fixation.

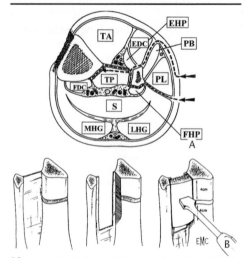

10 *Intertibiofibular graft for nonunion of the tibial diaphysis with soft tissue defect or scarred soft tissues on the anteromedial aspect of the leg. The tibiofibular space may be approached anteriorly or posteriorly (A) and a quadrangular corticocancellous iliac graft is impacted between tibia and fibula across the nonunion (B).*
(Fig. 10B is reprinted from: Burdin P., Favard L. Traitement des pseudarthroses de jambe. Editions Techniques. Encycl. Méd. Chir. (Paris-France), Techniques chirurgicales, Orthopédie, 44875, 1991, 6 p., with permission).

volume, they can be fixed by screws to the fragments, or one end may be inserted into the medullary canal. Complete revascularisation of the transplant requires several months and protection against fracture of the graft must be provided for several months.

Massive cortical grafts are now rarely used; cancellous grafts are preferred owing to their higher osteoinductive potential, and stability is provided by some form of internal or external fixation [48]. Cancellous bone grafting is usually performed through a surgical approach to the nonunion. Bahn and Mehara [10] however reported on percutaneous bone grafting and Kim et al [47] even used an endoscopic technique with which they reportedly performed accurate debridement and precise bone grafting with minimal injury to the soft tissues. They achieved healing in 6/8 nonunions of the femur or humerus, but they stressed the technical difficulty and the risk of compartment syndrome, and they have not extended the indications to the leg and forearm.

A few specific indications remain however for isolated bone grafting. One instance is the Russe technique for nonunion of the carpal navicular [79]. Another example is tibiofibular bone grafting for tibial nonunions with infection, segmental bone loss or soft tissue damage on the anterior aspect of the leg. The technique as originated by Jones and Barnett [41] in 1955 made use of cancellous bone grafts; Reckling and Waters [76] and others reported satisfactory results. The technique was modified by Evrard [29] who used a corticocancellous graft from the posterior iliac crest which was wedged between tibia and fibula in order to bridge the union *(fig 10)*. This technique of intertibiofibular grafting has reportedly given high success rates in several series of tibial nonunions with a history of sepsis [29, 68, 90]. Some authors have combined intertibiofibular bone grafting with open cancellous graft filling of a bone and soft tissue defect. The latter technique was advocated by Papineau et al [73], but it had important drawbacks when used on its own: time for healing of bone

and soft tissue was extremely long and the reconstituted bone was of poor mechanical quality; besides, it only applied to partial bone defects, less than 4 cm, with at least one tibial cortex left intact [56].

Bone grafting associated with internal or external fixation

When an ununited fracture is already fixed by effective internal or external fixation, the latter may be left intact and there may be an indication for simple bone grafting, either cancellous or corticocancellous, in cases with a partial defect or a circumferential defect less than 2 cm in length. More often, bone grafting is necessary in cases where pre-existing internal or external fixation was ineffective and must be replaced. If this involves opening the nonunion site, bone grafting should be done in the same setting, but it may be better to delay it if the new fixation is done without opening the nonunion site. Depending on the individual case, packing cancellous bone chips in and around the nonunion may suffice, or it may be combined with a structural corticocancellous graft.

A limited amount of cancellous grafts may in some cases be harvested from a metaphysis close to the nonunion, but when a large amount of graft material is required, this will usually be harvested from the anterior or posterior iliac crest, which may also provide strips of corticocancellous bone. A long corticocancellous graft may also be obtained from the medial aspect of the proximal tibia, taking care to leave the anterior and medial border intact. Such a graft may, in specific cases such as nonunion of the distal humerus, be fixed with screws across the nonunion, combined with intramedullary Rush pin or Ender nail fixation.

For defects less than 2 cm long, particularly in the forearm bones, a cancellous insert graft may be selected [70] using a solid block of cancellous bone which is trimmed for a tight fit and wedged in position between the bone ends; the latter are fixed with a compression plate (fig 9C).

When dealing with a larger bone defect, the fragments may be fixed with a unilateral external fixator or a long bridging plate and the defect may be filled with one or several corticocancellous grafts associated with a large volume of cancellous chips. Another option is a free or vascularised fibular graft.

Non-vascularised fibula

A non-vascularised segment of the fibula may be used as a graft to fill a large bone defect in the radius or ulna; this has also been done occasionally at the humerus, femur or tibia, but such reconstructions are fragile and must be protected from mechanical stress for a long period of time; despite this, fatigue fractures have occurred in a number of cases. In the adult, the transplanted fibula will not hypertrophy to a significant degree, but in children, it may well hypertrophy to approach the volume and strength of a normal tibia or humerus.

Fibula resection has been considered to induce no significant morbidity in the adult, but several studies have reported significant disability due to loss of the weight-bearing function of the fibula and to ankle instability [7, 53]. Potential donor site morbidity must therefore be taken into consideration in the decision to use the fibula to fill a large bone defect.

■ *Vascularised bone grafts*

With traditional bone autografting, reconstruction of a bone defect depends upon creeping substitution within an avascular graft, a process which requires capillary ingrowth and takes an extended period of time during which the graft is mechanically fragile. The process is somewhat faster in cancellous autografts which, in addition, may retain a certain proportion of living osteoblasts and display a higher osteoinductive potential than cortical autografts. The situation is worse with cortical allografts, which induce a cell-mediated immune response and are at risk for infection in a post-trauma context; their use in the treatment of nonunions is therefore very limited.

Vascularised autografts present a number of advantages, but their use was dependent on the development of microvascular techniques. Anterior or posterior vascularised rib grafts were used first, then free vascularised transfer of the fibula [86] and from the iliac crest. Composite osteocutaneous or osteomyocutaneous vascularised grafts may also be used, which makes it possible to treat a composite defect in one surgical session, a goal which however may also be achieved by combining cancellous bone grafting and a pedicled or free muscular transplant [62].

Tibial defects up to 10 cm have been bridged successfully [54] using a composite osteo(myo)cutaneous transplant from the iliac crest, based on the deep circumflex iliac vessels. Larger defects up to 18 cm may be bridged with a fibular transplant, which may also include part of the soleus muscle or flexor hallucis longus or a cutaneous flap. Free vascularised fibular transfer has also been used to bridge defects in the femoral diaphysis [63].

Techniques for bridging tibial defects with the ipsilateral vascularised fibula have in fact been developed over a century ago: tibialisation of the ipsilateral fibula was reportedly initiated by Albert in 1877 and it has been performed ever since, using a variety of techniques [1]. With some techniques, a tibiofibular synostosis is created proximally and distally to the tibial defect; with others, a segment of the fibula is transported into the defect as one or two segments following extensive dissection of the blood supply to the segment to be transported. An angiogram should be done prior to graft harvesting and caution is required when using a circular external fixator, as the wires may damage the vessels of the graft. Fixation of the fibula is usually done using K-wires or screws and spanning unilateral fixators. Atkins et al [6] have developed a method with which a fibular segment of adequate length is transported into the defect using pulling wires mounted on an Ilizarov frame; once it is in place, compression is applied to anchor the transplant. Contrary to other techniques, the latter permits weight-bearing which encourages bone union and fibular hypertrophy.

The development of microvascular surgery has now made it possible to use the contralateral fibula, which may be advantageous in cases where the ipsilateral fibula cannot be used; on the other hand, it introduces a risk of morbidity at the donor site on the otherwise undamaged limb. As previously stated, several studies have shown indeed that resection of a fibular segment may result in ankle instability in some cases.

SOFT TISSUE COVERAGE

Union of a fracture requires, among other conditions, an environment which promotes osteogenesis. In many cases with a long-standing nonunion, the condition of the soft tissue is far from satisfactory, as a result of severe initial trauma or complications of previous treatments (skin necrosis, scarring, compartment syndrome, infection, etc.). Before the development of microvascular surgery, these problems were addressed using techniques such as cross leg flaps or Papineau's open cancellous bone packing; such techniques may still be helpful for surgeons working in a suboptimal environment. Adequate soft tissue coverage is now usually restored using local (myo)cutaneous flaps or free flaps; the specific technique depends on the precise localisation of the area to be covered, on the condition of the potential donor area and also on the surgeon's preference. As mentioned earlier, osteo(myo)cutaneous flaps may also be obtained from the iliac crest or fibula, which makes it possible to address the bone and soft tissue problems simultaneously. In cases with extensive soft tissue scarring but no defect, it is also possible to leave this unchanged and to perform grafting through healthy tissues, such as posterolateral tibiofibular grafting at the leg.

On the other hand, when bone transport using Ilizarov's method is planned, it is possible to simultaneously achieve soft tissue transport, although some authors have found that the soft tissue recruitment thus achieved is of questionable value and it may be preferable to perform a soft tissue flap simultaneously [57]. The use of soft tissue spacers or expanders may be helpful in some cases before bone grafting [62].

The choice of a technique to achieve soft tissue coverage must be integrated in the general treatment scheme: for instance, transfixing pins or wires may endanger the vascular pedicle of a flap or vascularised bone graft, or some important blood vessel in a limb with an already compromised blood supply. A preoperative arteriogram should be done in all cases where there is a risk to damage a main artery or when a microvascular anastomosis is planned. When a further surgical approach is needed on a nonunion following soft tissue reconstruction by a free flap, the approach should be either at a distance from the flap or along its edge, and great care must be taken not to damage its pedicle.

General treatment strategy

Several major advances have been made in the surgical treatment of nonunions over the past few decades; furthermore, non-surgical treatments are presently under evaluation. Bone autografting has been for a long time the basic treatment for most cases of nonunion; its indications have decreased considerably and it may now be dispensed with in a number of cases. Well-aligned diaphyseal nonunions without infection and without bone and soft tissue defects may be considered good indications for nailing after reaming: interlocking nails have extended the indications to proximal and distal nonunions. Nailing after external fixation requires caution to minimise the risk of infection. Compression plating may still be considered in hypertrophic nonunions although one may wish not to open the fracture site when this can be avoided. These are the straightforward cases, of which less are seen now, owing to overall improvement in the primary treatment of simple fractures. It may well be that, a few years from now, the indications for surgery in such cases will further decrease if non-surgical treatments presently under evaluation are found to be effective and are applied more liberally.

We are now facing a majority of difficult nonunion cases as a result of several factors. A number of patients with severe multiple trauma now survive the initial phase and are left with complex fractures which, out of necessity, have received suboptimal initial treatment. As a result of high-energy trauma, such fractures are often compound, with variable degrees of bone and soft tissue damage, often leaving bone defects and poor-quality scarred soft tissues. Infection may be present as a result of the initial trauma or of previous operative treatment.

When it comes to treating nonunions with bone loss, a choice exists between methods which may essentially not be combined. Bone defects may be bridged by bone grafting, if necessary by repeat grafting; if the soft tissue coverage is inadequate, it must first be improved by local or free vascular myocutaneous flaps.

Classical alternative solutions remain available, such as posterolateral tibiofibular grafting or tibiofibular proximal and distal synostosis at the leg: such options may be less ambitious and less gratifying for the surgeon but they may achieve consolidation in a simpler and less risky way in patients with particular local or systemic risk factors. A microvascular graft from the iliac crest or fibula may be used to bridge large defects in major long bones, and it may also help in improving the vascularity of the recipient bed, but it is a more invasive procedure which may also entail donor site morbidity. Donor site morbidity is a factor which should not be overlooked. When repeated bone autografting is anticipated, one must keep in mind that the available supply is not unlimited and no graft should be decided upon without a clear indication. Using the ipsilateral fibula to treat a tibial nonunion has the advantage of restricting the added morbidity to the already damaged limb, but it eliminates the possibility of load sharing through an intact fibula throughout the period of graft hypertrophy. When using the contralateral fibula for a vascular graft, one clearly inflicts some damage to a normal limb, which may have clinical impact in some cases.

Most nonunion problems may also be addressed using one of the techniques derived from Ilizarov's principles, based upon a different philosophy. These techniques are of particular interest in cases with major bone defects, when bone transport or bifocal compression – distraction (acute shortening followed by lengthening at a healthy metaphysis) may achieve union without creating donor site morbidity in another area, with a reduced need for flap surgery and with preservation of load sharing through the fibula. Lengthening over a nail appears as an appealing composite technique.

The choice between such different methods is clearly influenced by the individual surgeon's preference and expertise. The methods available differ to a large extent in their invasiveness and in their potential for minor and major complications; a balance should be sought in every individual case between the necessity to address all components of the problem – deformity, shortening, bone loss, soft tissue scarring, infection, etc. – and to avoid excessive and undue risks. The simplest method should be preferred as long as it gives a fair chance of achieving union within a reasonable time period. "Overkill" should be avoided and the burden of the treatment to the patient should also be taken into consideration. Successful treatment of a nonunion often requires several consecutive surgical actions and a global strategy must be established from the beginning, taking care not to interfere with the next steps and to leave alternative treatments possible in case of failure of the initial plan.

Adjunctive nonsurgical means to enhance bone healing

Over the past 30 years, a large amount of investigative work has been devoted to mechanical, biophysical or biological enhancement of fracture healing, and has resulted in the development of a number of adjunctive treatments with potential applications to the treatment of nonunion of fractures.

Mechanical enhancement

Controlled micromotion has been used experimentally [33] and clinically in patients with tibial diaphyseal fractures treated by external fixation [45]; it was found to result in significantly faster healing. So far, the method does not seem to have been tested in healing of nonunions.

Biophysical enhancement

ELECTRICAL STIMULATION

Treatment of nonunions by electric current has been used anecdotally since the middle of the 19th century. The scientific basis for such treatments was gained through more recent studies [30], which resulted in the development of several types of electrical stimulation devices: constant direct-current stimulation using percutaneous or implanted electrodes (invasive), inductive coupling produced by a magnetic field (non-invasive) and capacitive coupling (non-invasive). The main clinical application has been the treatment of nonunions. Brighton et al [13] reported 78% solid osseous unions after treating 258 nonunions with constant direct current. Bassett et al [8] had 87% of osseous union after treating 127 ununited fractures of the tibial diaphysis. Scott and King [81] performed a prospective, double-blind study on nonunions treated with either capacitive coupling or a placebo unit and found significantly better consolidation with electrical stimulation. Sharrard made similar findings using pulsed electromagnetic fields in a double-blind study in patients who had delayed union of a tibial fracture [82].

Clinical experience has shown that the method is effective in hypertrophic nonunions, but less so in atrophic nonunions and in the presence of a gap. It also cannot correct deformity or shortening and its use is therefore restricted to diaphyseal hypertrophic nonunions with little or no deformity, gap or shortening.

Even for these typical indications, the method usually requires a long period of non-weight-bearing cast immobilisation, with a risk of joint stiffness and muscle atrophy. For these reasons, the method has never gained wide acceptance; another reason in some countries, is the fact that the health care system does not cover the cost of such treatments unless in highly selected cases.

ULTRASOUND STIMULATION

Low-intensity pulsed ultrasound, in the range of milliwatts per square centimetre, has shown substantial efficacy in accelerating healing of fractures of the upper and lower extremities. Duarte [26] reported such observations as early as 1983 on experimental cortical defects and fibular osteotomies and also clinically on ununited fractures. Acceleration of healing has been noted in double blind studies by Heckman et al [36] in tibial fractures and by Kristiansen et al [51] in fresh Colles fractures.

As regards nonunions, Duarte et al reported in 1996 [27] their results in 385 delayed unions and nonunions, with an 85% success rate in fractures which remained ununited after an average of 14 months. This is close to the results reported in a prescription use registry: the success rate was 91% in 951 delayed unions and 86% in 366 nonunions [67]. Mainard et al [58] reported healing in 44/50 nonunions (88%); Albers et al [2] in 35/37 nonunions (94.6%), with 100% hypertrophic nonunions healed, versus 92% of oligotrophic nonunions and 88% of atrophic cases.

Low-intensity ultrasound seems to influence positively different processes in all phases of fracture healing and its action does not seem to depend upon one singular mechanism [35]. At the intensity level used, which is in the same range as that used for diagnostic ultrasonography, it is considered athermal and non destructive. No untoward side-effects have been reported; the treatment requires patient compliance, which should not be a problem as the treatment only involves daily application of an external device for 20 minutes at home. Here again, the reimbursement issue is a major limiting factor, but further prospective randomised studies will hopefully demonstrate the value and cost-efficiency of the method, both in nonunions and in fresh fractures.

HIGH-ENERGY EXTRACORPOREAL SHOCK WAVES

Extracorporeal shock waves (ESW) have become an accepted method of treatment for urolithiasis. In orthopaedics, they have been used as a tool to facilitate bone cement removal in revision hip arthroplasty and, starting in the early nineties, an increasing number of reports have appeared regarding other applications to musculoskeletal conditions such as epicondylitis, rotator cuff calcifications, heel spurs and also nonunion of fractures. Valchanou and Michailov first

reported in 1991 [88] healing in 70 out of 79 cases of delayed union or nonunion, following a single application of 1000 to 4000 shock waves with a bone focus of 1000 to 1700 bars. Others reported healing in 41 to 91% of nonunions [9, 78], with better results in hypertrophic than in atrophic nonunions. ESW treatment thus appears to some authors as an alternative to surgery in the management of ununited fractures. Heller et al [37] made a meta-analysis of 55 papers reporting results with ESW in 4,825 cases with various indications and concluded that, although ESW therapy clearly has a potential to induce osteogenesis in ununited fractures, its mode of action has not been clearly established; they pointed out that only 4 papers with 210 nonunions reached the standards of a scientific investigation, and they concluded that ESW therapy should still be regarded as experimental until its efficacy has been indisputably demonstrated. The indications and contraindications must be defined, as well as the adequate energy density levels and impulse rates for specific groups of indications. Reimbursement is another issue, as the treatment is indeed considered experimental by most social health-care systems. There is a clear need for scientific investigations to establish the efficacy and also the cost-efficiency of the treatment. Obvious advantages are the non-invasiveness and low rate of complications, added to the fact that the treatment can be applied on an outpatient basis in many cases.

PERCUTANEOUS INJECTION OF AUTOGENOUS BONE MARROW

Autogenous bone marrow has been used clinically to augment the osteogenic response to implanted allografts; it has also demonstrated a similar potential when injected percutaneously into a nonunion. Using this technique, Garg et al [31] obtained healing of 17/20 ununited fractures (85%); Hernigou and Beaujean [39] reported healing of 21/26 ununited fractures (81%), using a technique of marrow centrifugation which eliminates plasma and erythrocytes while preserving white blood cells and mesenchymal cells among which the osteoprogenitor cells. Centrifugation makes it possible to deliver with 50 ml of concentrated marrow the amount of osteoprogenitor cells present in 300 ml of

non-centrifuged bone marrow. Clinical application of the method has been limited so far, but appears promising. Conolly, who reported the first clinical experience with percutaneous injections of bone marrow to stimulate fracture repair, later reported an 80% response to bone marrow injection in conjunction with adequate fracture stabilisation [22]; he noted that there are large individual variations in the colony-forming efficiency of the blood marrow in cultures. Hernigou and Beaujean [39] also noted that failures in their clinical series were related to poor cellularity and colony-forming capacity of the bone marrow.

OTHER NON-SURGICAL MEANS OF BIOLOGICAL ENHANCEMENT OF BONE HEALING

Several molecules have demonstrated an osteoinductive capacity in animal studies, when injected into bone defects or fractures: this is true for molecules of the TGF-β (transforming growth factor - β subfamily, BMP (bone morphogenetic protein) subfamily, or PDGF (platelet-derived growth factor). Human recombinant BMP-2 is presently under investigation in human trials [28]. The potential clinical applications of such biological enhancement of fracture healing are evident, but none of these molecules has yet reached routine clinical application. Besides, the physicochemical characteristics of the carrier system used have a high impact on the release kinetics of the molecule and the choice of an adequate carrier is therefore important [93].

A systemic approach of fracture healing enhancement appears even more remote. It has been known for a long time that patients who have sustained a head injury heal faster and with more callus, and there is some evidence that there may be a humoral mechanism for the enhanced osteogenesis after head injury [28]. Several growth factors may be involved in another phenomenon, i.e. mineral apposition at distant skeletal sites after localised direct or indirect injury to bone marrow in one part of the skeleton. Other clinical observations have shown that prostaglandins may stimulate cortical and trabecular bone formation, an effect which can be blocked by prostaglandin inhibitors such as indomethacin. So, there are several paths which seem worthwhile to pursue in research, but which have not yet resulted in any real clinical applications.

References

[1] Agiza AR. Treatment of tibial osteomyelitis defects and infected pseudarthroses by the Huntington fibular transference operation. *J Bone Joint Surg Am* 1981 ; 63 : 814-819

[2] Albers RG, Patka P, Janssen IM, Van DerKrans A. Effective therapy for nonunions. Low intensity ultrasound. Proceedings of 4th EFORT Congress, Brussels, 1999 : 127

[3] Alho A, Ekeland A, Stromsoe K, Benterud JG. Nonunion of tibial shaft fractures treated with locked intramedullary nailing without bone grafting. *J Trauma* 1993 ; 34 : 62-67

[4] Alonso JE, Regazzoni P. The use of Ilizarov concept with the AO/ASIF tubular fixator in the treatment of segmental defects. *Orthop Clin North Am* 1990 ; 21 : 655-665

[5] Aronson J, Harp JH Jr. Factors influencing the choice of external fixation for distraction osteogenesis. AAOS Instr Course Lect, 1990 ; 39 : 175-183

[6] Atkins RM, Madhavan P, Sudhakar J, Whitwell D. Ipsilateral vascularised fibular transport for massive defects of the tibia. *J Bone Joint Surg Br* 1999 ; 81 : 1035-1040

[7] Babhulkar SS, Pande KC, Babhulkar S. Ankle instability after fibular resection. *J Bone Joint Surg Br* 1995 ; 77 : 258-261

[8] Bassett CA, Mitchell SN, Gaston SR. Treatment of ununited tibial diaphyseal fractures with pulsing electromagnetic fields. *J Bone Joint Surg Am* 1981 ; 63 : 511-523

[9] Beutler S, Regel G, Pape HC, Machtens S, Weinberg AM, Kremeike I et al. Die extrakorporale Stosswellentherapie (ESWT) in der Behandlung von Pseudarthrosen des Rohrenknochens. Erste Ergebnisse einer prospektivenklinischen Untersuchung. *Unfallchirurg* 1999 ; 102 : 839-847

[10] Bhan S, Mehara AK. Percutaneous bone grafting for nonunion and delayed union of fractures of the tibial shaft. *Int Orthop* 1993 ; 17 : 310-312

[11] Bost FC, Larsen LJ. Experiences with lengthening of the femur over an intramedullary rod. *J Bone Joint Surg Am* 1956 ; 38 : 567-584

[12] Boyd HB. The bridging of bone defects. *AAOS Instr Course Lect* 1944 ; 2 : 522

[13] Brighton CT, Black J, Friedenberg ZB, Esterhai JL, Day LJ, Connolly JF. A multicenter study of the treatment of nonunion with constant direct current. *J Bone Joint Surg Am* 1981 ; 63 : 2-13.

[14] Brunner U, Kessler S, Cordey J, Rahn B, Schweiberer L, Perren SM. Treatment of large bone defects using segment bone transportation (Ilizarov) with intramedullary nailing. *Unfallchirurg* 1990 ; 93 : 244-250

[15] Brutscher R, Rahn BA, Ruter A, Perren SM. The role of corticotomy and osteotomy in the treatment of bone defects using the Ilizarov technique. *J Orthop Trauma* 1993 ; 7 : 261-269

[16] Burny F, Donkerwolke M. Elastic fixation of fractures: Biomechanics of fracture healing. In : Lane JM ed. Fracture healing. New York : Churchill Livingstone, 1987 : 123-137

[17] Campbell WC, Boyd HB. Fixation of onlay bone grafts by means of Vitallium screws in the treatment of ununited fractures. *Am J Surg* 1941 ; 51 : 748

[18] Carroll L, Heppenstall HP, Frey J, Ryaby J. Le traitement non invasif des pseudarthroses par ultrasons pulsés à faible intensité. *Rev Chir Orthop* 1999 ; 85 (suppl III) : 139

[19] Cattaneo R, Catagni M, Johnson EE. The treatment of infected nonunions and segmental defects of the tibia by the methods of Ilizarov. *Clin Orthop* 1992 ; 280 : 143-152

[20] Chacha PB, Ahmed M, Daruwalla JS. Vascular pedicle graft of the ipsilateral fibula for non-union of the tibia with a large defect: an experimental and clinical study. *J Bone Joint Surg Br* 1981 ; 63 : 244-253

[21] Cierny G, Zorn KE. Segmental tibial defects: Comparing conventional and Ilizarov methodologies. *Clin Orthop* 1994 ; 301 : 118-123

[22] Connolly JF. Clinical use of marrow osteoprogenitor cells to stimulate osteogenesis. *Clin Orthop* 1998 ; 355 : 257-266

[23] Danis R. Theory and practice of osteosynthesis. Paris : Masson, 1949

[24] DeBastiani G, Aldegheri R, Brivio LR. The treatment of fractures with dynamic axial fixation. *J Bone Joint Surg Br* 1984 ; 66 : 538-545

[25] Delee JC, Heckman JD, Lewis AG. Partial fibulectomy for ununited fractures of the tibia. *J Bone Joint Surg Am* 1981 ; 63 : 1390

[26] Duarte LR. The stimulation of bone growth by ultrasound. *Arch Orthop Trauma Surg* 1983 ; 101 : 153-159

[27] Duarte LR, Xavier CA, Choffie M. Review of nonunions treated by pulsed low intensity ultrasound. Sicot 20th World Congres, 1996 ; 111 : PDS 30

[28] Einhorn TA. Enhancement of fracture healing. *J Bone Joint Surg Am* 1995 ; 77 : 940-956

[29] Evrard J. Place de la greffe inter-tibio-péronière dans le traitement des fractures et pseudarthroses infectées de jambe. *Rev Chir Orthop* 1992 ; 78 : 389-398

[30] Friedenberg ZB, Brighton CT. Bioelectric potentials in bone. *J Bone Joint Surg Am* 1966 ; 48 : 915-923

[31] Garg NK, Gaur S, Sharma S. Percutaneous autogenous bone marrow grafting in 29 cases of ununited fracture. *Acta Orthop Scand* 1993 ; 64 : 671-672

[32] Gill AB. Treatment of ununited fracture of the bones of the forearm. *Surg Clin North Am* 1932 ; 12 : 1535

[33] Goodship AE, Kenwright J. The influence of induced micromovement upon the healing of experimental tibial fractures. *J Bone Joint Surg Br* 1985 ; 67 : 650-655

[34] Green SA. Skeletal defects: A comparison of bone grafting and bone transport for segmental skeletal defects. *Clin Orthop* 1994 ; 301 : 111-117

[35] Hadjiargyrou M, McLeod K, Ryaby JP, Rubin C. Enhancement of fracture healing by low intensity ultrasound. *Clin Orthop* 1998 ; 355 : 216-229

[36] Heckman JD, Ryaby JP, McCabe J, Frey JJ, Kilcoyne RF. Acceleration of tibial fracture healing by non-invasive, low intensity pulsed ultrasound. *J Bone Joint Surg Am* 1994 ; 76 : 26-34

[37] Heller KD, Wirtz DC, Birnbaum K, Niethard FU. Use of high-energy extracorporeal shock-wave therapy (ESWT) in pseudarthrosis. A meta-analysis of clinical studies. Proceedings of 4th EFORT Congress, Brussels, 1999 : 128

[38] Henderson MS. Bone graft in ununited fractures. *J Bone Joint Surg* 1938 ; 20 : 635

[39] Hernigou P, Beaujean F. Pseudarthroses traitées par greffe percutanée de moelle osseuse autologue. *Rev Chir Orthop* 1997 ; 83 : 495-504

[40] Ilizarov GA. Pseudoarthroses and defects of long tubular bones: treatment of marked defects. In : Ilizarov GA ed. Transosseous osteosynthesis. Berlin : Springer-Verlag, 1992 : 478-479

[41] Jones KG, Barnett HC. Cancellous-bone grafting for non-union of the tibia through the posterolateral approach. *J Bone Joint Surg Am* 1955 ; 37 : 1250-1260

[42] Judet J, Judet R. Ostéogenèse, retards de consolidation et pseudarthroses des os longs. 8th SICOT Congress, 1960 : 315

[43] Jurgens C, Wolter D, Queitsch C, Schultz JH. Treatment concepts and results in non-infected post-traumatic pseudarthroses of the femur and tibia. *Zentralbl Chir* 1994 ; 119 : 706-713

[44] Kempf I, Grosse A, Rigaut P. The treatment of noninfected pseudarthrosis of the femur and tibia with locked intramedullary nailing. *Clin Orthop* 1986 ; 212 : 142-154

[45] Kenwright J, Richardson JB, Cunningham JL, White SH, Goodship AE, Adams MA et al. Axial movement and tibial fractures. A controlled randomised trial of treatment. *J Bone Joint Surg Br* 1991 ; 73 : 654-659

[46] Khan MZ, Downing ND, Henry AP. Tibial reconstruction by ipsilateral vascularized fibular transfer. *Injury* 1996 ; 27 : 651-654

[47] Kim SJ, Yang KH, Moon SH, Lee SC. Endoscopic bone graft for delayed union and nonunion. *Arthroscopy* 1999 ; 15 : 324-329

[48] Kinzl L. Operative treatment of bone defects in traumatology. *Instr Course Lect EFORT* 1997 ; 3 : 133-143

[49] Klein MP, Rahn BA, Frigg R, Kessler S, Perren SM. Reaming versus non-reaming in medullary nailing : interference with cortical circulation of the canine tibia. *Arch Orthop Trauma Surg* 1990 ; 109 : 314-316

[50] Klemm KW. Treatment of infected pseudarthrosis of the femur and tibia with an interlocking nail. *Clin Orthop* 1986 ; 212 : 174

[51] Kristiansen TK, Ryaby JP, McCabe J, Frey JJ, Roe LR. Accelerated healing of distal radial fractures with the use of specific, low intensity ultrasound. *J Bone Joint Surg Am* 1997 ; 79 : 961-973

[52] Lammens J, Bauduin G, Driesen R, Moens P, Stuyck J, DeSmet L et al. Treatment of nonunion of the humerus using the Ilizarov external fixator. *Clin Orthop* 1998 ; 353 : 223-230

[53] Lee EH, Goh JC, Helm R, Pho RW. Donor site morbidity following resection of the fibula. *J Bone Joint Surg Br* 1990 ; 72 : 129-131

[54] Legré R, Samson P, Tomei F, Jouve JL. Traitement des pertes de substance du squelette jambier en traumatologie par transfert osseux libre vascularisé de crête iliaque. A propos de 13 cas. *Rev Chir Orthop* 1998 ; 84 : 264-271

[55] Lemaire R, Gillet P, Rondia J. Noninterlocked nailing after reaming in the treatment of tibial diaphyseal nonunions: A retrospective study of 102 cases. American academy of orthopedic surgery, 59th meeting, Washington, 1992 : 108

[56] Lortat-Jacob A, Koechlin PH, Benoit J, Lecestre P. Échecs et limites de l'opération de Papineau. À propos de 54 cas. *Rev Chir Orthop* 1977 ; 63 : 667

[57] Lowenberg DW, Feibel RJ, Louie KW, Eshima I. Combined muscle flap and Ilizarov reconstruction for bone and soft tissue defects. *Clin Orthop* 1996 ; 332 : 37-51

[58] Mainard D, Moyen B, Laurin C, Azoulai J. Un traitement efficace de pseudarthroses par l'ultrason de faible intensité. *Rev Chir Orthop* 1999 ; 85 (suppl III) : 139

[59] Marsch D. Concepts of fracture union, delayed union and nonunion. *Clin Orthop* 1998 ; 355 : 22-30

[60] Marsh DR, Shah S, Elliott J, Kurdy N. The Ilizarov method in nonunion malunion and infection of fractures. *JBone Joint Surg Br* 1997 ; 79 : 273-279

[61] Marsh JL, Prokuski L, Biermann JS. Chronic infected tibial nonunions with bone loss: Conventional techniques versus bone transport. *Clin Orthop* 1994 ; 301 : 139-146

[62] Masquelet A. Les pseudarthroses infectées de jambe. In : Cahiers d'enseignement de la SOFCOT. Paris : Expansion Scientifique Française, 1991 ; n° 40 :177-188

[63] Mathoulin CH, Gilbert A, Judet H, Judet TH, Siguier M, Brumpt B. Transfert libre de péroné vascularisé dans les pseudarthroses et pertes de substance fémorale. *Rev Chir Orthop* 1993, 79 : 492-499

[64] Matthews LS, Kaufer H, Sonstegard DA. Manual sensing of fracture stability: a biomechanical study. *Acta Orthop Scand* 1974 ; 45 : 373-381

[65] Maurer DJ, Merkow RL, Gustilo RB. Infection after intramedullary nailing of severe open tibial fractures initially treated with external fixation. *JBone Joint Surg Am* 1989 ; 71 : 835-838

[66] May JW, Jupiter JB, Weiland AJ. Current concepts review: clinical classification of post traumatic tibial osteomyelitis. *J Bone Joint Surg Am* 1989 ; 71 : 1422-1428

[67] Mayr E, Frankel V, Ruter A. Ultrasound: an alternative healing method for nonunions? *Arch Orthop Trauma Surg* 2000 ; 120 : 1-8

[68] Moyikoua A, Pena-Pitra B. Intérêt de la greffe inter-tibio-péronière dans les pseudarthroses de jambe à risque septique. A propos de 21 cas. *Rev Chir Orthop* 1998 ; 84 : 358-362

[69] Muller ME, Thomas RJ. Treatment of nonunion in fractures of long bones. *Clin Orthop* 1979 ; 138 : 141-153

[70] Nicoll EA. The treatment of gaps in long bones by cancellous insert grafts. *J Bone Joint Surg Br* 1956 ; 38 : 70

[71] Paley D. Treatment of tibial nonunion and bone loss with the Ilizarov technique. *Instr Course Lect* 1990 ; 39 : 185-197

[72] Paley D, Catagni MA, Argnani F, Villa A, Benedetti GB, Cattaneo R. Ilizarov treatment of tibial nonunions with bone loss. *Clin Orthop* 1989 ; 241 : 146-165

[73] Papineau LJ, Alfageme A, Dalcourt JP, Pilon L. Chronic osteomyelitis of long bones: resection and bone grafting with delayed skin closure. *J Bone Joint Surg Br* 1976 ; 58 : 138

[74] Phemister DB. Treatment of ununited fractures by onlay bone grafts without screw fixation and without breaking down of the fibrous union. *J Bone Joint Surg* 1947 ; 29 : 946-960

[75] Raschke MJ, Mann JW, Oedekoven G, Claudi BF. Segmental transport after unreamed intramedullary nailing. Preliminary report of a "Monorail" system. *Clin Orthop* 1992 ; 282 : 233-240

[76] Reckling FW, Waters CH. Treatment of non-unions of fractures of the tibial diaphysis by posterolateral cortical cancellous bone-grafting. *J Bone Joint Surg Am* 1980 ; 62 : 936-941

[77] Ring D, Jupiter JB, Gan BS, Israeli R, Yaremchuk J. Infected nonunion of the tibia. *Clin Orthop* 1999 ; 369 : 302-311

[78] Rompe JD, Eysel P, Hopf C, Vogel J, Küllmer K. Extrakorporeale Stosswellenapplikation bei gestörter Knochenheilung. Eine kritische Bestandsaufnahme. *Unfallchirurg* 1997 ; 100 : 845-849

[79] Russe O. Fracture of the carpal navicular. Diagnosis, non-operative treatment, and operative treatment. *J Bone Joint Surg Am* 1960 ; 42 : 759-768

[80] Saleh M, Rees AR. Bifocal surgery for deformity and bone loss-bone transport and compression distraction compared. *J Bone Joint Surg Br* 1995 ; 77 : 429-434

[81] Scott G, King JB. A prospective, double-blind trial of electrical capacitive coupling in the treatment of non-union of long bones. *J Bone Joint Surg Am* 1994 ; 76 : 820-826

[82] Sharrard WJ. A double-blind trial of pulsed electromagnetic fields for delayed union of tibial fractures. *J Bone Joint Surg Br* 1990 ; 72 : 347-355

[83] Simpson AH, Cole AS, Kenwright. Leg lengthening over an intramedullary nail. *J Bone Joint Surg Br* 1999 ; 81 : 1041-1045.

[84] Sowa DT, Weiland AJ. Clinical applications of vascularized bone autografts. *Orthop Clin North Am* 1987 ; 18 : 257-273

[85] Steen H, Field TO, Miller JA, Ludvigsen P. Biomechanical factors in the metaphyseal and diaphyseal lengthening osteotomy: an experimental and theoretical analysis in the ovine tibia. *Clin Orthop* 1990 ; 259 : 282-294

[86] Taylor GI, Miller GD, Ham FJ. The free vascularised bone graft: a clinical extension of microvascular technique. *Plast Reconstr Surg* 1975 ; 55 : 533-544

[87] Vail TP, Urbaniak JR. Donor-site morbidity with use of vascularized autogenous fibular graft. *JBone Joint SurgAm* 1996 ; 78 : 204-212

[88] Valchanou VD, Michailov P. High energy shock waves in the treatment of delayed and nonunion of fractures. *Int Orthop* 1991 ; 15 : 181-184

[89] Vidal J, Buscayret C, Connes H, Puran M, Allieu Y. Traitement des fractures ouvertes de jambe par le fixateur externe en double cadre. *Rev Chir Orthop* 1976 ; 62 : 433-448

[90] Vidal J, Buscayret C, Finzi M, Melka J. Les greffes intertibio-péronières dans le traitement des retards de consolidation jambiers. À propos de 47 cas. *Rev Chir Orthop* 1982 ; 68 : 123-132

[91] Weber GB, Czech O. Pseudarthrosis: pathology, biomechanics, therapy, results. Bern : Hans Huber Medical Publisher, 1976

[92] Weiland AJ. Current concepts review: vascularized free bone transplant. *J Bone Joint Surg Am* 1981 ; 63 : 166-169

[93] Winn SR, Uludag H, Hollinger JO. Carrier systems for bone morphogenetic proteins. *Clin Orthop* 1999 ; 367 (suppl) : S95-S106

Microvascular surgery

PN Soucacos

Abstract. – With the introduction of the operating microscope along with micro-instruments and microsutures, orthopaedic surgeons were able to achieve successful anastomoses of small vessels less than 1 mm in diameter, including digital arteries in complete and incomplete non viable, digital amputations. Although the use of microsurgery by orthopaedic surgeons, at least initially, was almost exclusively applied to replantation, the growing expertise in microsurgical techniques has evolved towards a role in the management of other traumatic injuries. Recently, the orthopaedic surgeon has been able to apply certain reconstructive microsurgical procedures, particularly free tissue transfers, such as free flaps, free vascularised bone and nerve grafts, in addition to toe-to-hand transfers. Fine work, with reliable accuracy, is made possible in microsurgery with an operating microscope, but the refined techniques and skills can only be acquired after many hours of practice. Therefore, before participating in complex cases of complete or incomplete amputations, surgeons need to demonstrate sufficient experience and skill acquired in the laboratory, where devotion of adequate time, practice and patience are prerequisites to performing small vessel anastomosis. Microsurgery in orthopaedics has made sweeping contributions to trauma and has shown a rapid growth in complicated reconstructive procedures for severe defects secondary to traumatic injury, as well as for congenital malformations.

© 2000, Editions Scientifiques et Médicales Elsevier SAS. All rights reserved.

Keywords: microvascular surgery, end-to-end anastomosis, end-to-side anastomosis, vein grafting, replantation, free flaps.

Introduction

With the introduction of the operating microscope and other means of magnification (i.e. loupes), along with micro-instruments and microsutures, orthopaedic surgeons were able to achieve successful anastomoses of small vessels less than 1 mm in diameter, including digital arteries in complete and incomplete non viable digital amputations [3]. Although the use of microsurgery by orthopaedic surgeons, at least initially, was almost exclusively applied to replantation, growing expertise in microsurgical techniques has evolved towards a role in the management of other traumatic injuries including brachial plexus injuries, peripheral nerve injuries and type IIIb and IIIc compound fractures. Furthermore, the orthopaedic surgeon has been able to perform certain reconstructive microsurgical procedures, particularly free tissue transfers, such as free flaps, free

Panayotis N Soucacos, MD, FACS, Professor and Chairman, Department of Orthopaedic Surgery, University of Ioannina, School of Medicine, Ioannina 451 10, Greece.

vascularised bone and nerve grafts, in addition to toe-to-hand transfers and a plethora of other microvascular reconstructive procedures.

Basic principles in microvascular surgery

Fine work with reliable accuracy is made possible in microsurgery with the aid of an operating microscope or magnifying loupes. However, the refined techniques and skills needed to perform microvascular procedures can only be acquired after many hours of practice. Training in the laboratory has therefore proven to be a key factor before a surgeon can make a successful clinical contribution. Before participation in complex cases of complete or incomplete non viable amputations, surgeons need to demonstrate that they have acquired adequate experience and skill in the laboratory, where devotion of time, practice and patience are prerequisites to performing small vessel anastomosis. The ability of a surgeon to obtain a patent anastomosis is dependent upon adequate magnification, proper

instruments, needles, suture material of appropriate size and meticulous microsurgical technique.

MAGNIFICATION AND INSTRUMENTATION

Microsurgical procedures are performed on small structures which require magnification. Magnification can be achieved by an operating microscope or ocular loupes *(fig 1)*. Although several types and models of operating microscopes are currently available, similar general principles apply to the use of most of them. In general, a magnification of 6x and 10x is used for dissection and exposure of small nerves and vessels, while microsurgical repair of vessels and nerves requires 16x and 25x magnification. The magnification on the operating microscope can be determined by the numbers marked on the knob. If, however, the manufacturer states that the selector knob represents only the objective magnification, then this value can be multiplied by the inscription on the eyepiece magnification, to obtain the final magnification. Double binocular (diploscope) microscopes are important tools

All references to this article must include: Soucacos PN. Microvascular surgery. Editions Scientifiques et Médicales Elsevier SAS (Paris). All rights reserved. Surgical Techniques in Orthopaedics and Traumatology, 55-030-G-10, 2000, 7 p.

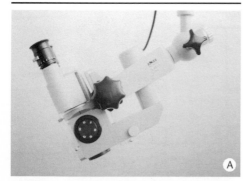

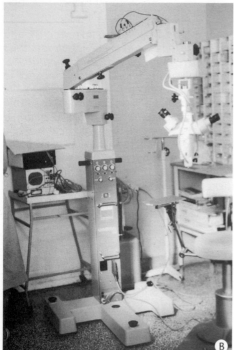

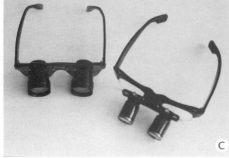

1 A. Operating microscope.
B, C. Diploscope with movable platform and foot
pedals for tracking (B), and magnifying loupes (C).

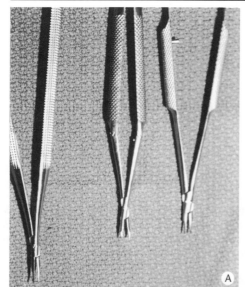

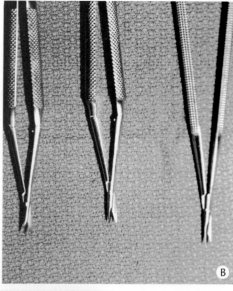

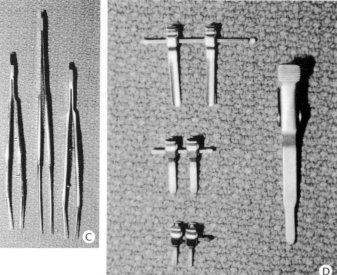

2 Instruments for microvascular surgery vary, but the basic armamentarium includes four types of micro-instruments.
A. Microneedle holders.
B. Straight and curved tip microscissors for adventitial cleaning and dissecting.
C. Microforceps for tying, fine tissue handling, needle manipulation and vessel manipulation.
D. Microclamps for holding vessels 0.3 mm to 2.0 mm in diameter. Some clamps have stay suture holding frames.

for microsurgical procedures requiring an assistant who must view the same surgical field.

While magnification from 16x to 40x is provided by the microscope and is essential when working with structures less than 2 mm in diameter, many procedures may be performed using magnifying loupes of up to 5x. Ocular loupes are invaluable tools for anastomosis of large vessels (diameter 3 mm) or for initial dissection. The magnification of loupes ranges from 2x to 8x. It is important to remember that movement is amplified when viewed through the microscope and thus, extraneous movement should be kept to a

minimum. Finally, practice in the microsurgical laboratory will assist the surgeon in keeping constant visual contact with the surgical field through the microscope and in being aware of the location of his unseen hand relative to the operating field and microscope.

Microvascular surgery usually entails long hours in one position. As a result, the surgeon's position and posture are important factors in determining the success of the outcome. Fatigue is a serious obstacle for time consuming procedures. Fatigue and tremor can be kept to a minimum by keeping elbows on a stable platform and maintaining a comfortable posture. Moreover, stabilisation of the elbow is imperative for fine control of wrist and finger movements. The absence of a stable elbow will result in accentuated and gross movements of the hand.

Microvascular instruments are extraordinarily delicate, so the surgeon can execute very precise procedures. Although a variety of specialised instrumentation exists, general requirements include simple, corrosion resistant instruments which should be made

of non-glare material and approximate accurately (*fig 2*). Microvascular procedures mainly require three or more straight and curved jeweller's forceps for manipulating fragile tissues and fine sutures. Broad tip forceps are also required for dilating the lumen and for patency testing after anastomosis. Microscissors for fine dissection are also required. Curved scissors with blunt points are better for dissection, while straight, sharp pointed scissors, with a serrated blade, are better for sectioning as they do not leave a ragged edge. Needle holders require either curved or straight fine tips. It is important, however, for the needle holders to have easy to handle round hand grips, with a continuous smooth spring action, rather than a stepped action which can produce uncontrolled movements and, subsequently, an "earthquake" phenomenon under the operating microscope. Sufficient length of scissors and needle holders will help minimise intrinsic fatigue and, in turn, decrease hand tremors and technical errors. Microvascular clamps should have a closing pressure of between 10g and 30g per square millimetre, to avoid damaging the vascular

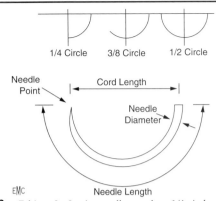

3 *Ethicon Inc® microneedles can be a 1/4 circle, 3/8 circle, 1/2 circle or straight, with a needle diameter which ranges from 30 to 130 microns and needle points which are classified as tapered (round), surgical needle (straight cutting tip) or cutting tip (Vas). The most frequently used suture materials are 10/0 and 11/0 with a 22 and 18 microdiameter monofilament nylon, respectively.*

intima of small vessels and causing subsequent thrombosis. Fine suture material is standard to the microsurgeon's armamentarium. Suture material ranges from 14 µm (8/0) to 45 µm (11/0) in diameter with atraumatic needles ranging from 30 µm to 130 µm in diameter (fig 3). Recent advances in needle design have resulted in a smaller needle-to-suture ratio. This has not only improved patency following fine microvascular procedures, but allows the surgeon to select the needle best suited for the suture material for each task. Additional instruments include irrigating tubes and bipolar cautery.

PATENCY OF MICROVASCULAR ANASTOMOSIS

The patency rate obtained in microvascular anastomosis depends on the skills learned in the laboratory and on careful attention paid to factors that influence its success. The factors which effect the patency of microvascular anastomosis include [6]:

■ *Adventitial stripping*

Minimal, no more than 1-2 mm, adventitial stripping is recommended to visualise the lumen and avoid an excess of adventitia which can invert and occlude the lumen. On the other hand, extensive stripping of the adventitia can lead to necrosis of the adventitial wall at the anastomosis site.

■ *Appropriate suture material and needles*

A tapered point needle, with a diameter of less than 75 microns, is the most suitable for vessel anastomosis and nerve suturing. Cutting or spatula type needles are inappropriate for vessel anastomosis as they can cause trauma to the intima and lead to intimal proliferation and thrombus formation.

■ *Suture technique*

Interrupted suturing is the technique of choice in contrast to a running suture which

can cause unacceptable constriction of the lumen. A few interrupted sutures symmetrically placed in both the anterior and posterior walls of the vessel are preferable to an excessive number, as the latter may produce increased areas of vessel wall necrosis which could lead to scar formation and necrosis of the intima. Excessive suturing may also cause added deformation of the ends of the vessel, causing exposure of collagen from the tunica media to blood flow, and in turn, producing clot aggregation and thrombus formation. A common technical error is to inadvertently suture a portion of both walls of the vessel together which will cause anastomotic failure. As the vessel wall, particularly the intima, is very susceptible to injury, particular care must be taken in handling the vessels: the surgeon must avoid picking up vessel edges with the forceps during suturing, and stretching the vessel. A microstapling technique for anastomosing vessels has recently been devised. This method, however, is still at the trial stage.

■ *Tension*

Suturing of the vessels must be done on healthy tissue and under no tension. The distance between the edges of the anastomosis must not exceed 1-2 mm or the transverse diameter of the vessel. Breakage of the suture during knotting and pulling of the vessel ends together, is indicative of excessive tension. On the other hand, sutures tied too loosely will project into the lumen and inevitably cause thrombus formation. In general, correct tension can be indicated by a small loop of suture visible through the opposed vessel walls. The diameter of this loop should be equal to the thickness of the wall [1].

■ *Perfusion*

Although perfusion of the lumen of the vessel is not always necessary as it may induce damage to the intima, irrigation of the edges of the vessel, to remove any residual traces of blood, is helpful.

Once anastomosis has been achieved, patency is evaluated. A simple patency test is to inspect the fullness and pulsatility of the vessel or to gently palpate the site of the anastomosis. However, the most reliable patency test is the "empty-and-refill" or "milking test" performed by clamping the artery with forceps, just distal or proximal to the anastomosis site and then milking the vessel distal to the anastomosis site using another forceps, and thus creating an empty vessel pocket (fig 4). Once an empty segment has been obtained, the proximal forceps are released. If the vessel is patent then the empty space should show blood flow and rapid filling.

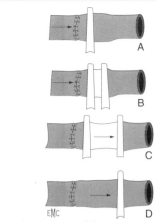

4 *A. The patency test following microvascular anastomosis involves first occluding the vessel just distal to the site of anastomosis with a clamp or forceps. (Arrow indicates direction of blood flow).*
B. Using forceps, the blood is gently milked from the vessel.
C. This causes the vessel walls to empty and flatten.
D. Once the proximal clamp or forceps is released, blood should fill the empty and flattened area, indicating a patent anastomosis.

Basic microvascular techniques

MICROVASCULAR DISSECTION

Careful microvascular dissection under magnification is used to expose the selected vessel. Magnification by a microscope is required when working with vessels less than 2 mm in diameter, while ocular loupes are valuable for the initial dissection and anastomosis of vessels greater than 3 mm in diameter. Proper exposure entails clearing enough room to be able to perform the procedure, and to visualise enough of the proximal recipient vessel so as to verify its condition. This allows the vessel to be placed in a better position for anastomosis and avoids technical errors attributable to unfavourable exposure. The proximal and distal ends are examined respectively, with care to avoid blind and extensive handling which can cause further damage. If the lumen can not be visualised, traction should be placed on the vessel stump with forceps and the vessel transsected about 0.3 to 0.5 mm from the end. Inspection of the ends will assess the condition of the intima and media and determine their suitability for anastomosis. Haemorrhage within the media, disruption of the intima and intimal tears are contra-indicated for suturing, and the damaged area should be excised. It is imperative that the anastomosis is only attempted on healthy tissue, and without tension.

Once the loose connective tissue surrounding the vessel has been removed with the jeweller's forceps and microscissors, each end of the vessel is mobilised to obtain adequate length so that both ends can be approximated without tension. This can be achieved by ligation, or by bipolar electrocautery of side branches which tether

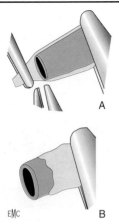

5 *Adventitial stripping using the "sleeve amputation" technique.*
A. The adventitia is gently pulled over the vessel ends and the sleeve which hangs over the vascular wall is transsected.
B. After excision of the adventitia, the remaining adventitia coils back showing the clean vascular wall, and the intima can be inspected under high magnification.

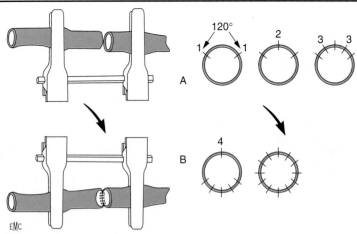

6 *End-to-end microvascular anastomosis.*
A. Once the vessel ends are placed in a bar clamp, the 2 stay sutures (1) can be placed 120 degrees apart. A suture (2) is then placed in-between the stay sutures in the anterior wall, followed by the even placement of subsequent sutures (3).
B. The clamped vessel is then turned 180 degrees to show the posterior wall. A stitch (4) is placed 120 degrees from the initial stay sutures in the posterior wall, followed by evenly spaced sutures in between.

the vessel. Branches are ligated or safely cauterised leaving about a 0.5 mm stump. Most microsurgeons find that visualisation is considerably augmented by placing a contrasting coloured plastic sheet underneath the vessel. To keep the vessel moist and pliable, and to prevent the suturing material from becoming sticky, the area should be continuously irrigated with heparinised, lactated Ringer's solution throughout the procedure

Adventitial tissue, or more specifically the collagen fibres, tissue thromboplastin and Hageman factor which it contains, is highly thrombotic when intruding into the lumen and needs to be excised to prevent clot formation and to promote visualisation of the lumen. Adventitia is removed from the vessel ends by circumferential trimming or by applying traction to the adventitia, pulling it over the vessel stump and then transsecting it ("sleeve amputation") (fig 5). By doing this, all layers of the vessel wall should be exposed, although the surgeon should always keep in mind that over cleaning may lead to trauma and devascularisation of the vessel wall. Upon inspection of the intima under high magnification (25x - 40x), the vascular wall can be cut until the normal tissue ends appear. The vessel ends can then be opposed with a clamp approximator. It should be noted that the dissection of a vein is similar to that of an artery, but since it has a thinner wall it requires more cautious handling.

END-TO-END MICROVASCULAR ANASTOMOSIS

Interrupted sutures which go through the full thickness of the vessel wall are used. The first stitch is of primary importance, as if it is incorrectly positioned, it can change the orientation of the vessel, twist the vessel or lead to stenosis. The point of needle entry must be carefully chosen, beforehand, by the

surgeon to avoid damage from several unnecessary attempts. Several points must be kept in mind during suturing. Forceps should not grip the vessel wall during suturing, but rather should create a counter force to facilitate needle passage by being inserted and gently expanded in the lumen. In general, stitches should be placed at a distance from the edge which is about twice the thickness of the vessel wall, and penetration of the needle tip should be perpendicular to the wall. The suture should involve only the deep layers of the vessel wall and not the adventitia (which should have been cleared away). Guiding the pull of the needle in a motion which follows the curvature of the needle, prevents unwanted lacerations of the vessel wall. The thread, however, should be drawn parallel to the vessel. Three single knots are usually enough for knotting the thread.

The first two sutures (stay sutures) are placed about 120 degrees, or in some cases 180 degrees, apart on the vessel's circumference. The suture ends are left long so that they can be used for traction during the anastomosis. The advantage of placing stay sutures 120 degrees apart is that the ends of the suture can be gently pulled to lightly lift the anterior wall from the posterior wall. This helps the surgeon to avoid suturing the anterior and posterior walls together inadvertently. After the two stay sutures are made, the remaining sutures are then placed symmetrically in the anterior wall (free surface). Once the clamp approximators are rotated to expose the posterior wall, a stitch, 120 degrees from the initial two stay sutures, can be placed. Additional stitches are placed in the remaining spaces. Stitches should be equally spread and numbered according to the diameter of the vessel. In general, arteries 1 mm in diameter usually need five to eight sutures, while veins need 7 to 10 sutures (fig 6).

Once the anastomosis is complete, the clamp distal to the anastomosis is removed first, followed by the upstream clamp. Some minimal bleeding between stitches is of no concern. A patency test should be performed as described above, and soft tissues are closed over the vessels so as to avoid exposure and drying of the vascular wall.

END-TO-SIDE MICROVASCULAR ANASTOMOSIS

Dissection and vessel mobilisation are performed as for end-to-end anastomosis. Once dissection and mobilisation have been carried out, a small elliptical portion is carefully excised from the recipient vessel using microscissors. The vessel which is to be connected is then cut at a 45 degree angle. Sutures with long suture ends for traction are placed in the proximal and distal ends of the ellipse of the receiving vessel, followed by sutures placed evenly between the traction sutures. First, sutures are placed in the anterior wall of the vessel, and then the side vessel is gently flipped over for the placement of the remaining sutures in the posterior wall (fig 7). Once anastomosis is complete, the procedures followed are similar to those described above.

MICROVASCULAR VEIN GRAFTING

Vein grafting is performed when the arterial gap is so large that it can not be bridged with end-to-end microvascular anastomosis without tension. In replantation procedures, this may also entail bone shortening. There are several candidate veins available for grafts which can approximate the diameter of the recipient vessel. Close approximation of sizes between vein graft and recipient vessel avoids thrombosis resulting from turbulence. Vein grafts are generally harvested from the upper and lower extremities. Upper extremity veins tend to be more flimsy because of the lower muscle

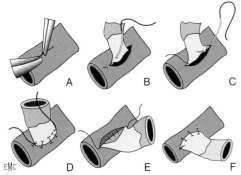

7 *End-to-side microvascular anastomosis.*
A. A small ellipse is excised with microvascular scissors from the wall of the recipient vessel. The excised ellipse is easily matched with an oblique cut on the anastomosing vessel.
B, C, D. Sutures are first placed at each end of the ellipse (B, C), followed (D) by evenly spaced sutures on the anterior wall.
E, F. The anastomosing vessel (E) is gently flipped to show the posterior wall, so that the remaining sutures can be placed (F).

content in the upper extremity, but as a result they also demonstrate fewer spasm problems. The foot and forearm are sources for veins 1 to 2 mm in diameter, although grafts can frequently be obtained from amputated parts. The graft should be handled minimally during harvesting.

When the vein is harvested, the small side branches are either ligated or cauterised far from the vein wall. A suture is placed on the proximal end. This provides an arbitrary convention for the surgeon for orienting the graft, knowing that the blood flow is always from the unmarked end of the graft towards the end with the suture. For arterial reconstruction using interposition grafts, the vein graft should be reversed end to end so as to avoid obstruction of blood flow by the valves in the veins (*fig 8*). This is not necessary for venous reconstruction. The suturing technique is similar to that used for end-to-end anastomosis described above, although size differences in vessel diameters often need to be overcome by cutting the vessel ends obliquely or in a fish-mouth pattern. The proximal anastomosis is performed once the vein graft has been gently perfused with heparinised Ringer's solution. Flow through the graft is confirmed by briefly releasing the vascular clamps. Once the distal anastomosis has been performed, flow through the graft is checked again, by removing the clamps.

Postoperative management

Although postoperative treatment and complications are diverse, and vary according to the microsurgical procedure used for the microvascular anastomosis, some general postoperative rules remain.

GENERAL CONSIDERATIONS

The patient's vital signs and vascularity of the area should be monitored continuously and regularly. The part (e.g. arm) should be

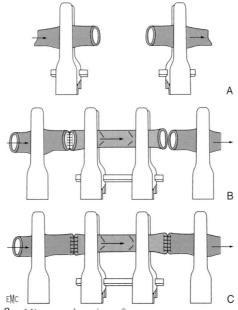

8 *Microvascular vein graft.*
A. Vessel ends which have been trimmed to healthy intima are held in microvascular clamps. (The direction of blood flow is indicated by the arrows).
B. The harvested vein graft is reversed, so as not to inhibit normal blood flow. First the proximal and then the distal anastomoses are performed, using a suturing technique similar to that described for end-to-end anastomosis.
C. The completed microvascular vein graft interposition.

kept elevated in a bulky dressing. Dressing changes should be performed every other day, so as to avoid dried blood building up and constricting the replanted part or reconstructed tissue. The room should be warm, as cooling can often lead to cold-induced vasospasm. In addition, the patient should be left in a quite room with limited visits. This avoids stress-induced vasospasm. Cigarette smoking by the patients and visitors is strictly forbidden, as nicotine is a potent inducer of vasospasm. Finally, cold drinks as well as those with caffeine are restricted.

Patients are administered antibiotics, sedative and analgesics depending upon each clinical case. Anti-coagulation therapy includes low molecular weight dextran, aspirin and Thorazine®, among others. The area is kept elevated to avoid venous congestion, although if the part appears ischaemic, it may be lowered to assist arterial flow.

ANTIBIOTIC PROPHYLAXIS AND THERAPY

Broad spectrum antibiotic (cephalosporins) are generally indicated for 5 to 10 days for patients with open injuries. They are administered parenterally or orally, and the duration of treatment is dependent on the clinical situation of the patient. For vessel repair in open injuries, antibiotic administration is considered therapeutic and the duration of administration can be somewhat longer. Prophylatic antibiotics are usually continued for about three days.

ANTI-THROMBOTIC PROPHYLAXIS AND THERAPY

Sharp lacerations of vessels usually require minimal anticoagulant therapy. In contrast, high energy crush or avulsion injuries with extensive vessel damage depend on adequate anticoagulant therapy for better patency. Among the agents commonly used are heparin, aspirin and low molecular weight dextran (dextran 40) [7].

Heparin is is usually administered intra-operatively from the time the initial anastomosis is performed until the dressing is applied. A dose of 2500-5000 units of heparin is given immediately after removal of the clamp per anastomosed artery. The role of heparin has diminished over the years, as it has become clear with experience, that patency is more a factor of suturing without tension, and on healthy tissue. The use of heparin postoperatively is also avoided because of potential excess bleeding.

POSTOPERATIVE MONITORING

Several methods of monitoring after microvascular surgery have developed over the past decade. Despite the method used, the most valuable and essential tool is the regular clinical evaluation by the surgeon and nurses. Clinical evaluation should include colour, capillary refill, temperature and turgor. Clinical evaluation should be performed continuously for the first three days postoperatively.

Among the mechanical monitoring techniques now available are: ultrasonic and Doppler probes and scanning, plethysmography, skin temperature probes, transcutaneous oxygen tension monitoring, radio-isotope clearance assays, fluorescein perfusion, among others. Overall, skin temperature monitoring probes have been found to be the simplest and most reliable adjunct to clinical evaluation. Continuous temperature monitoring is now widely used to assess temperature changes in replanted digits and vascularised free flaps. This method, which assesses the changes in relative and absolute temperature, requires three probes, one placed on the revascularised area, one on the normal adjacent area and one on the dressing. If the temperature of the revascularised area drops below 30°C or more than 3°C from the adjacent normal tissue, then vascular compromise is likely to be present.

Complications

CIRCULATORY COMPROMISE

Following microvascular repair, the area must be closely monitored to detect signs of inadequate circulation before detrimental ischaemic changes develop. Following most microvascular procedures used in replantation, free tissue transfer etc, the rule of thumb is that when the part or area develops pallor and loss of turgor (e.g. the area is pale with loss of capillary refill), then arterial insufficiency is present. On the other hand, when the area is cyanotic, congested and turgid, then venous insufficiency is present. If the problem is minor, it can sometimes be managed without having to re-operate. Ways of managing circulatory compromise are strictly dependent on whether arterial or venous insufficiency is present.

■ *Venous congestion*

The room should be warm following any type of microvascular surgery. Venous congestion is usually seen to appear gradually, 6 to 12 hours postoperatively, and shows a tendency to become progressively worse with time. If venous insufficiency is suspected, the area or part should be elevated to enhance drainage. In patients treated with free flaps, the skin of the flap develops a bluish discolouration in the segment of a flap which then rapidly spreads over the rest of the flap. It also exhibits rapid dark bleeding with a pin prick. Congestion can be relieved with the use of medicinal leeches or with small pricks in the area which are wiped with heparinised gauzes [2, 4, 5].

Once a patient demonstrates signs of venous congestion, leeches from a commercial supplier can be applied. Before leech application, the congested flap or digit is thoroughly cleaned to remove any antiseptics or old blood. The region should then be surrounded with gauze to inhibit the leech from moving to other areas. Gently handling the leeches with disposable gloves, they should be applied to the areas of skin with the greatest amount of venous insufficiency, recognised by their bluish color. To facilitate attachment, small nicks can be made in the congested region, producing a few drops of blood to stimulate the leech to bite. Once attached, the leech should be left undisturbed until it detaches voluntarily, usually about 20 minutes. Depending on its size, the leech consumes approximately 5-15 ml of blood, although blood can flow from the site of the leech's bite for 24 to 48 hours. In order to stimulate the egress of blood from the congested area, it is necessary to wipe the wound area with heparinised gauzes on a regular basis (approximately every hour). The estimated blood loss per leech applied is about 50 cc.

■ *Arterial insufficiency*

Once there are signs of arterial insufficiency present, conservative and, if necessary, surgical measures must be promptly considered. Initially, several conservative measures can be taken:
1. The part or area should be placed in a dependent position (e.g. lowered).

2. Possible constriction by splints and dressing should be examined, and removed accordingly.
3. Gentle milking of the artery from proximal to distal may also be helpful.
4. Heparin injected in a bolus of 3000-5000 units may be required.
5. Vessel spasm can be managed with the administration of about 5 ml of 0.25% bupivacaine or stellate sympathetic block when catheters are still present.

If theses conservative measures fail to correct the problem and if signs of vascular compromise persist, then the anastomosis site must be explored in a re-operation to assess patency. Exploration of the anastomosis site ranges from the removal of a few stitches, rinsing vessel ends and inspection for thrombus formation to remove the thrombus, to excision of the thrombotic area when extensive, and interpositioning of a vein graft. It is important for the surgeon to check that a strong, arterial pulse is present afterwards. If not, this may lead to renewed thrombus formation.

OTHER INTRA-OPERATIVE COMPLICATIONS

Thrombosis following vessel reconstruction can be attributed to intraoperative complications including technical errors and systemic problems. Close inspection of vessels under high-power magnification will assist the surgeon in correctly judging the extent of damage to the vascular wall and avoid repairing vessels which are irreversibly damaged. Common technical errors during anastomosis include sutures which catch the side or back wall of the vessel, sutures which fail to penetrate the wall, uneven opposition of the intima or spacing of sutures, discrepancy in size, damage to the intima from needle tears, false needle passes or probes and clamps (fig 9). Unintentional crushing of the vessels by clamps during the procedure frequently leads to postoperative thrombosis. Poor technique, including malalignment, intimal inversion, twisted anastomosis and excessive tension, requires careful assessment by the surgeon intra-operatively, to determine whether the repaired area should be resected, and the anastomosis redone. Histological examination of the anastomosis site has unequivocally demonstrated that extensive stripping of the adventitia, or suturing under tension, can seriously damage the vascular wall (fig 10).

Systemic complications which can occur intra-operatively include hypothermia, hypovolaemia and acidosis. These can result in excessive vasoconstriction which, in turn, promotes thrombus formation. In these cases, heparin has been found to be an effective prophylactic. Vascular spasm can be decreased by bicarbonates (if systemically induced), or by raising the room temperature, warm saline baths or adventitial stripping (if secondary to local

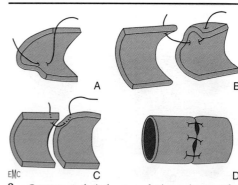

9 *Common technical errors during microvascular anastomosis include sutures catching on the back of the vessel (A), suturing the side wall of the vessel (B), sutures which are poorly placed and fail to penetrate the vessel wall fully (C), and uneven spacing of sutures with poor approximation of intima (D).*

factors). Vasoconstriction can also be controlled by local or intravascular agents, such as lidocaine, papaverine and nitroprusside.

OTHER POSTOPERATIVE COMPLICATIONS

Thrombosis of microvascular repair can be attributed to various postoperative causes including environment, oedema, haematoma, constriction and infection. Peripheral vasoconstriction or vasodilation is intimately affected by environmental conditions, such as cool air and anxiety. A decrease in tissue perfusion may be attributed to hypothermia, acidosis, hypovolaemia and shock, among others. Local pressure may increase from tight wound closure, oedema and external compression.

Salvage and revascularisation

Acute arterial thrombosis or evidence of inadequate tissue perfusion indicates the need for immediate re-exploration. If the patient shows early evidence of thrombosis following vascular anastomosis, then the wound is explored and the anastomosis is re-established after removal of the clot. Low molecular weight dextran is administered postoperatively at 20ml/hour for 1 to 5 days. During this period the patient is also given oral salicylates (325 mg twice daily). Afterwards, the patient is advised to take 325 mg aspirin per day for about 3 months.

Arterial vasospasm precipitated by changes in the local environment may mimic acute arterial thrombosis. Recognition and correction of the adverse environmental factors (e.g. cool draught) is usually sufficient to manage the problem effectively. Direct compression or reflex vasospasm may be induced by local mechanical problems, including oedema, haemorrhage or external compression. In these cases, relief of local

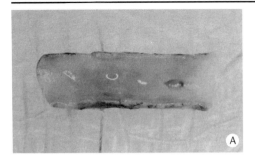

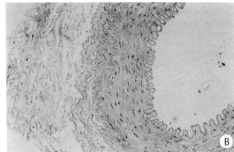

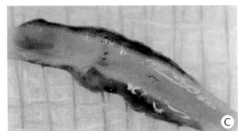

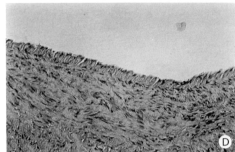

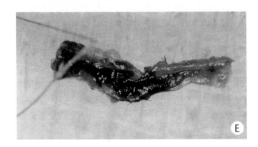

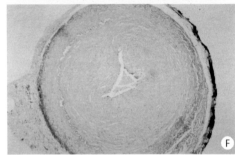

10 *Histological examination of the anastomosis site has unequivocally demonstrated that extensive stripping of the adventitia, or suturing under tension, can seriously damage the vascular wall.*

A. The appearance of the normal lumen in the longitudinal section of an intact vessel (the femoral artery of a rabbit) as it appears under the operating microscope.

B. Histological appearance of the normal vascular wall cytoarchitecture. (H& E, 50×).

C. A longitudinal section of the rabbit femoral artery following correct suturing technique. When suturing is done without tension and on healthy intima, the appearance of the lumen following an end-to-end anastomosis is close to normal (e.g. that in fig 10A).

D. This histological picture of the lumen following correct suturing technique is also similar to that of the intact vessel, showing only minimal (1 layer) proliferation of the intima. (H& E, 50×).

E. A longitudinal section of a typical example of end-to-end anastomosis under tension, and on damaged intima of the vessel which results in an abnormal vessel lumen.

F. Histological examination of a vessel anastomosed under tension and on unhealthy intima, reveals complete occlusion of the vessel lumen secondary to thrombus formation. (H& E, 50×). As a rule of thumb, suturing in microvascular surgery must be done on healthy intima and without tension.

pressure by loosening dressings, removing skin sutures or re-exploration to remove the haematoma, is usually sufficient.

Application of microvascular surgery to trauma and reconstructive orthopaedics

Microvascular surgery in orthopaedics has made sweeping contributions to trauma and has shown rapid growth in complicated reconstructive procedures for severe defects, secondary to traumatic injury, as well as for congenital malformations. Orthopaedic surgery has witnessed the growing role of microsurgical techniques in a variety of traumatic injuries. Major contributions of microvascular surgery to trauma include replantation or revascularisation of digits

and extremities, type IIIb and IIIc open fractures, and brachial plexus and peripheral nerve injuries. The application of microvascular techniques to secondary reconstructive procedures has been a relatively recent development, giving orthopaedic surgeons the ability to better manage various secondary complications associated with conventional orthopaedic surgery. Reconstructive methods primarily include: toe-to-hand transfer for treating either acquired or congenital anomalies of the hand; vascularised bone grafts for bridging large bony defects of long tubular bones in cases of septic pseudoarthrosis, and of the tibia in congenital pseudoarthrosis; following tumour resection, and in avascular necrosis of the femoral head; vascularised nerve grafts; free tissue flaps for covering large skin defects; and free muscle transfer for motor restoration.

References

[1] Daniller A, Strauch B. Symposium on microsurgery. St Louis : CV Mosby, 1976

[2] Malizos KN, Beris AE, Kabani CT, Korobilias AB, Mavrodontidis AN, Soucacos PN. Distal phalanx microsurgical replantation. *Microsurgery* 1994 ; 15 : 464-468

[3] Soucacos PN. Microsurgery in orthopaedics. In : Casteley N, Duparc J eds. Instructional courses of the european federation of orthopaedic surgery and traumatology. EFORT, Journal of Bone and Joint Surgery, 1995 ; vol 1 : 149-155

[4] Soucacos PN, Beris AE, Malizos KN, Kabani CT, Pakos S. The use of medicinal leeches, Hirudo Medicinalis, to restore venous circulation in trauma and reconstructive microsurgery. *Int Angiol* 1994 ; 13 : 251-258

[5] Soucacos PN, Beris AE, Malizos KN, Xenakis TA, Georgoulis AD. Successful treatment of venous congestion in free skin flaps using medical leeches. *Microsurgery* 1994 ; 15 : 496-500

[6] Urbaniak JR, Soucacos PN, Adelaar RS, Bright DS, Whitehurst LA. Experimental evaluation of microsurgical techniques in small artery anastomoses. *Orthop Clin North Am* 1977 ; 8 : 249-263

[7] Zoubos AB, Soucacos PN, Seaber AV, Urbaniak JR. The effect of heparin after microvascular repair in traumatically damaged arteries. *Int Angiol* 1994 ; 13 : 245-249

Approaches to the nerves of the upper extremity

C Oberlin
F Teboul
JY Beaulieu

Abstract. – A special technique is required to handle peripheral nerves for repair of traumatic lesions, decompression of compressive neuropathies and excision of tumours. It is based on the following principles: approach to the nerve from a normal zone to the site of pathology and atraumatic dissection. The main approaches to the brachial plexus, the spinal accessory nerve, the intercostal nerves and the terminal branches of the brachial plexus (musculocutaneous, radial, axillary, suprascapular, median and ulnar nerves) are described.

© 2002, Editions Scientifiques et Médicales Elsevier SAS. All rights reserved.

Keywords: nerves of the upper extremity, surgical approaches, brachial plexus, spinal accessory nerve, intercostal nerves, musculocutaneous nerve, radial nerve, axillary nerve, suprascapular nerve, median nerve, ulnar nerve.

Introduction

Surgical exposure of the peripheral nerves requires a good knowledge of the relevant anatomy, including the most common variations, as well as proper technique. Hence, prior dissection in fresh cadavers is highly recommended for surgeons who wish to practise repairs of the peripheral nerves.

Exposure of the peripheral nerves is required in various circumstances, e.g. traumatic lesions - isolated or combined with skeletal, tendinous or vascular injuries. It is also indicated in cases with syndromes of compressive neuropathy, e.g. thoracic outlet syndrome, compression of the ulnar nerve at the elbow, etc.

The final result of surgery depends equally upon the quality of the microsurgical repair and the surgical technique employed in the exposure of the nerves.

Principles

POSITION OF THE PATIENT

The site of pathology is always approached after exposure of the nerve in a normal zone. Hence, one must prepare for an adequately

Christophe Oberlin, M.D., Professor.
F Teboul, M.D., Chef de clinique, assistant des hôpitaux.
JY Beaulieu, M.D., Interne des hôpitaux.
Service de Chirurgie Orthopédique, Hôpital Bichat, 46, rue Henri Huchard, 75877 Paris cedex 18, France.

large incision at the outset. In the extremities, one must try to operate under a pneumatic tourniquet in as far as possible. If there is a possibility of the need for a nerve graft, both lower extremities must be prepared and draped before starting the operation.

SKIN INCISION

In as far as possible, it should directly overlie the affected nerve in order to avoid raising large skin flaps that could eventually result in the formation of a haematoma or produce problems in healing. These, in their turn, would lead to fibrosis that could interfere with the growth of the axons across the repair site.

It is advisable to include a Z-plasty wherever the incision crosses a joint crease.

EXPOSURE OF THE NERVE

One must always start by exposing the nerve at a distance from the lesion and progress from the normal to the pathological zones. A nerve stimulator is very useful in cases involving exposure of functioning motor nerves (absence of Wallerian degeneration). In such cases, care must be taken to avoid administration of muscle relaxant drugs. The plane of dissection should be in contact with the nerve and is better performed with a scalpel. As one reaches the pathological zone, the

disappearance of the plane of dissection indicates the beginning of the neuromatous zone that would need to be resected before the placement of a graft.

Lateral branch of the spinal accessory nerve

The spinal accessory nerve is frequently injured during biopsies of the lymph nodes in the posterior triangle in the neck. It then needs to be traced for repair. In cases with brachial plexus palsies, it is a very useful donor of axons for nerve transfers (neurotisations) [2].

APPROACH

The exposure of the spinal accessory nerve is rendered difficult by the numerous branches of the superficial cervical plexus that cross its path. In addition, it receives an anastomotic motor branch from the deep cervical plexus [1] (arising from the C2 and C3 spinal nerves). The spinal accessory nerve occupies the most posterior position in the supraclavicular region and is closest to the trapezius muscle. It is thinner than the overlying sensory nerves.

The skin incision (*fig 1A*) should follow a line joining the mastoid process to the inferolateral angle of the supraclavicular space (posterior triangle). The incision starts

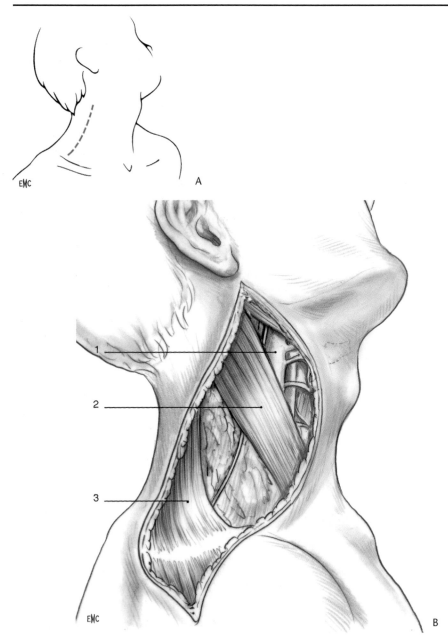

1 *A. Incision for approach to the spinal accessory nerve. The course of the spinal accessory nerve lies along the line joining the posterior border of the ascending ramus of the mandible to the anterior border of the trapezius.*
B. Approach completed. The nerve is visualised as it crosses the internal jugular vein anterior to the sternocleido-mastoid muscle and under the posterior belly of the digastric muscle. At its exit from the posterior border of the sternocleidomastoid muscle, the spinal accessory nerve must be differentiated from the numerous branches of the superficial cervical plexus.
On the other hand, it is easy to identify distally as the only nerve penetrating the anterior border of the trapezius muscle. 1. Internal jugular vein; 2. sternocleidomastoid muscle; 3. trapezius muscle.

around 4 cm below the tip of the mastoid process and extends inferiorly and laterally over a distance of 5-10 cm.

The skin and platysma are incised to expose the posterior border of the sternocleido-mastoid and the anterior border of the trapezius muscles. The spinal accessory nerve has to be traced at the superior angle between these two muscles (*fig 1B*). At this site, one finds numerous nerve branches winding round the posterior border of the sternocleidomastoid muscle. These are the branches of the superficial cervical plexus that provide sensation in the region of the ear and the mandible. The spinal accessory

lies posterior and inferior (with respect to the surgeon seated at the cephalic end of the patient) to all these branches.

In cases where it is difficult to identify the nerve at this site, it is exposed in the retrostyloid region (*fig 1B*), above the branches to the sternocleidomastoid muscle. This dissection is carried out with the help of a nerve stimulator. In 75% of the cases, the nerve passes superficial to the internal jugular vein, while the internal carotid artery lies in a deeper plane.

If the injury is more than 3 weeks old, stimulation of the distal stump will not produce any motor response in the

trapezius. In such cases, the distal portion of the spinal accessory nerve has to be traced over the deep and anterior aspects of the trapezius muscle, where it cannot be confused with any other nerve structure.

APPROACH UTILISED IN NEUROTISATIONS FOR BRACHIAL PLEXUS INJURIES

In these cases, the incision is that used for exposure of the supraclavicular portion of the brachial plexus. The phrenic nerve and the origin of the C5 root are traced and the dissection is extended posteriorly and laterally along the trapezius muscle. Here, the use of a nerve stimulator facilitates identification of the nerve.

Brachial plexus

Surgical exposure of the brachial plexus is most often indicated for traction injuries following motorcycle accidents [4, 5, 13]. In such cases, the plexus is always exposed with a view to "repair" the injured nerves. The pre-operative clinical examination, as well as the cervical myelogram combined with CT myelography or MRI, allows precise localisation of the site and extent of the lesions. At present, the surgical approach involves exposure of the anticipated sites of repair rather than exploration of the plexus. Hence, the incision and approach depend upon the surgical plan for nerve grafting or nerve transfers.

SURGICAL APPROACH TO THE BRACHIAL PLEXUS

■ *Position of the patient* (*fig 2A*)

The patient is under general anaesthesia with the exit of the endotracheal tube on the side opposite to the injured upper limb. The patient lies in a supine position with the cephalic end of the operating table being raised slightly. The head is turned to the opposite side and strapped in this position with a sticky elastic tape. The affected upper limb is placed on a side-table so that its position can be altered according to the requirement at different stages of the operation. Both the lower limbs are prepared up to the middle of the thighs so as to harvest nerve grafts if they are required.

The surgeon sits adjacent to the patient's head.

■ *Supraclavicular approach* [8]

Skin incision (*fig 2A*)

The skin is incised over the lower two-thirds of a line joining the mastoid process to the mid-point of the clavicle. This is

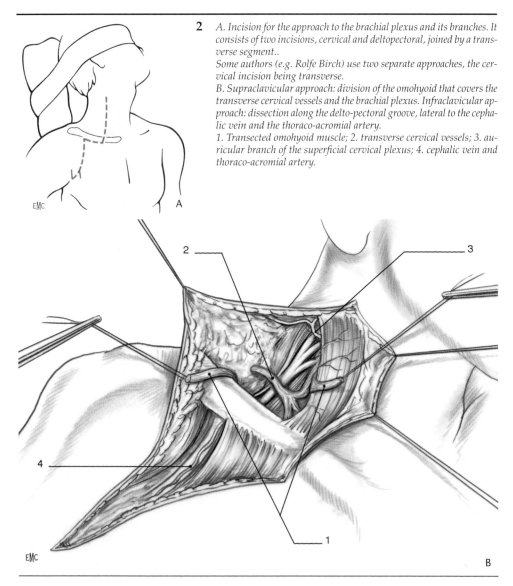

2 *A. Incision for the approach to the brachial plexus and its branches. It consists of two incisions, cervical and deltopectoral, joined by a transverse segment..*
Some authors (e.g. Rolfe Birch) use two separate approaches, the cervical incision being transverse.
B. Supraclavicular approach: division of the omohyoid that covers the transverse cervical vessels and the brachial plexus. Infraclavicular approach: dissection along the delto-pectoral groove, lateral to the cephalic vein.
1. Transected omohyoid muscle; 2. transverse cervical vessels; 3. auricular branch of the superficial cervical plexus; 4. cephalic vein and thoraco-acromial artery.

interscalene space is identified. The transverse cervical vessels that cross the path at this level are protected or divided between ligatures. The dissection proceeds upwards to the expected level of origin of the C5 root (spinal nerve). The phrenic nerve helps us identify this site as it crosses the C5 root before descending deep to the fascia covering the scalenus anterior muscle. The phrenic nerve can be easily identified clinically and with the help of a nerve stimulator. When a stump of the C5 root (extra-foraminal rupture) is found, stimulation usually evokes a motor response in the serratus anterior muscle, producing antepulsion of the shoulder. This confirms the absence of a lesion at a more proximal level (avulsion). On the other hand, if the plexus appears intact up to the intervertebral foramen with no response in the serratus anterior on stimulation, this usually corresponds to an avulsion of the roots with minimal displacement that is visible in a myelogram combined with CT-myelography.

It is then simple to expose the C6 root. It lies medial to the C5 root, i.e. below it (with respect to the surgeon). Lifting the C5 stump reveals the interscalene space and the C6 root along with some fibrosis.

The C7 stump, in the exceptional case that it exists, appears at a slightly inferior level in the same space. It is larger and has a course that is usually short and horizontal or, at least, much less vertical than that of the C5 and C6 roots. This explains the very low incidence of isolated C7 avulsions.

followed by a horizontal segment along and below the clavicle up to the superior end of the deltopectoral groove. The incision is then extended in the form of a classical delto-pectoral approach. It is prudent to incorporate a Z-plasty over the tendon of the pectoralis major, especially if it is necessary to extend the incision on to the arm.

The skin, subcutaneous tissue and platysma are incised. The latter must be carefully repaired at the end of the operation. The dissection proceeds lateral to the external jugular vein throughout the operation. The transverse veins that could obstruct the dissection are ligated. The omohyoid muscle that overlies the brachial plexus is then identified. For this, the assistant is asked to apply traction on the upper limb in order to depress the shoulder, and the overlying layer of the deep cervical fascia is incised in the supraclavicular fossa. This reveals the belly of the omohyoid as it passes downwards and laterally. The omohyoid muscle is divided between two ligatures

(fig 2B). One can then palpate the plexus or, in cases with avulsions of the roots, the fibrous tissue that replaces it.

The origin of the suprascapular nerve is located at the lateral border of the plexus. In the presence of ruptures with marked displacement of the distal stumps, the lateral border of the plexus and the origin of the suprascapular nerve are found at a lower level, behind the clavicle. Here, greater traction on the upper limb is required for exposure of these nerves.

It can be further facilitated by partial detachment of the trapezius muscle from the posterior border of the clavicle and by following the course of the lateral belly of the omohyoid muscle. The distal part of the suprascapular nerve can then be identified close to the suprascapular notch.

Exposure of the C5, C6 and C7 roots *(fig 2B)*

At this stage, the surgeon can proceed using one of the following two methods. He can dissect in a distal to proximal direction along the plexus or the fibrous tissue that has replaced it. In this way, the

Exposure of the C8 and T1 roots

This is a technically demanding procedure that is undertaken only in the absence of radiologically visible signs of root avulsions, i.e. in patients with retro- and infraclavicular lesions with clinical evidence of C8-T1 palsy.

An osteotomy of the clavicle is often necessary for this exposure (see figure 4).

In cases with compression of the plexus by a cervical rib or its equivalent, the incision is extended medially with partial detachment of the scalenus anterior muscle from the first rib. At this stage, one must take care to identify and protect the phrenic nerve, the thyrocervical trunk (branch of the subclavian artery) and the internal jugular vein (anterior and medial to the scalenus anterior). The C8 root is relatively large and has a course that is more transverse than vertical. The T1 root is generally small and has an ascending course. It can be readily visualised as it crosses the first rib. It is prudent to isolate the subclavian artery medial to the scalenus anterior with a linen tape before dissecting the C8 and T1 roots.

■ *Approach to the infraclavicular portion of the brachial plexus*

This is a routine step in cases where a nerve graft or nerve transfer for restoration of elbow flexion is envisaged.

Incision

It follows the deltopectoral groove and ends over the lateral part of the inferior border of the tendon of the pectoralis major. If it is necessary to extend the incision to the arm, a Z-plasty is incorporated at this level.

Exposure of the infraclavicular plexus *(fig 3)*

The deltopectoral groove is identified and the cephalic vein is retracted with the medial edge of the incision. The branch of the thoraco-acromial trunk to the anterior portion of the deltoid is ligated or cauterised. At the superior end of the groove, the clavicular insertion of the pectoralis major is detached over 2-3 cm. The deltoid and pectoralis major muscles are separated to reveal the coracoid process with the insertion of the pectoralis minor. Haemostasis is carefully achieved and the clavipectoral fascia is incised. The edges of the skin, fascia and muscles are separated with the help of a self-retaining retractor.

The plexus can be easily palpated after retracting the pectoralis minor superiorly. The origin of the musculocutaneous nerve from the lateral cord is usually found here. The nerve is traced distally through the coraco-brachialis muscle in order to confirm its integrity at this level (a secondary rupture of the musculocutaneous nerve is found at its entry into the coracobrachialis in 15% of cases).

In patients with extensive paralyses of the brachial plexus, the pectoralis minor should be left intact, as its subsequent re-innervation could provide useful function. On the other hand, in patients with isolated ruptures of the axillary nerve, division of the pectoralis minor would facilitate the dissection. In such cases, it is imperative to divide the muscle between two ligatures.

Dissection of the cords and of the terminal branches of the brachial plexus

The cords are traced in a distal to proximal direction. The lateral cord is usually dissected up to the origin of the ansa pectoralis, so that the distal suture of the nerve graft at a more proximal level would ensure restoration of the thoracobrachial grasp.

The axillary artery has to be isolated before dissecting the axillary and radial nerves distally. Distal dissection of the median nerve requires separation and isolation of the pectoralis major tendon. It is evident that

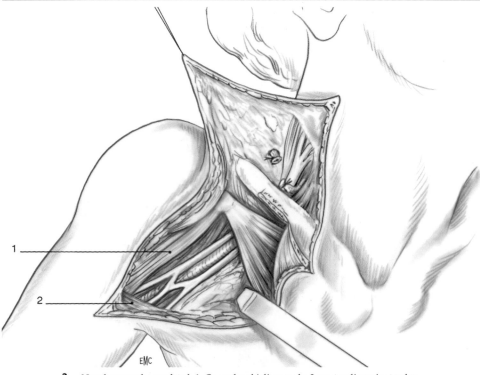

3   *Usual approach completed. 1. Coracobrachialis muscle; 2. pectoralis major tendon.*

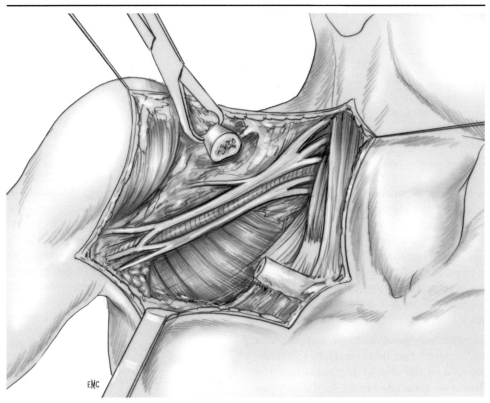

4   *Complementary approach with an osteotomy of the clavicle. A 6-holed plate is applied and the holes for the screws are drilled. Then, a transverse osteotomy is performed.*

if this tendon is divided, a strong repair must be carried out before closing the wound.

The dissection of the posterior and medial cords is more difficult. This is necessary in patients with retro- and infraclavicular lesions. In such patients, an osteotomy of the clavicle is required *(fig 4)*. The clavicle is isolated by passing anterior to the plexus

and deep to the subclavius muscle. A six-holed plate is applied over the anterior surface of the intact clavicle. The holes for the screws are prepared before performing the osteotomy to facilitate the stabilisation at the end of the procedure. The osteotomy is performed with the help of an oscillating saw. A plate is essential for stabilisation of the osteotomy in adults. The use of interosseous sutures is restricted to infants (obstetrical palsies).

In cases with associated ruptures of the musculocutaneous nerve at its passage through the coracobrachialis, the distal stump has to be located in the arm (see figure 7). The incision is extended over 5 cm distal to the tendon of the pectoralis major and along the biceps muscle. The skin and subcutaneous tissue are incised and the fascial envelope covering the biceps is opened. The biceps belly can then be retracted laterally to expose the space between the biceps and the coracobrachialis where the musculocutaneous nerve can be located by palpation. A distal stump of the nerve is always found and, paradoxically, the results of long nerve grafts to such stumps are better.

An extended form of this approach (over 10 cm) is utilised in the exposure of the nerve to the biceps and of the ulnar and median nerves for selective transfers.

EXPOSURE OF THE INTERCOSTAL NERVES

Usually, nerve transfers in extensive supraclavicular brachial plexus lesions involve the use of the lateral part of the spinal accessory nerve and of the 3rd to 6th intercostal nerves. The intercostal nerves [3] are dissected over a sufficient distance to allow a direct suture to the distal target nerve (usually the musculocutaneous or the branch of the radial nerve to the long head of the triceps).

Classically, the second intercostal nerve is left intact in order to preserve the vital intercostobrachial nerve that supplies sensation to the medial aspect of the arm.

■ **Incision** *(fig 5A)*

It follows the tendon and belly of the pectoralis major up to the sternum, passing 1-2 cm below the nipple. In women, the skin is incised along the inframammary groove.

One should avoid connecting this incision with the deltopectoral incision in order to retain a cutaneous bridge over the pectoralis major tendon. This helps to improve the eventual appearance of the scar.

■ **Approach to the intercostal nerves**

The costal insertions of the pectoralis major and minor muscles are detached by cauterisation along the 2nd to 6th ribs (for exposure of the 3rd, 4th and 5th intercostal nerves). The periosteum over the 3rd, 4th and 5th ribs is incised in the same manner from the mid-axillary line up to the costal cartilages. The lower border of the periosteum and, hence, the intercostal muscles, are gently stripped off the rib with

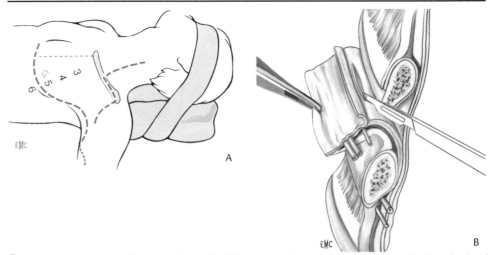

5   *A. Schematic drawing of incisions for transfer of the intercostal nerves. The incision follows the lower border of the pectoralis major and is extended along the medial aspect of the arm. Through this incision, the 3rd to 6th intercostal nerves can be exposed up to the costal cartilages (dotted line).*
This incision is not connected to the earlier deltopectoral approach so as to avoid the formation of a contracted scar.
B. Technique of harvesting the intercostal nerves. The costal periosteum is incised and elevated off the inferior aspect of the rib. The periosteal sleeve, along with the intercostal muscles, is then pulled downward strongly and incised on its deeper aspect. This reveals the intercostal nerve without any further dissection and without bleeding from the intercostal muscles.

a sharp periosteum elevator. The surgeon then tugs these muscles inferiorly while the periosteal sleeve is incised at the most superior level possible. Thus, the periosteum is incised from its deeper aspect *(fig 5B)*. This exposes the intercostal space without traversing the intercostal muscles and without significant bleeding. The intercostal nerve can then be visualised over the parietal pleura without any additional dissection. This can be confirmed by stimulation.

The nerve is first exposed over the anterior part of the intercostal space and then traced posteriorly by sharp dissection up to the mid-axillary line. The anterior and middle sensory branches are divided. The same dissection is repeated at each of the three levels. The nerves are divided anteriorly only after they have been completely freed.

It is advisable to dissect the target nerve first, in order to determine the exact length of the intercostal nerves required for a direct repair without tension.

Suprascapular nerve

Apart from the exposure of the suprascapular nerve as a part of the dissection of the supraclavicular portion of the plexus, it may be necessary to dissect this nerve in cases with compressive neuropathies. The site of compression could be the coracoid notch, below the suprascapular ligament and in the spinoglenoid notch (compression of the branch to the infraspinatus muscle alone, usually by a ganglion). Two surgical approaches can be used.

HORIZONTAL SUPRACLAVICULAR APPROACH

A transverse incision is made along the posterior border of the lateral half of the clavicle. It can be extended superiorly and medially in the direction of the C5 root. The insertion of the trapezius muscle is detached. Division of the omohyoid muscle exposes the lateral border of the plexus with the origin of the suprascapular nerve. The latter is then followed up to the suprascapular notch where the ligament is divided. Classically, the suprascapular vessels pass outside the suprascapular notch.

THE SPINAL APPROACH

The incision follows the posterior border of the spine of the scapula and, then, the acromion *(fig 6A)*. The trapezius muscle is detached from its superior border to expose the supraspinatus muscle and the suprascapular notch. Detachment of the posterior part of the deltoid from the inferior border of the spine of the scapular provides access to the infraspinatus muscle and the spinoglenoid notch *(fig 6B)*.

Musculocutaneous nerve

Exposure of the musculocutaneous nerve is indicated in patients with isolated paralyses of the flexors of the elbow following a direct contusion of the brachial plexus. Injuries of this nerve are also seen due to iatrogenic causes following operations on the shoulder or due to wounds by penetrating objects.

SURGICAL APPROACH

It is identical to the lower part of the exposure of the infra-clavicular brachial plexus. The tendon of the pectoralis major is

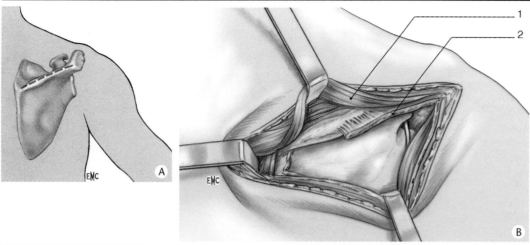

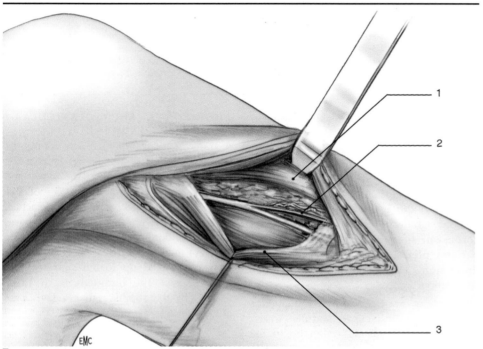

7 *Approach to the musculocutaneous nerve. The superficial fascia of the arm is incised and the fascial envelope of the biceps is opened. The biceps belly is retracted laterally to reveal the musculocutaneous nerve (the coracobrachialis muscle is retracted medially with a suture). 1. Biceps muscle; 2. nerve to the biceps muscle; 3. coracobrachialis muscle.*

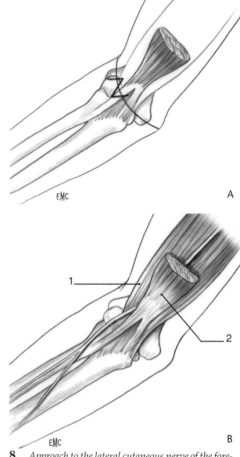

8 *Approach to the lateral cutaneous nerve of the forearm.*
A. Z-shaped incision at the elbow crease, lateral to the biceps tendon.
B. The nerve pierces the fascia just lateral to the biceps tendon. 5 cm of the nerve can be harvested as a graft. 1. Brachialis muscle; 2. biceps muscle.

preserved or, at the most, partly detached at its superior border. The musculocutaneous nerve is identified at its exit from the lateral cord. The distal stump is traced in a distal to proximal direction *(fig 7).*

APPROACH TO THE TERMINAL SENSORY PORTION OF THE MUSCULOCUTANEOUS NERVE *(fig 8)*

The musculocutaneous nerve, after its exit from the biceps and brachialis muscles, continues as the lateral cutaneous nerve of the forearm. This nerve is often used as a source of nerve graft for defects in the digital nerves in the hand. The incision is located at the lateral aspect of the biceps tendon and crosses the lateral oblique limb of the M-shaped venous arrangement at the elbow crease. The incision should be as short as possible in order to avoid a cosmetically

unappealing scar that often occurs at this site. One can thus harvest up to 5 cm of the nerve.

Axillary nerve

The axillary nerve is sometimes found to be ruptured following a dislocation of the shoulder or as a part of an infraclavicular brachial plexus injury [10, 11, 12].

PURE ANTERIOR APPROACH *(fig 9)*

This is the classical approach to the infraclavicular brachial plexus. The origin of the axillary nerve by bifurcation of the posterior cord is usually located posterior to the pectoralis minor tendon and, hence, it is necessary to divide this tendon. The nerve then passes posteriorly into the quadrilateral space.

One starts by isolation of the musculocutaneous nerve and of the axillary artery. The latter is retracted anteriorly. This may require ligature of the posterior circumflex humeral vessels. The radial nerve is retracted medially. The identity of the axillary nerve is confirmed by its oblique posterior direction and by the origin of the thoracodorsal nerve just above that of the axillary nerve. Usually, the thoracodorsal nerve is intact and gives a normal motor response in the latissimus dorsi on stimulation.

The axillary nerve can be traced over a distance of 3-4 cm by this approach.

DOUBLE (ANTERIOR AND POSTERIOR) APPROACH

This is the approach generally utilised in repairs of the axillary nerve.

The patient lies in a supine position with a sandbag placed under the scapula. The trunk is left free and the upper limb is prepared completely. This allows moving the upper limb anteriorly for the posterior incision.

■ *Anterior incision*

This is identical to the approach described above.

■ *Posterior incision* (fig 10)

The arm is held vertically and a longitudinal incision is made along the posterior border of the deltoid and lateral to the long head of the triceps. The center of the incision lies over the neck of the humerus.

The skin and subcutaneous tissue are incised and the posterior border of the deltoid is identified. The pale denervated belly of the deltoid can be easily differentiated from the triceps. The deltoid muscle is retracted towards the patient's head while the long head of the triceps is retracted inferiorly (fig 10). The distal portion of the axillary nerve is generally found more or less covered by fine vessels, particularly veins, which require careful haemostasis. The nerve can be identified by rolling it over the neck of the humerus. An extension of the incision allows identification of the branch to the teres minor.

For combined repairs of the axillary and suprascapular nerves, the deltopectoral and posterior approaches can be connected across the superior aspect of the shoulder.

INFERIOR APPROACH

Laurent Sedel described the use of this approach for the exploration of the axillary nerve in his series of patients. It is feasible only if full passive abduction of the shoulder is retained.

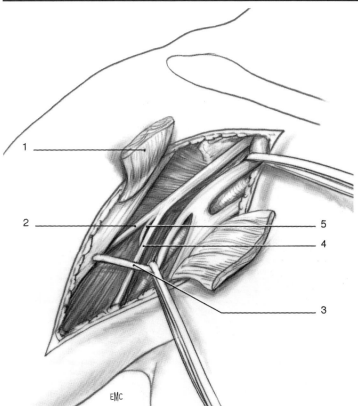

9 *The tendon of the pectoralis minor is divided. The musculocutaneous nerve (linen tape retractor) and then the axillary artery are retracted medially. The axillary nerve is usually found ruptured distal to the origin of the thoracodorsal nerve. 1. Pectoralis minor muscle; 2. axillary nerve; 3. musculocutaneous nerve; 4. radial nerve; 5. thoracodorsal nerve.*

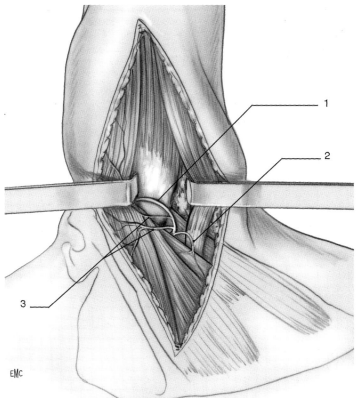

10 *Approach to the terminal part of the axillary nerve. Incision between the long head of the triceps and the depression corresponding to the paralysed deltoid muscle. The incision is centred over the neck of the humerus that is palpable.*
This approach allows identification of the branch to the teres minor, one or more sensory branches and the terminal motor branch to the deltoid. 1. Axillary nerve; 2. nerve to the teres minor muscle; 3. sensory branches of the axillary nerve.

The median nerve

The course of the median nerve is relatively superficial and it is hence vulnerable to direct injury in wounds, particularly over the volar aspect of the wrist and in the arm. It can also be injured in supracondylar fractures of the humerus with severe displacement of the shaft fragment. The need for exposure of the median nerve at the wrist is equally frequent in cases with carpal tunnel syndrome [7, 12].

APPROACH TO THE MEDIAN NERVE IN THE ARM

In the brachial canal, the median nerve gradually crosses in front of the brachial vessels from the lateral side proximally to the medial side distally.

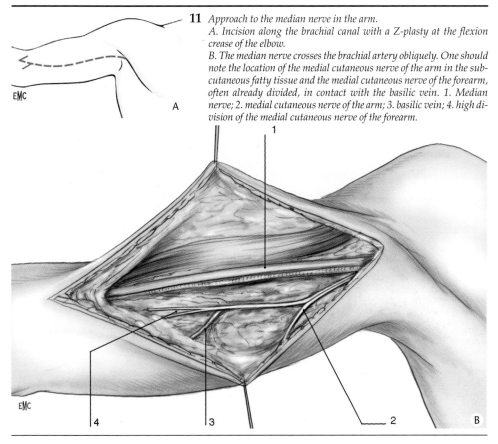

11 *Approach to the median nerve in the arm.*
A. Incision along the brachial canal with a Z-plasty at the flexion crease of the elbow.
B. The median nerve crosses the brachial artery obliquely. One should note the location of the medial cutaneous nerve of the arm in the subcutaneous fatty tissue and the medial cutaneous nerve of the forearm, often already divided, in contact with the basilic vein. 1. Median nerve; 2. medial cutaneous nerve of the arm; 3. basilic vein; 4. high division of the medial cutaneous nerve of the forearm.

■ *Incision* (fig 11A)

Its general direction follows the line joining the distal insertion of the pectoralis major tendon to the elbow crease, slightly medial to the biceps tendon. A Z-plasty is incorporated with the incision as it crosses the elbow crease.

■ *Approach*

The skin and subcutaneous tissue are incised to reveal the bicipital aponeurosis. The medial border of the biceps tendon is identified and the neurovascular bundle is exposed *(fig 11B)*. The medial cutaneous nerve of the forearm is found perforating the fascia at a variable level. It may or may not have divided at a higher level and proceeds along the forearm close to the basilic vein. The medial cutaneous nerve of the arm also varies in its size and distribution. At the medial aspect of the arm, it lies in the subcutaneous tissue.

APPROACH AT THE ELBOW CREASE

At this level, the median nerve passes between the two heads of the pronator teres

12 *Approach to the median nerve in the medial bicipital gutter and in the forearm.*
A. Incision.
B. Superficial approach. The aponeurotic expansion of the biceps is divided to expose the branches of the median nerve to the muscles of the common flexor origin.
C. Completed approach. The branches to the pronator teres, flexor carpi radialis and flexor digitorum superficialis muscles are visible. The branches to the radial two bellies of the flexor digitorum profundus and to the pronator quadratus are covered by the superficial group of muscles. 1. Pronator teres muscle; 2. flexor carpi radialis muscle; 3. palmaris longus tendon; 4. flexor digitorum superficialis muscle.

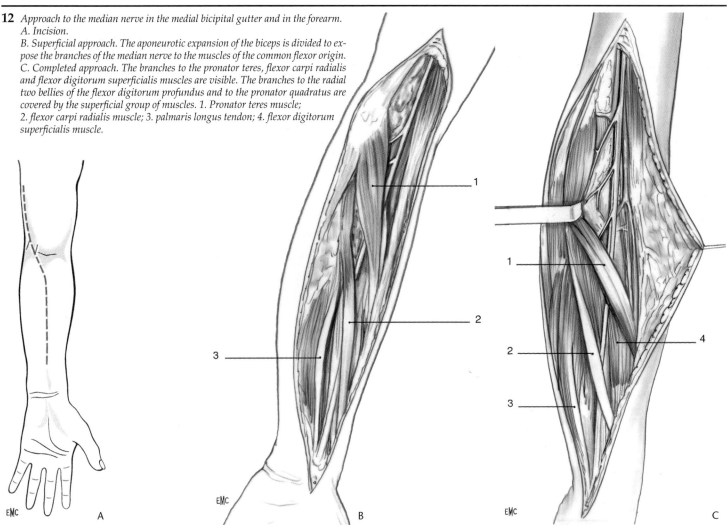

muscle and, then, under the flexor digitorum superficialis muscle.

■ *Incision* (fig 12A)

It follows a line joining the medial border of the biceps tendon to the mid-point of the volar aspect of the wrist. It includes a Z-plasty at the level of the elbow crease. The median basilic vein has to be ligated and the medial aponeurotic expansion of the biceps (lacertus fibrosus) has to be incised.

■ *Exposure of the nerve* (fig 12B)

The nerve is easily identifiable medial to the artery. It rapidly descends into a deeper plane. One must remember that the principal branches, particularly those to the muscles of the common flexor origin, leave the median nerve on its medial aspect. Hence, the nerve is approached from its lateral aspect. The superficial (humeral) origin of the pronator teres muscle has to be retracted distally to expose the median nerve (fig 12C). The nerve then passes under the fibrous arch connecting the radial and ulnar origins of the flexor digitorum superficialis muscle. This can be divided vertically, taking care to dissect in the direction of the nerve. The brachial artery divides into two branches - an ulnar-interosseous trunk that passes under the nerve at the elbow crease and the radial artery that remains lateral to the nerve. The radial artery subsequently becomes more and more superficial and accompanies the superficial branch of the radial nerve.

APPROACH TO THE MEDIAN NERVE IN THE FOREARM (fig 12A)

The incision grossly follows the anterior midline of the supinated forearm. After incision of the skin and subcutaneous tissue, the fascia covering the anterior compartment of the forearm is opened between the tendon of the flexor carpi radialis laterally and that of the palmaris longus on the medial side (fig 12B, C).

APPROACH AT THE WRIST AND IN THE HAND

The median nerve lies exactly along the midline at the wrist. The skin incision should allow exposure of the nerve without the eventual formation of a contracture and should avoid damage to the palmar cutaneous branch that arises from the anterolateral aspect of the nerve at 5-6 cm above the wrist crease.

■ *Short incision for release of carpal tunnel syndrome*

The incision is 15-20 mm long and starts at the distal wrist flexion crease. It extends

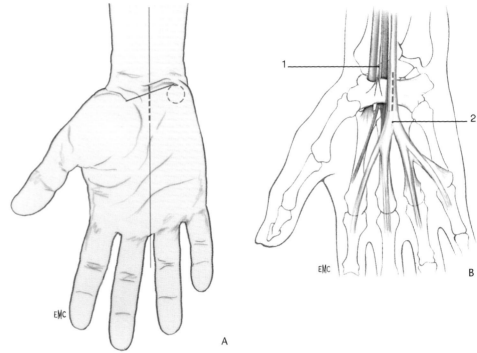

13 *Short approach for release of the carpal tunnel.*
A. Incision. It starts at the distal flexion crease of the wrist and runs in the direction of the axis of the 3rd web over a length of approximately 2 cm.
B. Details of subcutaneous approach for decompression of the median nerve in the carpal tunnel. The terminal aponeurosis of the palmaris longus is divided. It lies in a distinct plane superficial to the flexor retinaculum.
One should note the palmar cutaneous branch along the lateral border of the median nerve, which terminates anterior to the flexor retinaculum. 1. Cutaneous branch of the median nerve; 2. aponeurosis of the palmaris longus.

distally in the direction of the 3rd web space (fig 13A). It involves incision of the distal expansion of the palmaris longus tendon (fig 13B), division of some fibres of the palmaris brevis muscle, followed by opening of the flexor retinaculum. At this stage, the peritendinous synovium pouts into the incision, indicating the opening of the carpal tunnel. The incision is then completed, particularly distally where the terminal fibres of the flexor retinaculum provide the most compression of the median nerve. Proximal release of the forearm fascia is not necessary.

The radial nerve

The close approximation of the radial nerve to the humerus at the spiral groove renders it particularly vulnerable to injury with closed fractures. In such cases, the nerve function usually recovers spontaneously. Exploration of the radial nerve is indicated only after 6 weeks in the absence of clinical and electrical signs of recovery.

Sometimes, the injury to the radial nerve is iatrogenic in origin, e.g. during internal fixation of the humeral fracture, during removal of the plate or during stabilisation of fractures of the upper one-third of the radius.

Finally, paralysis of the radial nerve may result from phenomena of constriction or of torsion at the level of the lateral intermuscular septum.

The choice between the medial and the lateral approaches to the radial nerve depends upon whether one wishes to expose the nerve proximal or distal to the fibrous canal of the lateral head of the triceps. These two approaches can be combined if the lesion is located just posterior to the humerus, as is most common.

MEDIAL APPROACH

■ *Incision* (fig 14A)

It follows the axis of the brachial canal, starting from the tendon of the pectoralis major and extending distally over 10 cm. The skin and subcutaneous tissue are incised and the brachial vessels are located by palpating the arterial pulsations.

■ *Exposure of the radial nerve*

At the beginning of the brachial canal, the radial nerve lies posterior to the brachial vessels. It crosses the tendons of the latissimus dorsi and of the teres major close to their insertions on the humerus and then divides into its branches, particularly to the long head of the trixceps.

Hence, the radial nerve can be located at this level by identifying the tendons of the latissimus dorsi and teres major muscles and retracting the brachial vessels anteriorly (fig 14B).

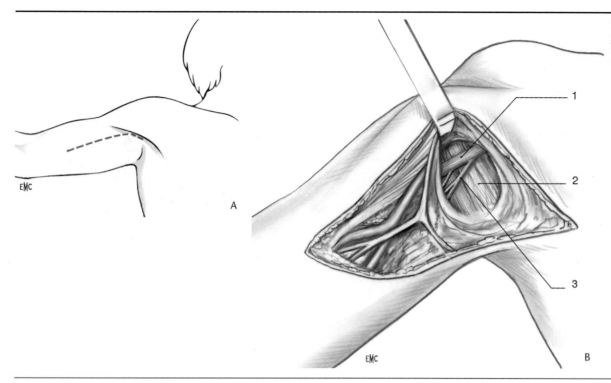

14 *Approach to the proximal part of the radial nerve at the medial aspect of the arm and in the axilla.*
A. Incision. It follows the posterior border of the brachial canal, curving medially at the inferior border of the pectoralis major tendon. B. Completed approach. The radial nerve lies posterior to the brachial neurovascular bundle (under the retractor). The nerve crosses the conjoint tendon of the latissimus dorsi and teres major muscles. At this level, the branch to the long head of the triceps separates from the radial nerve, followed by the other branches to the triceps. This division helps us identify the radial nerve at this site. 1. Radial nerve; 2. tendon of the teres major and latissimus dorsi muscles; 3. nerve to the long head of the triceps muscle.

■ *Lateral approach in the arm and at the elbow*

After its exit from the spiral groove, the radial nerve pierces the lateral intermuscular septum and courses between the brachialis and brachioradialis muscles, supplying branches to both these muscles (lateral one-third of the brachialis). The radial nerve terminates just distal to the elbow crease by dividing into the superficial branch and the posterior interosseous nerve. The terminal branches can be traced by extending the incision distally, passing lateral to the brachioradialis for the motor component.

■ *Incision* (fig 15A)

The lateral approach to the humerus continues along the lateral border of the biceps.

■ *Exposure of the nerve* (fig 15B)

The anterior border of the brachioradialis muscle is identified and retracted laterally. The lateral cutaneous nerve of the forearm (terminal portion of the musculocutaneous nerve emerging between the biceps and the brachialis) and the terminal cutaneous branches of the radial nerve are identified and protected. The radial nerve is then isolated between the brachialis and brachioradialis muscles.

■ *Approach to the motor component of the radial nerve*

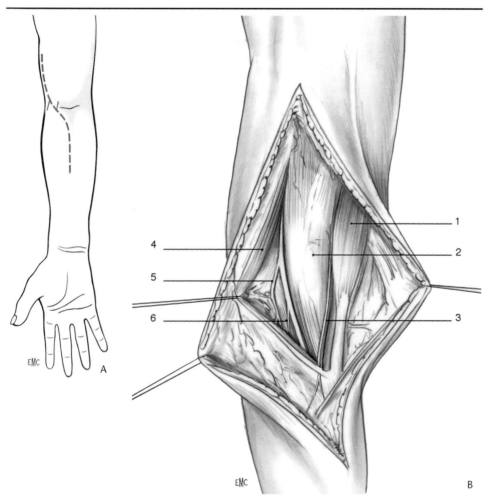

15 *Approach to the radial nerve in the lateral bicipital gutter.*
A. Incision. It is a lateral incision in the arm that extends distally in the lateral bicipital gutter. A Z-plasty is incorporated at the flexion crease of the elbow.
B. Completed approach. The radial nerve is accompanied by the anterior branch of the profunda brachii artery and gives minute cutaneous branches. Please note the lateral cutaneous nerve of the forearm lying medially. It is the terminal branch of the musculocutaneous nerve that pierces the fascia at the elbow crease. 1. Biceps muscle; 2. brachialis muscle; 3. lateral cutaneous nerve of the forearm; 4. brachioradialis muscle. 5. sensory branch of the radial nerve; 6. nerve to the brachioradialis.

The incision is extended into the forearm in a slightly posterior direction *(fig 16A)*. The dissection passes lateral to the brachioradialis and between this muscle and the radial extensors of the wrist. The supinator muscle is exposed and the

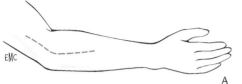

16 *Approach to the distal part of the radial nerve, at the dorsal aspect of the forearm.*
A. Incision. It starts at the lateral aspect of the arm and follows the upper one-third of the radius (the nerve crosses the neck of the radius).
B. The trunk of the radial nerve is exposed proximally at the medial aspect of the brachioradialis muscle (linen tape). The posterior interosseous nerve (motor branch) appears between the two heads of the supinator muscle. 1. Brachioradialis muscle; 2. supinator muscle; 3. extensor digitorum communis muscle; 4. extensor carpi radialis muscle.

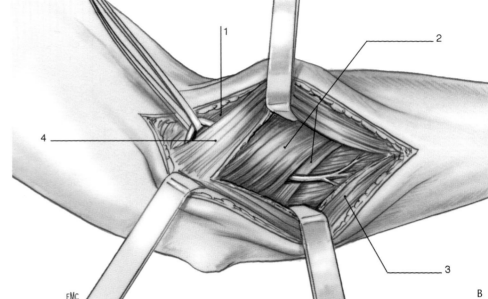

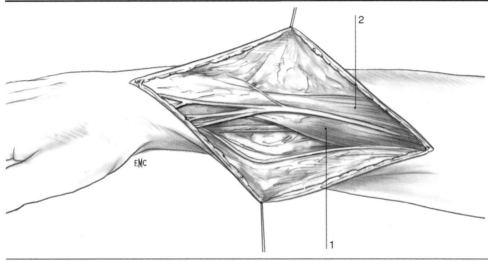

17 *Approach to the sensory branch of the radial nerve. A longitudinal incision is made along the anterolateral aspect of the forearm. The nerve emerges between the tendon of the brachioradialis and the lateral aspect of the radius. 1. Brachioradialis muscle; 2. extensor carpi radialis longus and brevis muscles.*

superficial portion is incised. The motor branch of the radial nerve follows an oblique course, passing distally and posteriorly and winding around the neck of the radius.

■ **Approach to the superficial branch of the radial nerve**

This involves a lateral incision over the junction of the middle and lower thirds of the forearm *(fig 17)*. The nerve passes posteriorly below the brachioradialis muscle and can be compressed at this site (Wartenberg's neuritis). It is not uncommon to find injuries of the superficial branch of the radial nerve at this site following plate osteosynthesis for fractures of the radius *(fig 16B)*.

Ulnar nerve

APPROACH AT THE ELBOW

It is often required in cases with compression of the ulnar nerve at this level.

■ **Incision** *(fig 18A)*

A curved incision with an anterior concavity is made on the medial aspect of the elbow. The apex of the incision lies over the medial epicondyle. Distally, the incision continues anteromedially over the belly of the flexor carpi ulnaris muscle.

■ **Exposure of the nerve** *(fig 18B)*

The nerve is located by rolling it over the humerus through the anterior portion of the triceps. It is then traced distally, posterior to the medial epicondyle. At this level, care is taken to avoid injury to the posterior branch of the medial cutaneous nerve of the forearm. The nerve follows a curved course with an anterior concavity till it reaches the fibrous arch connecting the two heads of the flexor carpi ulnaris muscle. Here it provides 1 or 2 branches to this muscle.

In cases with isolated compression of the ulnar nerve under this fibrous arch, the nerve is sometimes left in its place after

decompression. In most cases, however, it is transposed anterior to the medial epicondyle after dividing the distal portion of the medial intermuscular septum completely. An incomplete release of this septum would create a risk of secondary compression of the nerve at that site.

APPROACH IN THE FOREARM

■ **Incision** *(fig 19A)*

The incision follows a line joining the medial epicondyle to the pisiform bone along the course of the flexor carpi ulnaris [6, 9].

■ **Approach to the nerve**

The deep fascia is incised *(fig 19B)* and the flexor carpi ulnaris muscle is retracted medially. The nerve is visualised under the muscle, where the ulnar vessels that appear from a deeper plane join it. The medial bellies of the flexor digitorum profundus lie posterior to the ulnar nerve.

The dorsal cutaneous branch of the ulnar nerve arises at approximately 5 cm above

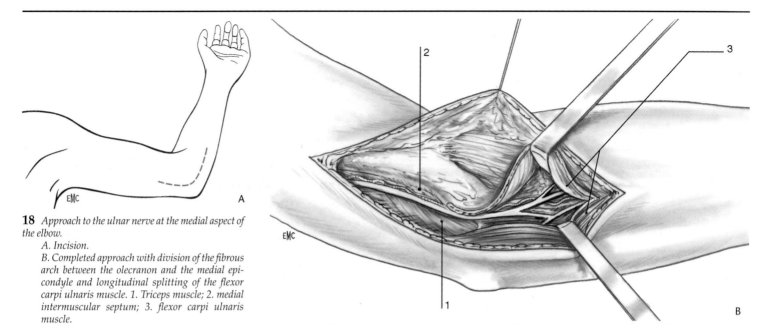

18 *Approach to the ulnar nerve at the medial aspect of the elbow.*
A. Incision.
B. Completed approach with division of the fibrous arch between the olecranon and the medial epicondyle and longitudinal splitting of the flexor carpi ulnaris muscle. 1. Triceps muscle; 2. medial intermuscular septum; 3. flexor carpi ulnaris muscle.

19 *Approach to the ulnar nerve in the forearm.*
A. Incision.
B. One passes lateral to the flexor carpi ulnaris. The flexor carpi radialis and palmaris longus are retracted laterally. The ulnar vessels emerge from a deeper plane. 1. Flexor carpi radialis muscle; 2. ulnar vessels; 3. flexor carpi ulnaris muscle; 4. palmaris longus muscle.

the wrist and passes between the ulna and the flexor carpi ulnaris tendon. It courses in the subcutaneous plane and crosses the ulnar aspect of the wrist in contact with the head of the ulna.

APPROACH AT THE WRIST

■ *Incision*

The incision is curved gently or straight with a Z-plasty at the level of the flexion crease of the wrist *(fig 20A)*. It follows a line extending from the lateral border of the tendon of the flexor carpi ulnaris.

■ *Exposure of the ulnar nerve and of its terminal branches (fig 20B)*

This is indicated in cases with benign tumours (ganglion, lipoma) in Guyon's canal, pseudarthrosis of the hook of the hamate or in traumatic lesions of the ulnar nerve at this level.

One must always start by isolating the trunk of the ulnar nerve proximal to the pisiform bone. At this level, it lies lateral to the tendon of the flexor carpi ulnaris. It then enters Guyon's canal. This is a fibro-osseous space covered by anterior expansion of the flexor retinaculum that is attached to the pisiform and extends distally down to the

hook of the hamate. The nerve is accompanied by the ulnar vessels that lie lateral to it. The nerve divides at its exit from Guyon's canal *(fig 20B)*.

The motor branch arises from its posteromedial aspect and passes posteriorly under the fibrous arch of the insertion of the flexor digiti minimi brevis muscle. This deep branch can be traced distally by division of the fibrous arch and medial retraction of the long flexor tendons along with the lumbricals.

The superficial (sensory) branch continues in the same direction as the main trunk of the ulnar nerve and passes anterior to the flexor

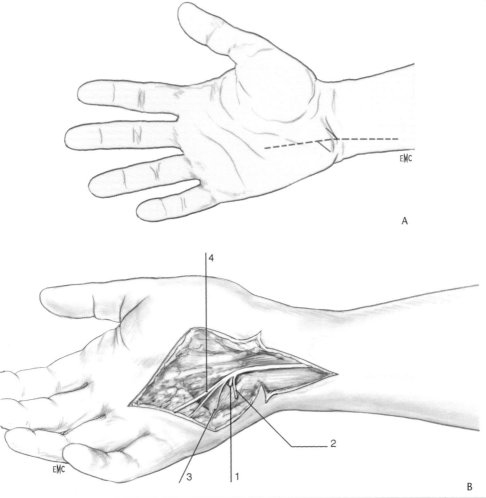

20 *Approach to the ulnar nerve at the wrist*
A. Incision. It is longitudinal and lateral to the pisi-form bone. A Z-plasty is incorporated at the flexion crease of the wrist.
B. Completed approach. The nerve to the hypothenar muscles and the digital nerves are immediately visible, medial to the ulnar artery. Division of the fibrous arch between the pisiform and the hook of the hamate, which forms the site of insertion of the hypothenar muscles, is necessary for exposure of the deep motor branch of the ulnar nerve. 1. Deep branch of the ulnar nerve; 2. nerve to the hypothenar muscles; 3. proper ulnar digital nerve to the little finger; 4. common digital nerve to the 4th web.

digiti minimi brevis. It rapidly divides into the proper medial digital nerve to the little finger and the common digital nerve to the 4th web.

References

[1] Aboujaoude J, Alnot JY, Oberlin C. Le nerf spinal accessoire. I : Étude anatomique. *Rev Chir Orthop Repar Appar Mot,* 1994 ; 80 (4) : 291-296

[2] Alnot JY, Oberlin C. Nerves available for neurotization: the spinal accessory nerve. In: Alnot JY, Narakas A, eds.Traumatic brachial plexus injuries. 1996 : 33-38

[3] Asfazadourian H, Tramond B, Dauge MC, Oberlin C. Morphometric study of the upper intercostal nerves: practical application for neurotisations in traumatic brachial plexus palsies. *Chir Main* 1999 ; 18 (4) : 243-253

[4] Bauer R, Kerschbaumer S, Poisel S. Voies d'abord en chirurgie orthopédique et traumatologique. Paris : Masson, 1988

[5] Birch R, Bonney G, WynnParry CB. Surgical disorders of the peripheral nerves. Edinburgh : Churchill Livingstone, 1998

[6] Breidenbach W, Terzis JK. The anatomy of free vascularized nerve grafts. *Clin Plast Surg* 1984 ; 11 (1) : 65-71

[7] Cadenat FM. Les voies de pénétration des membres. Paris : Doin, 1978

[8] Hovelacque A. Anatomie des nerfs crâniens et rachidiens et du système grand sympathique. Paris : Doin, 1927

[9] Lebreton E, Oberlin C, Alnot JY. Nerves which can be used as grafts: the ulnar nerve at the arm and forearm. In: Alnot JY, Narakas A, eds. Traumatic brachial plexus injuries. 1996 : 28-32

[10] Ochiai N, Nagano A, Mikami Y, Yamamoto S. Full exposure of the axillary and suprascapular nerves. *J Bone Joint Surg* 1997 ; 79B (4) : 532-533

[11] Sunderland 5. Nerves and nerve injuries. Edinburgh : Churchill Livingstone, 1972

[12] Tubiana R. Traité de chirurgie de la main, vol 2. Paris : Masson, 1990

[13] Tubiana R, McCullough CJ, Masquelet AC. Surgical exposure of the upper extremity. London : Martin Dunitz, 1990

Single-stage tissue transfer: free flaps

C Cedidi
R Hierner
AC Berger

Abstract. – *Severe trauma and radical tumour resections frequently lead to complex defects with loss of different tissue qualities. The use of microsurgical techniques now makes it possible to reconstruct complex defects as microvascular free flaps with a wide variety of tissues from sites that are distant from the defect. New concepts of early single-stage reconstruction have replaced the strategy of defect coverage using a small selection of reliable flaps and a stepwise reconstruction of the underlying functional structures. Microvascular flaps can be raised at several donor sites, such as the forearm, back, groin or leg. The subscapular vascular system from the back offers the greatest variety of flaps and tissue qualities, because muscle, skin, fascia and bone are linked in a common vascular tree. Several clinical series and case reports have demonstrated their high reliability due to the large vessel calibre of the subscapular artery.*

Keywords: free flaps, fasciocutaneous flaps, myocutaneous flaps, osteocutaneous flaps, compound flaps, soft tissue reconstruction.

General principles [3, 11, 12, 14, 18]

The stable immobilisation of fractures is an essential pre-requisite for successful soft tissue closure. If there is a fracture, it must be immobilised to ensure necessary mechanical stability and prevent further soft tissue damage. The method of fracture management applied will be determined by the extent and location of the soft tissue and bone damage.

A thorough analysis of the transplant recipient site must take place before preparation of a microsurgical transplant can begin. There is a fundamental distinction between acute and chronic soft tissue defects: acute soft tissue injuries with combined tissue defects are usually the result of high velocity trauma and, because of diagnostic and therapeutic problems, they represent a special form of multiple trauma. Chronic soft tissue defects are frequently the result of chronic osteomyelitis arising as a late complication of internal fixation.

Can Cedidi, M.D.
Robert Hierner, M.D., Ph D.
Alfred C Berger, M.D., Ph D.
Clinic for Plastic, Hand and Reconstructive Surgery, Burn Center (Head: A.C. Berger, M.D., Ph D.), Hannover Medical Center, School of Medicine, Podbielskistrasse 380, 30659 Hannover, Germany.

Criteria for successful reconstruction [3]

Nowadays, defect coverage alone is not sufficient. To fulfil the criteria of successful reconstruction, there must be:

– complete wound closure;

– durable wound closure;

– stable functional reconstruction allowing early mobilisation;

– acceptable length of time for rehabilitation and return to normal life;

– acceptable cosmetic results [3].

AIMS OF RECONSTRUCTION [3, 6, 9, 11, 18]

The aims of soft tissue reconstruction are:

– to cover soft tissue defects;

– to clear up infection;

– to prepare for further surgical procedures.

By using a free (microvascular) flap, a simultaneous reconstruction of any coexisting bone defect can also be achieved in special cases. The soft tissue lesion is covered, using skin for superficial defects and viable muscle tissue to fill cavities [3, 18]. Experimental and clinical studies have shown that chronic infections can be successfully treated by transplantation of well-vascularised tissue, usually muscle. In

dealing with acute infections, the basic principles of conservative treatment (specific antibiotic therapy) and surgical debridement are applicable. In such cases, reconstruction by flaps is chiefly of value for covering a defect. It is also an effective tool in preventing an acute infection from becoming chronic. In chronic infections, the main objective of reconstructive surgery with flaps is to clear up the infection. By covering the area with healthy well-vascularised tissue, the vascularity at the site of infection is enhanced. Improved local perfusion enables adequate levels of systemically administered antibiotics to reach the site of infection. In addition, the enhanced transport of oxygen enriched blood, together with some improvement in the body's intrinsic defence against infection in the area of the bony lesion, will convert a "non-osteogenic" or "partially osteogenic" site into a "highly osteogenic" site. This is of great value in promoting fracture union and in the reconstruction of coexisting bone defects [3].

DIAGNOSIS [3, 11, 12, 14, 18]

The history of the patient provides information which will be relevant to future treatment: this includes aetiology, how long the lesion has existed, previous therapeutic attempts, general health and chronic morbid conditions. The clinical examination is to assess the extent of damage to blood vessels, bone, nerves, muscles, tendons and skin.

Preoperative planning should include a thorough general medical work-up for preoperative optimisation of the overall conditions as well as banked blood, since this kind of procedure may require transfusions. In elective cases, preoperative autologous blood donation should be offered to the patient.

Preoperative radiography in two planes is required. A digital subtraction angiography (DSA) should be considered preoperatively if there is any doubt in delineating the anatomy of the recipient site vessels in areas altered by trauma, previous surgery, radiation or arteriosclerosis. Besides aiding the diagnosis of arterial injuries, DSA provides important information on the actual status of the arterial system. This is extremely useful in the planning of a free flap procedure. In addition, as adequate perfusion is mandatory for satisfactory wound healing, this also emphasises the importance of evaluating its quality in the distal segments of the limb. Phlebography is now more widely used, especially in trauma and chronic inflammatory conditions. The visualisation of the quality and quantity of venous drainage channels seems to be of value to minimise postoperative venous complications which may result in flap necrosis.

Magnetic resonance imaging may give additional information about the extent of a neoplastic infiltrating process and bone involvement. A detailed assessment of the real extent of soft tissue damage, especially of muscle, tendons, and nerves, is often impossible without surgical exploration.

TIMING [3, 11, 12, 14, 18]

When dealing with soft tissue defects, exposed vessels and nerves and areas of bone denuded of periosteum must be covered as soon as possible. Any accompanying vascular injuries and sub-total or complete amputations must be dealt with within 4 to 6 hours of cold ischaemia time. During this period, the soft tissue is in good condition and acute soft tissue repair ("primary closure") may be considered. However, the clinically visible soft tissue damage is usually less than the true extent of the lesion.

Delayed acute soft tissue closure, carried out 3-14 days after injury, appears to be the better option. The actual extent of the soft tissue lesions can be reliably assessed after demarcation has taken place over the following 24 to 72 hours. Absolute indications for this procedure are cases in which the extent of the soft tissue damage is initially uncertain, and those with extensively contaminated wounds. Delayed soft tissue closure is employed primarily to clear up infection and to improve the soft tissue condition in preparation for further operations. Definitive soft tissue closure is performed only after the infection site has been successfully treated, usually by

adequate wound debridement. Low-grade residual infection can be successfully treated by performing a muscle flap.

OPERATIVE TECHNIQUE

The harvesting of a microsurgical flap can only begin after a thorough analysis of the transplant recipient site (defect). During the operative procedure, an acute post-traumatic or chronic wound, whatever its origin, or a neoplasm has first to be widely resected and debrided to healthy tissue. Following ablation, the condition defines the requirements for the necessary reconstruction, either at the time of resection or at a second stage. Depending on the extent of tissue components lost after debridement to viable tissue, a suitable microvascular flap is chosen, harvested and grafted simultaneously or at a second stage. If there is any doubt about free margins after resection of a neoplasm, or of the viability of the recipient site tissue (in high voltage injury or long-standing infection), a two-stage procedure is advisable. These complex defects might be best handled by resection and temporary dressing while the specimen is thoroughly studied to determine the adequacy of resection. Once the recipient site is judged clear or healthy, a microvascular flap can be performed.

A microsurgical grafting procedure requires careful planning including preoperative design of the flap site and size, as well as determining the vascular pedicle, transplantation site and adequate placement of the patient on the operating table. The defect and the flap require positioning in such a way that enables two teams to prepare the recipient site and harvest the flap simultaneously. Additional fields for vein grafts and skin grafts should be prepped and draped.

POSTOPERATIVE CARE

Following a microvascular procedure, patients are generally placed in intensive care for close monitoring of the patient and flap. A microvascular flap can be monitored for circulatory competence by clinical judgement of capillary refill, while sophisticated techniques of laser Doppler flow measurement are currently under investigation. Other techniques, such as quantitative fluorometry, pulse oximetry or metabolic measurements associated with perfusion (temperature probes or pH monitors), have not proven reliable. If there are any persistent signs of arterial or venous insufficiency, prompt exploration of the anastomosis site is mandatory. The ability of tissue to survive a second ischaemia-re-perfusion cycle is less than its ability to survive a first episode. Vascular occlusion following initial successful transplantation produces a secondary ischaemia episode. Postoperative monitoring and prompt detection of circulatory interruption should minimise secondary ischaemia and improve

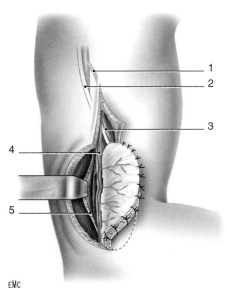

1 *Lateral upper arm flap. 1. Radial collateral artery; 2. radial nerve; 3. anterior radial collateral artery; 4. posterior radial collateral artery; 5. lateral head of triceps muscle partially divided and separated from the septum.*

the salvage rate of flaps. Patients with an uncomplicated postoperative follow-up leave the intensive care unit in 1 to 2 days and the hospital after 14 to 21 days.

Microvascular flaps

FASCIOCUTANEOUS, FASCIAL, AND CUTANEOUS FLAPS

■ *Lateral upper arm flap* [10, 11, 14]

The lateral arm flap consists of skin, subcutaneous tissue, and fascia. The flap territory reaches from the insertion of the deltoid muscle to the lateral epicondyle of the humerus and can measure up to 6 cm in width in an adult and still permit primary closure of the donor site. A wider harvested flap requires skin grafting of the donor site. The posterior radial collateral artery (a terminal branch of the profunda brachii artery) and its accompanying vein are the vascular pedicle and are dissected from the fascial layer between the biceps and triceps muscles. The pedicle vessels can measure up to 8 cm in length and be 1 to 1.5 mm in diameter. The inferior lateral cutaneous nerve of the arm can be taken with the flap for sensory reinnervation *(fig 1)*.

■ *Radial forearm flap* [10, 11, 14]

The radial forearm flap is a very thin unit of skin, subcutaneous tissue, and fascia. The pedicle is based on the underlying radial artery, its accompanying veins or subcutaneous veins. The flap can be designed to include all skin of the distal volar forearm. Its thinness makes it an ideal choice for intra-oral defects. A segment of radius can be taken with the flap as a vascularised bone graft. The donor site

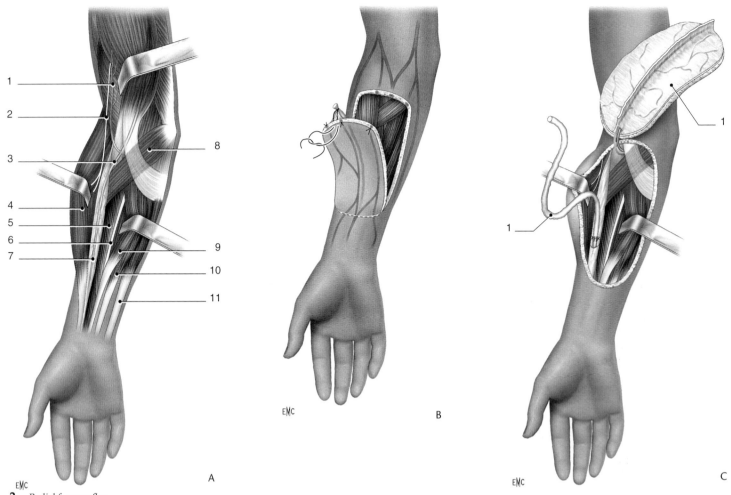

2   *Radial forearm flap.*
A. Anatomy and planning of the flap. 1. Radial recurrent artery; 2. radial nerve; 3. radial artery; 4. brachioradialis muscle; 5. flexor digitorum profundus muscle; 6. median nerve; 7. intermuscular septum and radial artery; 8. pronator teres; 9. flexor carpi radialis muscle; 10. flexor digitorum superficialis; 11. flexor carpi ulnaris.
B. Raising the flap. Superficial view.
C. Raising the flap. 1. Fasciocutaneous radial forearm flap isolated on radial artery and cephalic vein; 2. vein graft for radial anastomosis.

usually requires a skin graft. Prior to harvesting this flap, it is necessary to ensure that the patient has intact and sufficient ulnar circulation to the hand by an Allen test or, after trauma, by arteriography *(fig 2)*.

■ *Scapular/parascapular flap*
[7, 10, 11, 12, 13, 14]

The scapular or parascapular flap can be taken as a large (10 x 20 cm) cutaneous unit oriented horizontally or perpendicularly over the central portion of the scapula. The circumflex scapular vessels coming through the triangular space from their origins on the subscapular vessels, or the parascapular vessels as an extension of these vessels caudally, serve as the vascular recipient pedicle. The lateral border of the scapula can be taken with these flaps as a vascularised bone graft. The origin of the circumflex scapular vessels allows the flap to be raised as a unit with other tissue based on the thoracodorsal vessels, i.e. the latissimus dorsi and serratus flaps. For defects involving skin, muscle and other soft tissues, scapular and parascapular flaps based on the subscapular artery can be used for complex reconstructions together with a

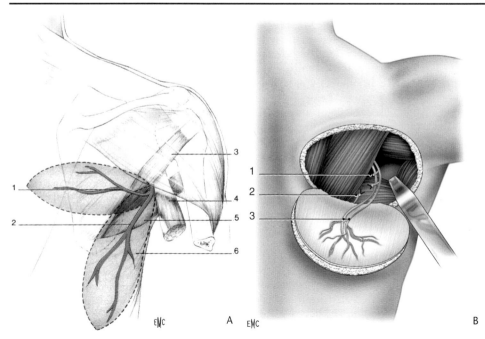

3   *Parascapular flap.*
A. Anatomy and planning of the flap. 1. Scapular artery; 2. parascapular artery; 3. teres minor muscle; 4. long branch of the triceps; 5. teres major muscle; 6. latissimus dorsi muscle.
B. Raising the flap. 1. Descending branch of circumflex scapular artery and vein (muscular branches cut); 2. parascapular cutaneous branch (ligated); 3. scapular cutaneous artery and vein.

latissimus dorsi and/or serratus anterior flap, such as the "axillary mega-flap" described by Haydn [7]. The most striking advantages of the scapular flap are its constant anatomical relationships, easy dissection technique, large diameter of the vessels, good skin quality, good cosmetic results and minimal damage to the donor area. However, the absence of sensory supply to the scapular flap must be seen as a disadvantage. These flaps are suitable for fasciocutaneous defects where bulk is to be avoided, as in head and neck reconstructions (*fig 3*).

■ **Temporoparietal fascial flap** [11, 14]

The temporoparietal fascia flap is a thin fascial unit in the scalp, superficial to the temporalis muscle and fascia and deep to the fat. The flap is harvested after raising the overlying scalp layers as anterior and posterior flaps with careful preservation of the hair follicle integrity. The pedicle of the temporoparietal fascia is represented by the superficial temporal vessels. Above the temporal muscle, the temporoparietal fascia has extensive vascular connections to the underlying skull permitting incorporation of cranial bone segments with the flap. Since the temporoparietal fascia has no cutaneous unit, it must be grafted with split-thickness skin. This flap is an attractive flap for coverage of facial and hand defects or reconstruction of earlobe defects. The donor site is usually closed by approximating the scalp flaps.

■ **Groin flap** [1, 8]

The groin flap is a bulky unit of skin and fat. The pedicle is based on the superficial circumflex iliac vessels. These small and variable vessels are dissected to the femoral vessels along the medial border of the sartorius muscle. Their suitability as a flap pedicle should be determined before the flap is completely mobilised. A cutaneous branch of T12 can be incorporated with the flap for restoration of sensation. The flap can be designed as a large unit (up to 8 x 20 cm in adults) parallel to the groin crease, and the donor site can be closed. Besides filling large cutaneous defects, the flap can be de-epithelialised for the reconstruction of subcutaneous contour defects (*fig 4*).

■ **Dorsalis pedis flap** [5, 11, 14]

The dorsalis pedis flap is a thin cutaneous flap and is mostly innervated by the deep superficial peroneal nerves. The flap is based on the dorsalis pedis artery which can be harvested in continuity with the anterior tibial artery to provide a long pedicle. The venous drainage is obtained by including a subcutaneous vein in the flap. The vein can usually be taken in continuity with the

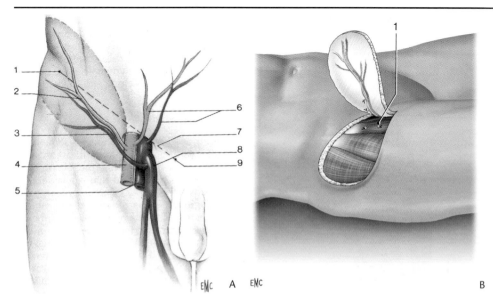

4   *Groin flap.*
A. Anatomy and planning the flap. 1. Anterosuperior iliac spina; 2. superficial circumflex iliac artery; 3. superficial circumflex iliac vein; 4. femoral artery; 5. femoral vein; 6. subcutaneous abdominal artery and vein; 7. inguinal ligament; 8. saphenous arch; 9. pubic spina.
B. Raising the flap. 1. Muscular branches of superficial circumflex iliac artery to sartorius muscle (cut).

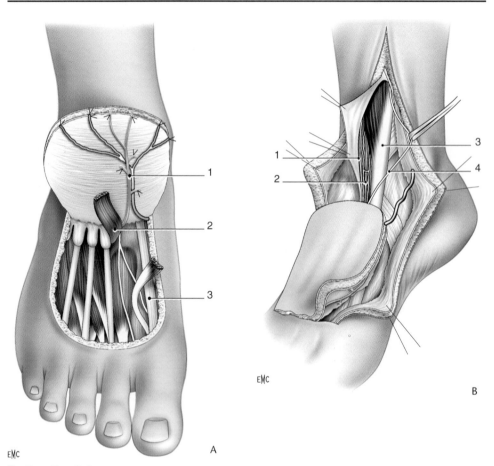

5   *Dorsalis pedis flap.*
A. Anatomy. 1. First dorsal metatarsal arch; 2. extensor hallucis brevis tendon; 3. extensor hallucis longus tendon.
B. Raising the flap. 1. Deep peroneal nerve; 2. dorsalis pedis artery and veins; 3. extensor hallucis longus; 4. superficial peroneal nerve.

saphenous vein. The underlying second metatarsal bone can be included as vascularised bone. The long pedicle of this flap makes it useful in difficult defects of the face and hands that would otherwise require vein grafts for flap insertion. The donor site of this flap requires a skin graft. Frequent donor site instability and dysaesthesia are recognised problems which limit the liberal use of this flap (*fig 5*).

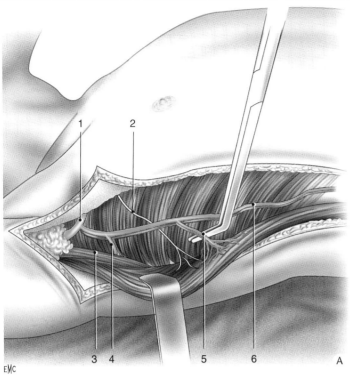

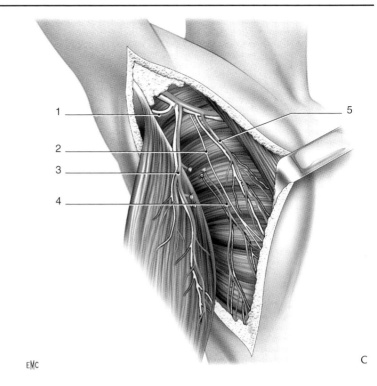

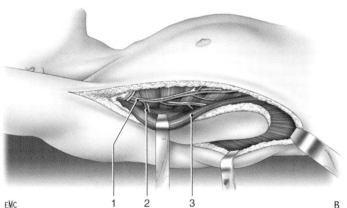

6 *Latissimus dorsi flap.*
A. Anatomy and planning the flap. 1. Axillary artery and vein; 2. long thoracic nerve; 3. teres major muscle; 4. circumflex scapular vessels; 5. vascular pedicle of the latissimus dorsi muscle; 6. vascular pedicle of the serratus muscle.
B. Raising the flap. 1. Subscapular artery; 2. thoracodorsal artery and vein; 3. latissimus dorsi muscle.
C. Proximal end of the flap. 1. Circumflex scapular artery; 2. long thoracic nerve; 3. thoracodorsal artery and vein; 4. branch of the thoracodorsal artery to serratus anterior (ligated and divided); 5. lateral thoracic artery and vein.

MYOCUTANEOUS FLAPS

■ *Latissimus dorsi flap* [7, 11]

A free latissimus dorsi flap is the graft of first choice for extensive defects involving skin, muscle and other soft tissues and for soft tissue and bone defects requiring a multi-stage treatment plan. The advantages are constant anatomy, easy dissection, large diameter of vessels, good skin quality, minimal donor site morbidity, possibility of segmenting the muscle component and of taking an auxiliary anastomosis. The latissimus dorsi is a large fan-shaped muscle that originates in the posterior layer of the lumbodorsal fascia and inserts on the humerus. Its large, reliable pedicle consists of the thoracodorsal vessels which, when taken in continuity with the subscapular vessels, yield a long pedicle with vessel diameters up to 4 mm. The thoracodorsal nerve travels with the vascular pedicle and can be used for muscular reinnervation. The overlying skin can be reliably taken with the muscle while the muscle will support a skin graft. The donor site is closed over suction drains. This large muscle is a reliable flap for complex defects of the extremities and scalp *(fig 6)*.

■ *Serratus anterior flap* [7, 11, 14]

The serratus anterior muscle is located beneath the latissimus dorsi, rising from the first nine ribs and anchoring in the scapula. The most caudal four slips of this muscle can be transplanted and fed by vessels which are continuous with the thoracodorsal vessels which, in their turn, can be incorporated into the pedicle for extra length. The distal segment of the long thoracic nerve is taken with the flap and can be used for restoration of muscular function. The proximal segment of the nerve must be protected to preserve the innervation of the upper serratus slips and prevent scapular winging. The serratus muscle flap is a malleable piece of tissue that can be fitted into irregular defects. This flap has been used for functional reconstruction of the face and hand. The long vascular pedicle makes flap positioning very flexible. Underlying ribs can be harvested as a vascularised bone graft *(fig 7)*.

■ *Rectus abdominis flap* [10, 11, 12, 13, 14]

The rectus abdominis flap is a long muscle flap that can cover defects with dimensions up to 10 x 25 cm. Overlying skin can be taken, either parallel to the muscle or transversely oriented over the distal third and extending to the iliac crest. The muscle is mobilised out of the rectus sheath and the inferior epigastric vessel pedicle. The myocutaneous flap, using the transverse abdominal skin, is increasingly used for breast reconstruction. The muscle flap is a very reliable cover for limited size defects of the extremities and head. Careful closure of the rectus sheath is necessary to prevent herniation or diffuse bulging at the donor site.

■ *Gracilis muscle flap* [10, 11, 12, 13, 14]

The gracilis muscle originates from the pubic tubercle and inserts in the tibia underneath the medial condyle. The gracilis flap is

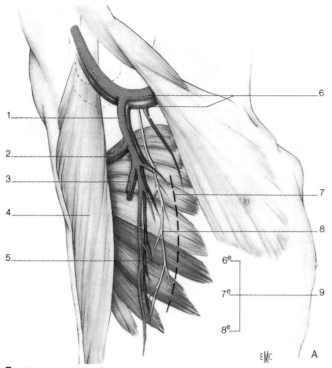

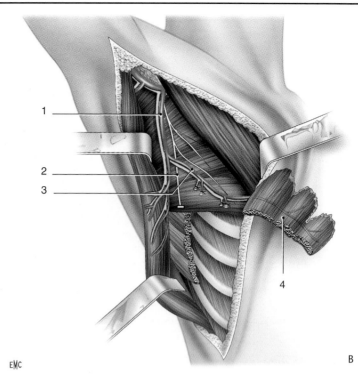

7 *Serratus anterior flap.*

A. Anatomy and planning of the flap. 1. Suprascapular artery; 2. circumflex scapular artery and vein; 3. thoracodorsal artery and vein; 4. latissimus dorsi muscle 5. artery and vein of the serratus muscle; 6. axillary artery and vein; 7. skin incision; 8. nerve of serratus muscle; 9. branches of the serratus muscle.

B. Raising the flap. 1. Thoracodorsal artery and vein; 2. long thoracic nerve; 3. serratus anterior branch of the thoracodorsal artery and vein; 4. serratus anterior muscle.

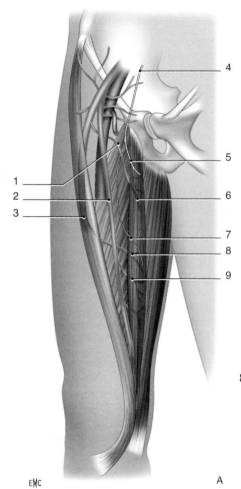

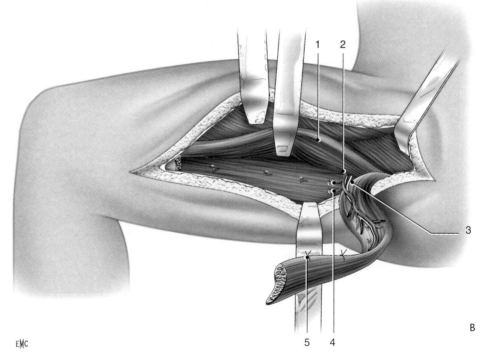

8 *Gracilis (myocutaneous) flap.*

A. Anatomy and planning the flap. 1. Medial femoral circumflex artery; 2. deep femoral artery; 3. superficial femoral artery (under sartorius muscle); 4. obturator nerve; 5. muscular branch of the obturator nerve; 6. perforating branch of the medial femoral circumflex artery; 7. cutaneous branch of the obturator nerve; 8. deep femoral perforating artery; 9. perforating branch of the superficial femoral artery.

B. Raising the flap. 1. Adductor longus muscle; 2. medial femoral circumflex artery; 3. muscular branch of the obturator nerve; 4. branches to adductor longus and magnus muscles (ligated); 5. five centimetre markers on gracilis muscle.

useful as a functional muscle in facial and extremity reconstruction. This long muscle can also be used for general coverage of small- to medium-sized defects with minimal donor site morbidity. The muscle is harvested through a medial thigh incision. The primary vascular pedicle is composed of terminal branches of the medial femoral circumflex vessels. The terminal obturator nerve is taken with the gracilis for restoration of muscular function. A cutaneous component can be reliably taken over the proximal third of the muscle (fig 8).

OSTEOCUTANEOUS FLAPS

Several of the flaps described above can be designed to include components of vascularised bone. These multi-component flaps can solve a combined skeletal-soft-tissue defect with a single transplant. The most commonly used combination flaps are temporoparietal fascia/calvarial bone, radial forearm flap/radius, scapula flap/scapula and serratus/rib.

■ *Anterior iliac crest flap* [1, 11, 14]

A vascularised anterior iliac crest graft or deep circumflex iliac artery (DCIA) flap is indicated for bone defects < 10 cm in size when there is a small soft tissue defect which requires coverage simultaneously in a "single stage" operation. The iliac crest can be transplanted with the deep circumflex iliac vessels. Flap elevation may involve division of the inguinal ligament if the pedicle vessels originate from the iliac vessel. Careful donor site reconstruction is necessary to prevent herniation. The iliac crest yields a thick flap of bicortical bone that can be 14 cm long in adults. Osteotomes can be safely used to shape this bone flap. A skin component, based on periosteal perforators, can be included with the flap.

In cases of bone defects due to chronic osteomyelitis in particular, vascularised anterior iliac crest grafts have proved superior to vascularised fibular grafts and they achieve bony incorporation into the tibia in a higher percentage of cases. The superiority of vascularised anterior iliac crest grafts lies in their good resistance to unfavourable conditions in the graft bed and the high incidence of successful bony incorporation even at "partially osteogenic" or "non-osteogenic" sites. This emphasises the fact that tissue coverage can be carried out at the same time as bone grafting. The constancy of the anatomical relationships, the large diameter of the artery and the acceptable defect of the donor area are advantages of this flap. The disadvantage is the unsatisfactory cosmetic result due to the large proportion of subcutaneous adipose tissue (fig 9).

■ *Fibular flap* [2, 4, 11, 14, 15, 16, 17]

The use of a vascularised fibular graft is indicated mainly for bone defects greater than 10 cm in size. As in an illiac crest graft,

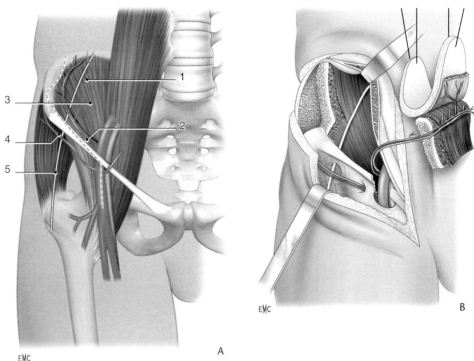

9 Anterior iliac crest flap.
  A. Anatomy and planning the flap. 1. R. ascendens; 2. deep circumflex iliac artery; 3. iliac muscle; 4. superficial circumflex iliac artery; 5. lateral cutaneous nerve of the thigh.
  B. Raising the flap.

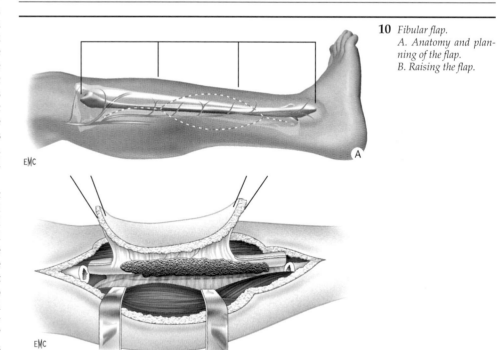

10 Fibular flap.
  A. Anatomy and planning of the flap.
  B. Raising the flap.

a medium-sized soft tissue defect can be reconstructed at the same time in a single stage operation. Other advantages are the good resistance of the graft to unfavourable conditions at the host site, the high rate of bony consolidation even when local vascularity is poor, constant anatomy, easy dissection, large vessel diameter, minimal damage in the donor area and the relatively high initial load-bearing capacity of the vascularised cortical bone graft. Furthermore, vascular defects involving a considerable length of artery can be reconstructed by a second anastomosis based on the "flow through" principle. The disadvantages are: hypertrophy of the graft is often unsatisfactory, the 10% to 25% incidence of stress fractures after remobilisation, the unaesthetic cosmetic result in the donor area after raising an osteomyocutaneous fibular graft and the possibility of a progressive valgus deformity in the donor area in children after removal of the fibula (fig 10).

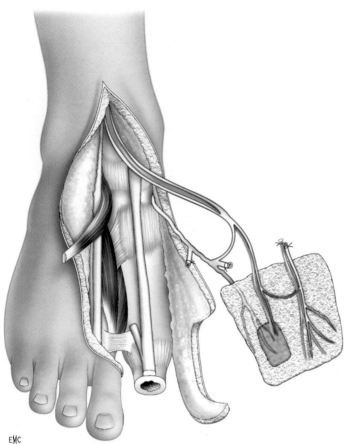

11 *Wrap around flap. Raising the flap.*

arterial supply for the toe and a subcutaneous vein provides venous return. If there is doubt about the dorsalis pedis supplying the great toe, either because of trauma or the existence of a dominant plantar arterial system, the foot should be studied by arteriography. Dissection of the recipient site should provide measurements for the toe transplant, including skeletal, tendon, vessel, and nerve length. The donor defect of the foot requires careful closure and mobilisation with occasional secondary revision for soft-tissue problems or neuroma. Most patients recover with minimal or no functional defect.

The second toe has been used for thumb reconstruction, but is best suited as a transplant for an ulnar digit to provide pinch. An arteriography is recommended to delineate recipient site vessels in the palm. The second toe may receive a dominant blood supply from either the dorsal first metatarsal artery or plantar arteries, and the largest pedicle vessel must be chosen after carefully dissecting both options. The donor site is closed as a ray amputation with negligible morbidity.

Combined second and third toe transplants can provide two digits in a single unit. These units are suitable for replacing fingers that have been amputated proximal to the web space. This transplant is also based on either the dorsal metatarsal artery or plantar vessels.

Subtotal toe or "wrap-around" flaps use only a segment of the great or second toe. For example, a partial thumb amputation can be reconstructed by taking only part of the donor toe, e.g. the distal phalanx, nail bed, and a portion of the pulp from the toe. The stump of the great toe can then be covered by skin grafts or local flaps *(fig 11)*.

COMPOUND FLAPS

■ *Toe transplants: wrap around flap* [4, 10, 11, 12]

Toe transplantation offers a single-stage reconstruction for missing digits. Most often applied to thumb reconstruction, toe transplantation can also provide multiple opposable digits for a severely injured or mal-developed hand. Great toe transplantation can be used to replace a missing thumb if at least one third of the metacarpal shaft remains. Thumb amputation at the metacarpophalangeal or proximal phalangeal level can be reconstructed with a great toe amputated at the appropriate level. The dorsal radial vessels in the snuff box are preferred as recipient vessels, and if doubt exists about their availability, the recipient area should be studied by angiography.

The terminal segment of the dorsalis pedis artery (the dorsal metatarsal artery) is the

References

[1] Allieu Y, Gomis R, Bonnel F et al. The free composed cutaneous-osseous iliac flap (FCCOIF). *Anat Clin* 1980 ; 2 : 83-88

[2] Baudet J, Panconi P, Schoofs M et al. The composite fibula and soleus transfer. *Int J Microsurg* 1983 ; 5 : 10-26

[3] Berger A, Hierner R. Neue Entwicklungen bei der Deckung posttraumatischer Weichteildefekte. *Orthopäde* 1997 ; 26 : 470-480

[4] Chen ZW, Yan W. The study and clinical application of the osteocutaneous flap of the fibula. *Microsurgery* 1983 ; 4 : 11-16

[5] Foucher G, Marin-Braun F, Smith DJ Jr. Custom-made free vascularized compound toe for traumatic loss of the thumb. *Plast Reconstr Surg* 1991 ; 87 : 310-314

[6] Gustilo RB. Management of open fractures and their complications. Philadelphia : WB Saunders, 1982

[7] Haydn RE. The mega-flap, Lecture at the international congress for microsurgery in Brescia, 27-21 July 1987

[8] Irons GB. An overview: Indications for complete skin coverage in the lower limb. *Microsurgery* 1990 ; 11 : 48-53

[9] Kerrigan CL, Zelt RG, Daniel RK. Secondary critical ischemia time of experimental skin flaps. *Plast Reconstr Surg* 1984 ; 74 : 522-526

[10] Mantkelow RT. Microvascular reconstruction. Heidelberg : Springer-Verlag, 1986

[11] Mathes SJ, Nahai F. Reconstructive surgery. Edinburgh : Churchill Livingstone, 1997

[12] O'Brien BM, Morrison WA, Gumley GJ. Principles and techniques of microvascular surgery. In : Plastic surgery. Philadelphia : WB Saunders, 1990 : 413

[13] Raine T. Microvascular techniques. In : Jurkiewicz MJ ed. Plastic surgery: principles and practice. St Louis : Mosby-Year Book, 1990 : 1573

[14] Serafin D. Atlas of microsurgical composite tissue transplantation. Philadelphia : WB Saunders, 1996

[15] Siegert JJ, Wood MB. Thrombosed vascularized bone graft: viability compared with conventional bone graft. *J Reconstr Microsurg* 1987 ; 3 : 99-103

[16] Wei FC, Colony LH, Chen H, Chuang CC, Noordhoff MS. Combined second and third toe transfer. *Plast Reconstr Surg* 1989 ; 84 : 651-661

[17] Wood MB, Cooney WP. Vascularized bone segment transfer for management of chronic osteomyelitis. *Orthop Clin North Am* 1984 ; 15 : 461-471

[18] Yaremchuk MJ, Brumback RJ, Manson PM, Burgess AR, Poka A, Weiland AJ. Acute and definitive management of traumatic osteocutaneous defects of the lower extremity. *Plast Reconstr Surg* 1987 ; 80 : 1-14

[19] Zwipp H, Flory P, Borger A, Tscherne H. Kombination von Spongiosaplastik und freier mikrovaskulärer Knochentransplantation bei grossen knöchernen Defekten. *Handchir Mikrochir Plast Chir* 1989 ; 21 : 235-245

Vascularised bone transfers

R Hierner
G Felmerer
A Berger

Abstract. – Pedicled bone grafts (local vascularised bone transfers) have been used since the beginning of the twentieth century, but microvascular bone grafts (free vascularised bone transfers) have only been known since the beginning of the 1970s.

Vascularised bone grafts have been compared to non-vascularised grafts in numerous experimental and clinical studies. As they have their own uninterrupted blood supply and thus nearly normal vitality in the recipient site, compared to their non-vascularised analogues, vascularised bone grafts show:

– more rapid fracture healing;

– better adaptation to the new mechanical loadings (e.g. graft hypertrophy);

– a higher survival and consolidation rate in poor recipient bed conditions (infection, poor vascularisation);

– some neovascularisation potential on the surrounding bone tissue.

Given these properties, it became possible to successfully treat a large segmental bone defect with a reduced number of operations. Severely damaged extremities which would have been amputated before could now be functionally reconstructed. However, during the 1980s, the initial enthusiasm to treat all complex combined soft tissue/bone defects by a free vascularised composite flap subsided, because of high complication rates of up to 40%-60%. Over the following years, as a result of large clinical studies, indications and contraindications were better defined and the complication rate was lowered to approximately 10%. It was found that even for vascularised bone grafts, the functional status of the surrounding soft tissue plays a major role in successful bone healing. Thus, bone reconstruction must never precede soft tissue repair. With this increased knowledge, it became possible to choose the best-suited vascularised bone graft for each individual case. This type of graft should be limited to a few specialised centres, because of its long operation time and the absolute need to master microsurgical techniques.

Cancellous bone grafting, callus distraction and free vascularised bone grafts have often been described as competing reconstruction techniques, but they are now viewed as complementary procedures, with every technique having a so-called main indication, i.e. a situation in which the use of that specific technique will lead to the best functional and cosmetic results at the lowest risk for the patient [8, 10, 34, 37, 38, 43, 48].

Keywords: free vascularised bone transfers, fibula bone grafts, iliac crest graft, scapula bone graft, humerus bone graft, radius bone graft, pisiform transfer.

General considerations

BLOOD SUPPLY OF BONE
[2, 4, 5, 7, 17, 25, 27, 28, 29, 39]

In long bones in particular, two main systems of internal blood supply can be distinguished:

– the central medullary blood supply;

– the peripheral musculoperiosteal blood supply.

Robert Hierner, M.D., Ph D.
G Felmerer, M.D.
Alfred Berger, M.D., Ph D.
Clinic for Plastic, Hand and Reconstructive Surgery, Burn Center, Hannover Medical Center, School of Medicine, Podbielskistrasse 380, 30659 Hannover, Germany.

Both systems are connected through multiple anastomoses and are, to different degrees, responsible for the nutrition of the cortical bone (fig 1A, C). According to the "concept of the dual blood supply" described by Berggren et al [4], the intraosseous blood vessels correspond to a system of rigid tubes in which the blood flow is directed following the pressure gradient. In physiological circumstances, the internal two-thirds of the cortex are mainly supplied from the medullary space, the outer third is supplied from the musculoperiosteal vascular system (fig 1A). A reverse flow is possible. If the blood pressure in the bone marrow drops below the pressure in the periosteum (e.g. after insertion of an intramedullary nail), then a centripetal pressure gradient rises and causes a centripetal blood flow. The cortex is then vascularised almost completely from the periosteal vascular system ("musculoperiosteal blood supply") (fig 1B). The missing medullary blood supply can be compensated for by the periosteal blood supply. On the other hand, if the blood pressure in the musculoperiosteal system decreases markedly, e.g. following burn injuries, then the whole cortex can be nourished almost completely from the medullary vascular system ("medullary vascular supply") (fig 1C). Animal experiments and clinical studies have shown that medullary as well as periosteal blood supplies alone provide a sufficient blood supply to a vascularised bone graft.

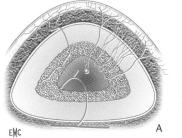 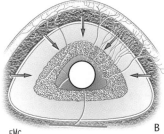 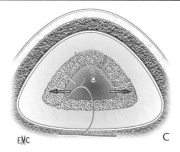

1 *Concept of the dual blood supply according to Berggren [4].*
A. Physiological blood supply (in the diaphyseal region).
B. Musculoperiosteal (centripetal) blood supply during blockade of the medullary central vascular system.
C. Medullary (centrifugal) blood supply during blockade of the musculoperiosteal peripheral vascular system.

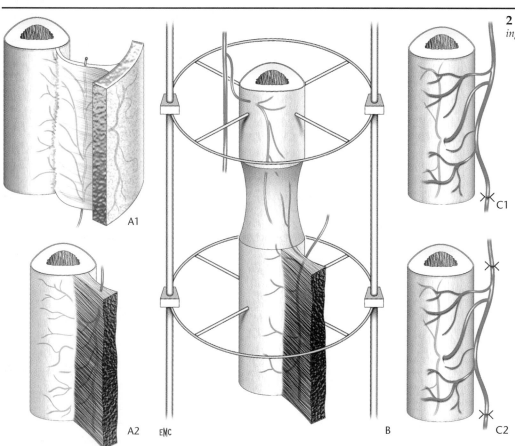

2 *Classification of vascularised bone grafts according to their external vascularisation pattern.*
A. Type I: Random pattern flaps. A1. Skin-pedicled flap; A2. muscle-pedicled flap.
B. Type II: Segmental bone transfer.
C. Type III: Axial pattern flaps. C1. Vascular pedicled flap. C2. free microvascular transplantation flap.

CLASSIFICATION

Vascularised bone grafts are defined as grafts which are transplanted to their host site with their own blood supply. With regard to the macroscopic external blood supply, several types of vascularised bone graft can be distinguished (*fig 2*).

Skin- (type Ia) and muscle-pedicled (type Ib) transplants belong to "random pattern flaps", because their blood supply comes through vessels which are not anatomically classifiable and localisable. The blood supply comes according to a circuit change from the periosteal vascular system of the bone in a centripetal direction to the bone marrow. Because of their vascularisation, the "random pattern flaps" take an intermediate position, concerning biological and mechanical properties, between the conventional or non-vascularised bone graft and the vascularised ones. Skin-pedicled bone grafts have been largely superseded by

muscle-pedicled bone grafts, because they often provided a poor blood supply to the bony component.

From a pathophysiological point of view, callus distraction to lengthen extremities or to cover bone defects with segmental transport is a special form of local vascularised bone transposition (type II). According to the level of the osteotomy, it is a vascular and/or muscle-pedicled local vascularised bone graft. In contrast to the above transplants, there is also a further vascular connection over the callus envelope.

Vessel-pedicled bone transplants (type IIIa) have a macroscopically defined supply and drainage which should not be harmed during preparation and rotation. In free vascularised bone grafts (type IIIb), the blood supply is interrupted for a short time and restored with microsurgical techniques in the host area. Both are considered as "axial pattern flaps".

INDICATIONS AND CONTRAINDICATIONS
[1, 3, 6, 11, 12, 14, 19, 33, 36, 44, 45, 46, 47]

The indications are summarised in table I. Indications concern the delay of fracture healing in a poorly vascularised recipient site, where cancellous bone grafting is not reliable. Given the higher success rate and lower complication rate of the vascularised iliac crest transfer in bone defects after osteomyelitis, the iliac crest should be preferred to the fibula in tibial defects of more than 4 cm but less than 10 cm, even in the area of the diaphysis. Vascularised osteoperiostal anterior iliac crest transplants offer additional advantages for tibial reconstruction. In defects of more than 10 cm, only the vascularised fibula transplant can be used.

Over the past few years, vascularised bone transfers have been used to stimulate the neovascularisation of avascular bone necrosis in the wrist, femur head and talus areas (*table II*).

Table I. – Indications for microvascular bone transfers for bone defect coverage in the upper and lower extremities.

Upper extremity
1. Bone defect > 4 cm after trauma and osteomyelitis.
2. Bone defect after tumour resection with consecutive irradiation or chemotherapy.
3. Bone defect < 4 cm with additional non-osteogenetic host site.
4. Additional vascular defect.
5. Additional radius and bone defect of the ulna.

Lower extremity
1. No possibility of callus distraction in bone defects. After trauma (> 4 cm) and osteomyelitis.
2. Partial or half-shaft defects with no possibility of non-vascularised bone transfer.
3. Bone defect after tumour resection with consecutive irradiation or chemotherapy.

Table II. – Indications for (free) vascularised bone transfers for neovascularisation of avascular bone necrosis in the wrist, hip and talocrural area.

Necrosis of the lunate	Grades II and IIIa according to Decoux
Scaphoid pseudarthrosis	Persistent pseudarthrosis Poor perfusion Last possibility of therapy before partial arthrodesis
Femur head necrosis	Extensive grade I according to Ficat All grades II according to Ficat (possibly combined with derotation osteotomy) Rarely grade III (possibly combined with derotation osteotomy)
Talus	Extensive area of necrosis in the load area

Table III. – Contraindications for free microvascular bone grafts.

1. Extensive vascular changes in the donor or host area.
2. Systemic haemostasis disorders.
3. Lack of operability or limited operability of the patient.
3. Nicotine abuse.
4. Alcohol abuse.
5. Diabetes mellitus with extensive macro-angiopathic lesions.
6. Age (limited or restricted operability).

General contraindications for vascularised bone transfers are: considerable vascular changes in the donor and recipient areas, diabetes mellitus, systemic coagulation disease, patient inoperability, nicotine and alcohol abuse and age over 65 (relative contraindication) *(table III)*.

The main techniques

Numerous free vascularised muscle or vessel-pedicled bone grafts have been described in the literature. The most often used donor sites for a vascularised bone graft are described in this chapter *(table IV)*. Large and small vascularised bone grafts can be distinguished. For reconstruction of large bone defects in long bones of the upper and lower extremity and the spine, the

Table IV. – Donor areas for vascularised bone grafts.

Large microvascular bone grafts
1. Fibula [9, 17, 44]
2. Anterior iliac crest [38, 22, 36]
3. Posterior iliac crest [26, 20, 33]

Small microvascular bone grafts
1. Scapula [40]
2. Ribs [25]
3. Humerus [21]
4. Radius [6, 31]
5. Metacarpal bones [7]
6. Pisiform [3]
7. Femur [23]
8. Second metatarsal

vascularised anterior iliac crest transplant (DCIA flap), the vascularised posterior iliac crest transplant, and the vascularised fibula transplant have demonstrated their value. Vascularised rib grafts were used initially, but they do not play any role in orthopaedic reconstructions. The so-called small vascularised bone grafts are taken from the scapula, humerus, radius, femur, second metacarpal bone and second metatarsal bone. Due to limitations in length and volume, small vascularised bone grafts are most often used for skeletal reconstructions at the hand and foot. Furthermore, they are often harvested as compound microvascular transplants with a bony part and a soft tissue part.

FIBULA (A. FIBULARIS FLAPS)
[9, 13, 15, 18, 24, 41, 42, 44, 45, 46]

The fibula gives rise to two different microvascular bone grafts: the diaphyseal bone graft supplied by the peroneal artery and the fibular head graft including the proximal epiphysis which receives its vascular supply from a branch of the anterior tibial artery or lateral genicular artery. The fibular head graft will not be described in this chapter.

■ ***Anatomy***

All three main arteries of the lower leg supply the fibula *(fig 3)*. The anterior tibial artery supplies the proximal epiphysis and contributes to the supply of the upper two-thirds of the diaphysis. The diaphyseal blood supply mainly comes from the peroneal artery. The peroneal vessels run along the ventral aspect of the muscles to the medial aspect of the fibula after they have perforated the posterior tibial muscle. The muscle separates the bundle proximally from the interosseous membrane. In the distal part, the muscle is the medial border of the deep layer. The vessel bundle comes to the interosseous membrane and divides into three terminal branches: the communicans branch anastomoses with the posterior tibial artery, the perforating branch anastomoses with the anterior tibial artery and the malleolar branch to the vascular network of the ankle joint. Along almost its whole length on the lower leg, the vascular bundle is covered by the flexor hallucis longus muscle. The peroneal veins are emptied forcibly by the contractions of the flexor hallucis longus muscle.

Normally, the peroneal artery and its branches have two accompanying veins. The peroneal veins go into the posterior tibial vein, on average 52 mm below the head of the fibula and 21 mm distal to the lower border of the popliteus muscle. At the proximal site, the diameter of the veins is slightly bigger than that of the peroneal artery. The outer diameter averages 4.5 mm (1.7 to 6.5 mm).

The common peroneal nerve runs just distal to the fibula head from the laterodorsal side into the peroneal compartment and divides into a deep and a superficial peroneal nerve. The deep peroneal nerve and its branches to the anterior tibial and extensor digitorum muscles leave the peroneal muscle

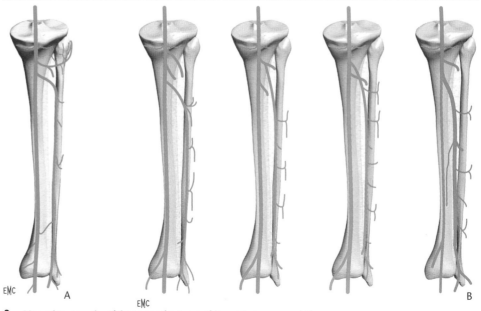

3 *Normal topography of the peroneal artery and its most common variations.*
A. "Textbook" topography.
B. Variations.

compartment through the anterior intermuscular septum. The superficial peroneal nerve runs distally through the long and short peroneus muscles which it supplies. Before perforating the sural fascia, in the distal third of the lower leg, it divides into the dorsal medial cutaneous nerve and the intermedial dorsal cutaneous nerve supplying the skin of the dorsum of the foot and toes.

■ Operative technique

The operation is carried out with the patient in a supine position and with a tourniquet at the thigh. A pillow is put under the ipsilateral buttock. For a vascularised bone graft, the skin incision begins dorsally from the neck of the fibula and continues straight along the dorsal bone edge distally. The length of the incision depends on the length of the bone to be removed (*fig 4*). The sural fascia is opened between the soleus and the peroneal muscles in the area of the lateral intermuscular septum. The divided perforating fasciocutaneous arterial branches must be ligated. They are used as a guide to find the peroneal vessels. If only a vascular bone graft is harvested, then 2 or 3 neurovascular pedicles at the upper end of the soleus muscle must be ligated in the proximal third of the leg. The soleus muscle is then cut transversely under the neck of the fibula. It can then be flipped to the dorsal side, if the proximally based fibres are to be divided. The peroneal vessels are found where they go under the flexor hallucis longus muscle and the posterior tibial nerve should be carefully pulled away from the pedicle. The anterior dissection is done next. When harvesting a longer bone graft, the peroneal muscles and the extensor digitorum longus are also divided close to the bone. The anterior and posterior intermuscular septa are divided about 0.5 cm from their tibial origin. The superficial peroneal nerve and its muscle branches are dissected carefully from the muscle layer. The anterior tibial neurovascular bundle, which lies in front of the interosseous membrane, is retracted to the medial side and it is then possible to expose the interosseous membrane over its whole length. The periosteum is divided 1 cm above the site of the osteotomy and stripped by sharp dissection. This procedure allows an effective musculoperiosteal blood supply on both ends of the graft. After proximal and distal osteotomy, the fibula transplant is gently pulled to the lateral side to stretch the interosseous membrane, which is divided in a caudocranial direction, about 0.5 cm from its fibular insertion. The next step is the posterior dissection. The proximal part of the flexor hallucis muscle is left in place to prevent damage to the peroneal vessels. The separation of the posterior muscles is performed so that the graft is only connected to the leg by its vessel pedicle. The graft is then gently pulled laterally; the pedicle can be shown at its

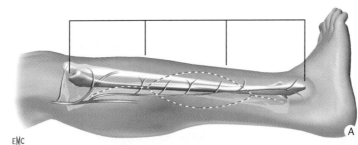

4 *Vascularised osteocutaneous fibula transfer.*
  A. Anatomy and planning of the flap.
  B. Anterior dissection.
  C. Harvesting the graft.

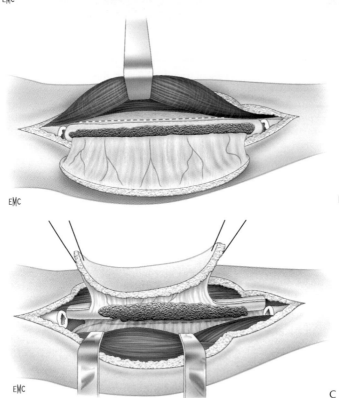

origin with the peroneal artery (*fig 4B*). The pedicle is ligated to the proximal side and the graft is harvested. After releasing the tourniquet with careful haemostasis and placement of a drain without suction, suturing is performed layer by layer. Postoperatively, the leg is held in a resting position with a dorsal splint for 7 to 14 days. Physiotherapy should be prescribed after removal of the sutures.

■ Variations

Given their anatomical relationship with the skin (osteocutaneous) and muscle (myoosseous, osteomyocutaneous), compound flaps including fibular diaphyseal bone can be harvested (*fig 5*).

■ Indications

The vascularised fibula diaphysis graft can be used to cover congenital or acquired bone (soft tissue) defects of the long bones of the lower and upper extremities, the pelvic ring and the spine.

■ Complications

Given the close topographical relationship of the common peroneal nerve to the fibula,

paraesthesia is possible. Furthermore, muscle weakness of the extensor hallucis longus muscle after harvesting of the fibula has been described. A claw toe deformity of the big toe may be found, mainly after extensive dissection of the extensor hallucis longus muscle. In growing children, after harvesting fibular grafts, a progressive valgus deformity of the talocrural joint can occur. It seems that the valgus deformity after fibula harvesting is due to disruption of growth of the distal epiphysis, and the severity of the valgus deformity depends on the number of years left before closure of the physis. A valgus deformity does not occur when the harvesting is carried out on patients older than about 12 years. This complication can be avoided by conservation of the distal one-third of the fibula or by implantation of a tibiofibular screw.

ANTERIOR ILIAC CREST (DEEP CIRCUMFLEX ILIAC ARTERY (DCIA) FLAPS) [16, 20, 22, 26, 30, 35]

■ Anatomy

The area of the anterior iliac crest is supplied by deep and superficial circumflex iliac

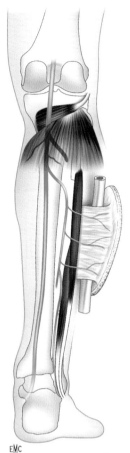

5 *Possible soft tissue components after a vascularised fibula transplant.*

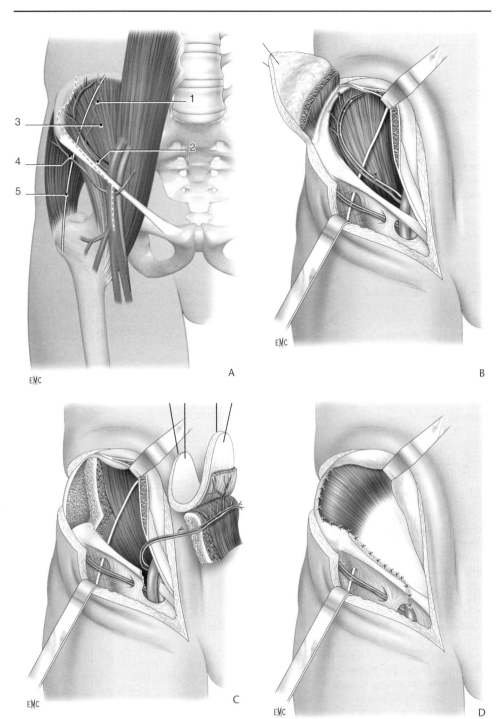

6 *Anterior iliac crest graft according to Taylor.*
A. Anatomy and planning of the flap. 1. R. ascendens; 2. a. circumflexa iliaca profunda; 3. m. iliacus; 4. a. circumflexa iliaca superficialis; 5. n. femoris cutaneus lateralis.
B. Dissection of the deep circumflex iliac artery.
C. Harvesting of the flap.
D. Closure of the donor area, layer by layer.

vessels, which supply a common musculoperiostal vessel system. The deep circumflex iliac artery arises from the external iliac artery on its posterior lateral side, just above the inguinal ligament, and runs parallel to the inguinal ligament to the anterior superior spine in the layer between the transverse and iliac fasciae. About 1 cm medial to the anterior superior spine, the artery has a constant ascending branch (r. ascendens), which perforates the transverse abdominis muscle and runs cranially on the dorsal side of the internal oblique muscle. Several variations of this ascending branch are described. After the bifurcation of the ascendant branch, the deep circumflex iliac artery perforates the transverse fascia and goes under the fascia of the iliac muscle about 0.5 to 2 cm under the iliac crest along the medial edge, between the iliac muscle and the transverse fascia. In this muscle groove several perforating branches arise to the bone, the periosteum and the covering skin. These arteries perforate through the external oblique muscle. The deep circumflex iliac artery perforates the transverse abdominis muscle again, approximately in the middle of the iliac crest to anastomose finally with the iliolumbar artery and branches of the superior gluteal artery. Along the iliac crest, the artery gives

out numerous branches to the periosteum, to the neighbouring muscles and to the skin. The superficial circumflex iliac artery arises laterally from the femoral artery about 1 to 3 cm below the inguinal ligament, and numerous anatomical variations are described. At its origin, the diameter of the vessel is about 1 to 2 mm. Distally, the artery has a regular course with a slight ascent, parallel to the inguinal ligament. First, it runs below the fascia, then a perforating point can be found in the area of the fascia of the sartorius. After perforating the fascia,

the vessel runs for about 2.5 cm underneath the anterior superior spine and gives out branches to the surrounding skin and the iliac crest in the area. Above the iliac spine, the vessel runs for a length of about 5-6 cm to finally join a plexiform vessel network *(fig 6A)*.

The deep circumflex iliac artery is accompanied along the inguinal channel and the iliac crest by two concomitant veins. The veins cross the external iliac artery in most cases. The superficial iliac artery is also accompanied by two concomitant veins which drain centrally into the venous plexus of the lacuna vasorum, which, in turn, drains into the femoral vein.

The nerve supply of the skin in the area of the anterior iliac crest comes from the subcostal and iliohypogastric nerves (fig 6A).

■ *Operative technique*

The operation is carried out with the patient in a supine position and under general anaesthesia. For a better exposure of the anterior part of the iliac crest, a support is positioned under the buttock. To harvest a simple bone graft, the incision begins parallel to the femoral vessels, continues along the upper border of the inguinal ligament and the iliac crest and extends laterally, according to the needed length of the graft. The abdominal wall must be stretched to the cranial side, because the abdominal muscles shift over the iliac crest in the relaxed patient (fig 6A). After the skin incision, the abdominal external oblique muscle is divided about 1 cm above the inguinal ligament and parallel to it, from the middle of the inguinal ligament to the anterior superior iliac spine. By holding apart the spermatic duct or the teres uteri ligament, the dorsal wall of the inguinal channel and the transverse fascia become visible. After exposing and holding the internal iliac vessels, the deep iliac circumflex artery and vein are searched. They are usually found on the posterolateral side. The deep circumflex iliac artery and vein run between the internal oblique and transverse abdominis muscles about 1 cm above and medial to the anterior superior iliac spine. After division of the muscle fibres of the oblique internal and transverse abdominis from the inguinal ligament, the pedicle can be dissected. The lateral cutaneous femoral nerve, which is occasionally found in this region, just underneath the vessels, must be protected carefully. Further dissection of the pedicle is carried out along the inner side of the iliac crest (fig 6B). According to requirements and size, a suitable bone graft is harvested using an oscillating saw or chisel. To prevent functional and cosmetic complications, the anterior superior iliac spine must be left in place. Generally, the inner lamella of cortical bone with the cancellous bone are sufficient for coverage of bone defects alone (monocortical bone graft). The outer cortical bone should be left intact, in situ, to preserve the contour of the iliac crest and to improve the quality of the donor area closure, avoiding abdominal wall weakness and hernias. After completing the graft harvesting, control of the perfusion of the vascularised anterior iliac crest bone graft is carried out (fig 6C). After division of the pedicle and positioning, meticulous haemostasis is performed, because bleeding in this area can lead to considerable blood loss (500-1500 cc). Bleeding from the cancellous bone can be reduced by compressing the cancellous bone and

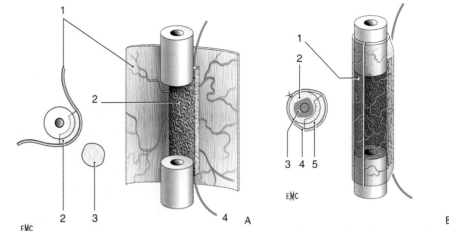

7 A. Primary reconstruction of a bone tube with a osteoperiostal vascularised bone transplant from the anterior iliac crest. (The missing bone tube is initially reconstructed by a tube with one-third of the circumference being the vascularised bone graft and the other two-thirds, the vascularised periosteal flap. The space within the tube can be filled with cancellous bone chips.) 1. Bone formation coming from both fracture stumps; 2. cancellous bone graft; 3. fracture haematoma; 4. vascularised periosteal flap; 5. vascularised bone graft.
B. Vascularised periosteal flap. 1. Vascularised periosteal flap; 2. vascularised bone graft; 3. cancellous bone graft; 4. deep circumflex iliac vessels.

inserting a collagen sponge. The abdominal wall is closed layer by layer. First the fascia of the iliac muscle is sutured with the transverse abdominal muscle and the transverse fascia. The first drainage (without suction) is placed here. The internal and external oblique abdominal muscles are sutured on the remaining outer cortex or, if harvested, on the gluteal and the tensor fasciae latae muscles. The inguinal channel and the inguinal ligament must also be closed layer by layer. After positioning a second drain (with suction), the skin closure takes place (fig 6D).

Postoperatively, at least one day of bed rest is recommended. Mobilisation is encouraged but depends on the amount of pain in the donor area.

■ *Variations*

Given their anatomical relationship, skin (osteocutaneous), muscle (myo-osseous, osteomyocutaneous) and periosteum compound flaps can be harvested (fig 7, 8).

Osteocutaneous anterior iliac crest graft

In addition to a pure bone graft in the area of the iliac crest, a fasciocutaneous flap can be harvested with it. The following incision should be chosen in such a case: the pubic bone, the iliac crest and the inguinal ligament are palpated and marked. The perforating branches to the skin enter the soft tissue about 1 to 2 cm above the iliac crest and run about 6 cm lateral to the superior iliac spine. Under slight tension in the direction of the umbilicus, the midline of the skin flap, which lies on a line between the femoral artery and the inferior angle of the scapula, is marked. The skin flap is optimally vascularised when it is harvested slightly above the iliac crest. If a skin area bigger than 8 x 4 cm is needed, the superficial circumflex iliac artery must be harvested with it. For an osteocutaneous flap

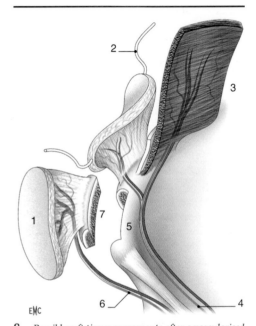

8 *Possible soft tissue components after a vascularised bone transplant from the anterior iliac crest.*
(Two individual skin pads, a periosteal flap and the internal oblique muscle can be harvested simultaneously on the deep circumflex iliac artery pedicle.) 1. Skin; 2. nerve; 3. m. obliquus internus; 4. a. v. circumflexa iliaca profunda; 5. periosteum; 6. a. v. circumflexa iliaca superficialis; 7. bone.

which is only pedicled on the deep circumflex iliac artery, the muscles of the abdominal wall are divided lateral to the anterior superior iliac spine with a distance of 2 to 3 cm to protect the perforating and anastomosing branches to the overlying soft tissues. The inferior border of the skin flap can be harvested to the fascia lata at the thigh. If a strip of fascia is needed for fixation in the recipient area, a strip of the tensor fascia lata muscle can be harvested together with the transplant. Even after harvesting of a relatively big osteocutaneous graft, the donor defect can be closed primarily in most cases.

Osteomyocutaneous anterior iliac crest graft

The lower part of the internal oblique muscle can be harvested together with the vascularised bone graft as a compound graft. To achieve this, the ascending branch of the deep circumflex iliac artery is dissected and preserved. It maintains the supply of the lower parts of the internal oblique abdominis muscle. This muscle can be harvested with the graft, after dissection from the rectus sheath and the iliac crest.

■ Indications and contraindications

The free vascularised iliac crest transfer is indicated in extensive bone and soft tissue defects in the metaphyseal area of the long bones, especially in defects after tumour resection with consecutive irradiation and/or chemotherapy. In the area of the radiocarpal or talocrural joints, when arthrodesis is necessary, the vascularised iliac crest graft is the procedure of choice. In patients with pre-existing hernias, another donor site should be used.

■ Complications

The donor defect is directly dependent on the area, type and size of the harvested bone. The superior anterior spine should be spared for the following reasons:

– Loss of this bony landmark results in a disturbing loss of contour in slim patients, which is noted in about 77% of all cases.

– Dissection in this region always risks damaging the lateral femoral cutaneous nerve. Injuries to this nerve lead to very disturbing paraesthesias in the area of the lateral thigh. They are reported in about 5-20% of cases.

– There are about 10% sensibility disturbances in the area of the inner thigh and scrotum or the big labia. These are caused by damage to the iliohypogastric and genitofemoral nerves which probably occurs by exposure of the inner cortex of the iliac wing.

– The occurrence of lateral abdominal wall hernia after harvesting of bigger grafts is reported in about 10% of cases. The number of complications can be reduced if the outer cortex of the iliac bone is left in situ and if the inguinal ligament is reconstructed anatomically.

– The donor site defect rate is higher after bicortical graft harvesting. Following monocortical dissection, 5% persistent paraesthesia and 40% anaesthesia have been reported; for bicortical harvesting, the rates are 37% and 42%, respectively.

The a. and v. circumflexa iliaca superficialis should be harvested in every case in which an osteocutaneous iliac crest transplant is used, because they are the main source of blood supply to the soft tissues in the groin region. If only the deep pedicle (a. and v. circumflexa ilium profunda) is anastomosed,

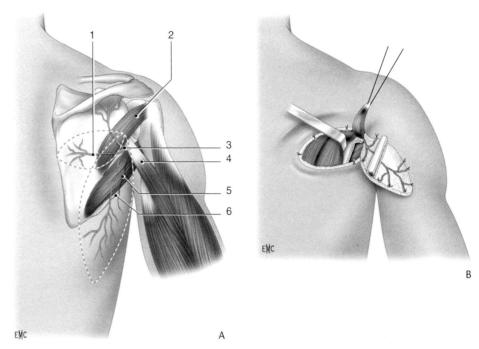

9   *Osteocutaneous parascapular flap.*
A. Anatomy and planning of the flap. 1. R. horizontalis; 2. m. teres minor; 3. a. circumflexa scapulae; 4. m. triceps brachii, caput longum; 5. m. teres major; 6. r. descendens.
B. Dissection of the vascular pedicle in the axial region and harvest of the flap.

it can lead to necrosis of the skin part in about 10% of cases, especially if a large skin pad over the iliac crest has been harvested.

SCAPULA (A. CIRCUMFLEXA SCAPULAE FLAPS) [40]

■ Anatomy

The subscapular artery (diameter: 3 to 4 mm) has its origin in the axillary artery. Two to six centimetres from its origin, the circumflex scapula artery arises (diameter: 2.5 to 3.5 mm) and from that point it is called the thoracodorsal artery. In less than 5% of cases, the circumflex scapula artery arises directly from the axillary artery. The thoracodorsal artery continues caudally and divides into two main branches to nourish the serratus anterior and latissimus dorsi muscles. A third branch (diameter 1.5 to 2 mm) runs in the space between the serratus anterior and the latissimus dorsi. A fourth branch (angular branch) which comes either from the thoracodorsal artery (42%) or from the serratus branch (58%) goes directly to the lateral border of the scapula.

The circumflex artery of the scapula goes from its origin to the dorsal side through the medial gap of the axilla. The medial axillary gap is limited cranially by the teres minor and subscapular muscles, caudally by the teres major muscle and laterally by the long head of the triceps muscle. On its way to the medial axillary gap, the circumflex scapular artery gives numerous branches to the surrounding muscles and direct osteoperiosteal branches to the lateral scapula rim. The localisation of the perforating points projected to the skin of

the dorsum can be determined by the formula D (cm) = L (cm) - 2 (cm), where D is the distance between the spine of the scapula and the perforating point, and L is the distance between the spine of the scapula and the inferior apex *(fig 9A)*. The circumflex scapular artery finally divides into 2 to 3 branches to the skin and these perforate the deep fascia in the subcutaneous tissue. One branch goes horizontally parallel to the spine of the scapula (diameter: 0.8 to 1.5 mm). This vessel provides the blood supply to the scapula flap. The second branch runs obliquely in a cranial direction to the spine of the scapula *(fig 9A)*. The circumflex artery with its three skin branches reliably supplies a skin territory which lies just underneath the inferior angle of the scapula and can cross the midline in the medial direction.

The circumflex artery of the scapula is accompanied by two veins of different calibres (3.5 - 4.5 mm). Both veins run into the thoracodorsal vein. In 12% of cases they drain into the axillary vein.

The nerve supply of the skin in the area of the parascapular and scapular flaps comes from different nerves: laterally, there are branches from the cervical plexus, axillary nerve and intercostal nerves; medially, there are dorsal branches of the spinal nerves.

■ Operative technique

The operation is done under general anaesthesia. The patient is in a lateral position. The upper extremity is draped and left free to facilitate the dissection of the pedicle in the area of the medial axillary triangle. Abduction of more than 90° at the shoulder should not be done to prevent traction on the brachial plexus. To shorten the operation time, two surgical teams should work simultaneously to harvest the flap, dissect the recipient area and prepare the vessels. The landmarks for harvesting the flap are the angle of the scapula, the spine of the scapula, the lateral border of the scapula and the dorsal median line. The medial axillary gap is localised either by bimanual palpation or with the aid of a Doppler.

The parascapular flap is drawn in the form of an ellipse over the descending branch of the circumflex scapula artery. A primary wound closure in the donor area (up to 9-10 cm in width) is possible (*fig 9A*). In the area of the lower half of the flap, the skin is divided to the fascia of the muscle. The dissection is conducted beneath the superficial fascia of the dorsum and the flap is harvested from caudal to cranial. The dissection is carried out in the layer between the superficial fascia of the dorsum and the fascia of the latissimus and teres major muscles (*fig 9B*). In the region of the medial axillary gap, on the undersurface of the flap, the descending branch with its two accompanying veins is visible. After dissection of the perforating point of the circumflex scapular artery from the axillary gap, the cranial section of the flap is cut around and harvested completely. The dissection of the vascular pedicle in the area of the medial axillary gap is the same as for the scapula flap. By retraction of the deltoid muscle, the view to the medial axillary gap is improved. The exit of the pedicle lies generally at the cutting point of the teres major muscle with the lateral scapula rim (about 4-7.5 cm above the scapular angle). In the area of the lateral border of the scapula, there is a close network of veins and arteries. This is the area of division of the circumflex scapular artery, which gives numerous muscular end branches and goes directly to the scapula. These branches disrupt easily when the muscles are torn apart. If there is dissection to the axillary artery, a pedicle length of 4 to 6 cm can be obtained. If it is to the branching of the thoracodorsal artery, a pedicle length of up to 8 cm, with a diameter of 2 to 5 mm, can be obtained. The donor site is closed in layers after insertion of one or two suction drains. Postoperative physiotherapy begins with initial movement exercises, i.e. walking up the wall with the fingers. Six weeks later, exercises to strengthen the shoulder muscles can be initiated.

■ *Variations*

Due to their anatomical relationship, skin (osteocutaneous) and muscle (myo-osseous, osteo-myocutaneous) compound flaps including the lateral scapula margin can be harvested.

Osteocutaneous flap

If the muscle branches to the teres major muscle and the osteoperiosteal branches to the lateral scapula rim are protected, the lateral scapula rim from the angle of the scapula up to the insertion of the long head of the triceps can be harvested as a vascularised bone graft. Anatomical and clinical studies have demonstrated the good vascularisation of this mainly cortical bone graft, which can be harvested up to a length of 10-14 cm and a width of 2 to 4 cm. Dissection starts with an incision of the teres major, minor and infraspinatus muscles to the periosteum. The muscles are then dissected by sharp dissection, until the thickness of the scapula diminishes. The bone part is harvested with an oscillating saw. To preserve the mobility of the scapula and to avoid damaging shoulder function, the reinsertion of the detached muscles is required.

Bipedicled osteocutaneous scapula flap

With preservation of the angular branch of the thoracodorsal artery and associated veins, it is possible to modify the scapula osseous flap as a bipedicled flap (*fig 9A*). The lateral scapula may be split into two parts: a superior half based on the circumflex scapular artery and an inferior half based on the angular branch of the thoracodorsal artery with a common proximal pedicle, the subscapular artery and veins. Furthermore, with the cutaneous portion of the flap based on the circumflex scapular artery and the lateral scapular bony portion of the flap based on the angular-thoracodorsal system, the vascularised bone portion of the flap will have a separate pedicle length of 13 to 15 cm, allowing greater mobility for the inset of the cutaneous flap and the separate osseous component with this pedicle design (*fig 9B*).

Chimer flap (mega-flap variants)

By combining a scapula flap with other flaps of the subscapular artery system, tissue defects of up to 35 x 25 cm can be covered.

■ *Indications and contraindications*

The osteocutaneous flap is especially indicated for combined bone/soft tissue defects at the hand and foot. It should not be used for reconstruction of bone defects in long bones because of its insufficient quantity and stability. A contraindication for parascapular and scapular flaps as fasciocutaneous flaps is a severe infection of the soft tissues as found in osteomyelitis and Grade III open fractures. In these cases, the soft defect coverage should be performed with a muscle flap.

■ *Complications*

The muscles detached from the scapula must be reattached to prevent loss of function in the scapulothoracic gliding space.

HUMERUS (A. PROFUNDA BRACHII FLAPS) [21]

■ *Anatomy*

The deep brachial artery (diameter 1.2 to 3.5 mm) arises from the brachial artery just distal to the insertion of the latissimus dorsi muscle, and continues parallel to the radial nerve between the medial and lateral muscle bellies of the triceps muscle around the humerus to the distal side. The artery mainly divides underneath the insertion of the deltoid muscle into a dorsal (posterior collateral radial artery) and ventral (collateral anterior radial artery) branch. The anterior branch, often smaller, accompanies the radial nerve in the biceps groove between the brachioradialis and brachialis muscles. The posterior branch goes into the septum which separates the brachioradialis and triceps muscles and gives numerous fasciocutaneous, musculotendinous and osseous branches. The fasciocutaneous branches supply the skin area of the lateral brachial and the proximal part of the lateral forearm regions. Many branches leave the artery to supply the triceps muscle as well as its tendon and the brachioradialis muscle. The distal part of the humerus is supplied on its lateral side from periostal arteries which also come from the posterior branch of the deep brachial artery. The artery is accompanied by one or two veins and by the posterior antebrachial cutaneous nerve. Distal to the epicondyle, it anastomoses in a fatty tissue layer with the posterior recurrent artery, an ascending branch of the posterior interosseous artery (*fig 10A*).

Venous drainage is over the superficial skin veins which drain in the cephalic vein, as well as over the deep accompanying veins of the deep brachial artery (diameter 2.0 to 5.0 mm) and their branches. Both systems are connected by anastomoses.

The radial nerve runs on the anterolateral side of the humerus in its groove together with the deep brachial artery along the lateral intermuscular septum. The posterior cutaneous brachial nerve (diameter 1-2 mm), which supplies the skin of the lateral upper arm, separates from the radial nerve in the anterior upper arm compartment, where the radial nerve goes into the septum (*fig 10A*). The posterior antebrachial cutaneous nerve arises about 1-5 cm posteriorly on the lateral border of the brachioradialis muscle, perforates the deep fascia of the upper arm proximal to the lateral epicondyle and innervates the posterolateral side of the forearm.

■ *Operative technique*

Preoperatively, the localisation of the fasciocutaneous perforating branches ("perforans") can be precisely determined by Doppler. The operation is done with the patient in a supine position and under general anaesthesia. The flap design is made on the upper arm with the elbow joint flexed

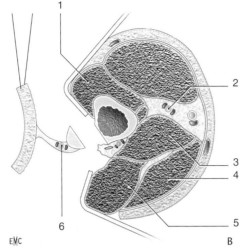

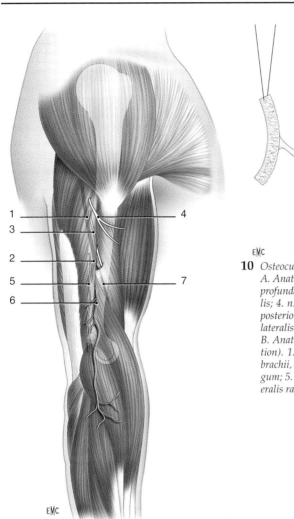

10 *Osteocutaneous upper lateral arm flap.*
A. Anatomy and planning of the flap (overview). 1. A. profunda brachii; 2. a. collateralis radialis; 3. n. radialis; 4. n. cutaneus brachii; 5. n. cutaneus antebrachii posterior; 6. a. collateralis radialis posterior; 7. a. collateralis radialis anterior.
B. Anatomy and planning of the flap (transverse section). 1. M. brachialis; 2. a. brachialis; 3. m. triceps brachii, caput medialis; 4. m. triceps brachii, caput longum; 5. m. triceps brachii, caput medialis; 6. a. collateralis radialis posterior.

at 90°. The area extends from the insertion of the deltoid muscle to the upper part of the forearm, 3-6 cm below the epicondyle. When planning the flap, it is important to note that the subcutaneous tissue gets thinner from proximal to distal.

After marking the acromion and the insertion of the deltoid muscle on the humerus and lateral epicondyle, a line is drawn on the lateral side of the upper arm between the acromion and the lateral epicondyle. This line is the axis of the flap in form of an ellipse which can be harvested. Direct donor site closure is possible up to a width of 6 cm (up to 10 cm in elderly patients). For bigger flaps, continuous skin stretching using a tissue expander is necessary before flap transplantation (pre-expansion) can be done *(fig 10A, B)*. Harvesting the flap is made easier by positioning a sterile tourniquet. The incision begins at the posterior part of the flap. The fascia which covers the triceps muscle is sutured on the subcutaneous tissue and the dissection is done quickly to the septum which inserts on the humerus. The same technique is used for the anterior part, where the dissection exposes the brachialis and the brachioradialis muscles. The flap remains connected to the septum which contains the supplying vessels. The

tourniquet is released to allow dissection of the deep brachial artery in the groove of the humerus, and is followed by the isolation of the pedicle between the deltoid and triceps muscles. These are retracted to expose the vascular pedicle of the flap and the radial nerve. The profunda brachii artery and its accompanying veins are carefully separated from the nerve. The distal humerus is supplied by periostal vessels which run over the intermuscular septum, and musculoperiostal vessels come from the surrounding muscles and perforate the bone. A vascularised bone graft up to 10 cm long and 1.5 cm wide can be harvested between the insertion of the deltoid muscle and the lateral epicondyle. To secure the periosteal blood supply, a sleeve of 1 cm from the insertion of the triceps muscle (dorsally) and the brachialis and brachioradialis muscles (ventrally) of the septum should be left in place *(fig 10B)*. The radial nerve trunk must be identified and protected when the bone is cut using an oscillating microsaw.

After meticulous haemostasis and positioning of a Redon drain without suction, wound closure is done layer by layer. Only in exceptional situations is a skin graft necessary for wound closure. A

postoperative arm brace is recommended for 4-6 weeks depending on the width of the harvested piece of bone.

■ *Variations*

Given their close anatomical relationship, skin (osteocutaneous), muscle (myo-osseous, osteomyocutaneous), and tendon (osteomyotendineous) compound flaps including a humeral diaphyseal bone segment can be harvested (see above).

■ *Indications and contraindications*

The osteocutaneous flap is especially indicated for combined bone/soft tissue defects at the hand and foot. It should not be used for reconstruction of bone defects in long bones because of its insufficient quantity and stability.

■ *Complications*

The harvesting of bone of the distal humerus can lead to a fracture in the donor area if more than half of the bony circumference is taken, and if long grafts are harvested. Postoperative protection in an upper arm brace is recommended when harvesting a long bone graft. The radial nerve must be protected during dissection and osteotomy. Postoperative loss of function has been reported.

RADIUS (A. RADIALIS (CHINESE) FLAPS) [22, 31]

■ *Anatomy*

The radial artery normally arises from the brachial artery and supplies the whole palmar side of the forearm distally to about the height of the styloid process and proximally to the crease of the elbow, as well as to the parts on the radial side of the dorsal aspect. Along its course, the radial artery gives out many branches. About 1 cm distal from its origin, the biggest skin branch arises. In the proximal area of the forearm the radial artery gives several muscle branches to the brachioradialis muscle (usually 2 vessels) and to the flexors. In the middle and distal areas, 4 to 18 skin branches leave the radial artery, perforate the fascia of the forearm and end in a epifascial plexus of the skin. On its course, the branches give ramifications to the flexor tendons, as well as to the superficial branch of the radial nerve running parallel. The lateral third of the distal radius, between the insertion of the pronator teres muscle proximally and the brachioradialis muscle distally, is supplied by two direct osteoperiostal branches, which run in the lateral intermuscular septum to the radius. Finally, the radial artery branches shortly before its entrance into the anatomical snuff box; the superficial palmar branch continues towards the palm. The variable and usually thin vessel runs on top of or inside the thenar muscles and anastomoses with the superficial palmar arch *(fig 11A)*.

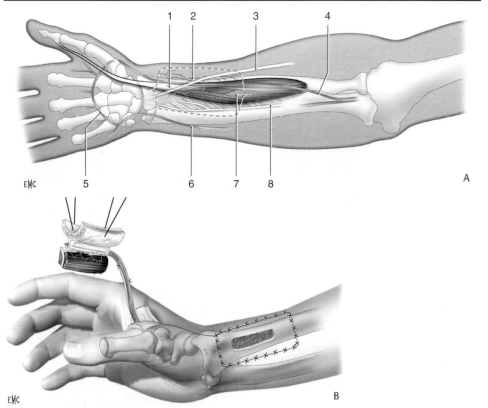

11 *Osteocutaneous Chinese flap.*
A. Anatomy and planning of the flap (overview). 1. Fasciocutaneous perforans; 2. musculoperiosteal perforans; 3. n. cutaneus antebrachii lateralis; 4. a radialis; 5. arcus palmaris superficialis; 6. a ulnaris; 7. m. flexor pollicis longus; 8. n. cutaneus antebrachii medialis.
B. Harvesting the osteocutaneous flap.

The venous drainage *(fig 11A)* of the forearm flap is through deep (two accompanying veins) and/or superficial veins (radial side: branches of the cephalic vein, ulnar side: branches of the basilic vein). Both systems are in continuity with functionally important anastomoses. Under physiological circumstances, the blood flows from the deep to the superficial system by muscle contractions in the hand and forearm region. For distally pedicled flaps, the direction of the blood flow can be reversed because of the denervation of the vessel, rise of intravenous pressure and the architecture of the veins ("cross-over pattern").

The palmar side of the forearm is supplied by the medial and lateral cutaneous antebrachial nerves *(fig 11A)*. These are recommended for microsurgical nerve coaptation because of their diameter of about 2 mm. The static two point discrimination in the area of the forearm flap is about 15-25 mm.

■ *Operative technique*

The operation is carried out with the patient in a supine position under general anaesthesia and with the upper arm in a tourniquet.

The skin flap is centred according to the needs of the defect which must be assessed on the course of the radial artery. The flap size, both functional and cosmetic, its thickness and the required length of the

pedicle must be respected. A cortico (cancellous) vascularised radius bone graft of 10 to 12 cm length can be harvested between the insertion of the pronator muscle proximally and that of the brachioradialis muscle distally *(fig 11A, B)*. To diminish the danger of fracture when harvesting the graft, a burr hole is drilled at the proximal and distal ends of the radius. The bone graft is taken using an oscillating saw and preserving the supplying vessels. To cover the donor defect, the muscle bellies of the brachioradialis and/or flexor carpi radialis muscles can be approximated over the donor area. After releasing the tourniquet, meticulous haemostasis must take place. Postoperatively, the forearm is immobilised for 10 to 14 days. Intensive physiotherapy of the whole extremity as well as careful skin care of the graft area are then necessary. A forearm splint is applied for 4 - 6 weeks on fracture-risk patients, after reduction of swelling and healing of the skin graft. The frequent mechanism of fracture is to push on the forearm while pushing up from a sitting position.

■ *Variations*

Due to their close anatomical relationship, skin (osteocutaneous), muscle (myoosseous, osteomyocutaneous), and tendon (osteomyotendineous) compound flaps including the distal radial part of the radius can be harvested (see above).

■ *Indications and contraindications*

The osteocutaneous flap is especially indicated for combined bone/soft tissue defects at the hand and foot. It should not be used for reconstruction of bone defects in long bones because of its insufficient quantity and stability. Contraindications for the Chinese flap are pre-existing disturbances of perfusion in the area of the hand as well as known injuries of the anatomical snuff box. With a negative Allen test, lack of blood stream reversal in the ultrasound examination and/or lack of visualisation of the palmar arches under angiography, the radial forearm flap should not be used because of the higher risk of donor defect morbidity. In obese patients with a thick subcutaneous fat layer, this flap should be second choice because of the considerable cosmetic donor defect morbidity. Given the higher incidence of fractures in menopausal women, the harvesting of the radial forearm graft is relatively contraindicated.

■ *Complications*

The incidence of fractures of the distal radius diaphysis after graft harvesting is about 10% to 20%. In longer transplants, immobilisation in an upper arm splint is recommended to prevent pronation and supination.

DISTAL RADIUS [6, 19, 47]

Based on the anatomical studies of Kuhlmann, a variety of vascularised bone grafts have been described at the distal radius. They are harvested either from the palmar, dorsal or dorsoradial side. The most reliable and most frequently used is the innominate artery flap.

■ *Anatomy*

The dorsoradial surface of the radius is supplied by a constant branch of the radial artery which arises at the level of the radiocarpal joint in the anatomical snuff box. This branch is known as an innominate artery, because it is not named in standard anatomical textbooks. It ascends deep into the radiocarpal ligament at the level of the radiocarpal joint and turns to lie on the dorsoradial aspect of the distal radius at the level of the radial styloid. In many cases, there is anastomosis with the perforating branch of the posterior interosseous artery *(fig 12A)*.

The venous drainage is over the one to two fine accompanying veins.

■ *Operative technique*

The operation is performed with the patient in a supine position under plexus anaesthesia and using a tourniquet. By a dorsoradial incision, the radial artery is exposed and its branch, the innominate artery, is dissected. The sensible branches of

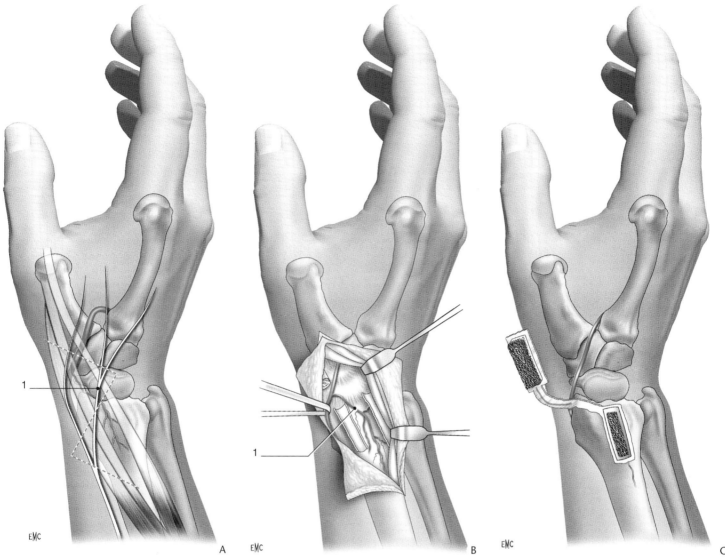

12 *Innominate artery flap.*
 A. Anatomy and planning of the flap. 1. R. superficialis of n. radialis.
 B. Dissection of the vascular pedicle. 1. A. innominata.
 C. Transposition of the flap into a scaphoid non-union.

the superficial branch of the radial nerve must be preserved. Through the same incision, the scaphoid bone can be exposed, as, for example, in the treatment of scaphoid non-union. For a better exposure and correction of the non-union, as well as for preservation of the blood supply, the exposure of the scaphoid bone is recommended through an additional volar incision. The first extensor tendon compartment is then opened and the tendons of the extensor pollicis brevis and the abductor pollicis longus are held to the radial side, and those of the extensor carpi radialis and extensor communis are retracted to the ulnar side. The innominate artery can now be identified on the dorsoradial side of the radius (*fig 12B*). According to the size of the scaphoid defect, the corticocancellous bone graft is centred on the periostal vessel. For reasons of stability, a distance of about 1 cm from the radiocarpal joint facet should be kept. After cutting the periosteum with a scalpel, the bone area is lifted with a sharp chisel. No shearing should be done between the periosteum and the bone underneath. The pedicle stays on the periosteum and can

be dissected to the radial artery. If necessary, a skin pad can also be harvested to facilitate the postoperative diagnosis of vitality. The vascularised bone graft can be placed in the anatomical snuff box in the scaphoid bone (*fig 12C*).

After releasing the tourniquet, the vascularity is checked and meticulous haemostasis is carried out. The vascularised bone graft is fixed in the recipient site with K-wires or with a (Herbert) screw. After loose closure of the capsule to avoid squeezing the pedicle and positioning of a drain without suction, the wound is closed. Postoperatively, immobilisation in a split forearm cast with inclusion of the thumb for 6 -12 weeks is necessary.

■ *Indications and contraindications*

The innominate artery bone graft from the dorsoradial radius is indicated in the therapy of established non-union of the scaphoid bone, which cannot be healed by simpler operative procedures. In pre-existing injuries of the radial wrist area, a locally pedicled bone transfer is contraindicated.

■ *Complications*

With the pedicled bone transplant in the hand area, care must be taken not to stretch or squeeze the pedicle too much.

SECOND METACARPAL (DORSAL METACARPAL ARTERY/DMCA FLAPS) [7]

The dorsal part of the first intermetacarpal space and the radial side of the second metacarpal bone are supplied by the first dorsal metacarpal artery. Two branches can be distinguished: one superficial, on top of the fascia of the first dorsal interosseous muscle and one deep subaponeurotic intramuscular artery network. Both are suitable for a transposition of the second metacarpal bone, because selective injections of the supplying vessels lead to colouring of the whole bone in all cases, despite numerous anatomical variations (*fig 13A*).

One to two veins accompany the supplying vessel and secure the venous drainage of the graft.

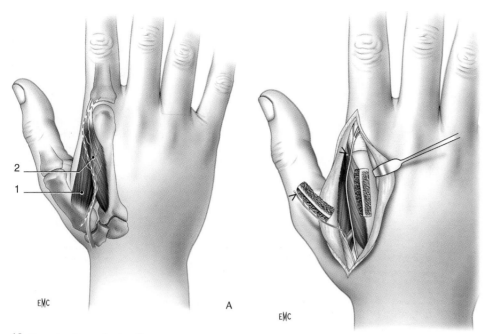

13 *Second metarcapal artery flap.*
A. Anatomy and planning of the flap. 1. M. interosseus dorsalis; 2. a. metacarpalis dorsalis.
B. Transposition of the harvested flap.

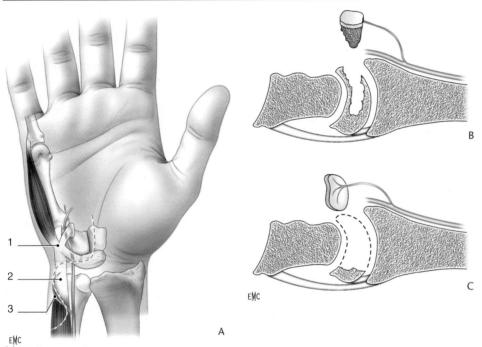

14 *Pisiform transfer.*
A. Anatomy and planning of the flap. 1. Os pisiformis; 2. m. flexor carpi ulnaris; 3. r. cubitodorsalis.
B. Pisifom transfer for neovascularisation of the lunate according to Beck.
C. Pisiform transfer for replacement of the lunate according to Saffar.

saw followed by a fine chisel, and the preparation is then continued in a proximal direction to the base of the second metacarpal bone *(fig 13B)*. The perfusion of the graft is checked after releasing the tourniquet. With a vascular pedicle of about 5 cm in length, the graft can easily be placed in the radial carpal bones.

■ *Indications and contraindications*

The second metacarpal flap with preservation of index finger function is indicated in established scaphoid non-unions. In these cases, the corticocancellous bone graft is anchored using a modification of the Matti-Russe technique. In avascular conditions of the carpus, the partial second metacarpal bone flap is an alternative procedure. The complete transfer of the second metacarpal bone is suitable for thumb-bone reconstruction after complex hand injuries with loss of the index finger. The cost of the operative technique is lower compared to vascularised grafts of the forearm, and no big vessel of the hand is sacrificed.

PISIFORM TRANSFER [3, 11]

■ *Anatomy*

The vessel which nourishes the pisiform arises from the ulnodorsal branch or directly from the ulnar artery, which crosses the pisiform in a radial direction through Guyon's canal. Numerous variations have been described *(fig 14A, B)*. The artery to the pisiform is accompanied by one to two veins.

■ *Operative technique (Beck's technique)*

The patient is in a supine position, under plexus anaesthesia and with a tourniquet applied. The incision, in the form of an "S", starts on the linea vitalis, then obliques in an ulnar direction, to be continued to the forearm in a proximal direction. After dissection of the ulnar vessel nerve bundle, the flexor retinaculum is cut and mobilised to the radial side. By positioning the flexor tendons to the radial side of the carpal channel, a volar approach is made to the lunate. After identification of the lunate, the volar aspect is opened. The necrotic bone is removed, preserving the cortical structures of the lunate and its ligamentous attachments. Intraoperatively, X-rays in AP and lateral projections should be taken. The pisiform is dissected with the aid of magnifying glasses. The pedicle for the pisiform is dissected from its origin from the ulnodorsal branch of the ulnar artery and prepared for the pisiform. The pisiform is then divided by sharp dissection on its proximal, ulnar and distal sides from the tendons of the flexor carpi ulnaris, and the abductor digiti minimi. The ligamentous structures of the pisohamate ligament are

■ *Operative technique*

The operation is done with the patient in a supine position under plexus anaesthesia and using a tourniquet. The radial artery is exposed by an incision in the form of a double-S in the anatomical snuff box at the dorsal side of the first intermetacarpal space. As in some cases the superficial system of the first dorsal metacarpal artery is missing, a broad pedicle is harvested with fascia and subcutaneous fat tissue, which includes both first dorsal metacarpal arteries. The

dissection of the 1.5 cm wide pedicle goes from the angle to the head of the second metacarpal bone distally. In doing so, the passage from fascia to periosteum must not be harmed, because it contains the supplying vessels. The entry point of the last bone branches of the vessel is at the area of the proximal insertion of the radial collateral ligament. A maximum of one-third of the second metacarpal bone can be harvested without loss of stability. The corticocancellous graft is exposed using an oscillating dissected. The pisiform is mobilised from the ulnar side and turned in a hanging position under the ulnar nerve to the area of the lunate. Proximal, distal and ulnar cortices as well as the cartilaginous surfaces of the pisiform are now prepared to fit into the hollow space of the lunate (*fig 14B*). While doing this, the pedicle must not be twisted. After releasing the tourniquet, the vascularisation of the bone graft is checked and haemostasis is performed. Fixation of the pisiform in the lunate with two K-wires is recommended until the bone has completely healed. The tendon of the flexor carpi ulnaris is sutured to the origin of the abductor digiti minimi, the pisohamate ligament and the pisometacarpal ligament. After positioning of a suction drain, the wound is closed. Postoperatively, the hand is held in a split forearm cast for 4 to 6 weeks. After removal of the K-wires, intensive physiotherapy is necessary. Exercising with a full load should not be done before three months, because initial resorption of the bone through neovascularisation of the lunate increases the risk of fracture.

■ Variations

Complete substitution of the lunate with a vascular pedicled pisiform transfer

The incision is the same as for Beck's technique. The pisiform is left pedicled on the tendon of the flexor carpi ulnaris muscle and the branches of the ulnar artery. The absence of the flexor carpi ulnaris only slightly weakens the force of flexion in the wrist. Alternatively, the tendon can be divided about 1 cm proximal to the pisiform bone and fixed to the capsule apparatus of the triquetrum. The lunate is then identified and removed. The dorsal part of the corticalis of the lunate should be left intact. This prevents the dislocation of the graft in a dorsal direction and preserves the dorsal ligament structures. The pedicled pisiform is placed (with its pisotriquetral joint surface showing) in the capitate and fixed with two K-wires (*fig 14C*). Aftertreatment is as above.

■ Indications and contraindications

Beck's technique [2] is indicated for revascularisation in necrosis of the lunate, stage II. It is contraindicated if fracture of the lunate (stage III) has already occurred. In this case, Saffar's modification can be used.

Contraindications for both transpositions are cases of pre-existing injuries of the ulnar wrist area.

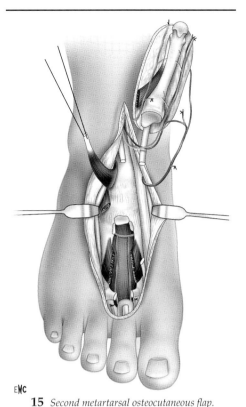

15 *Second metartarsal osteocutaneous flap.*

■ Complications

Up until now, nothing has been reported about donor defect site pathology following pedicled vascularised bone transplants in the hand.

SECOND METATARSAL (SECOND TOE FLAPS) [22]

■ Anatomy

The second metatarsal bone is supplied in the majority of cases from branches of the first dorsal metatarsal artery which runs medial to the bone, in the muscle itself, or underneath the first interosseous muscle. A number of anatomical variations have been described.

The venous drainage is provided by the accompanying veins of the dorsalis pedis artery, the first dorsal metatarsal artery, or, if a osteocutaneous graft is harvested, by the superficial vein system.

■ Operative technique

The harvesting of the flap should start after the debridement in the recipient hand area has been completed. The operation is done with the patient in a supine position, under general anaesthesia and using a tourniquet (children: 300 mm Hg, adults: 500 mm Hg). If only the second metatarsal is harvested as

a vascularised bone graft, then this can be done from a skin incision from the distal lower leg to the dorsum of the foot in the direction of the second ray (*fig 15*). After exposure and identification of the dorsalis pedis artery with its accompanying vessels medial to the tendon of the extensor hallucis longus muscle, the pedicle is dissected distally until the branch of the deep plantar artery, taking into account the change of direction of the dorsalis pedis artery in the tarsometatarsal area. To do this, the division of the tendon of the extensor hallucis brevis, which crosses from proximal lateral to distal medial, is necessary. As for a dorsalis pedis flap harvest, the different branches and branch patterns of the vessels in the area of the first intermetatarsal space are to be respected. After amputation of the second toe and approximation of the neighbouring metatarsal bones, the donor defect is closed. Fixation of the third and first metacarpal bones can be obtained by suturing both deep intermetatarsal ligaments together and/or by making a tendon loop from the second long extensor tendon. Temporary fixation can be achieved by a K-wire. The foot is held in a resting position for about four weeks, while the would is healing. Physiotherapy and walking exercises are indicated.

■ Variations

Due to their close anatomical relationship, skin (osteocutaneous), muscle (myoosseous, osteomyocutaneous), and tendon (osteomyotendineous) compound flaps including the second metatarsal bone can be harvested.

■ Indications and contraindications

The vascularised second metacarpal bone graft is indicated in the adult to cover bone defects in the carpal and metacarpal areas with poor or badly vascularised recipient sites (e.g. infection, irradiation). According to the concept of "single stage reconstruction" a combined soft tissue/bone defect in the metacarpal region can be covered quickly and reliably by an osteocutaneous graft. In children with congenital hypoplasia of the thumb, the vascularised second metacarpal bone graft can be used to substitute the hypoplastic first metacarpal bone, while preserving the epiphyses for further growth.

■ Complications

After harvesting the second metatarsal bone, there are temporary distortions in gait. Disturbances of the architecture of the longitudinal arches of the foot are described. Paraesthesia in the forefoot area is possible.

References ➤

References

[1] Abe M, Doi M, Ishizu T, Hasegawa T, Onomura T. Replacement of the lunate by the pisiform in Kienböck's disease. In : Nakamura R, Linscheid RL, Miura T eds. Wrist disorders, current concepts and challenges. Berlin : Springer-Verlag, 1992 : 135-140

[2] Barth A. Histologische Untersuchungen über Knochenimplantationen. *Beitr Pathol Anat* 1895 ; 17 : 65-142

[3] Beck E. Die Verpflanzung des Os pisiforme am Gefäbstiel zur Behandlung der Lunatummalazie. *Handchir* 1971 ; 3 : 64-67

[4] Berggren A, Weiland AJ, Östrup LT. Bone scintigraphy in evaluating the viability of composite bone grafts revascularized by microvascular anastomoses, conventional autogenous bone grafts, and free non-revascularized periosteal grafts. *J Bone Joint Surg Am* 1982 ; 64 : 799-809

[5] Berggren A, Weiland AJ, Östrup LT, Dorfman H. Microvascular free bone transfer with revascularization of the medullary and periosteal circulation or the periosteal circulation alone. A comparative experimental study. *J Bone Joint Surg Am* 1982 ; 64 : 73-87

[6] Braun RM. Viable pedicle bone grafting in the wrist. In : Urbaniak JR ed. Microsurgery for major limb reconstruction. St Louis : CV Mosby, 1987 : 220-229

[7] Brunelli F, Mathoulin CH, Saffar PH. Description d'un greffon osseux vascularisé prélevé au niveau de la tête du deuxième métacarpien. *Ann Chir Main* 1992 ; 11 : 40-45

[8] Davis PK, Mazur JM, Coleman GN. A torsional strength comparison of vascularized and non-vascularized bone grafts. *J Biomech* 1982 ; 15 : 875-880

[9] De Boer HH. Vascularized fibular transfer. [thesis], Leiden, 1988

[10] Dell PC, Burchardt H, Glowczewskie FP Jr. A roentgenographic, biomechanical and histological evaluation of vascularized and non-vascularized segmental fibular canine autografts. *J Bone Joint Surg Am* 1985 ; 67 : 105-112

[11] Erbs G, Böhm E. Langzeitergebnisse der Os pisiforme-Verlagerung bei Mondbeinnekrose. *Handchir Mikrochir Plast Chir* 1984 ; 16 : 85-89

[12] Ganz R. Pedicled autografts and osteotomy in revascularization of the femoral head. In : Aebi M, Regazzoni P eds. Bone transplantation. Berlin : Springer-Verlag, 1989 : 240-244

[13] Gidumal R, Wood MB, Sim FH, Shives TC. Vascularized bone transfer for limb salvage and reconstruction after resection of aggressive bone lesions. *J Reconstr Microsurg* 1987 ; 3 : 183-188

[14] Gilbert A, Razaboni RM. Free vascularized bone transfer in children. In : Brunelli G ed. Textbook of microsurgery. Paris : Masson, 1988 : 361-367

[15] Gore DR, Gardner GM, Sepic SB, Mollinger LA, Murray MP. Function following partial fibulectomy. *Clin Orthop* 1987 ; 220 : 206-210

[16] Harbon S, Chartounni M, Ricbourg B. Morbidité des prises de greffes osseuses iliaques. *Ann Chir Plast Esthét* 1991 ; 36 : 45-50

[17] Hierner R. Der vaskularisierte Fibulatransfer - Literaturüberblick und tierexperimentelle Modifikation. Med. Diss. Ludwig-Maximilians-Univ. München, 1992

[18] Hierner R, Wood MB. Comparison of vascularized iliac crest and vascularized fibula transfer for reconstruction of segmental and partial bone defetcs in long bones of the lower extremity. *Microsurgery* 1995 ; 16 : 818-826

[19] Hirasé Y, Kojima T. Vascularized bone graft pedicled on the dorsal innominate artery for scaphoid non-union. In : Nakamura R, Linscheid RL, Miura T eds. Wrist disorders, current concepts and challenges. Berlin : Springer-Verlag, 1992 : 187-191

[20] Huang GK, Hu RQ, Miao H. Microvascular free transfer of iliac bone based on the deep superior branches of the superior gluteal vessels. *Plast Reconstr Surg* 1985 ; 75 : 68-73

[21] Kincaid B, Banis CJ. Lambeau brachial externe S. In : Gilbert A, Masquelet AC, Hentz RV éd. Les lambeaux artériels pédiculés du membre supérieur. Paris : Expansion Scientifique Française, 1990 : 45-51

[22] Leung PC. Current trends in bone grafting. Berlin : Springer-Verlag, 1989

[23] Masquelet AC, Nordin JY, Guinot A. Vascularized transfer of the adductor magnus tendon and its osseus insertion: A preliminary report. *J Reconstr Microsurg* 1985 ; 1 : 110

[24] Mathoulin CH, Gilbert A, Judet H, Judet T, Siguier M, Brumpt B. Transfert libre de péroné vascularisé dans les pseudarthroses et pertes de substance fémorale. *Rev Chir Orthop* 1993 ; 79 : 492-499

[25] McCullogh DW, Frederickson JM. Neovascularized rib graft to reconstruct mandibular defects *Can J Otolaryngol* 1973 ; 2 : 96

[26] Mialhe C, Brice M. A new compound osteo-myocutaneous free flap: the posterior iliac artery flap. *Br J Plast Surg* 1985 ; 38 : 30-37

[27] Östrup LT. Free bone transfer, some theoretical aspects. *Scand J Plast Reconstr Surg [suppl]* 1982 ; 19 : 103-104

[28] Östrup LT, Fredrickson IM. Distant transfer of a free, living bone graft by microvascular anastomoses: An experimental study. *Plast Reconstr Surg* 1974 ; 54 : 274-285

[29] Papanastasiou VW, Lalonde DH, Williams HB. The vascular pattern and viability of microvascularized rib grafts based on periosteal circulation. *Ann Plast Surg* 1984 ; 13 : 375-380

[30] Pechlaner S, Hussl H, Künzel KH. Alternative Operationsmethode bei Kahnbein pseudarthrosen Prospektive Studie. *Handchir Mikrochir Plast Chir* 1987 ; 19 : 302-305

[31] Ray AK, Soutar DS. The forearm flaps. In : Hallock GG ed. Fasciocutaneous flaps. Oxford : Blackwell Scientific Publications, 1992 : 63-88

[32] Ruff G, Serafin D. Intercostal osteocutaneous flap. In : Brunelli G ed. Textbook of microsurgery. Paris : Masson, 1988 : 263-268

[33] Schwetlick G. Hüftkopfnekrose und gefäbgestielter Beckenkammspan Hefte zur Unfallheilkunde. Berlin : Springer-Verlag, 1991

[34] Shaffer JW, Field GA, Goldberg VM, Davy DT. Fate of vascularized and nonvascularized autografts. *Clin Orthop* 1985 ; 197 : 32-43

[35] Stock W, Hierner R. Applications and techniques of vascularized bone transfer. *Injury* 1994 ; 25 (suppl 1) : A35-A45

[36] Stock W, Hierner R, Wolf K. The iliac crest region, donor site for vascularized bone, periosteal and soft tissue flaps. *Ann Plast Surg* 1991 ; 26 : 105-109

[37] Takato T, Harii K, Nakatsuka T, Ohtake T. Experimental study of vascularized bone: quantitative analysis of bone scintigraphy and histology. *J Reconstr Microsurg* 1988 ; 4 : 391-396

[38] Taylor GI, Buncke HJ Jr, Watson N, Murray W. Vascularized osseus transplantation for reconstruction of the tibia. In : Serafin D, Buncke HJ Jr eds. Microsurgical composite tissue transplantation. St Louis : CV Mosby, 1979 : 713-742

[39] Teissier J, Bonnel F, Allieu Y. Vascularization, cellular behaviour and union of vascularized bone grafts: Experimental study in the rabbit. *Ann Plast Surg* 1985 ; 14 : 494-504

[40] Teot L, Bosse JP, Tassin X. La crête scapulaire. Rappel anatomique et technique de prélèvement. *Ann Chir Plast Esthét* 1993 ; 38 : 100-106

[41] Tho S, Harata S, Ohimi Y, Tsubo K, Nakahara K, Nishikawa S. Dual vascularized fibula transfer on a single vascular pedicle: a useful technique in long bone reconstruction. *J Reconstr Microsurg* 1988 ; 4 : 217-221

[42] Ueba Y, Fujikawa S. Nine years follow-up of a vascularized fibular graft in neurofibromatosis: a case report and literature review. *Orthop Trauma Surg* 1983 ; 26 : 595

[43] Weiland AJ. Fate of vascularized bone grafts. In : Aebi M, Regazzoni P eds. Bone transplantation. Berlin : Springer-Verlag, 1989 : 29-50

[44] Wood MB. Free vascularized bone transfer for nonunions, segmental gaps, and following tumor resection *Orthopedics* 1986 ; 9 : 810-816

[45] Wood MB. Upper extremity reconstruction by vascularized bone transfer: Results and complications. *J Hand Surg Am* 1987 ; 12 : 422-427

[46] Wood MB. Femoral reconstruction by vascularized bone transfer. *Microsurgery* 1990 ; 11 : 74-79

[47] Zinberg EM, Wood MB, Brown ML. Vascularized bone transfer: evaluation of viability by postoperative bone scan. *J Reconstr Microsurg* 1985 ; 2 : 13-19

[48] Zwipp H, Flory P, Berger A, Tscherne H. Kombination von Spongiosaplastik und freier mikrovaskulärer Knochentransplantation bei groben knöchernen Defekten. *Handchir Mikrochir Plast Chir* 1985 ; 21 : 235-245

Surgical repair of peripheral nerves

A Ferreres
J Fores
M García-Elias

Abstract. – Repair of peripheral nerves does not result in a complete recovery of function. This is the main reason for trying different methods of suture. The type of suture will depend on several factors, such as the type of nerve injured and, if there is loss of substance or excessive tension applied to the suture, a graft has to be interposed. Other methods for repair such as fibrin glue have been tested, but no definitive conclusion can be made from the published data. Lesions in continuity constitute an important challenge for the surgeon. Intra-operative neurophysiological recordings will help in determining which part of the nerve must be repaired.

Keywords: *nerves, peripheral nerves, nerve injuries, nerve repair.*

Introduction

NERVE INJURY

For a better understanding of the goals of the techniques commonly used for nerve repair, it is important to keep in mind what natural changes take place after a nerve injury. Following nerve transsection, changes occur proximal and distal to the lesion. The distal stump rapidly disintegrates due to a proteolytic process (Wallerian degeneration) that has the ultimate purpose of facilitating axon growth. Changes in the proximal part, where the cell body is located, will affect the nucleus and cytoplasm, as sectioning of the axon causes a leak of axoplasm with interruption of axonal transport. The first signs of Wallerian degeneration occur within 24 hours following section. The degradation process is carried out by calcium-activated proteolytic enzymes. Schwann cells (SC) produce the leukaemia inhibitor factor which attracts macrophages that will contribute to phagocyting myelin and taking away detritus from inside the microtubuli. The latter are also producers of growth factors (fibroblast growth factor, platelet derived growth factor, glial growth factor).

Angel Ferreres, M.D., PhD, Hand Unit, Institut Clínic Aparell Locomotor, Hospital Clinic Universitar; Institut Kaplan, Hand and Upper Extremity Surgery, Barcelona, Spain.
Joaquim Fores, M.D., PhD.
Hand Unit, Institut Clínic Aparell Locomotor, Hospital Clínic Universitari Barcelona, Spain.
Marc García-Elias, M.D., PhD.
Institut Kaplan, Hand and Upper Extremity Surgery, Barcelona, Spain.

The cytoplasm of these cells will show aggregates of FFA, cholesterol, and phospholipides that will be used in regeneration phases [34]. The cell is affected by axoplasm loss. Retrograde axonal transport stops and calcium concentrations increase at the site of injury. The cell body swells and the nucleus displaces to the periphery. Basophilic material (Nissl granulations) disappears from the cytoplasm (chomatolysis). These changes are due to the expression of different groups of genes [18, 21]. Changes in RNA reflect the increase in protein synthesis, necessary to axon regeneration. Axons also degenerate proximal to the lesion until the nearest node of Ranvier, leaving an empty cylinder. After a period of time, proximal sprouts will develop and will advance inside the endoneural tube. Neuronal sprouts appear after a few hours as a response to local factors [17]. These sprouts will find SC in a longitudinal disposition on connective tissue and basal lamina of endoneural tubes. They constitute the Bügner bands [37]. SC create a gradient of neurotrophic factors that will guide new axons to the denervated target organs [12]. SC, in the presence of growth factors (GF), such as glial GF, platelet derived GF, or fibroblastic GF, will transform into immature SC that will grow around peripheral axons [36]. Generally, surgical techniques have to take advantage of these processes when suturing, grafting or applying neural guides.

INSTRUMENTATION FOR NERVE REPAIR

Only basic instruments are strictly necessary for nerve repair (needle holder, forceps, scissors). We will discuss some aspects of design that can facilitate handling of the nerve. Instruments have to roll between fingers when used for suturing, tying, grasping and dissecting, and cylindrical holding is useful, especially for needle holders and forceps. The needle holder must also maintain the needle firmly, avoiding rotation. This is best accomplished by means of concave-convex jaws that conform to the curvature of the needle (*fig 1*). Another aspect of the needle holder is whether "to lock or not to lock". We think that for a surgeon who is unused to using it, a locking needle holder offers no handling advantages, as the pressure needed to unlock it may cause a loss of precision.

Forceps have two main functions, grasping and tying. They must grip without damage. Among the alternatives to toothed or notched ends that hold tissues firmly but risk injuring them, a ring end (which overcomes the disadvantages without losing the advantages) has been advocated by some surgeons. Tying with toothed forceps can be difficult and may cause damage to the suture.

Also, when cutting, the tissues are pushed away by the blades of the scissors, and the cutting action has to be repeated to be totally accomplished. Serrations will help in retaining the tissue between the blades and

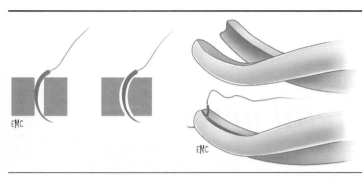

1 *The flat jaws of the needle holder have only three contact points with the needle, so it may rotate. Concave-convex tips achieve complete contact and stability.*

facilitate cutting but, at the same time, serrations leave an irregular cutting edge. If serrations are parallel to the bevel, scalloping in the cutting edge is avoided.

Magnification with a microscope (of which there are a great variety) is needed, although for some procedures, loupes may be helpful if the surgeon is used to them. The microscope offers the advantage of allowing the assistant to observe. It also permits the use of a camera for documentation.

BASIC CONSIDERATIONS

The purpose of all nerve repair techniques is to restore continuity of the nerve trunk, in order to achieve reinnervation of correct peripheral targets as rapidly as possible. According to Millesi and Terzis [27], the four basic steps of nerve repair can be defined as follows :

– Preparation of the stumps, which often involves resection or interfascicular dissection with separation of individual fascicles or groups of fascicles. In this step, the zone of injury is removed as completely as possible by microscopic dissection.

– Approximation, with special reference to the length of the gap between the stumps as well as the amount of tension present.

– Coaptation of the nerve stumps. Coaptation describes the opposition of corresponding nerve ends with special attention paid to bringing the cross-section of the fascicles into optimal contact. Neurorrhaphy can oppose stump to stump, fascicle to fascicle, or fascicle group to fascicle group in the corresponding ends. An indirect coaptation can be performed by interposing a nerve graft.

– Maintenance of coaptation, involving the use of stitches, glue or a natural fibrin clot.

There are two anatomical considerations in the surgical procedure for nerve repair: the type of nerve and its excursion. Nerves are subdivided into three types depending on the number of intraneural structures:

– monofascicular, when its cross-section contains a large fascicle;

– oligofascicular, when the cross-section consists of few fascicles;

– polyfascicular when the cross-section consists of many small fascicles [27].

The same nerve trunk may have different intraneural organisations at different levels.

For example, the ulnar nerve is classified as polyfascicular in the arm and as monofascicular after the division of the motor branch in the hand.

Another consideration is excursion. During limb movement, peripheral nerves accommodate to changes in the length of their bed. Wilgis and Murphy [41], using 15 fresh cadaver arms noted that the brachial plexus had an average excursion of 15 mm as the arm moves from full abduction to full adduction. The median and ulnar nerves at the elbow moved an average of 7.3 mm and 9.8 mm respectively, with elbow motion. The greatest excursion of peripheral nerves occurred at the wrist. Through a full arc of flexion and extension in the sagittal plane, the median and ulnar nerves had 15.5 mm and 14.8 mm of longitudinal sliding, respectively. The surgeon must consider the internal elastic tension of the nerve, but also the need for longitudinal excursion during limb movement.

■ *The right time for repair*

Deciding the right time for repair depends on several factors. The aspect of the wound and surrounding tissue injury are the most important ones. If there is a great deal of damage, and a gross debridement must be done, it may be wise to wait for a improvement of the wound and to perform a delayed repair. In a clean wound, where both ends of the nerve are easily identified and peripheral nerve vessels are seen, immediate repair, generally achieved without tension, is the best choice and also has the best prognosis.

The length of the delay depends on histological and biochemical changes that occur. In two weeks, distal degeneration and neurotrophic factors accumulate that will facilitate regeneration, as studied by Dahlin [7]. This means that, after a nerve section, there is a two week period in which to perform a repair in the best conditions. Bolesta et al [2] reported that, in a rabbit model, the best results are obtained after immediate neurorrhaphy, compared to a delayed nerve repair 3 weeks to 6 months later.

■ *Pre-operative care*

If motor function is involved by the injury, no joint stiffness must be present at the time of surgery. This means that the patient with stiff joints must undergo a period of physical

therapy to recover passive joint motion. Patients must be informed that recovery will take a long time as they may expect rapid improvement and feel disappointed with a normal evolution.

■ *Intraoperative care*

The duration of procedures varies considerably and the anaesthesiologist must be aware of this. Electrophysiologists may also be required for nerve action potential recordings. Additional important help during procedures may come from the pathologist. Normal tissue often has to be identified with the help of a microscope and with special staining.

■ *Sutures*

Material for sutures must fulfil several conditions. Induced inflammatory reaction has to be minimal, so as not to interfere with the degeneration-regeneration processes. Material resistance together with ease in tying knots are also important, not so much because of suture strength, but because the diameter needs to be the smallest possible. Non-absorbable sutures usually develop less inflammatory response than absorbable material. Among the former, monofilament nylon is the most frequently recommended. The size of the filament has been under discussion: 10/0 seems to be too fine, while 8/0 has been said to pull out of nerve tissue. So 9/0 has been advocated by Giddens et al [13]. Needles are also a matter for discussion. They are characterised by their arch length, diameter and point shape. A short arch (3/8) and triangular point are suitable for sutures, as nerve end handling is easier with a triangular pointed needle. Needle diameter will, however, always be greater than suture material because of the characteristics of stainless steel used in their manufacture.

End to end nerve repair

EPINEURAL REPAIR

Coaptation of the nerve stumps by suturing the external epineurium is the classic method of repair [29] and remains the gold standard with which other new techniques must be compared [40]. It is simple and non-traumatic, but as Edshage [11] demonstrated, the epineural suture may cause malalignment of fascicles in spite of a perfect superficial appearance. It is indicated in monofascicular or polyfascicular nerves where a fascicular dissection for fascicular repair would add trauma and fibrosis.

■ *Technique*

The first step is the initial debridement of nerve ends which can be carried out using soft membranous material wrapped circumferentially around the nerve to make

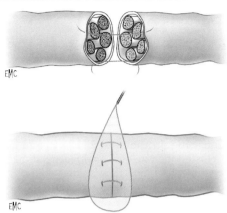

2 *Stitches only go through the epineurium. Some authors recommend sealing the suture.*

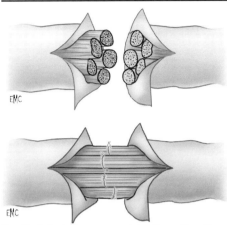

3 *Each fascicular group matches its continuation on the other stump. Some epineural dissection is needed.*

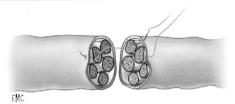

4 *If the same stitch goes through the epineurium and the fascicular epineurium, suture strength is increased.*

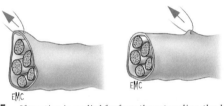

5 *If traction is applied far from the suture line, the deformity and stress do not affect the fascicular structure and suturing can be accomplished without traction.*

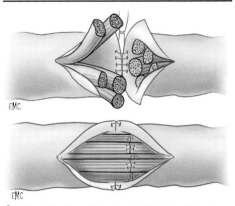

6 *Applying the splint principle. Suturing the epineurium enables the fascicular suture to be performed without tension. If the epineural suture is performed at another level, scar formation is also decreased.*

the end firm enough to be cut with a scalpel or a pair of scissors. Frequently, the nerve has been sharply cut (glass, knife) and then, there is no reason for further debridement. The cut surface of the nerve may show protrusion of fascicular contents. If not too extensive, this should be accepted in order to avoid further trauma. Landmarks such as longitudinal epineural blood vessels or big fascicles are identified to ensure correct rotation of the nerve stumps. The sutures are initially placed circumferentially in the epineuriun of both stumps, at points of external landmarks. Further stitches are then placed around the circumference, to secure and maintain the initial orientation. It is important to make the sutures very loose owing to postoperative swelling of the nerve ends during the first few days, because if the sutures are too tight, the ends will be strangulated. The number of sutures should be as few as possible, and no more than are needed to hold the ends close enough together with sufficient strength (*fig 2*).

FASCICULAR REPAIR

The objective of this technique is to achieve a better coaptation and orientation by adapting fascicles or groups of fascicles individually [26, 38]. It is indicated in oligofascicular nerves.

■ *Technique*

The epineural tissue is resected over a short distance from the cut nerve end, followed by careful identification of the fascicles in the cross-sectional anatomy of the nerve stumps under high magnification. The exact matching of the fascicular groups is accomplished by placing 9-0 or 10-0 sutures in the perineurium or in the interfascicular perineurium (*fig 3*). The repair does not resist much tension, and it can therefore be carried out when no resection is required. With this technique the axons remain in the same group of fascicles across the juncture, but it has the potential disadvantage of adding surgical trauma to the original injury. Some authors recommend cutting fascicles at different levels in order to keep different scars apart.

Peri-epineural sutures, proposed by Bourrel [3] (*fig 4*) can provide a better alignment than epineural repair and improve the strength of the stitches without increasing surgical trauma.

EPINEURAL SPLINT

An epineural bridge to splint the nerve can be used in both primary and secondary repairs. A contraindication to the technique is a long length of neuroma formation or retraction of the nerve ends. The bridge itself takes up the tension, allowing accurate fascicular coaptation without tension. The principle was described by De Medinaceli and Seaber [9]. "In order to manipulate and displace an elastic body without inflicting stress at the tip of the structure, it suffices to apply mechanical traction at a distance from the tip equal to at least one-and-a-half times the diameter of the structure" (*fig 5*).

■ *Technique*

The nerve ends are identified and mobilised at a short distance. If the transsection results from a sharp instrument, it usually does not inflict damage on adjacent nerve tissue.

Using magnification, a longitudinal incision is made through the external epineurium which is then trimmed of the underlying fascicles for about 1 cm to 1.5 cm. A few sutures (three or four) of 7-0 or 8-0 nylon, are used to construct the bridge (*fig 6*). The epinerium may be excised from one side while the other end is left at its original length. The effect is to offset the epineural suture line from the fascicular coaptation. When the epineural splint is done, the fascicular ends are driven toward each other without tension, and the coaptation is not difficult. Sutures of 9/0 or 10/0 nylon are placed in the internal epineurium. The fascicles can be held by a fibrin seal [16].

ANCHORING FUNICULAR SUTURES

The indication for anchoring funicular sutures is to reduce the tension of the conventional technique in nerve repair [39]. For example, when a nerve defect is at, or just beyond, the critical limits for direct approximation (e.g. 3 cm for the cubital nerve in the forearm) and the gap is too large for primary repair.

■ *Technique*

A 5-0 or 6-0 nylon suture, designed with the needle fitted on the end of a loop, is used for nerves larger than 4 mm in diameter.

The superficial loop stay is fitted at a distance from the stump 1.5 - 2 times the diameter of the nerve. After making the loop, the radius of the needle is enlarged, so that it can easily pass through the longitudinal axis of the epineurium. The stay suture on the opposite nerve end is put at the same distance, taking the funicular pattern into consideration. One of the two sutures is cut, and drawn in and out of the epineurium again so that the knot can be tied. A second anchoring suture is inserted 180° from the first. Grouped fascicular sutures are performed using 9-0 filament (*fig 7*).

TISSUE ADHESIVE

Nerve repair using tissue adhesive is a generally successful technique for experimental repair, including the use of

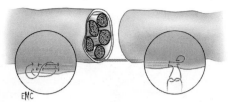

7 *The same principle again of diminishing the tension at the suture line. In this case, for larger nerves.*

plasma glue [23] and fibrin sealant [42]. The theoretical advantages are: the absence of foreign material (sutures), avoidance of nerve trauma and saving operative time. They have been analysed by Moy et al [30]. In spite of these advantages, this technique has failed to gain popularity, because it does not provide enough suture resistance, the material may cause local tissue reactions, and there is a theoretical risk of acquired immunodeficiency syndrome or hepatitis from pooled blood products. Clinical experience, although limited to Europe, has shown good results [25, 31].

Elimination of the tension is basic for successful neurorrhaphy and may be most appropriate for reconstruction by nerve grafting.

■ *Technique*

The nerve stumps are resected sharply until normal fascicles are noted. Neurorrhaphy without tension is performed using fibrin alone. However, if the repair is subjected to any tension, one to three epineural stay sutures are added. Nerve stumps are isolated from blood with a thin transparent foil placed beneath the repair site. Fibrin glue is then applied as a thin layer and over a distance four times longer than the diameter of the nerve to create a cylinder sufficiently strong to resist shear. Foil wrapped around the nerve repair site for 30 seconds ensures distribution of the fibrin glue and separation from surrounding tissues. Postoperative immobilisation for at least two weeks is required, as fibrin glue may start to break down after only three days.

Nerve grafting

Direct suture of the ends of a severed nerve is not always possible to perform without considerable tension. Although tension can to some extent be overcome by mobilisation of the nerve ends and flexion of the adjacent joints, it has been demonstrated that tension at the suture line increases scar tissue and decreases the quality of axonal regeneration [26]. On the other hand, minimal tension is not necessarily disadvantageous [19].

NERVE GRAFT

■ *Technique*

After grafts have been decided on, the dissection procedure is performed from

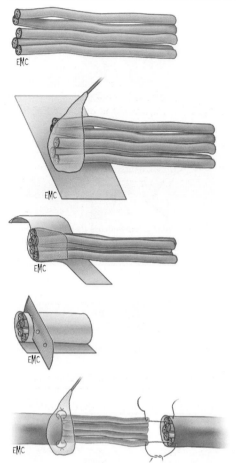

8 *After cutting the nerve grafts, these are packed together at their tips, trimmed in the usual way and sutured to the nerve stumps. Sutures may be reinforced by fibrin glue if desired.*

normal to abnormal tissues. The epineurium is incised to make the identification of groups of fascicles possible. At the point where fascicles lose their normal appearance, the group is transsected. The epineurium may be excised over a distance of several millimetres from the ends *(fig 8)*. The nerve grafts are packed together just at the tips with fibrin glue, then wrapped and regularised in the usual way, and sutured to nerve stumps. A frequent error is packing together the nerve grafts all along their length. This makes revascularisation difficult and increases fibrosis.

Mechanical considerations are the key to the success of free nerve grafts. The length of a nerve graft must be 10% longer than the distance between the two stumps in the respective extended positions of the adjacent joints. Coaptation is performed with the limb in an extended position without tension. If the trajectory of the graft is crossed by scar tissue, a longer graft must be used to avoid this area. All efforts must be made to define the two nerve stumps perfectly, to recognise the original orientation, and to apply existing knowledge of intraneural topography.

VASCULARISED NERVE GRAFTS

Theoretically, vascularised nerve grafts improve results by increasing the number of

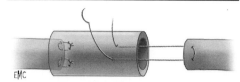

9 *Anchoring nerve stumps to the tube with epineural stitches.*

Schwann cells surviving the procedure, by decreasing intraneural fibrosis, and by increasing the rate of axonal regeneration [4]. Experimental blood flow studies show that nonvascular nerve grafts undergo 72 hours of ischaemia [4], but by the seventh day, flow is superior and maintained until the sixth week. It then returns to normal levels.

The indication for a vascularised nerve graft is a poorly vascularised recipient bed, with large gaps, proximal nerve lesions and compromised recipient beds [4].

The sural nerve [10] represents the best choice for peripheral nerve reconstruction. In brachial plexus injuries, with preganglionic lesions of C8-T1, a vascularised ulnar nerve graft is indicated.

TUBE REPAIR

A number of experimental studies have been carried out on animals to delineate the effect of nerve repair, using a tube as a guide, on different aspects of nerve function after peripheral nerve lesion [1, 5]. In human subjects, with nerve lesions in the forearm (median and ulnar nerves), a treatment attempt with either silicone tube repair or direct end-to-end has been carried out in Sweden [20]. This study showed that the recovery of hand function was similar in both cases

■ *Technique*

The proximal and distal ends of the nerve are inserted into the tube with a sleeve overlap length equal to the internal diameter of the collagen nerve conduit, and are anchored by two sutures of nylon 8-0 passed through the tube and into the epineurium *(fig 9)*. The nerve guide tube has an internal diameter slightly larger (30%) than that of the nerve, to allow for the nerve ends to be easily inserted into the nerve guide and to avoid compression. The maximal distance between nerve stumps must be 3 cm. The space between the nerve ends inside the guide is then filled with physiological serum.

DONOR NERVES

The sural nerve, thanks to its length and facility for harvesting, is the most common nerve used for grafting. Although its length is a favourable condition, it also can facilitate traction injury during harvesting. This should be avoided. It is localised through a longitudinal incision between the lateral malleolus and Achilles tendon and followed proximally to the level of the proximal gastrocnemius muscle. The antebrachial cutaneous nerve may also be used for grafting. It runs in the internal part of the arm with the basilic vein. For digital nerves, the distal branch of the posterior interosseous nerve in the distal forearm, where no motor fibres remain, is a good graft as it matches collateral nerves in diameter [35]. Other possible donor nerves are: the arterial antebrachial cutaneous nerve, the lateral femoral cutaneous nerve and the nerves of amputated parts.

Nerve lesions in continuity

Peripheral nerve lesions with preserved continuity of the nerve trunk, but with partial loss of function, might result from subtotal nerve transsection, blunt nerve trauma, or traction injuries. Some axons may be transsected or ruptured; others may be compressed by intraneural scarring or compromised by vascular insufficiency. The surgical approach for this lesion, also called "neuroma in continuity", must be performed by an experienced surgeon. The challenge of approaching this type of lesion is to preserve undamaged fascicles. This is best done with the use of compound nerve action potentials (CNAP), proximal and distal to the lesion site, because a single inspection, even under high magnification, may not be helpful and may lead to errors. This is very important, not only in assessing which fascicles are not conducting in a partial lesion, but also in assessing the length of a complete lesion if a traction injury has occurred. The techniques of applying CNAP are clearly exposed in a

chapter written by Happel and Kline [15], devoted to lesions in continuity, in Gelberman's textbook on operative nerve repair and reconstruction. After identifying injured fascicles, they must be repaired either by direct suture if the damage is short, leaving the intact fascicles like a sagging rope, or by graft interposition, if too much tension is suspected at the repair point.

NEUROLYSIS

It may happen that, after resecting the epineural scar of a lesion in continuity and applying CNAP, the nerve transmits stimulus. In this case, only neurolysis is necessary if the time elapsed since the injury is less than 9 months and pain is not a major problem. If pain is a more significant problem, internal neurolysis has been said to help. After carrying out internal neurolysis, each fascicular group should be tested to determine which may be injured. There should be no place for neurolysis without CNAP.

Postoperative care

Wound care is the same as that for other soft tissue operations. Collections of blood or serum should be minimised because they lead to severe scarring around the repaired nerve. We give antibiotic coverage during the intervention and three days postoperatively.

Prior to wound closure, the repair site is visually inspected while adjacent joints are moved. The surgeon selects a position of slightly more flexion so as to relieve any tension on the suture. The limb is splinted

in that position for 3 weeks because the tensile strength of nerves appears to be maximal at this time. Patients are allowed to flex their joints actively. This decreases the likelihood of adherence of the repair site to surrounding tissue. If the end-to-end has been performed under some tension, extension of the limb, even after 3 weeks postoperatively, should be performed gradually. At 3 weeks, joints are allowed to extend to neutral, and a protective splint to prevent too much extension without restricting flexion is left in place. At 6 weeks, a full active range of motion is permitted.

Tinel's sign is the best way to monitor progress in a recently repaired nerve. Digital percussion has to begin distally and proceed proximally towards the area of repair. The other ways of assessing progress are: clinical muscle function, sensory testing and electrodiagnostic studies. If the Tinel's sign does not progress, the surgeon should re-explore the nerve and perform a reparation, as indicated.

Evaluation of results

Erik Moberg [28], in 1962, pioneered the idea of validating measures for the evaluation of sutured peripheral nerves. He concluded that the Weber 2 point discrimination correlated best to function. Dellon and Kallman [8] introduced the term "moving 2 point discrimination". Other authors have pursued this analysis, developing several ways of assessing outcomes [6, 22]. These studies are very commonly addressed to a single disease, for instance, carpal tunnel syndrome. Outcome research has developed important tools for surgeons, so they can evaluate their surgical acts scientifically.

References

[1] Archibald SJ, Krarup C, Shefner J, Li ST, Madison RD. A collagen-based nerve guide conduit for peripheral nerve repair: an electrophysiological study of nerve regeneration in rodents and nonhuman primates. *J Comp Neurol* 1991; 306: 685-696

[2] Bolesta MJ, Garret WE, Ribbeck BM, Glisson RR, Seaber AV, Goldner JI. Immediate and delayed neurorrhaphy in a rabbit model: A functional, histologic, and biochemical comparison. *J Hand Surg Am* 1988; 13: 364-369.

[3] Bourrel P. Sections nerveuses traumatiques sans paralysie motrice de la main. *Ann Chir* 1974; 47-48: 2015-2023

[4] Breidenbach WC, Graham B. Vascularized nerve grafts. In: Gelberman RH ed. Operative nerve repair and regeneration. Philadelphia: JB Lippincott, 1991: 569-585

[5] Buti M, Verdu E, Labrador RO, Vilches JJ, Fores J, Navarro X. Influence of physical parameters of nerve chambers on peripheral nerve regeneration and reinnervation. *Exp Neurol* 1996; 137: 26-33

[6] Chung KC, Pillbury MS, Walters MR, Hayward RA, Arbor A. Reliability and validity testing of the Michigan Hand Outcomes Questionnaire. *J Hand Surg Am* 1998; 23: 575-587

[7] Dahlin LB, Danielsen N, Lundborg G, Ochi M. Axonal growth in mesothelial chambers: effects of a proximal preconditioning lesion and or predegeneration of the distal segment. *Exp Neurol* 1988; 99: 655-663

[8] Dellon AL, Kallman CH. Evaluation of functional sensation in the hand. *J Hand Surg Am* 1983; 8: 865-870

[9] De Medinaceli LD, Seaber AV. Experimental nerve reconnection: Importance of initial repair. *Microsurgery* 1989; 10: 56-70

[10] Doi K, Kuwata N, Sakai K, Tamaru K, Kawai S. A reliable technique of free vascularized sural nerve grafting and preliminary results of clinical applications. *J Hand Surg Am* 1987; 12: 677

[11] Edshage S. Peripheral nerve injuries-diagnosis and treatment. *N Engl J Med* 1968; 278: 1431-1433

[12] Fawcett JW, Keynes RJ. Peripheral nerve regeneration. *Annu Rev Neurosci* 1990; 13: 43-60

[13] Giddens GE, Wade PJ, Amis AA. Primary nerve repair: strength of repair with different gauges of nylon suture material. *J Hand Surg Br* 1989; 14: 301-302

[14] Hallin RG. Somatosensory and autonomic deficiencies following trauma in man; evaluation of symptomatology by studying peripheral neural correlates and induced tissue reactions. *Int J Tiss Reac* 1992; 14: 37-46

[15] Happel LH, Kline DG. Nerve lesions in continuity. In: Gelberman RH ed. Operative nerve repair and regeneration. Philadelphia: JB Lippincott, 1991: 599-616

[16] Jabaley ME. Technical aspects of peripheral nerve repair. *J Hand Surg Br* 1984; 9: 14-19

[17] Kato S, Ide C. Axonal sprouting at the node of Ranvier of the peripheral nerve disconnected with the cell body. *Restor Neurol Neurosci* 1994; 6: 181-187

[18] Leah JD, Herdegen T, Bravo R. Selective expression of Jun proteins following axotomy and axonal transport in peripheral nerves in the rat: evidence for a role in the regeneration process. *Brain Res* 1991; 566: 198-207

[19] Lundborg G. Nerve repair: clinical aspects. In: Lundborg G ed. Nerve injury and repair. London: Churchill Livingstone, 1988: 196-216

[20] Lundborg G, Rosén B, Dahlin L, Danielsen N, Holmberg J. Tubular versus conventional repair of median and ulnar nerves in the human forearm: Early results from a prospective, randomized, clinical study. *J Hand Surg Am* 1997; 22: 99-106

[21] Lunn ER, Brown MC, Perry VH. The pattern of axonal degeneration in the peripheral nervous system varies with different types of lesion. *Neuroscience* 1990; 35: 157-166

[22] Marsh D. The validation of measures of outcome following suture of divided peripheral nerves supplying the hand. *J Hand Surg Br* 1990; 15: 25-34

[23] Matras H. Fibrin Seal: The state of the art. *J Oral Maxillofac Surg* 1985; 43: 605-611

[24] McNamara MJ, Garrett WE, Seaber AV, Goldner JL. Neurorrhaphy, nerve grafting, and neurotization: A functional comparison of nerve reconstruction techniques. *J Hand Surg Am* 1987; 12: 354-360

[25] Merle M, Becker C, Pankovic C, Bagot D'Arc M. La réparation microchirurgicale des nerfs périphériques et des vaisseaux par le Tissucol: étude clinique et expérimentale. *Rev Laryngol Otol Rhinol* 1987; 108: 13-14

[26] Millesi H. The current state of peripheral nerve surgery in the upper limb. *Ann Chir Main* 1984; 3: 18-34

[27] Millesi H, Terzis JK. Nomenclature in peripheral nerve surgery. *Clin Plast Surg* 1984; 11: 3-8

[28] Moberg E. Criticism and study of methods for examining sensibility of the hand. *Neurology* 1962; 12: 8-19

[29] Moberg E. Evaluation and management of nerve injuries in the hand. *Surg Clin North Am* 1964; 44: 1019-1029

[30] Moy OJ, Peimer CA, Koniuch MP, Howard C, Zielezny M, Katikanemi PR. Fibrin seal adhesive versus nonabsorbable microsuture in peripheral nerve repair. *J Hand Surg Am* 1988; 13: 273-278

[31] Narakas A. The use of fibrin glue in repair of peripheral nerves. *Orthop Clin North Am* 1988; 19: 187-199

[32] Navarro X, Rodriguez FJ, Labrador RO, Buti M, Ceballos D, Gómez N et al. Peripheral nerve regeneration through bioresorbable and durable nerve guides. *J Periph Nerv Syst* 1996; 1: 1-12

[33] Palazzi S. The use of fibrin sealant in nerve adhesions. In: Schlag G, Redl H eds. Fibrin sealant in operative medicine. Ophtalmology-Neurosurgery. Berlin: Springer-Verlag, 1986; 2: 186-191

[34] Perry VH, Brown MC. Macrophages and nerve regeneration. *Curr Opin Neurobiol* 1992; 2: 679-682

[35] Reissis N, Stirrat A, Manek A, Dunkerton M. The terminal branch of the posterior interosseous nerve: a useful donor for digital nerve grafting. *J Hand Surg Br* 1992; 17: 638-640

[36] Reynolds ML, Woolf CJ. Reciprocal Schwann cell-axon interactions. *Curr Opin Neurobiol* 1993; 3: 683-693

[37] Selzer ME. Regeneration of peripheral nerve. In: Summer AJ ed. The physiology of peripheral nerve disease. Philadelphia: WB Saunders, 1980: 358-431

[38] Sunderland S. Nerves and nerve injuries. Edinburgh: Churchill Livingstone, 1978: 32-35

[39] Tsuge K, Mizuseki T. New approaches in nerve suture. In: Gelberman RH ed. Operative nerve repair and regeneration. Philadelphia: JB Lippincott, 1991: 327-333

[40] Tupper JW, Crik JC, Matteck LR. Fascicular nerve repairs: a comparative study of epineural and fascicular (perineurial) techniques. *Orthop Clin North Am* 1988; 19: 57-69

[41] Wilgis EF, Murphy R. The significance of longitudinal excursion in peripheral nerves. *Hand Clin* 1986; 2: 761-776

[42] Young JZ, Medawar PB. Fibrin suture of peripheral nerves. *Lancet* 1940; 2: 126-128

Traumatic brachial plexus injuries in the adult

JY Alnot

Abstract. – *Knowledge about traumatic brachial plexus injuries has considerably increased over the past 15 years, and diagnostic and therapeutic approaches have greatly evolved. Lesions may occur at all levels, from the medulla to the divisions of the brachial plexus in the axillary region. Thus we distinguish:*
– palsies due to supraclavicular lesions of nerve roots (75% of the cases);
– palsies due to retro- and infraclavicular lesions (10%);
– palsies due to lesions of the terminal branches (15%).
In the absence of clinical recovery, the indications for surgery must be determined early. Paraclinical examinations (myelography, CT scan and electromyography) will help to evaluate the lesions and should be performed as of the sixth week after the injury. Surgical treatment, currently carried out in specialised centres, must not be envisaged without accurate determination of the anatomical lesions and a precise preoperative plan.
Surgical treatment provides very good results in partial palsies of C5 and C6, or C5, C6, C7. However, in the case of total paralysis, the results obtained justify the continuation of current therapeutic orientations, which should be associated with assistance aimed at the social and professional reintegration of injured young people.

© 2000, Editions Scientifiques et Médicales Elsevier SAS. All rights reserved.

Keywords: brachial plexus, injuries, traumatic nerve lesions, nerve repair.

Introduction

Although a certain number of patients spontaneously recover within a few months, it appears that after an important trauma following a motorcycle or car accident, there is no recovery in many cases.

Over the past 15 years, therapeutic approaches have changed much and they depend on an accurate evaluation of the pathological lesions. An update was published in a monograph by Alnot and Narakas in 1996 [6]. A better comprehension of the pathological lesions [1] leads to a clearer classification of injuries, and therefore to a better evaluation of results. There have been many attempts to classify these injuries, notably by Millesi [13] and Narakas [21]. While these appear to be complex and take into account a great number of elements, classifications are essential if we want to evaluate the results, particularly after nerve repair. The use of charts and diagrams describing nerve injuries and types of repair is a great help for further follow-up.

Jean-Yves Alnot, M.D., Professeur, Service de Chirurgie Orthopédique et Traumatologique, Département de Chirurgie de la Main et des Nerfs Périphériques, Centre Urgences Mains, Hôpital Bichat, 46, rue Henri Huchard, 75877 Paris cedex 18, France.

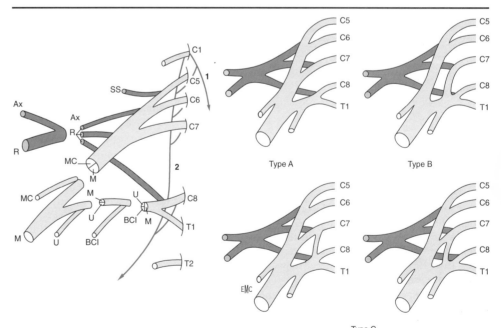

1 *Plexus anatomy with two anterior and posterior plans. C7 is a divided root bringing more nevre fibres but without a specific territory, and this explains the possibility of performing contralateral C7 neurotisation. 1. Phrenic nerve; 2. long thoracic nerve.*

Lesions can be situated at any level (*fig 1*), from the base of the nerve roots to the division of the brachial plexus in the axillary region. Several types of lesions can be differentiated:

– Supraclavicular lesions at the root or primary trunk level (75% of cases).

– Infra- and retroclavicular lesions of the secondary trunk (10% of cases).

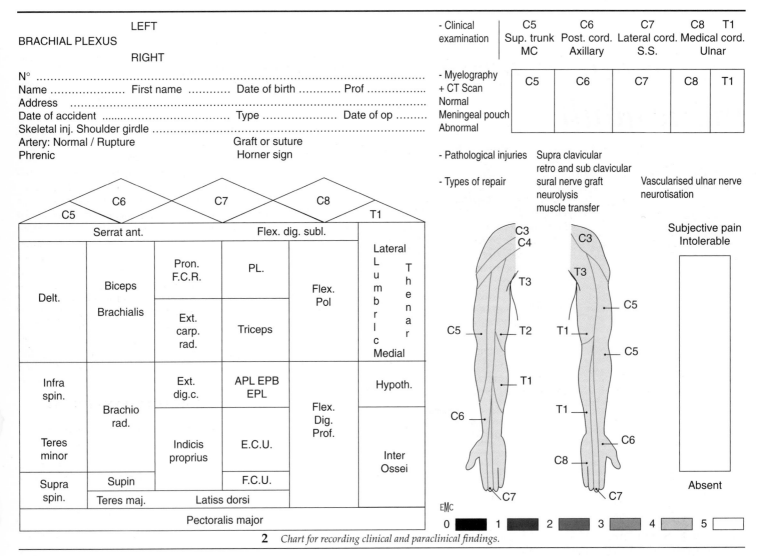

2 *Chart for recording clinical and paraclinical findings.*

– Lesions to terminal branches (15% of cases).

Diagnosis and treatment

Traumatic brachial plexus injuries present numerous problems. They are characteristic of young adults, aged 18-20, who have sustained a motorcycle or car accident. Whatever the clinical presentation (fig 2), a patient showing no recovery at 4 or 6 weeks after a traumatic palsy must undergo investigation (myelography combined with CTS and EMG) to identify surgical indications early enough.

Our experience at the Bichat Hospital includes more than 1,200 cases operated between 1975 and 1998; the results have been published in several papers [2-8]. Many other authors have also published their experience [1, 9, 13, 15, 20, 22].

Palsies due to supraclavicular lesions (75% of cases)

Among these lesions, which account for 75% of all cases and which occur at two levels in 15%, the following can be distinguished:

– C5, C6 or C5, C6, C7 palsies, which occur in 20%-25% of cases.

– C8 and Tl, which occur in 2% to 3% of cases;

– C5, C6, C7, C8, Tl lesions, which are the most frequent, occurring in 75% to 80% of cases.

It is important to determine the exact site of the lesions as this will weigh greatly on the prognosis and on the patient's future. Careful clinical as well as paraclinical examinations should be rapidly undertaken, to obtain an exact diagnosis and to allow for intervention within a period of 6 weeks to 3 months after trauma. These investigations permit evaluation of nerve lesions according to the roots which have been affected, after which therapeutic indications and a prognosis can be made.

Some factors can be considered favourable, for example, a patient with a brachial plexus palsy secondary to dislocation of the shoulder after a minor trauma has a 90% chance of recovery (Sunderland grades 1 to 3).

In contrast, the following factors carry a poor prognosis:

– severe trauma involving the upper limb as well as the plexus. Multiple bone fractures and other traumatic lesions are frequent in the injured upper limb (21% of all cases), bone lesions are found in 58% of these cases and vascular lesions in 11%;

– serratus anterior involvement and presence of Horner's syndrome, both of which indicate a proximal lesion;

– presence of pain and medullary signs suggesting injury to the cord.

Repeated clinical examination shows the evolution over time, and if there is no clinical recovery within a period of 30 days, paraclinical investigations, such as CT scan myelography and electromyography, should be carried out. The value of CT scan-myelography is to establish the existence of root lesions and especially root avulsion with pseudomeningocele (rupture of the dura sheath and rootlets).

In peripheral mechanisms (fig 3), depending on the direction of traction, the forces have an action on the anterior and posterior rootlets.

Avulsion is a very specific injury at the level of spinal rootlets, and is beyond surgical repair. The rootlets are avulsed from the spinal cord, notably C7, and mostly C8 and Tl, which become horizontal with abduction of the arm. Superior C5 and C6 roots, because of their oblique route, are often

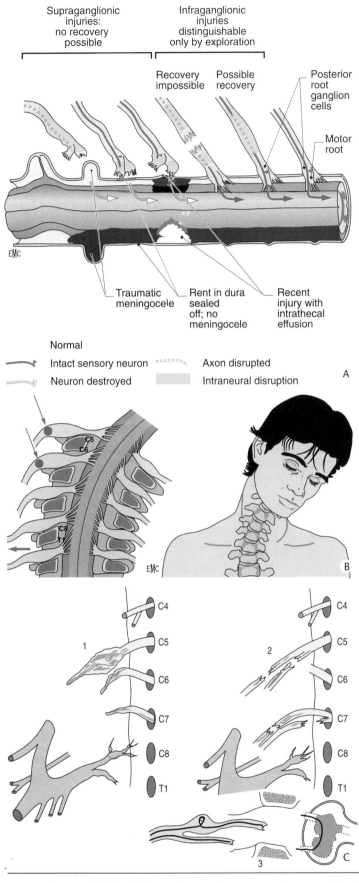

3 *A. Types of injuries suffered by roots of brachial plexus.*
B, C. The traction mechanism with, generally, C5-C6 ruptures in the scalenic interval and C8-T1 avulsion. 1. "Good" neuroma, good aspect of the root; 2. lengthwise disrupton, fibrous aspect of the root.

cell in the posterior ganglion. This is equivalent to avulsion.

Rupture can be more distal in the supraclavicular area, between the scalene muscles and beyond, preserving a proximal stump of root or trunks of variable lengths and quality which could possibly be available for nerve repair.

Electromyography is also part of the assessment and is particularly useful in C5, C6 and C5, C6, C7 palsies.

The surgical indications depend on the clinical evolution and can be decided on the basis of all the factors discussed above. In our experience, there is no indication for immediate nerve repair; the palsy is assessed by repeated motor and sensory examinations, and CT scan-myelography is carried out if there is no clinical and electrical recovery after 4 to 8 weeks, depending on the general condition of the patient.

The prognosis depends on the anatomy and type of lesions, and early therapeutic indications (first to third months) also depend on knowledge of the anatomical lesions.

CLINICAL PRESENTATIONS

■ *Total palsy with spontaneous recovery*

In cases where the immediate evolution is favourable, several clinical situations may be encountered:

Recovery from proximal to distal

In some cases, evolution can be towards a more or less complete recovery, starting from the shoulder, then to the elbow and finally to the hand. In total palsies after shoulder dislocation, this favourable result is frequent (80% to 90%). In other cases, the improvement is from proximal to distal, but some facts must be kept in mind: the absence of distal progression of Tinel's sign may be due to a distal rupture or, more rarely, to fibrosis. Some muscles can be saved in some specific radicular territories. There are usually traction injuries which may be improved by neurolysis, if there is nerve continuity (Sunderland grade 2 or 3). In some cases, there is rupture at the level of terminal branches and this must be repaired.

Recovery from distal to proximal

In some total palsies, recovery is rapid at C8 and T I, less so at C7, and absent in C5 and C6. Exploration must take place early because, in most cases, there is a reparable extrascalene lesion of the proximal roots or the upper trunk.

■ *Total palsy without recovery*

Total palsies with avulsion of the lower roots (64% of cases)

CT scan-myelography shows pseudomeningoceles at C8 and T1, and often C7. C6 may have an abnormal aspect and C5 is usually

ruptured more distally in the scalene region. Nerve injury can also be located immediately next to the transverse canal with frequent longitudinal disruption injuries and staged ruptures of the nerve fascicular groups, from the transverse canal, to the interscalene space. Nerve repair remains possible in some cases, but the proximal stump may, to some extent, have lost its potential for axonal regeneration. Damage to the fascicular groups in the transverse canal can also cause retrograde degeneration of nerve fibres, involving the motor cell in the ventral horn, or the sensory

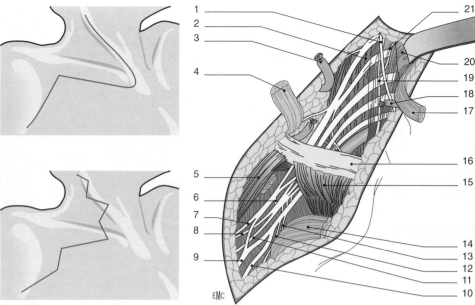

4 *Skin incisions and exploration above, below and under the clavicle. 1. Phrenic nerve; 2. scalenus medius muscle; 3. transverse cervical artery and vein; 4. omohyoid muscle; 5. deltoid muscle; 6. lateral pectoral nerve; 7. musculocutaneous nerve; 8. axillary nerve; 9. median nerve; 10. ulnar nerve; 11. radial nerve; 12. medial antebrachial cutaneous nerve; 13. medial brachial cutaneous nerve; 14. pectoralis minor muscle; 15. pectoralis major muscle; 16. clavicle; 17. omohyoid muscle; 18. transverse cervical artery; 19. long thoracic nerve; 20. internal jugular vein; 21. scalenus anterior muscle.*

normal on the CT scan. In these total palsies with avulsion of the lower roots (C7 C8 T1) and only one or two roots ruptured in the scalenic area, it is not possible to graft all the plexus. Surgery must be performed early (6 weeks to 3 months), and our approach is to strive for reinnervation of the proximal territories. The patients must be informed that they will have definitive paralysis of the hand.

• *Surgical procedure*

While each plexus is particular, there are common procedures for exploration, with specific problems concerning the site and type of lesions.

The patient is in a supine position under general anaesthesia. The cervical spine and the face are turned towards the opposite side. The upper extremity is placed on an arm table and the neck, shoulder girdle and chest must be exposed.

In certain cases, the ipsilateral hemithorax must be prepared and draped if an intercostal neurotisation is scheduled. Pneumatic tourniquets are applied to the thighs, and the two lower limbs are draped so that the sural nerve can be harvested.

The surgeon sits facing the axillary area, beside the patient's head.

The use of loupes (magnification from 2.5x to 4.5x) is suggested and a operating microscope must be available for the nerve grafts.

The operation is carried out through a long zigzag cervico-axillary incision and the entire plexus must be explored (*fig 4*).

Two types of skin incision are described, according to the literature:

– A large Z-incision including a vertical cervical incision at the posterior border of the sternocleidomastoid (SCM) muscle; a horizontal subclavicular incision, and a vertical incision in the deltopectoral groove.

– A multiple zigzag incision at the level of the cervical area to avoid a retractile scar, and open V-incisions in the subclavicular area and deltopectoral groove.

The key to the cervical approach is the omohyoid muscle. It must be located at the beginning of the dissection, transsected in its middle and retracted laterally to expose the supraclavicular plexus. The approach is performed at the posterior border of the SCM; the external jugular vein must be preserved with the posterior SCM muscle belly. The lateral transverse branches must be ligated, but the nerve branches of the superficial cervical plexus must be preserved.

At the upper part of the triangle made by the SCM and the trapezius muscle, the C4 loop must be preserved on the SCM muscle belly. It represents an important topographical landmark.

The scalene outlet must then be exposed and the phrenic nerve, at the anterior aspect of the anterior scalenus muscle, must be located and stimulated. The transverse cervical artery and vein must be ligated to complete the exposition of the plexus.

The suprascapular nerve is an essential landmark as there is no nerve element lateral to it. It is also important to locate the Charles Bell nerve, which must be preserved.

Finally, the spinal accessory nerve must be dissected if a neurotisation is scheduled. It is important not to dissect it too proximally, so as not to destroy the branches for the upper and mid trapezium. If neurotisation must be carred out with the distal accessory

spinal nerve, the latter can be divided distal to the branches for the upper trapezius muscle.

The key to the subclavicular and axillary approach is the pectoralis minor muscle. The approach in the deltopectoral groove must be wide and respect the cephalic vein. Desinsertion of the lateral part of the clavicular insertion of the anterior pectoralis major may be convenient. The pectoralis minor must be dissected and exposed, and in certain cases, it may be necessary to divide it. Communication between the cervical area and the axillary area is then established under the clavicle, using a sponge held with a clamp. In the majority of cases, it is not necessary to cut the clavicle; this additional step which has been systematically recommended by some authors, is now only performed in sub- and retroclavicular brachial plexus palsies.

The musculocutaneous nerve is identified as it enters the coracobrachialis muscle. This identification must be systematic in all explorations, to avoid a double level lesion. The other nerves are identified and the dissection is performed distal to proximal and proximal to distal. The axillary artery can also be located. A thorough evaluation of the lesions is made after exploration of the entire plexus. However, if there are meningoceles on C8 and T1, it is not necessary to explore these roots which are located in a deep area, making dissection dangerous.

At the end of the procedure, depending on the type of exploration and repair, closure is carried out plane by plane without a drain, or, in certain cases, with only a superficial drain at the distal part of the incision, at a distance from the nerve grafts.

In the immediate postoperative period, the patient is immobilised, with the elbow against the thorax, for a period of 3 weeks, associated with a cervical collar if nerve grafts have been performed at the level of the roots.

The type of repair depends on the localisation of the lesions. In a majority of cases, there is a C7, C8 and T1 avulsion. The C5 and C6 roots are vertical, having lost their oblique direction, and they will then be explored in the scalene outlet. Nerve grafts (the sural nerve or, more rarely, the ulnar nerve as a free or vascularised graft) are performed depending on root rupture in the scalene area.

Neurotisations must also be performed (spinal accessory nerve, intercostal nerves, etc.). For intercostal nerve neurotisation, a skin incision is performed below the pectoralis major muscle. Three intercostal nerves (T3, T4, T5) are transsected anteriorly to perform a direct suture with, for example, the musculocutaneous nerve.

The type of repair depends on anatomopathological lesions. When only one root (C5) can be grafted (*fig 5A*), our choice is to repair the anterior part of the

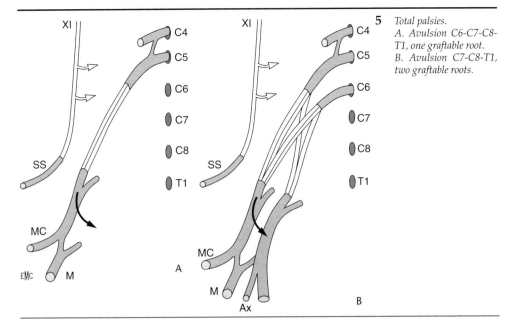

5 *Total palsies.*
A. Avulsion C6-C7-C8-T1, one graftable root.
B. Avulsion C7-C8-T1, two graftable roots.

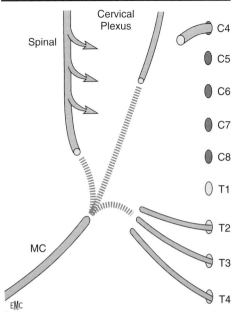

6 *Total palsies with avulsion of all the roots. Possibilities of neurotisation.*

first trunk with the C5 root, and the suprascapular nerve by neurotisation (direct suture) with the spinal accessory nerve, which is divided distal to the origin of the branches for the superior and middle parts of the trapezius.

The goal is to obtain stabilisation of the shoulder, an active pectoralis major to adduct the arm, flexion of the elbow and some palmar sensibility in the forearm and palm. When there are two roots (C5 and C6) (fig 5B) which can be grafted, it is also possible to graft some parts of the posterior cord to restore radial or axillary nerve function. Every effort is made to connect the anterior plane of the root grafts with the anterior plane of the plexus, and the posterior plane of the root with the posterior plane of the plexus, so as to respect the cortical representation and to avoid co-contractions between antagonist muscles. One must try not to graft everything, and if the roots are thin, the technique is similar to that used for one graftable root. From the technical view point, we most frequently use the sural nerve, but when Tl, C8, and C7 are avulsed, it is possible to use a vascularised ulnar nerve, either free or pedicled, when the aspect and size of C5 or C5 and C6 are good, and when the length of the nerve defect is longer than 15 cm.

• *Results*

Results must be analysed critically, evaluating motor and sensory functions. They can be evaluated only after sufficient time has elapsed, because reinnervation after nerve grafting is always delayed. This requires 2 to 3 years, depending on the type of lesion and its location (roots, trunk, cord, and terminal branches). The result must be evaluated according to the function of the structures repaired, and the therapeutic objectives to be achieved. Finally, the pain syndrome must be considered, and it is important to stress that surgical interventions with nerve repair for any

given region considerably modify the afferents originating in the upper limb.

The final functions [1, 3, 4, 6, 9, 14, 16, 19, 20, 22] must be studied according to the nerve repair, and depend on the number of grafted roots. A useful result means that at least elbow flexion is possible. 75%-80% of patients have satisfactory results with good elbow flexion ($M_3 + M_4$). Pectoralis major function is obtained in 60% of cases, allowing for objects to be held against the thorax. The shoulder poses problems, but it is possible to obtain stabilisation of the shoulder, with some active abduction and external rotation, by spinal accessory nerve neurotisation in 50% of cases. Some authors perform shoulder arthrodesis. It is rare to obtain function in the hand, but in the majority of cases, a "shovel hand" or "paper-weight hand" is still useful to stabilise an object on a table. Finally, some sensation in the forearm and hand is obtained, and this in fact may explain why 80% of patients suffer little or no pain.

TOTAL PALSIES WITH AVULSIONS OF ALL ROOTS (24% OF CASES)

CT scan-myelography shows meningocele or lacuna on all the roots, and there is no root available for repair. In these cases (fig 6), neurotisations are indicated using the spinal accessory nerve, the cervical plexus, the intercostal nerves, and, more rarely, the hypoglossus nerve or the contralateral C7 root [1, 4, 9, 14]. The goal is to provide elbow flexion by neurotisation of the musculocutaneous nerve; this can be associated with shoulder arthrodesis. When using the spinal accessory nerve associated with the superficial cervical plexus, an intervening autograft is necessary with two strands of sural nerve. The spinal motor fibres are connected to the lateral part of the musculocutaneous nerve trunk, and we add sensory fibres from the cervical plexus, connected to the medial part of the musculocutaneous nerve.

When using intercostal nerves, the neurotisation can be performed by direct suture between intercostal nerves 3, 4 and 5, divided in their anterior portion, and the musculocutaneous nerve (Hara's Technique).

■ *Results*

The results are good in 75% of cases with elbow flexion at $M_3 + M_4$. The problem is to know if we can do better by using other associated neurotisations,

PARTIAL PALSIES OF C5, C6 OR C5, C6, C7 (25% OF CASES)

The prognosis is dominated by the fact that the hand is normal, or only partially involved but useful. Surgery must be performed early because the lesions are often in the scalene area, on the roots or upper trunk, with a good possibility of nerve repair giving a satisfactory result.

■ *Surgical procedure*

The musculocutaneous nerve is identified as it enters the coracobrachialis muscle and dissection from distal to proximal then allows for dissection of the lateral cord and the anterior component of the upper trunk, as well as the posterior trunk and the posterior component of the upper trunk. The lesions must then be located, and repaired in the scalene space between the anterior and middle scalene muscles. Lesions of C5 and C6 and possibility C7 roots, are evaluated, and if there are ruptures in the scalene area, it is possible to perform grafts. On the other hand, in C5-C6 avulsion, we prefer a medial approach to the upper arm, approximately 120 mm distal to the acromial process, so as to perform a neurotisation of the biceps nerve with a bundle of the ulnar nerve [17].

Nerve reconstruction and muscle transfer are studied according to a global scheme

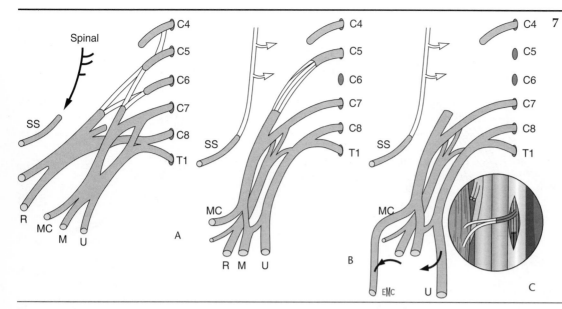

7 *C5-C6 palsies.*
A. Two graftable roots with good aspect and size. It is possible to graft all the lesions.
B. One graftable root C5, possibilities of repair associated with accessory nerve neurotisation. A similar repair is performed if there are two graftable roots of small size.
C. C5-C6 avulsion. Accessory nerve neurotisation and ulnar biceps neurotisation. Muscle transfers are also possible.

[7, 8, 18] and the indications are derived from the anatomopathological lesions *(fig 7)*. In C5-C6 palsies, when the two roots are disrupted in the scalene area *(fig 7A)*, if they are of a good size and aspect, it is possible to graft all the lesions. However, if the size of the roots is too small or when only one root is available *(fig 7B)*, the nerve fibres must not be dispersed, and the graft must be performed to the anterior part of the first trunk. Neurotisation of the spinal accessory nerve on the suprascapular nerve is added, with better results than after grafting C5 with one strand of sural nerve. A graft can also be performed on the axillary nerve with the use of ulnar biceps neurotisation. Finally, in C5-C6 palsies when no roots are available *(fig 7C)*, we neurotise the spinal accessory nerve to the suprascapular nerve and, in the same session, perform a neurotisation using a fascicular group of the ulnar nerve, with direct suture to the biceps nerve [11, 12, 17], or, perhaps, after end to side neurorraphy [10, 23]. Concerning C5, C6, C7 palsies, the overall plan is similar but is complicated by the severity of the lesions. When all the roots are avulsed and when there are no acceptable possibilities of muscle transfer, we perform associated neurotisations to restore elbow flexion and shoulder stability.

■ *Results*

Our results have been published in several papers [5, 6, 7, 18]; they depend on correct indications.

The present results of ulnar biceps neurotisation are good in C5 and C6 palsies, but the results are still uncertain in C5, C6, C7 palsies. Muscle transfer must be decided upon and performed during the same operative sesion.

In C5-C6 palsies, active elbow flexion must be obtained in all cases by nerve surgery or muscle transfer. The shoulder can be stabilised after spinal accessory nerve neurotisation. Restoration of active anteposition and active external rotation is essential in order to allow for more functional elbow flexion. However, the shoulder remains the main problem, with 73% good results in C5 and C6 cases, and only 49% in C5, C6, C7 cases because of the greater severity of the lesions. Rotation osteotomy of the humerus, ligamentoplasty and arthrodesis can all be used.

For the axillary nerve, end to side neurorraphy is a possible new technique [10, 23].

Finally, concerning the wrist and hand in C5, C6, C7 palsies, there is always the possibility of muscle transfers which can be decided early.

PARTIAL PALSIES OF C8 AND T1

In these cases, a decision regarding surgery will be based on the results of the clinical examination and other diagnostic studies. Here again, the prognosis is determined by the degree of hand function and the severity of the nerve lesions. Myelography will reveal the presence or absence of pseudomeningoceles. According to the degree of diagnostic certainty of the existence of avulsion of different roots, the clinical status should be re-evaluated and a decision regarding surgical exploration made.

If pseudomeningoceles involves the lower roots, exploration is not justified and muscle transfers are carried out [2, 6].

However, if the myelograms are normal but spontaneous regeneration has not occurred, surgery is appropriate for assessment and possible nerve repair. It is important to remember that although C8 and Tl roots, or even some more distal lesions of the trunk and cords, can be repaired by nerve grafts, the distance between the nerve lesions and the hand precludes reinnervation of the intrinsic muscles.

Palsies due to retroclavicular and infraclavicular lesions (25% of cases)

Retro- and infraclavicular lesions represent 25% of cases and nerve lesions are frequently associated with bone and vascular lesions [6]. Diagnosis and prognosis are based on the results of the clinical examination. CT scan-myelography is normal and electromyography often shows diffuse signs that are difficult to evaluate.

The lesions can be divided into two groups:

LESIONS AFFECTING THE SECONDARY TRUNK BEHIND AND UNDER THE CLAVICLE

Diagnosis is most difficult in these cases, with frequent associated bone and vascular lesions. Treatment is complex and a clavicle osteotomy is necessary to make an adequate assessment. The associated vascular lesions increase the problem, and it appears judicious to repair not only the nerves but also the vessels, even if there is an adequate vascular supply. This gives a better chance of nerve regeneration. In our experience, in brachial plexus palsies with vascular ruptures, the nerve lesions are severe and two situations may arise: a severe ischaemic syndrome in which emergency vascular repair is necessary with very difficult technical problems to be expected during secondary nerve repair. In the other situation, there is no acute ischaemia and it is judicious to repair nerves and vessels secondarily in the same operating session.

The surgical approaches will require transsection of the pectoralis minor muscle belly, and clavicle osteotomy.

Prior to performing the osteotomy, the fixation plate must be contoured on to the anterior edge of the clavicle and used for predrilling the screw holes. When the nerve lesions are very important, posterior cord injuries, either isolated or associated with concomitant lesions (posterior + lateral + medial cord), are the most frequent and may account for a more complex clinical picture and treatment. Exploration is long and difficult and because of multiple and diffuse lesions, repair presents problems owing to the length of the lesions and a limited stock of nerve graft [6].

Results are difficult to evaluate because of the wide variety of anatomopathological lesions (Sunderland grades 1-5) and are further complicated by proximal nerve trunk lesions. The main problems concern the median and the ulnar nerves.

DISTAL LESIONS AFFECTING THE TERMINAL BRANCHES OF THE PLEXUS [5, 6]

Clinically, the sensory and motor signs are established, and in the majority of cases, the lesions involve the axillary nerve. The clinical picture is characterised by a paralytic shoulder in typical cases, but the diagnosis can be difficult, because a complete palsy of the deltoid muscle may exist without any functional loss, except loss of power. This is due to the compensatory action of the rotator cuff muscles and explains the frequent delay of diagnosis and treatment.

In injuries caused by stretching, the nerve lesion is usually located at a level of relative fixation (quadrilateral space for the axillary nerve, coracoid notch for the suprascapular nerve and entry into the coracobrachialis muscle for the musculocutaneous nerve).

There may be a Sunderland grade 1 or 2 lesion which recovers spontaneously, but the nerve is ruptured in about 20% of cases and operation is indicated if there is no clinical and electrical recovery at 4 to 6 months.

Surgical approach in the deltopectoral groove allows location of the proximal stump of the axillary nerve posteriorly, and the musculocutaneous nerve anteriorly. An additional posterior approach is then necessary at the posterior edge of the posterior deltoid, to dissect the distal stump.

The nerve graft, generally performed with two strands, is pulled out anteriorly from the posterior approach through the quadrilateral space using strong nylon. The distal microsuture is performed first and the posterior approach is closed immediately; the proximal suture is performed secondarily.

Axillary nerve injury is often associated with lesions of other terminal branches. The musculocutaneous nerve lesion is easy to expose through the anterior approach, but the problem is much more difficult in cases of suprascapular nerve injury. In some cases, it will be necessary to dissect the nerve distally until it crosses the coracoid fossa which represents a fixed level where rupture can occur. In these cases, it is very difficult, or even impossible, to expose the distal stump and an additional posterior approach is required, at the level of the scapular spine and of the supraspinatus fossa.

The results after graft are, on the whole, good because of the proximity of the muscle and we obtain 90% recovery ($M_3 + M_4$) after axillary or musculocutaneous repair.

Conclusion

Pre-operative diagnosis is fundamental, and clinical evaluation and other investigations (CT scan-myelography, electromyography) must be used to establish coherent therapeutic indications.

If surgery is indicated, the preoperative assessment must anticipate any pathological lesions that may be encountered, so that a specific surgical plan can be drawn up. Early surgical exploration (6th week to the 3rd month) will allow evaluation of these lesions and determine the possibilities of neurolysis, nerve grafts or neurotisation.

The best results obviously occur in the upper root partial palsies, with C5 and C6 supraclavicular lesions, and also in the terminal branch lesions. However, in total root paralysis, the increasing percentage of useful return of function, depending upon the roots grafted and the structures repaired, suggests that this type of surgery must be carried out with precise and early indications.

References

[1] Allieu Y, Chammas M, Picot MC. Paralysie du plexus brachial par lesions supraclaviculaires chez l'adulte. Résultats comparatifs à long terme des greffes nerveuses et des transferts nerveux. *Rev Chir Orthop* 1997 ; 83 : 51-59

[2] Alnot JY. La main plexique. Atteinte du poignet et de la main dans les paralysies traumatiques du plexus brachial de l'adulte. In : Cahier des conférences d'enseignement de la sociéte française de chirurgie de la main (GEM). Paris : Expansion scientifique française, 1993 : 129-143

[3] Alnot JY. Traumatic brachial plexus lesions in the adult. Indications and results. *Hand Clin* 1995 ; 11 : 623-633

[4] Alnot JY, Daunois O, Oberlin C et al. Total palsy of brachial plexus by supra-clavicular lesions. *J Orthop Surg* 1993 ; 7 : 58-66

[5] Alnot JY, Liverneaux PH, Silberman O. Les lésions du nerf axillaire. *Rev Chir Orthop* 1996 ; 82 : 579-590

[6] Alnot JY, Narakas A. Les paralysies du plexus brachial. In : Monographie du GEM. (1re et 2nd éd). Paris : Expansion Scientifique française, 1989, 1995 : 1-297

[7] Alnot JY, Oberlin C. Tendon transfers in palsies of flexion and extension of the elbow. In : Tubiana R ed. The hand, vol IV. Philadelphia : WB Saunders, 1993 : 134-146

[8] Alnot JY, Rostoucher P, Oberlin C, Touam C. Les paralysies traumatiques C5-C6 et C5-C6-C7 du plexus brachial de l'adulte par lésions supraclaviculaires. *Rev Chir Orthop* 1998 ; 84 : 113-123

[9] Brunelli G, Monini L. Neurotization of avulsed roots of brachial plexus by means of anterior nerves of cervical plexus. *Clin Plast Surg* 1984 ; 11 : 144-153

[10] Franciosi LF, Modestti C, Mueller SF. Neurotization of the biceps muscle by end to side neurorraphy between ulnar and musculocutaneous nerves. A series of five cases, *Ann Chir Main* 1998 ; 17 : 362-367

[11] Leechavengvongs S, Witoonchart K, Uepairojkit CH, Thuvasethalkul PH, Ketmalasiri W. Nerve transfer to biceps muscle using a part of the ulnar nerve in brachial plexus injury (upper arm type): a report of 32 cases, *J Hand Surg Am* 1998 ; 23 : 711-716

[12] Loy S, Bhatia A, Asfazadourian H, Oberlin C. Ulnar nerve fascicle transfer on the biceps motor nerve in C5-C6 or C5-C6-C7 avulsion of the brachial plexus bared on a series of 18 cas. *Ann Hand Uper Limb Surg* 1997 ; 16 : 275-284

[13] Millesi H. Brachial plexus injuries. Management and results. *Clin Plast Surg* 1984 ; 11 : 115-121

[14] Narakas A. The surgical management of brachial plexus injuries. In : Daniel RK, Terzis IK eds. Reconstructive surgery. Boston : Little Brown, 1977

[15] Narakas A. Surgical treatment of traction injuries of the brachial plexus. *Clin Orthop* 1978 ; 133 : 71-90

[16] Narakas A. Les neurotisations ou transferts nerveux dans le traitement des lesions traumatiques du plexus brachial. In : Tubiana R éd. Traité de chirurgie de la main. Chirurgie des tendons, des nerfs et des vaisseaux, Tome 3. Paris : Masson, 1986 : 542-568

[17] Oberlin C. Nerve transfer to biceps muscle using a part of ulnar nerve for C5-C6. Avulsion of the brachial plexus. Anatomical studies and report of four cases. *J Hand Surg Am* 1994 ; 19 : 232-237

[18] Rostoucher P, Alnot JY, Oberlin C, Touam C. Tendon tranfers to restore elbow flexion after traumatic paralysis of the brachial plexus in adults. *Int Orthop* 1998 ; 22 : 255-263

[19] Rusch DS, Friedman A, Nunley JA. The restoration of elbow flexion with intercostal nerve transfer. *Clin Orthop* 1995 ; 314 : 95-103

[20] Sedel L. Résultats des réparations microchirurgicales du plexus brachial. À propos d'une série de 170 cas. In : Tubiana R éd. Traite de chirurgie de la main. Chirurgie des tendons, des nerfs et des vaisseaux, tome 3. Paris : Masson, 1986 : 568-571

[21] Sunderland S. Nerves and nerve injuries. Edinburgh : Churchill Livingstone, 1978 : 854-900

[22] Terzis JK. Microreconstruction of nerve injuries. Philadelphia : WB Saunders, 1987

[23] Viterbo F, Trindade JC, Hoshino K, Mazzoni Neto A. End to side neurorraphy with removal of the epineural sheath. Experimental study in rat. *Plast Reconstr Surg* 1994 ; 94 : 1038-1047

Peripheral nerve tumours

JY Alnot
G Chick

Abstract. – *Tumours of the peripheral nerves are largely benign, and nerve preservation is the main concern. As regards isolated benign tumours, it is necessary to distinguish resectable tumours (schwannomas and intraneural lipomas) and non-resectable tumours (neurofibromas, neurofibrolipomas and intraneural haemangiomas). The definitive treatment depends on the resectable character of the tumour, which is usually only known after epineurotomy. For resectable tumours, enucleation is performed, with an excellent prognosis. For non-resectable tumours, only epineurotomy is performed. An interfascicular biopsy should confirm the histological type. The problem is primarily one of the persistence of diminished paraesthesia. Multiple tumours of the peripheral nerves are seen in neurofibromatosis. These tumours must be treated in the same manner as single lesions, and assessment should determine whether they are resectable (schwannoma) or non-resectable (neurofibroma). The clinical presentation of peripheral nerve mucoid degeneration (PNMD) is often completely different from a benign tumour. Growth is rapid, with associated neurological disorders. Malignant nerve tumours are very rare with a poor prognosis and conservative surgery is no longer the primary concern.*

Keywords: *peripheral nerve, nerve tumours, schwannoma, neurofibroma, neurofibrolipoma.*

Introduction

Peripheral nerve tumours develop from nerve components *(fig 1)*. They are rare, accounting for 2% of soft tissue tumours [3, 11], and are benign in 90% of cases [3].

Isolated benign tumours

As regards surgical management, it is necessary to distinguish resectable tumours (schwannomas and intraneural lipomas), which push the fascicular groups towards the periphery without penetrating them, and non-resectable tumours (neurofibromas, neurofibrolipomas and intraneural haemangiomas) which infiltrate all the nerve components. This difference is absolutely essential for selecting the appropriate surgical procedure. However, irrespective of the type of tumour, the main therapeutic concern is to respect nerve continuity, and nerve resection must not be performed [4]. MRI, although non-specific, is the best

Jean-Yves Alnot, M.D., Orthopaedic Hand Surgeon, Head of Department.
Grégoire Chick, M.D., Attending Orthopaedic Hand Surgeon.
Orthopaedics and Traumatology Surgery, Hand Surgery Unit, Hôpital Bichat, 46, rue Henri Huchard, 75877 Paris Cedex 18, France.

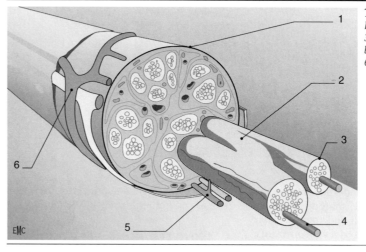

1 *Nerve components. 1. Epineurium; 2. perineurium; 3. nerve fascicles; 4. nerve fibres; 5. intrinsic vessels; 6. extrinsic vessels.*

investigation for the diagnosis of a nerve tumour. Schwannoma generally presents as a round lesion, whereas neurofibroma has a more oval shape.

The operation is performed under pneumatic tourniquet through a surgical approach which allows dissection of the nerve trunk, its divisions and branches. If the tumour is localised in, or close to, a compressive tunnel, the fibro-muscular arch should be opened. The definitive treatment depends on the resectable character of the

tumour which is usually only known after anterior epineurotomy.

ISOLATED RESECTABLE TUMOURS

Their macroscopic appearance is very typical, presenting as round and encapsulated lesions. Schwannomas are the most common resectable tumours (95%) [3], and intraneural lipomas are extremely rare (5% in our experience).

After epineurotomy under an operating microscope *(fig 2A)*, enucleation of the

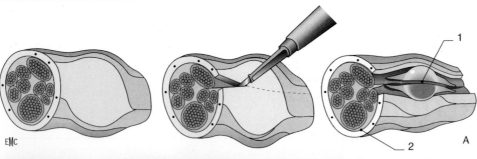

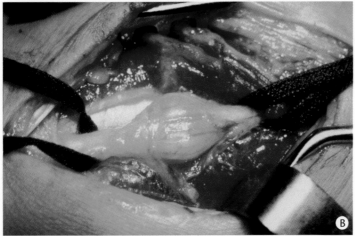

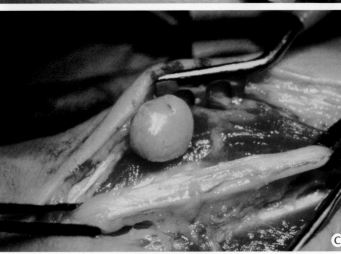

2 *A. Resectable tumour (schwannoma) : epineurotomy under operating microscope. 1. Fascicular group displaced around the tumour mass must be dissected and kept in continuity. 2. epineurium.*
B. Schwannoma can be completely excised without injury to the nerve.
C. Enucleation preserves fascicular group.

tumour [3, 5, 10, 11, 13] is made possible by the existence of a constant anatomical plane between the tumour wall and the fascicular groups. This preserves nerve continuity during surgery (fig 2B, C). However, in certain cases, the tumour is suspended from a small nerve fascicle from which it cannot be separated, and which will therefore be sacrificed. This should cause no additional deficit, since such nerve fascicles are already non-functional [3].

Clinical examination frequently reveals paraesthesia, without objective motor or sensitive deficits. If the rules regarding dissection are respected, no iatrogenic deficit should be noted in the immediate postoperative period in relation to contusion of the fascicular groups. When a nerve deficit does occur, it is generally transient [13]. When pre-operative nerve deficits are present, their regression is a function of the age of the lesion [3, 5, 10, 13]. The prognosis is

excellent. The surgeon should check whether there are any other lesions in the vicinity.

ISOLATED NON-RESECTABLE TUMOURS

Solitary neurofibroma is the most common non-resectable nerve tumour (10% of isolated nerve tumours in our experience). Most of the time, the macroscopic appearance of solitary neurofibroma is in the form of an oval dilatation, and after epineurotomy (fig 3A), it presents as a tumour infiltrating the nerve. Tumour resection is impossible without sacrificing nerve tissue but the nerve itself should not be sacrified (fig 3B, C). In the most frequent cases, where there is no objective neurological deficit, the epineurotomy is performed under microscope. The patient should be informed that the paraesthesia will improve only progressively in the post-operative period [4, 5]. Interfascicular biopsy

should confirm the histological type. When there is an incomplete motor deficit, muscle transfer should be performed. Exceptionally, in the presence of a complete motor deficit, nerve resection may be performed, immediately followed by a nerve graft. If the tumour is localised on a minor nerve (e.g. sensory branch of radial nerve or sural nerve), nerve resection can be carried out without grafting. There is no recorded study indicating malignant transformation in this type of solitary neurofibroma. The problem is primarily that although paraesthesia is reduced, it still persists to some degree.

Neurofibrolipoma is a particular form of non-resectable tumour, probably of congenital origin, and is most commonly linked to the median nerve [18]. It begins in childhood and is associated with macrodactyly in most cases.

Intraneural haemangiomas are very rare, non-resectable tumours. Differenciation of intraneural haemangiomas from classical haemangiomas is made by their presence in nerve tissue. These tumours infiltrate the nerve, and treatment remains the same as for neurofibromas.

MULTIPLE TUMOURS

Multiple tumours of the peripheral nerves are seen in neurofibromatosis. They are hereditary and present and develop in a variety of different ways.

■ *Von Recklinghausen, type 1 neurofibromastosis (NF1)* [15]

The diagnostic criteria appear in Table I [15]. These tumours must be treated in the same manner as isolated lesions, and assessment should determine whether the tumours are resectable (schwannoma) or non-resectable (neurofibroma). The average number of tumours is variable (one to several dozen per patient) [17] and their size is often greater in cases of multiple tumours than in isolated tumours [14]. A particular form of neurofibroma is specific to NF1 [15]: plexiform neurofibroma (7.5% of neurofibromas) [17]. It presents as multiple dilatations along the nerve and has a chain-like appearance. In the event of asymptomatic tumours, continued follow-up is advised. Any new and rapid changes noted at clinical examination should lead to surgery, because of potential malignant transformation of the neurofibroma into neurofibrosarcoma (3 to 13%) [17, 19]. The interval between neurofibromatosis diagnosis and transformation varies from 10 to 30 years [19].

■ *Type 2 neurofibromatosis (NF2) or bilateral neuro-acoustic neurofibromatosis* (table I) [8]

Type 2 is characterised by the existence of a vestibular schwannoma (bilateral presentations are pathognomonic). The number of tumours is variable, with a higher incidence of schwannomas as opposed to

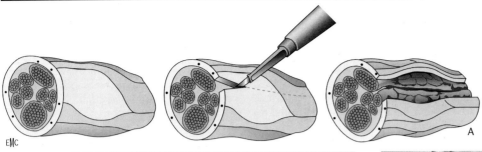

3
A. Non-resectable tumour: epineurotomy under operating microscope.
B. Neurofibroma.
C. Neurofibroma presents as a tumour infiltrating the nerve.

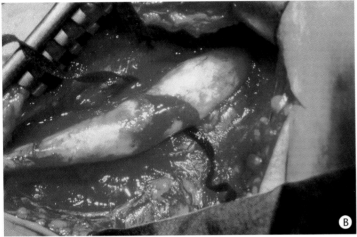

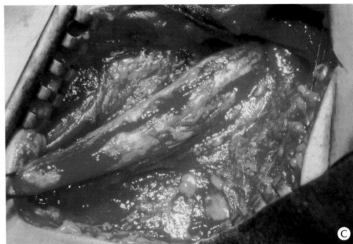

Table I. – Diagnostic criteria for neurofibromatosis [8, 9, 15].

Type 1: von Recklinghausen
minimum of 2 criteria:
- at least 6 café-au-lait maculae over 15 mm in diameter (5 mm if pre-pubertal)
- 1 plexiform neurofibroma or 2 or more neurofibromas
- multiple freckles in the axillary or inguinal regions
- bilateral optic nerve gliomas
- 2 or more iris Lisch nodules on slit lamp examination
- sphenoid wing dysplasia or congenital bowing or thinning of long bone cortex with or without pseudarthrosis
- a first-degree relative with von Recklinghausen NF, by the above criteria

Type 2: Bilateral acoustic neurofibromatosis
- bilateral vestibular schwannoma
          or
- a first degree relative with bilateral acoustic neurofibromatosis and one of the following:
     a) unilateral vestibular schwannoma
     b) any 2 of the following: meningioma, glioma, schwannoma or juvenile posterior subcapsular lenticular opacities juvenile cortical cataract.

Type 3: Schwannomatosis
- 2 or more pathologically proved schwannomas
          and
- lack of radiographic evidence of vestibular nerve tumour, at age > 18 years

---

neurofibromas. The surgical treatment is similar. Malignant degeneration has never been reported.

■ *Type 3 neurofibromatosis (NF3) or schwannomatosis*

This presents as multiple schwannomatosis with unilateral lesions [9]. Tumour enucleation [11, 12, 16] should be performed in the event of symptomatic dysfunction with an average of 5 tumours per intervention [11, 16]. The possibility of a chain-like tumour should be checked by palpation of the nerve to search for subclinical nodules. The persistence of clinical dysfunction or the occurrence of new symptoms suggests new localised tumours, or pre-existing lesions which have gone unrecognised because of their small size [3, 5, 16].

Peripheral nerve mucoid degeneration (PNMD)

The clinical presentation is often completely different from a benign tumour. Growth is rapid with associated neurological disorders. PNMD is a rare benign nerve tumour (between 8% and 15% of benign isolated tumours of the peripheral nerves) [2]. The connective origin is characterised by the infiltration into the neural sheath of a mucoid substance which forms an intraneural tumour, compressing the nerve fascicles towards the periphery. There is no epithelial lining as with a synovial cyst. The pathogenesis remains controversial. It is most commonly localised (80%) [2, 7] on the common fibular nerve at the neck of the fibula. Other localisations are near a joint or

a narrow compression tunnel like the arch of the flexor carpi ulnaris at the elbow. These tumours are associated with neurological deficits in the corresponding nerve territory.

The treatment is exclusively surgical with an approach allowing dissection of the nerve trunk and its branches. Macroscopically, the pseudocyst presents either in the form of a single and bulky mass or as several translucent masses embedded in the nerve trunk. After epineurotomy under microscope [7], the content is evacuated; the appearance is similar to yellowish jelly. The fibromuscular arch should be opened. Although a connection between the pseudocyst and the joint is rarely found, it must nevertheless be sought. As regards the nerve, it is often impossible to remove the wall of the cyst fully. Intrafascicular dissection is contraindicated considering the risk of injury to the fascicular groups.

For long-standing tumours, the average time for neurological recovery, which occurs in most cases, is prolonged (average 10 months). Recurrences are rare [7], but may present with reappearance of a new nodule. Successful outcome following surgical treatment is dependent on early diagnosis of the lesion, before neurological damage has occurred.

Malignant tumours

These are rare, accounting for 10% of all nervous tumours [1, 3], and 10% of soft tissue sarcomas [6], with a poor prognosis: 50% survival at 5 years [3]. 50% of malignant tumours occur in patients with pre-existing von Recklinghausen's disease. Malignant tumours are generally locally malignant, and rarely metastasise, except for fibroblastic tumours (20% to 50%) [6]. Evolution is rapid with associated neurological disorders.

Conservative surgery is no longer the primary concern. Surgical biopsy and pathology remain the cornerstone of diagnosis. The tumour is approached without dissection and a biopsy is carried out after epineurotomy to confirm the histological diagnosis. Histologically, the malignant character is easy to confirm. However, the diagnosis of tumour type and assertion of its nervous origin may be difficult due to frequent metaplasia (immediate pathology remains less precise than final pathological assessment). Malignant tumours of the peripheral nerves include tumours derived from the neural sheath called MPNST (Malignant Peripheral Nerve Sheath Tumour) and fibroblastic tumours of connective tissue origin with intraneural development. In MPNST, malignant schwannoma (with an epithelioid variety) and neurofibrosarcoma must be distinguished.

All patients undergo chemotherapy. Following chemotherapy, management includes large surgical resection (including the nerve and the surrounding tissue) as usually performed for soft tissue malignant tumours. Any conservative surgery carries a risk of recurrence. In certain cases, amputation may be recommended, particularly in the event of recurrence. Chemotherapy is administered to those patients who show a positive response to the first course of chemotherapy. Local radiotherapy is ineffective and a prolonged surgical follow-up is essential.

Conclusion

Tumours of the peripheral nerves are largely benign and nerve preservation is the main concern. Malignant tumours are very rare, with a poor prognosis, and conservative surgery is then no longer the primary concern.

References

[1] D'Agostino AN, Soule EH, Miller RH. Primary malignant neoplasm of nerves (malignant neurilemmomas) in patients without manifestations of multiple neurofibromatosis (Von Recklinghausen's disease). *Cancer* 1963 ; 16 : 1003-1014

[2] Allieu Y, Cenac PE. Peripheral nerve mucoid degeneration of the upper extremity. *J Hand Surg Am* 1989 ; 14 : 189-194

[3] Allieu Y, Chammas M, Jacoulet P. Tumeurs primitives des nerfs périphériques. *Encycl Méd Chir* (Éditions Scientifiques et Médicales Elsevier SAS, Paris), Appareil locomoteur, 15-007-A-10, 2000 : 1-10

[4] Artico M, Cervoni L, Wierzbicki V, D'Andrea V, Nucci F. Benign neural sheath tumors of major nerves: characteristics in 119 surgical cases. *Acta Neurochir* 1997 ; 139 : 1108-1116

[5] Donner TR, Voorhies RM, Kline DG. Neural sheath tumors of major nerves. *J Neurosurg* 1994 ; 81 : 362-373

[6] Doorn PF, Molenaar WM, Buter J, Hoekstra HJ. Malignant peripheral nerve sheath tumor in patients with and without neurofibromatosis. *Eur J Surg Oncol* 1995 ; 21 : 78-82

[7] Giele H, Le Viet D. Intraneural mucoid cysts of the upper limb. *J Hand Surg Br* 1997 ; 22 : 805-809

[8] Gutmann D, Aylsworth A, Carley J, Korf B, Marks J, Pyeritz R, Rubenstein R et al. The diagnostic evaluation and multi-disciplinary management of neurofibromatosis 2. *JAMA* 1997 ; 278 : 51-57

[9] Jacoby LB, Jones D, Davis K, Short P, Gusella J, MacCollin M. Molecular analysis of the NF 2 tumor-suppressor gene in Schwannomatosis. *Am J Hum Genet* 1997 ; 61 : 1293-1302

[10] Kehoe NJ, Reid RP, Semple JC. Solitary benign peripheral nerve tumours. Review of 32 year's experience. *J Bone Joint Surg Br* 1995 ; 77 : 497-500

[11] Le Viet D, Lantieri L. Tumeurs extirpables des nerfs périphériques. À propos de 73 tumeurs nerveuses chez 53 patients. *Ann Chir Plast Esthét* 1993 ; 38 : 172-179

[12] Lewis RC, Nannini LH. Multifocal neurilemomas of median and ulnar nerves of the same extremity: a case report. *J Hand Surg* 1981 ; 6 : 406-408

[13] Oberle J, Kahamba J, Richter HP. Peripheral nerve schwannomas - an analysis of 16 patients. *Acta Neurochirurgica* 1997 ; 139 : 949-953

[14] Pou Serradell A. Lésions centrales dans les neurofibromatoses : corrélations cliniques, d'IRM et histopathologiques. Essai de classification. *Rev Neurol* 1991 ; 147 : 17-27

[15] Riccardi VM, Eichner JE. Neurofibromatosis: phenotype, natural history and pathogenesis. Baltimore : Johns Hopkins University Press, 1992

[16] Rosberg HE, Ekerot L. Multifocal neurilemmomas in the same upper extremity. Case report. *Scand J Plast Reconst Surg* 1996 ; 30 : 153-156

[17] Rubenstein AE. Neurofibromatosis. *Ann NY Acad Sci* 1986 ; 486 : 1-14

[18] Salon A, Guero S, Glicenstein J. Fibrolipomes du nerf médian. Revue de dix cas opérés avec un recul moyen de huit ans. *Ann Chir Main* 1995 ; 14 : 284-295

[19] Sorensen SA, Mulvihill JJ, Nielsen A. Long-term follow-up of Von Recklinghausen neurofibromatosis: survival and malignant neoplasms. *N Engl J Med* 1986 ; 314 : 1010-1015

Computer-assisted surgery

LP Nolte
F Langlotz
P Regazzoni

Abstract. — Since the mid-90s, freehand navigation systems and medical robots are in routine clinical use, and today, a large variety of interventions in orthopaedics can be assisted by computer. These devices can be classified according to the amount of autonomy they are given during the operation. Active navigators or robots act on the patient under supervision of a surgeon. Passive navigation systems provide visual positional feedback to the surgeon who actually performs the operation. A third class of semi-active navigators is still in an experimental phase. They let the surgeon carry out the intervention and ensure that a pre-operatively defined plan is followed. While the first generation of navigation systems relied solely on computed tomography scans for planning and visualisation purposes, alternatives have recently been introduced which aim at overcoming the disadvantages of CT-based navigation. They feature the integration of intra-operatively available imaging means, namely fluoroscopy, or replace radiological images by so-called "surgeon defined anatomy", in cases when neither preoperative nor intra-operative imaging is common. Ongoing prospective and retrospective clinical studies clearly indicate that computer assisted navigation provides significant improvements in accuracy in orthopaedic surgery.

Keywords: computer assisted surgery, navigation, robotics, virtual fluoroscopy.

Introduction

In the past decade, a new field of research and development, now commonly known as "Medical Robotics and Computer Assisted Surgery" (MRCAS) has evolved from areas such as medical imaging, image processing, robotics, motion analysis, virtual reality, etc. A number of studies outlining the deficiencies of classical approaches in several areas of orthopaedic surgery have led researchers to seek technological aids which improve accuracy and safety during interventions. Two pioneer applications representing the two major philosophies of MRCAS must be mentioned. For total hip replacement surgery, an apparatus called ROBODOC was first used in the operating theatre in 1991. This device was derived from a successful industrial robot. Today, first generation medical robots are used to prepare femoral cavities during cementless total hip arthroplasties in about 100 European centres. In parallel, several

Lutz-Peter Nolte, Ph.D., Maurice E. Müller Institute for Biomechanics, University of Bern, Bern, Switzerland.
Frank Langlotz, Ph.D., Maurice E. Müller Institute for Biomechanics, University of Bern, Bern, Switzerland.
Pietro Regazzoni, M.D., Department of Traumatology, Kantonsspital Basel, Switzerland.

research groups have independently developed visualisation systems for conventional surgery that allow surgeons to get real time feedback of surgical action on a computer screen, even if there is no direct insight into the surgical field. This approach adapts stereotactic concepts which are well established in neurosurgery. The implantation of pedicular screws in the sacral and lower lumbar spine has been chosen as the first field for these freehand navigation systems.

The early MRCAS systems relied upon pre-operative computed tomography (CT) scans of the patient, for preoperative planning and intra-operative navigation purposes. Derivatives of both robotic and freehand navigation systems are now available for various orthopaedic interventions. An increasing number of retrospective and prospective studies are proving their clinical benefits.

In this article, the general concept and underlying principles of this technology will be outlined; an overview of their clinical usage will be given. New developments that are currently being introduced clinically, and which aim at overcoming the restrictions and disadvantages of classical CT-based navigation, will also be presented.

General concept

ABSTRACT MODEL

All navigation systems currently being used clinically can be represented by one common abstract model [3]. A tool or instrument is used to treat a part of a patient's anatomy. The target of this procedure is termed "therapeutic object" or "surgical object". The position and orientation that the tool or instrument occupies in space are controlled in real time by a so-called "navigator". In addition, this navigator geometrically links the treated anatomy to an image or model, thus allowing this duplicate, termed "virtual object", to be used for precise planning or visualisation. To illustrate this rather theoretical description better, the two aforementioned pioneer applications may serve as examples. For the ROBODOC, a CT scan of the hip to be treated (therapeutic object) is acquired pre-operatively. This data is loaded into a planning computer, and in a three-dimensionally reconstructed model of the hip (virtual object), the surgeon plans the optimal position of the femoral component of the prosthesis within the bone. Intra-operatively, the robot (navigator) is linked to the patient, and is loaded with the planning data. It then guides a revolving high-speed cutter to mill the femoral cavity according to the plan.

In a freehand spinal navigation system, a CT scan also represents the virtual object. It is calibrated intra-operatively to match the patient's position on the operating table. A motion tracking device (navigator) follows the position and orientation of an instrument in the hand of the surgeon. This data is used to display an image of the instrument and its actual position on the CT scan, on a computer monitor.

CLASSIFICATION OF NAVIGATORS

The large number of different orthopaedic navigation systems developed during the last six to eight years may be classified according to the type of navigator incorporated. Three categories can be identified:

■ *Active*

Robots are also termed "active navigators" since they actively perform an operation or a part of an operation without any interaction on the part of the surgeon. They allow for a highly precise execution of a pre-operative plan, but they have to include a considerable number of redundant safety features, to protect patient and surgical staff from potential dangers in case of system failure. This complexity makes them rather inflexible and difficult to adapt to new applications, which may be the reason why the majority of the existing navigation systems are so-called freehand systems.

■ *Passive*

In contrast to the active robots, these devices use "passive navigators" that trace hand guided instruments in space while leaving the execution of surgical tasks to the surgeon. Technically, a number of possible solutions can be considered that allow measuring the position of an object remotely, most of which have been implemented in different navigation systems. Ultrasonic devices measure the time the sound waves travel between an emitter attached to the instrument to be tracked and an array of microphones. Knowing the speed of sound allows distances and thus positions from the recorded data to be calculated. Since the speed of sound greatly depends on air temperature, and it is a complex task to account for reflecting sound waves, this category of navigators is almost non-existent in MRCAS systems. A small number of orthopaedic navigation systems relies on magnetic trackers. These devices generate an electromagnetic field in which the position of sensitive coils attached to surgical instruments can be measured. As for ultrasonic devices, magnetic navigators suffer from inherent system inaccuracies, because the homogeneity of the magnetic field can easily be disturbed by metallic

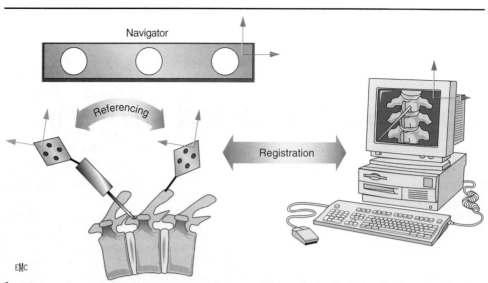

1 *The general concept of computer-assisted surgery is exemplified by a freehand spinal navigation system. Local co-ordinate systems are established on all relevant parts. Referencing allows the determination of instrument positions relative to the anatomy. Registration matches virtual and therapeutic objects.*

objects. The majority of the currently known freehand navigation systems is based on opto-electronic tracking devices that work with infra-red light emitting diodes (LEDs), or infra-red light reflecting spheres.

■ *Semi-active*

A third category is currently represented by laboratory set-ups only. These semi-active navigation systems may be classified as hybrids since they let a surgeon guide the instrument in a freehand manner, but a robot restricts the area in which the instrument may be moved safely. Semi-active navigators should potentially contribute to an advanced second generation of MRCAS systems.

■ *Analogy of classification*

Drawing an analogy with modern car technology, a GPS navigation system that displays the current position of the car on a street map can be seen as a passive navigator. An anti-blocking system, which allows the driver to put on the brake, but interacts by quickly releasing it again to avoid dangerous situations, represents a semi-active navigation system. Finally an auto-pilot which drives a car autonomously to a predefined destination can be seen as an active navigator.

MATHEMATICAL BACKGROUND

The underlying strategies that allow the merging of tool position, navigator, therapeutic object, and virtual object into one system are identical for robotic and freehand navigation. The steps described in the following subsections are illustrated *(fig 1)*.

■ *Calibration of instruments*

Local co-ordinate systems (COS) are established on each instrument. The spatial

relationship between different instruments can then be expressed by means of co-ordinate transformations. Special points of interest, e.g. the tip of a drill bit mounted on a drilling machine, are defined in respect to this COS.

■ *Referencing*

To enable the navigator to track not only surgical instruments but also operated anatomy, a local COS must also be established on the therapeutic object. In the case of robotic surgery, this is accomplished by means of a clamping mechanism rigidly attached to the treated bone. Freehand navigation systems require the bone to be instrumented with a special probe holding LEDs, reflecting spheres, magnetic or acoustic sensors – depending on the navigator's tracking technology. This probe is also known as the dynamic reference base.

■ *Registration*

Registration or matching is one of the most critical steps in each navigation system. Its purpose is to establish the link between the COSs of therapeutic and virtual objects. In the case of a freehand system, this allows instrument positions measured relative to the anatomy to be transformed into image space and displayed on the screen. For robotic surgery, registration is required so that the preoperative plan defined in the virtual object can be applied to the therapeutic object. A number of matching strategies have been reported in the literature, and Lavallée [20] gives an excellent overview of the different algorithms. Two of the most common registration approaches will be described here.

Paired points matching

At least three different points are identified on both the therapeutic and virtual object. The relationship between these pairs is given by the co-ordinate transformation to be found. Since these points serve as representatives for the entire region of interest, they should be well distributed over the accessible anatomy, and should be selected so that they are easily and precisely identifiable. Pre-operatively, each point is interactively marked on the virtual object with the computer mouse. During the operation, a digitisation probe of the navigator is used to identify the counterparts on the therapeutic object. In many cases, the intra-operatively accessible structures do not provide a sufficient number of clearly recognisable feature points. During total hip replacement for example, both pelvis and femur offer only rather regular surfaces without many prominent feature points. In these cases, pre-operatively inserted artificial markers such as screws, pins, or spheres can be used for paired point matching. However, this insertion is an invasive process requiring additional surgery prior to the main intervention, resulting in a major disadvantage of this matching strategy.

Surface matching

Surface registration is often used in combination with paired point matching when the latter alone is unable to yield an accurate matching of virtual and therapeutic objects. By means of image processing techniques, a three-dimensional model of the bony surface is pre-operatively generated from the CT data. During the operation, a cloud of points arbitrarily distributed over the accessible anatomy are digitised and mathematically fitted onto the model. The advantage of this approach is that the locations to be identified in the situs are not prescribed. Any group of surface spots are suitable as long as they are spread over a reasonable area. On the other hand, finding the right co-ordinate transformation is mathematically much more challenging than for paired point matching. To minimise computation times and to maximise reliability of the algorithm, both methods are usually used in conjunction with each other.

Clinical applications

CT-BASED APPLICATIONS

Computed tomography scans provide a relatively easy way of generating geometrically exact three-dimensional representations of bony structures. For this reason, they were the first images to be used as virtual objects in computer assisted orthopaedic surgery.

As mentioned before, robotic surgery based on CT scans was first applied to total hip replacement [2, 24]. In the ROBODOC system, for the first time, CT scans enabled precise pre-operative planning of implant placement in all three dimensions in a non-experimental set-up. Until now, more than

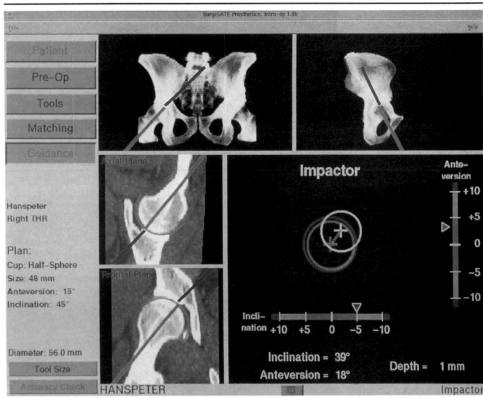

2 *During total hip replacement, the current position of an impactor is visualised together with a pre-operative CT scan. A flight-simulator-like display guides towards the planned position of the acetabular cup.*

1,600 hips have been implanted with ROBODOC in one clinic alone [30], and the success of this active navigation system must at least partly be attributed to its operative planning capacities. Meanwhile, a similar robot has been developed and introduced clinically [5]. First introduced for milling the femoral cavity during uncemented total hip replacement, robotic systems are now employed to drill attachment tunnels during anterior cruciate ligament (ACL) replacement, and to prepare femura and tibiae in total knee arthroplasty surgery.

In contrast to active robots, freehand navigation systems use CT scans as a visualisation basis. The implantation of transpedicular screws was identified as the first clinical application by several developers since it offered a large potential for improved accuracy. A number of research groups simultaneously developed freehand systems for this type of intervention. Although their first laboratory setting was based on a robot holding a laser as a guide [28], Lavallée et al presented a complete freehand navigation system in 1995 [21]. It featured an opto-electronic tracking system, pre-operative planning of screw trajectories, and a combination of paired points and surface matching. In the same year the first clinical experiences on another CT-based spinal navigation system were reported [26]. Subsequent clinical trials [29] performed with this set-up and its commercial version [17] initiated a sequence of studies [1, 10, 23] comparing computer assisted and conventional instrumentation of the spine.

All authors report drastically reduced misplacement rates, down to 2%-5%.

CT-based freehand navigation also has its domain in hip surgery. The first of these systems was developed and clinically tested by DiGioia et al [7]. Constant improvements of their HipNav® system have turned it into a complete surgical assistant, covering pre-operative planning and simulation, intra-operative navigation, and post-operative evaluation. Another CT-based freehand navigation system (*fig 2*) was presented by Langlotz et al [19]. This uses modules which were initially developed for a spinal CAS system. It can be used with a variety of different implant models and does not dictate any surgical approach or special positioning of the patient. Moreover, it demonstrates the usability of MRCAS technology for several orthopaedic applications.

Another class of orthopaedic interventions interesting researchers is that of repositioning osteotomies. Ellis et al [8] presented a planning and guidance system for high tibial osteotomies which is based on pre-operative CT scans and uses radio-opaque markers for matching. The domain of pelvic osteotomies has been covered by a system developed for peri-acetabular osteotomy [18]. It allows for precise intra-operative navigation during osteotomy of the acetabulum and subsequent re-orientation of the fragment.

In the area of CT-based computer assisted trauma surgery, applications for ilio-sacral

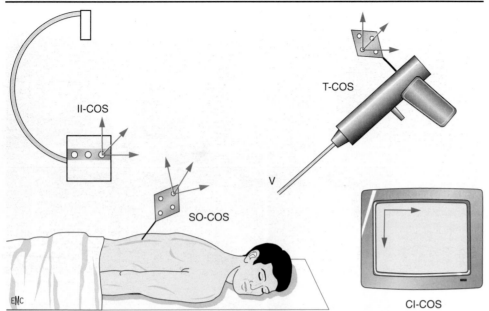

3 *Fluoroscopy-based navigation establishes local co-ordinate systems (COS) on the surgical tool (T), the surgical object (SO), the image intensifier unit (II), and in the resulting C-arm image (CI).*

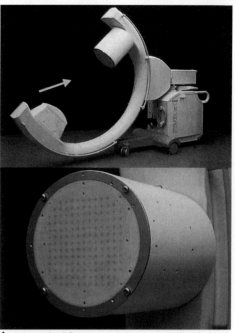

4 *A standard fluoroscope is instrumented with an additional calibration grid allowing for automatic undistortion of the acquired images.*

fixation and the treatment of pelvic fractures [33] have recently been presented.

FLUOROSCOPY-BASED SURGICAL NAVIGATION SYSTEMS

The CT-based computer aided surgery system provides a direct link between the pre-operative plan and its intra-operative surgical execution. Despite the described convincing early results, there has been a certain lack of widespread enthusiasm for CT-based navigation systems. Current criticism focuses on limited medical benefits in cases of normal morphology, costs for additional tomographic image data, and the difficulty and additional time spent intra-operatively for the registration procedure.

Based on their experience with CT-based freehand navigation systems, various research groups started a search for alternatives, looking at different imaging means, particularly those which were intra-operatively available. Recently, a novel freehand navigation system has been proposed [12, 13], which in practice achieves combining intra-operative fluoroscopy-based imaging, using widely available C-arm technology, with modern freehand surgical navigation (fig 3).

The key to this novel solution was the inherent calibration of commercially available C-arms adequate for use in the operating theatre, which for the first time allowed the digital X-ray image registration [4, 11, 15, 22] to be fully automated. This is in contrast to existing CT-based navigation systems, which require an often difficult registration procedure. Fluoroscopic image calibration requires slight modifications to the C-arms (fig 4). Cross-referencing the image intensifier with the surgical object produces the real time image and interactive navigation of surgical tools, based on one single registered X-ray image with no

further image updates. This is equivalent to the use of a C-arm unit in constant mode during the intervention, which implies high radiation exposure for the patient and the surgical staff. Furthermore, these systems allow for acquisition and real-time use of multiple registered images, which provide an advanced multi-directional control (pseudo three-dimensional) during surgical action (fig 5).

The next step was to develop concepts for radiation-free positioning of the C-arm during the intervention [14]. Using navigated pointing instruments the surgeon can

effectively predetermine the direction of the X-ray beam. Subsequently, the OR technician will adjust the C-arm relative to the patient using "flight simulator" type graphical user interfaces without any radiation.

Further research led to effective modules for intra-operative measurements on the patient's anatomy [14]. Using the back projection parameters of the C-arm model, anatomical landmarks, bone axes, anatomical angles (e.g. the femoral

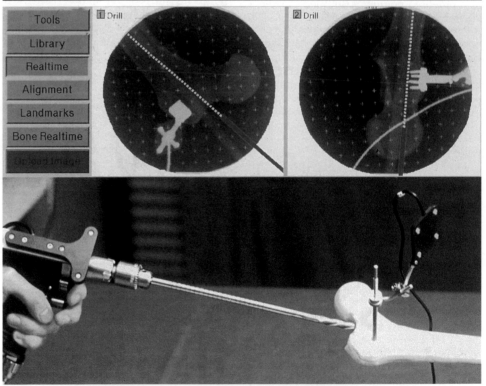

5 *The position of this drill is simultaneously displayed in two different fluoroscopic images providing pseudo three-dimensional visualisation. The white crosses are calibration markers needed for an undistorted image.*

antetorsion), and distances (e.g. the leg length) can be determined by the surgeon.

Today, stereotactic instrument sets and associated graphical user interfaces exist for fluoroscopy-based, image interactive spine surgery [9, 25] and various trauma applications, such as intramedullary nailing of the femur and the tibia [15, 31]. The elegance of this technology is best illustrated by the never solved problem of distal nail locking, which can now be performed easily, based on two orthogonal C-arm images [31].

Fluoroscopy navigation systems are currently in routine use in various European and North American clinics, and provide effective support in spinal and trauma procedures. Based on the resulting data, this novel technique holds promises for improved accuracy and safety in a broad range of open and percutaneous approaches.

NAVIGATION USING "SURGEON DEFINED ANATOMY"

In a variety of orthopaedic surgical procedures, it is quite uncommon to use pre-operative CT scanning as well as intra-operative imaging such as ultrasound or fluoroscopy. Issues such as related costs and additional OR time have made it difficult for existing navigation concepts to provide the missing link between the usually pre-operative X-ray based plan and the resulting intra-operative surgical actions in these cases. A potential solution is a non-imaging computer-based technique, the so-called "surgeon defined anatomy". It was originally introduced to this field by Dessenne et al [6]. This technique involves the use of computerised pointing instruments to define anatomical structures and viewpoints of these structures freely and interactively. This is important for the surgical plan and its intra-operative execution.

The first application of this technology was the computer-assisted arthroscopic reconstruction of the anterior cruciate ligament (ACL) [6, 27]. At the beginning of the procedure, dynamic reference bases are fixed onto the femur and tibia to track the knee's movement. No pre- or intra-operative imaging is required, but can be incorporated into the hybrid system if available [27]. Using a computerised palpation hook *(fig 6)* potential ligament attachment sites and other important functional anatomical structures, such as the femoral notch, are digitised under endoscopic control.

Impingement of the planned ligament placement can be predicted by the position of the virtual ligament with respect to the digitised notch entrance surface geometry. The virtually planned ligament can be seen to impinge where it graphically intersects with the digitised notch surface. The diameter of the simulated ligament must be interactively set by the knee surgeon to the equivalent of the harvested graft width,

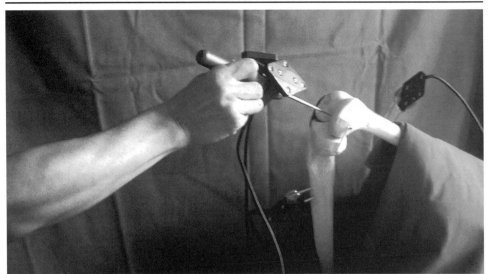

6   *An instrumented palpation hook is used to digitise structures in the knee to generate a virtual representation of the joint.*

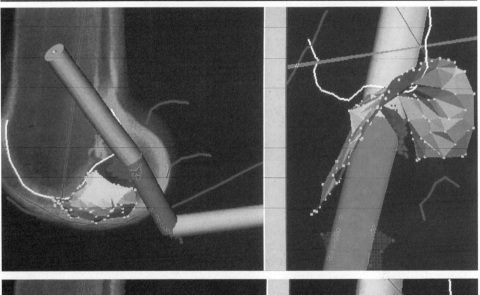
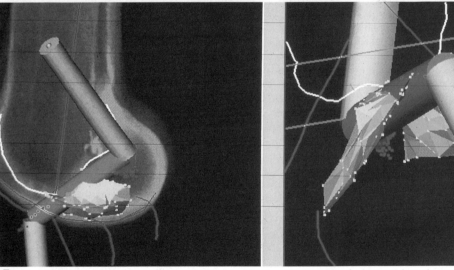

7   *Simulation of a virtual ACL graft allows for the determination of impingement for a potential attachment site.*

because ligament diameter has a significant effect on impingement *(fig 7)*.

Virtual analysis of the intra-operative plan also includes the graft elongation pattern as a function of knee flexion angle [27]. This information is either given numerically or represented as a coloured map on the potential attachment areas on the femur and tibia.

The surgical plan, with appropriate ligament attachment sites and orientations of the tibial and femoral tunnel, is finally executed using

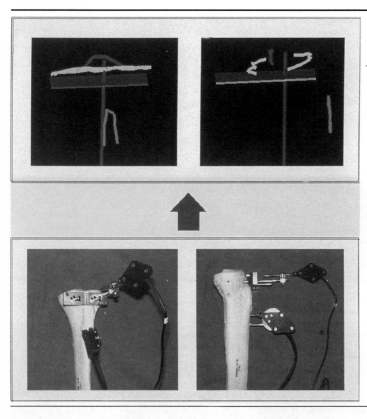

8 *Instrumented cutting jigs can be precisely aligned with the help of on-screen feedback.*

a drilling mode, which is similar to classic CT-based freehand navigation systems.

Built into these technologies is the capacity to record knee anatomy, ligament placement, and knee kinematics and to save this information for later analysis. Comparison between pre-operative knee instability and kinematics can therefore be carried out to assess the benefit of surgical reconstruction.

"Surgeon defined anatomy" systems have been designed to be flexible for different orthopaedic interventions. Following ACL reconstructive surgery their functionality was extended towards computerised total knee replacement (TKR) surgery. In this case pivoting techniques in combination with computerised pointing techniques are used to determine the mechanical axes accurately [32]. Recently, this approach was further extended to take in the complete process of ligament balancing, with special adaptation to functional constraints, arising from the specific prosthetic design [16].

Computerised cutting jigs (fig 8) are used to perform the resulting tibial and femoral cuts accurately.

After successful validation in different laboratory settings, freehand navigation systems for ACL and TKR are now in routine use in many centres throughout Europe.

Discussion

There has now been ten years of technological research and development and nearly six years of clinical experience in the area of computer assisted orthopaedic surgery - a novel area which has evolved through consequent technology transfer. The transition from the laboratory to the operating theatre was due to a few early clinical prototypes in the areas of total hip replacement and spinal surgery. They paved the way, through a variety of successful prospective and retrospective studies, to reveal the striking potential of this technology for improving accuracy and safety in orthopaedic surgical procedures. As a consequence, it must be stated that surgery assisted by computers is no longer a subject of laboratory settings or science fiction authors. A considerable number of robotic and freehand navigation systems are currently available, and numerous studies have doubtless proven the short-term clinical benefit of this technology. Further

investigations are necessary to prove the positive long-term outcome of Medical Robotics and Computer Assisted Surgery applications. Most of these systems are devices of the first generation of MRCAS, i.e., dominated by pre-operative CT scans and designed to fulfil the needs of one single clinical application. The great advantages of CT as imaging (easy availability, good hard/soft tissue contrast, geometrically precise three-dimensional representation) can be compared with a number of significant disadvantages. CT scans are not performed routinely for all operations; they result in radiation exposure; they are not suitable if soft tissue is to be operated on and, last but not least, they are cost intensive. Moreover, the complete domain of traumatology with its large potential for improvements of accuracy seems unsuitable for CT-based navigation, since referencing and registration are necessary for each bony fragment.

Current medical robots allow for an extremely precise execution of pre-operative plans. However, it still has to be proven that their long-term clinical benefits ultimately justify the immense investment costs.

Alternative imaging means such as fluoroscopy and "surgeon defined anatomy" are new approaches to overcoming the problems of CT-based navigation. This expansion must be positive because it provides researchers and developers with a broader base of technological modules when creating solutions for clinical problems. However, this flexibility increases the need for continuing experimental and clinical studies that evaluate new MRCAS systems and, in the end, prove their benefit.

In addition, some of these systems represent new tools for measuring anatomical structures, thus allowing biomechanical analyses to be performed in a novel way.

Conclusion

From a careful review of the current status of MRCAS technology, it is evident that computerised technologies will change the way we design, plan, simulate, and execute orthopaedic surgical procedures in the future. Provided that additional costs and training with computer-assisted orthopaedic surgery can be justified, this technology will find wide use in modern orthopaedics. Freehand navigation treatment platforms which allow the use of different surgical modules have already gained distinct acceptance among the orthopaedic community.

References

[1] Amiot LP, Lang K, Putzier M, Zippel H, Labelle H. Comparative results between conventional and computer-assisted pedicle screw installation in the thoracic, lumbar, and sacral spine. *Spine* 2000 ; 25 : 606-614

[2] Bauer A, Lahmer A, Börner M. Robot-assisted surgery in total hip replacement: concept and clinical experience. *Int Soc Comput Aided Surg* 1996 ; 3 : 13-17

[3] Bowersox JC, Bucholz RD, Delp SL, Grönemeyer D, Jolesz FA, Nolte LP et al. Excerpts from the final report for the second international workshop on robotics and computer assisted medical interventions, June 23,1996, Bristol, England ; *Comput Aided Surg* 1997 ; 2 : 69-101

[4] Brack C, Götte H, Gossé F, Moctezuma J, Roth M, Schweikardt A. Towards accurate X-ray-camera calibration in computer-assisted robotic surgery. In : Lemke HU, Vannier MW, Inamura K, Farman AG eds. Computer assisted radiology and surgery. Amsterdam : Elsevier Science, 1996 : 721-728

[5] Decking J, Eckardt A, Schöllner C, Heine J. The CASPAR system for cementless THR: surgical technique and early results. Proceedings of the 4th annual North American symposium on computer assisted orthopaedic surgery (CAOS/USA), 2000 : 175-176

[6] Dessenne V, Lavallée S, Julliard R, Orti R, Martelli S, Cinquin P. Computer-assisted knee anterior cruciate ligament reconstruction: first clinical tests. *J Image Guid Surg* 1995 ; 1 : 59-64

[7] Digioia AM 3rd, Simon D, Jaramaz B, Blackwell M, Morgan F, Kladakis S et al. HipNav: a system for preoperative planning and intraoperative navigational guidance of acetabular implant placement in total hip replacement surgery. Proceedings of the 1st annual North American Symposium on Computer Assisted Orthopaedic Surgery (CAOS/USA), 1997 : 147-150

[8] Ellis RE, Tso CY, Rudan JF, Harrison MM. A surgical planning and guidance system for high tibial osteotomy. *Comput Aided Surg* 1999 ; 4 : 264-274

[9] Foley KT, Simon DA, Rampersaud YR. Virtual fluoroscopy. *Oper Tech Orthop* 2000 ; 10 : 77-81

[10] Girardi FP, Cammisa FP Jr, Sandhu Hs, Alvarez L. The placement of lumbar pedicle screws using computerised stereotactic guidance. *J Bone Joint Surg Br* 1999 ; 81 : 825-829

[11] Hamadeh A, Sautot P, Lavallée S, Cinquin P. Towards automatic registration between CT and X-ray images: cooperation between 3D/2D registration and 2D edge detection. Proceedings of the 2nd International Symposium on Medical Robotics and Computer Assisted Surgery, 1995 : 39-46

[12] Hofstetter R, Slomczykowski MA, Bourquin I, Nolte LP. Fluoroscopy based surgical navigation - concept and clinical applications. In : Lemke HU, Vannier MW, Inamura K, Farman AG eds. Computer assisted radiology and surgery. Amsterdam : Elsevier Science, 1997 : 956-960.

[13] Hofstetter R, Slomczykowski MA, Sati M, Nolte LP. Fluoroscopy as an imaging means for computer assisted surgical navigation. *Comput Aid Surg* 1999 ; 4 : 65-76

[14] Hofstetter R. Fluoroscopy based computer guidance in trauma surgery. [thesis], University Bern, 1999

[15] Joskowicz L, Milgrom C, Simkin A, Tockus L, Yaniv Z. FRACAS: a system for computer-aided image-guided long bone fracture surgery. *Comput Aided Surg* 1998 ; 3 : 271-288

[16] Kunz M, Sati M, Langlotz F, Nolte LP. Grundlagen der computer-gestützten Prothesenimplantation. In : Eulert J, Hassenpflug J eds. Praxis der Knieendoprothetik. Heidelberg : Springer-Verlag, 2000

[17] Laine T, Lund T, Ylikoski M, Lohikoski J, Schlenzka D. Accuracy of pedicle screw insertion with and without computer assistance: a randomised controlled clinical study in 100 consecutive patients. *Eur Spine J* 2000 ; 9 : 235-240

[18] Langlotz F, Bächler R, Berlemann U, Nolte LP, Ganz R. Computer assistance for pelvic osteotomies. *Clin Orthop* 1998 ; 354 : 92-102

[19] Langlotz U, Lawrence J, Hu Q, Langlotz F, Nolte LP. Image guided cup placement. In : Lemke HU, Vannier MW, Inamura K, Farman AG eds. Computer assisted radiology and surgery. Amsterdam : Elsevier Science, 1999 : 717-721

[20] Lavallée S. Registration for computer-integrated surgery: methodology, state of the art. In : Taylor RH, Lavallée S, Burdea GC, Mösges R eds. Computer-integrated surgery. Cambridge : The MIT Press, 1996 : 77-97

[21] Lavallée S, Sautot P, Troccaz J, Cinquin P, Merloz P. Computer-assisted spine surgery: a technique for accurate transpedicular screw fixation using CT data and a 3D optical localizer. *J Image Guid Surg* 1995 ; 1 : 65-73

[22] Martins HA, Birk JR, Kelley RB. Camera models based on data from two calibration planes. *Comput Graph Image Process* 1981 ; 17 : 173-180

[23] Merloz P, Tonetti J, Eid A, Faure C, Lavallée S, Troccaz J et al. Computer assisted spine surgery. *Clin Orthop* 1997 ; 337 : 86-96

[24] Mittelstadt B, Kazandizes P, Zuhars J, Williamson B, Cain P, Smith F et al. The evolution of a surgical robot from prototype to human clinical use. In : Taylor RH, Lavallée S, Burdea GC, Mösges R eds. Computer-integrated surgery. Cambridge : The MIT Press, 1996 : 397-407

[25] Nolte LP, Slomczykowski MA, Berlemann U, Strauss MJ, Hofstetter R, Schlenzka D et al. A new approach to computer-aided spine surgery: fluoroscopy-based surgical navigation. *Eur Spine J* 2000 ; 9 (suppl 1) : 578-588

[26] Nolte LP, Zamorano L, Visarius H, Berlemann U, Langlotz F, Arm E et al. Clinical evaluation of a system for precision enhancement in spine surgery. *Clin Biomech* 1995 ; 10 : 293-303

[27] Sati M, Stäubli HU, Bourquin Y, Kunz M, Käsermann S, Nolte LP. Clinical integration of computer-assisted technology for arthroscopic anterior cruciate ligament reconstruction. *Oper Tech Orthop* 2000 ; 10 : 40-49

[28] Sautot P, Cinquin P, Lavallée S, Troccaz J. Computer assisted spine surgery: a first step towards clinical application in orthopaedics. IEEE Proceedings in medicine and biology, 1993 : 1071-1072

[29] Schwarzenbach O, Berlemann U, Jost B, Visarius H, Arm E, Langlotz F et al. Accuracy of computer assisted pedicle screw placement: an in vivo computed tomography analysis. *Spine* 1997 ; 22 : 452-458

[30] Skibbe H, Börner M, Lahmer A, Wiesel U. Computerunterstützte Operationen in der Hüftgelenkendoprothetik. *Trauma Berufskrankh* 1999 ; 1 : 104-107

[31] Slomczykowski MA, Hofstetter R, Strauss M, Bourquin Y, Sati M, Nolte LP et al. Fluoroscopy-based surgical navigation: concept and possible clinical applications. In : Nolte LP, Ganz R eds. Computer assisted orthopaedic surgery. Seattle : Hogrefe and Huber, 1999 : 206-217

[32] Stulberg SD, Picard F, Saragaglia D. Computer-assisted total knee replacement arthroplasty. *Oper Tech Orthop* 2000 ; 10 : 25-39

[33] Zura RD, Kahler DM. A transverse acetabular nonunion treated with computer-assisted percutaneous internal fixation. A case report. *J Bone Joint Surg Am* 2000 ; 82 : 219-224

Algodystrophy

F Schuind

Abstract. – Algodystrophy remains one of the most severe and least predictable complications in orthopaedic surgery. It is defined as a local or regional pain syndrome with dysaesthesias, frequent allodynia, vasomotor disturbances and dystrophic changes involving all tissues. The syndrome associates diffuse pain, diminished function, joint stiffness, skin and soft-tissue trophic changes, with varying amounts of vasomotor instability. These typical clinical signs are associated with a bone scintigram demonstrating peri-articular radioactive marker uptake, corresponding to an increase in bone turnover. The pathophysiology of the affection remains unclear. There are many arguments against the classical theory of Leriche, calling for the existence of an abnormal sympathetic short circuiting reflex arc. The present hypothesis is that algodystrophy corresponds to an exaggerated inflammatory reaction, with persistent low capillary flow and increased venous pressure. In many patients, it can be prevented by atraumatic surgery, control of the increased venous pressure (elevation, avoidance of constrictive casts and dressings, early active mobilisation), and control of post-traumatic pain.

© 2000, Editions Scientifiques et Médicales Elsevier SAS. All rights reserved.

Keywords: algodystrophy, post-traumatic algodystrophy, algoneurodystrophy, Sudeck's atrophy, reflex sympathetic dystrophy, staging, pathophysiology, aetiology, prevention, medical treatment.

Introduction

Algodystrophy, also called algoneurodystrophy, reflex sympathetic dystrophy, Sudeck's atrophy, Sudeck-Leriche's syndrome, or type I complex regional pain syndrome [15], among other terms, is one of the most severe and least predictable complications in orthopaedic surgery, and it remains a diagnostic and therapeutic challenge. It is particularly frequent after plaster cast immobilisation of distal radius fractures (incidence as high as 37% according to Atkins et al [4, 5]), malleolar and calcaneal fractures. It is therefore essential that orthopaedic surgeons set clear definitions of the syndrome, understand its pathophysiology in the light of the physiological postoperative changes, and develop strategies to prevent its occurrence [63]. This chapter will focus on these aspects. The treatment of algodystrophy will then be briefly discussed, as in several countries it is usually treated by other specialists, including physiotherapists, rheumatologists, anaesthesiologists or pain clinicians.

Frédéric Schuind, M.D., PhD, Service d'Orthopédie-Traumatologie, Cliniques Universitaires de Bruxelles, Hôpital Erasme, 808, route de Lennik, B-1070 Brussels, Belgium.

DEFINITION

A precise clinical definition of algodystrophy is needed to avoid errors in both over and under diagnosis. Algodystrophy is defined as "a local or regional pain syndrome with dysaesthesias, frequent allodynia, vasomotor disturbances, and dystrophic changes involving all tissues" [63]. The syndrome is an association of diffuse pain, diminished function (particularly in the hand), joint stiffness, skin and soft-tissue trophic changes, with varying amounts of vasomotor instability [48]. The diffuse pain, usually much greater than ordinarily expected for the clinical condition, often non anatomical, is present in an area larger than the primary site of injury and is usually described as burning. It increases with limb dependency ("orthostatism") and movement. Allodynia, hyperalgesia, hyperpathia, and dysaesthesia on light touch are frequent. Motor signs, including difficulty initiating movement, weakness, dystonia, and tremor, are common [12, 15, 21, 35, 60, 68, 73, 77]. Vasomotor instability is characterised by temperature increase or decrease, abnormal colour of the extremities and/or inappropriate responses to changes in environmental temperature. Hyperhidrosis and oedema are usual in the early stages. Later, shiny and atrophic skin, disappearance of skin wrinkles, fusiform fingers or toes, increase or decrease in hair and nail growth, and palmar fasciitis without nodules in the hand, are frequent. These typical clinical signs are associated with a bone scintigram demonstrating peri-articular radioactive marker uptake (*fig 1*), corresponding to an increase in bone turnover [29, 48, 58, 59]. If these typical abnormalities are not seen on the bone scan, the painful condition of the limb is not algodystrophy (it may either correspond to neurotonic compulsive posture or self-mutilation, or be related to psychological problems, post-traumatic arthritis, causalgia, nerve lesion, or pseudodystrophy [28, 29]). Osteoporosis is not specific to algodystrophy, and is not always present, especially in the early stages. Disuse osteoporosis, observed after any joint immobilisation, should not be confused with patchy peri-articular osteoporosis (*fig 1*), which is frequently associated with algodystrophy (or with other conditions associated with increased bone turnover such as hyperparathyroidism).

Clinical presentation and staging

Algodystrophy most frequently involves the hand and wrist or the ankle and foot.

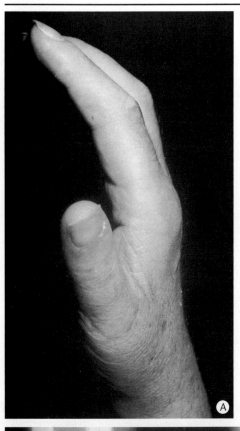

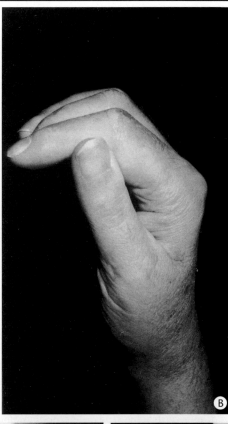

1 *Typical stage I algodystrophy, two months after osteosynthesis of a fracture of the distal radius by anterior plate and plaster cast. Diffuse hand pain, increasing with limb dependency, diminished hand function, joint stiffness, oedema and vasomotor instability. (Reproduced with permission from Schuind F and Burny F, Can algodystrophy be prevented after hand surgery?, Hand Clin 1997, 13 ; 455-476).*

A, B. Maximal active finger motion.
C. Patchy peri-articular osteoporosis, particularly at the level of the carpus and of the metacarpal metaphyses.
D. Peri-articular uptake on bone scintigram.

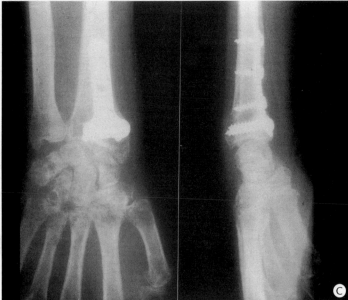

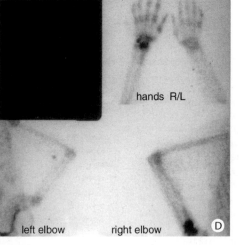

Another frequent clinical presentation is the shoulder-hand syndrome [70]. Extensive as well as limited forms have been reported, for example algodystrophy affecting one single finger [28, 29]. According to some authors, adhesive capsulitis of the shoulder is a localised form of algodystrophy [25, 50]. The clinical features are variable and often incomplete. Many cases do not present the classical signs, and the only striking symptom is pain of an abnormally long duration [25, 28].

The course of algodystrophy over time is classically divided into three stages according to the evolution of the symptoms and the vascular scintigram [29, 61, 70]. The vascular scintigram and the bone scan are usually performed at the same time and should not be confused. Although technetium pyrophosphate used for the bone scan may be chosen ("three-phase bone scan"), Driessens [29] recommends the injection of labelled serum albumin, because this tracer remains intravascular. Images are obtained immediately after the intravenous injection so that the arterial inflow can be evaluated semi-quantitatively (relative to the contralateral "normal" side). Over the next 20 minutes, the scan assesses the equilibrium phase ("blood pool" or limb blood volume). The vascular scan is needed for staging, whereas, as already explained, the bone scan, demonstrating peri-articular radiomarker uptake pathognomonic to algodystrophy, remains positive at all stages, except in late stage III [29, 58, 59].

Stage I, also called the warm, hypertrophic or traumatic stage, can last several months following the onset of the problem, and is characterised clinically by a progressive increase in pain, oedema, and the presence of inflammatory signs. Laboratory tests, however, do not show abnormally elevated parameters. The joints progressively become stiff. The vascular scan demonstrates an increase in arterial blood flow and in the blood pool. After several months, the inflammatory signs progressively disappear while trophic changes and cyanosis develop, leading to stage II or the atrophic stage, characterised by persistent pain, cyanosis, skin atrophy, marked joint stiffness, motor signs, and frequently hypersudation and hypertrichosis. The vascular bone scan at this stage demonstrates hypovascularisation. Stage III corresponds to the stabilisation of the condition, either with definitive sequelae, or, in rare instances in severe algodystrophy, by healing. The pain decreases or disappears. The skin usually remains atrophic with a thin, translucent character. Cyanosis and coldness of the extremities are frequent. The joints remain stiff. The vascular scan may have normalised, although some hypovascularisation frequently persists.

Pathophysiology

RISK FACTORS

Several factors increase the risk of postoperative or post-traumatic algodystrophy. There is clearly an individual predisposition to developing algodystrophy. Common experience shows that some patients use their injured limb even though it is painful. These patients do not develop algodystrophy. Other patients are extremely sensitive and suffer disproportionate pain, resulting in immobility and algodystrophy. Many authors believe that algodystrophy occurs more frequently in patients suffering from psychological problems, and in cases involving personal injury lawsuits, work related compensation, or other forms of secondary gain [75, 78]. Significant emotional dysfunction is especially found in the rare children affected by algodystrophy [6]. Rauïs [56] presented 104 adults suffering from post-traumatic algodystrophy and noted that all patients were over 30 years of age; there was no relationship between the degree of trauma and the severity of the algodystrophy; the condition nearly always emerged at the time of primary healing of the injury, and that 96% of the patients showed signs of chronic depression and 49% of alcohol abuse. The socio-professional context always revealed either a state of inactivity (jobless or disabled persons, childless housewives, retired persons) or an opportunity for inactivity. Schuind, Burny et al [63], in a prospective study of 164 patients treated by distraction-external fixation for distal radius fractures, with an overall rate of algodystrophy of 9.8%, found that the incidence of the complication was significantly higher in work compensated injuries (42.9%). Algodystrophy was not related to the type of fracture, gender, or age of the patient, nor to the type of treatment [63]. Other authors believe that observed psychological and sociological abnormalities are the consequences, rather than the causes, of the syndrome. It is well known that severe pain engenders emotional suffering and promotes behavioural changes. These frequently disappear after symptom relief [18, 22, 23, 41].

The risk of algodystrophy is increased in the case of an associated nerve lesion, whether central or peripheral (for example, a brachial plexus injury [38, 49]). Algodystrophy may also be favoured in cases of significant post-traumatic or postoperative inflammation (severe crush injuries, persistence of necrotic or infected tissues). Any trauma or surgical procedure results in a regional inflammatory reaction, characterised by increased arteriolar dilatation and capillary permeability, with subsequent oedema, related to the local release of various mediators [63, 66]. The risk of algodystrophy, an exaggerated inflammatory reaction being the initial manifestation, is therefore increased in the case of significant initial inflammation. Algodystrophy is also clearly more common in patients with immobilised extremities, either because of paralysis, excessive pain precluding motion, or because a plaster cast is applied [5, 10]. It starts with a massive oedema. External fixation is classically believed to be frequently complicated by algodystrophy. This has not been our experience, either in the upper or in the lower extremity. We have, however, empirically observed that prolonged transarticular distraction by external fixation, especially at the wrist, is responsible for a high rate of algodystrophy. In distal radius fractures, we avoid overdistraction and release the distraction in all patients after three weeks [62, 63, 64, 65].

PATHOPHYSIOLOGY

The pathophysiology of algodystrophy is not well understood. Many theories have been suggested, but conclusive evidence is lacking. The classical theory of Leriche [47] calls for the existence of an abnormal sympathetic short circuiting reflex arc, also called a nociceptive loop [47, 57]. There are many arguments against this theory which the author has reviewed in previous publications [63, 66]. Therefore, the terms "reflex sympathetic dystrophy" and "sympathetic-maintained pain syndrome" should be avoided. "Algodystrophy" is a better term, because it is shorter and it emphasises the painful nature of the condition without implying a pathogenesis which is not very well understood yet [25].

The initial and principal disturbance seen in algodystrophy is a vasomotor disorder of the microcirculation, characterised by

– modifications of the arterial inflow to the extremity,

– associated changes of capillary and venous flows,

– inappropriate vasomotor responses.

These alterations are now believed to correspond to an exaggeration of the normal post-traumatic inflammatory response, characterised by vasodilatation and increased capillary permeability related to the local release of vasoactive peptides [11, 19, 66, 73, 74, 77]. This hypothesis had already been suggested by Sudeck [7]. There is no clear distinction between marked inflammation and early algodystrophy. Algodystrophy is also initially characterised by pain, inflammation and oedema. With algodystrophy, however, the pain is said to be "out of proportion to trauma." There is probably a continuum in cases of severe postoperative inflammation and algodystrophy [10, 16, 77]. Factors thought to maintain this persistent state of inflammation with capillary sludge are numerous and include: individual hypersensitisation to vasoactive mediators, oversecretion of mediators, local release of free radicals [73, 74], failure of inhibitors, persistent immobility of the limb [11, 16, 37, 80], and increased venous pressure [34, 81]. Resistance to capillary outflow with increased venous pressure may be related to the associated dilatation of arteriovenous shunts, as suggested by the abnormal elevation of oxygen concentration in peripheral veins of algodystrophy patients [72]. In the upper extremity, an increase in venous resistance can also be related to subclavian venous stenosis [81]. More frequently, the increase in venous pressure is related either to a tourniquet effect caused by too constrictive plaster casts or dressings, immobility (paralysis, or if the patient is unable, unwilling or forbidden to move as, for example, in cases of unstable osteosynthesis, excessive pain or psychological problems), or to increased hydrostatic pressure from dependence in patients who do not elevate the inflamed extremity [63]. A series of vicious circles appears, in which vasodilatation, low capillary flow, and persistent stimulation of nociceptors all play their part [16]. Low capillary flow and precapillary shunting, allowing blood to be short-circuited, increase tissue hypoxia with further vasodilatation and stimulation of nociceptors. Increased venous pressure results in increased capillary pressure with further plasma extravasation and oedema. Efforts to produce vasoconstriction as a response to abnormal vasodilatation are ineffective, possibly because of a lowering in noradrenaline release from sympathetic nerve terminals, due to a depletion of locally stored noradrenaline. This is caused by the diversion of the regional flow by precapillary shunting, thus decreasing the inflow of circulatory inhibitors, and because of a hypothetical receptor conversion, causing a paradoxical vasodilatory response to noradrenaline. Persistent pain interferes with active mobilisation of the limb. Chronic oedema and ischaemia finally cause cellular damage and death.

Prevention

The prevention of algodystrophy is based on the knowledge of the already discussed risk factors and of the assumed pathophysiology of the condition. No trauma and no surgery is benign, and a procedure should not be undertaken if not possibly beneficial to the patient. In the pre-operative period, the risk of algodystrophy should be evaluated, and the individual's predisposition considered. Surgery should be avoided if possible in patients with a previous episode of algodystrophy (incidence of recurrence around 15% [37]), in depressed individuals, and in patients with work compensated injuries or with other forms of secondary gain. Surgery should be performed with the aim of minimising postoperative inflammation. The operative procedure should be as atraumatic as can be. Drainage is used to prevent the formation of haematomas. All contused wounds are debrided and covered by healthy tissue, using skin flaps when necessary. Antibiotics are used in infected cases. Anti-inflammatory and analgesic drugs are used to control postoperative pain. Long lasting peripheral nerve blocks may also be helpful. Any cause of persistent pain, particularly peripheral nerve compression, should be treated. It is important to recognise that in many cases, postoperative pain is related to distension of soft tissues by the postoperative oedema. In the first postoperative days, it is essential to increase the venous return, by decreasing the hydrostatic pressure (elevation of the affected extremity above the level of the heart). In the upper extremity, a sling may be used to raise the hand to the level of the heart. However, the prolonged use of this sling may in itself be dangerous, as it discourages the patient from mobilising his hand, and flexion of the elbow and immobilisation of the shoulder may decrease the venous flow. A more efficient technique, also applicable to the lower extremity, is the temporary suspension of the extremity. It is also important to prevent any tourniquet effect, avoiding, when possible, postoperative plaster immobilisation or even fluffy dressings. Early active mobilisation, within the patient's pain threshold, is encouraged. In the case of a fracture, the osteosynthesis should be stable enough to allow for immediate mobilisation. It is psychologically important for the patient to realise that, despite recent surgery, he is able to move without pain. Changes in microcirculation in early algodystrophy seem to be reversible in many patients by active exercise, despite the increase in pain that it may initially produce. Decongestive massage is helpful, starting at the proximal level of the oedema. Intermittent pneumatic compression is recommended by some authors [8]. Communication with the patient, reassurance, and relief of anxiety and pain are important points in prevention. When transarticular wrist or ankle external fixation is used, distraction release after some weeks is recommended. Finally, if there is any sign of algodystrophy, vascular and bone scintigraphies should be obtained, and immediate medical and physical treatment instituted. It is well known that early recognition and prompt treatment provide the best chances of a successful outcome [1, 2, 25, 31, 48, 82].

Principles of treatment

When an algodystrophic syndrome complicates orthopaedic trauma or an operative procedure, the surgeon has an important co-ordinating role, while the actual medical and physical treatments are carried out by other specialists. The treatment options depend on the stage of evolution. It is important to realise that the natural course of mild cases of algodystrophy is toward spontaneous healing, as the patient progressively regains motion. It is possible that the success of many forms of treatment is actually related to their analgesic effects which allow for active mobilisation of the limb.

Many therapeutic modalities have been described. The published series are difficult to interpret, as the criteria for diagnosing algodystrophy, including the patients in the studies, and measuring possible improvements, are variable and frequently not clearly defined. Measuring pain, usually based on visual analogue scales, is quite subjective. Most of the studies are also not controlled (no randomisation, no placebo control), and their results should be considered with caution.

The treatment of stage I algodystrophy includes physiotherapy, psychological support and medication. Many physical therapies have been described [8]. It is important to re-institute active motion. In the hand, the author uses the stress-loading programme developed by Watson and Carlson [80], consisting of active traction and compression exercises that provide stressful stimuli to the immobilised extremity. No passive joint mobilisation takes place until the pain and swelling begin to subside, and care is taken to avoid any added pain. The patient is seen daily or preferably twice daily by a hand physiotherapist. Contrast baths (placing the affected extremity in hot and cool water successively) seem to give very efficient pain relief [8]. The first-choice medication in stage I algodystrophy seems to be calcitonin at high doses (around 100 U/d subcutaneously for 4 weeks. Results with nasal administration have been disappointing [31]). Calcitonin is a hormone with antiosteoclastic properties. In algodystrophy, however, it seems to act on the microcirculation [3]. Calcitonin is the only treatment which has been shown in controlled studies to offer an unquestionable benefit in algodystrophy [26]. Unfortunately, treatment with calcitonin presents undesirable side effects, including flushes, nausea, and malaise occurring after the injection and lasting several hours. If for these reasons the treatment has to be discontinued or, in case of failure, the second choice medical treatment (especially in stage II) seems to be regional guanethidine (or reserpine or phentolamine) intravenous blocks. Many other treatments have been described, and are especially helpful in case of failure of calcitonin or intravenous blocks and in stages II and III. These include sympathetic blockade by pharmacological agents, and surgical or chemical (stellate ganglion block) sympathectomy (a sympathetic phenomenon, although not responsible for the algodystrophy, seems to be present in stages II and III), methylprednisolone and lidocaine intravenous blocks, "neuro-augmentation" by transcutaneous electrical nerve stimulation (TENS), spinal cord or peripheral nerve stimulation, various forms of physical and occupational therapy, acupuncture, beta-blockers, biphosphonates, analgesic and anti-inflammatory agents, corticosteroids, or tricyclics (calcitonin is contraindicated in stages II and III). The place of these various treatments is controversial and beyond the scope of this chapter on surgical techniques. The interested reader will, however, find excellent articles describing the various methods and their results in the reference section [8-10, 13, 14, 17, 20, 27, 30-33, 36, 39, 40, 42-46, 51-55, 67, 69-71, 76, 79, 83]. The surgeon should know that many patients do not totally recover from algodystrophy, and about one quarter of the patients fail to demonstrate permanent improvement [63]. End stage algodystrophy may even necessitate amputation [24].

Conclusions

Algodystrophy is a devastating orthopaedic complication. As the physical and medical treatments of the condition are long and frequently disappointing, the surgeon should concentrate his efforts on developing strategies of prevention. The present hypothesis is that algodystrophy corresponds to an exaggerated inflammatory reaction, with persistent low capillary flow and increased venous pressure. Simple means allow for efficient prevention. We recommend atraumatic surgery, reducing postoperative inflammation, control of increased venous pressure by elevation, avoidance of constrictive casts and dressings, early active mobilisation, and control of post-traumatic pain. If there is any sign of algodystrophy, a scintigram should immediately be carried out, and if confirmed, early physical, psychological and medical treatment, according to the stage of evolution, should be instituted.

References

[1] Amadio PC. Pain dysfunction syndromes. *J Bone Joint Surg Am* 1988 ; 70 : 944-949

[2] Amadio PC, Mac Kinnon SE, Merritt WH, Brody GS, Terzis JK. Reflex sympathetic dystrophy syndrome. Consensus report of an ad hoc committee of the American association for hand surgery on the definition of reflex sympathetic dystrophy syndrome. *Plast Reconstr Surg* 1991 ; 87 : 371-375

[3] Arlet J, Mazières B. Medical treatment of reflex sympathetic dystrophy. *Hand Clin* 1997 ; 13 : 477-483

[4] Atkins RM, Duckworth T, Kanis JA. Algodystrophy following Colles' fracture. *J Hand Surg Br* 1989 ; 14 : 161-164

[5] Atkins RM, Duckworth T, Kanis JA. Features of algodystrophy after Colles' fracture. *J Bone Joint Surg Br* 1990 ; 72 : 105-110

[6] Barbier O, Allington N, Rombouts JJ. Reflex sympathetic dystrophy in children – Review of a clinical series and description of the particularities in children. *Acta Orthop Belg* 1999 ; 65 : 91-97

[7] Baron R, Blumberg H, Jänig W. Clinical characteristics of patients with complex regional pain syndrome in Germany with special emphasis on vasomotor function. In : Jänig W, Stanton-Hicks M eds. Reflex sympathetic dystrophy: a reappraisal. Progress in pain research and management. Seattle : IASP Press, 1996 ; vol 6 : 25-48

[8] Bengtson K. Physical modalities for complex regional pain syndrome. *Hand Clin* 1997 ; 13 : 443-454

[9] Betcher AM, Casten DF. Reflex sympathetic dystrophy: criteria for diagnosis and treatment. *Anesthesiology* 1955 ; 16 : 994-1003

[10] Bickerstaff DR, O'Doherty DP, Kanis JA. Radiographic changes in algodystrophy of the hand. *J Hand Surg Br* 1991 ; 16 : 47-52

[11] Blair SJ, Chinthagada M, Hoppenstehdt D, Kijowski R, Fareed J. Role of neuropeptides in pathogenesis of reflex sympathetic dystrophy. *Acta Orthop Belg* 1998 ; 64 : 448-451

[12] Bullens P, Daemen M, Freling G, Kitslaar P, Van Den Wildenberg F, Kurvers H. Motor dysfunction and reflex sympathetic dystrophy – Bilateral motor denervation in an experimental model. *Acta Orthop Belg* 1998 ; 64 : 218-223

[13] Calvillo O, Racz G, Didie J, Smith K. Neuroaugmentation in the treatment of complex regional pain syndrome of the upper extremity. *Acta Orthop Belg* 1998 ; 64 : 57-63

[14] Christensen K, Jensen EM, Noer I. The reflex dystrophy syndrome: response to treatment with systemic corticosteroids. *Acta Chir Scand* 1982 ; 148 : 653-655

[15] Classification of chronic Pain. Descriptions of chronic pain syndromes and definitions of pain terms. In : Merskey H, Bogduk N eds. Seattle : IASP Press, 1994 : 40-43

[16] Cooke ED, Ward C. Vicious circles in reflex sympathetic dystrophy - a hypothesis: discussion paper. *J R Soc Med* 1990 ; 83 : 96-99

[17] Cooney WP. Electrical stimulation and the treatment of complex regional pain syndromes of the upper extremity. *Hand Clin* 1997 ; 13 : 519-526

[18] Covington EC. Psychological issues in reflex sympathetic dystrophy. In : Jänig W, Stanton-Hicks M eds. Reflex sympathetic dystrophy: a reappraisal. Progress in pain research and management. Seattle : IASP Press, 1996 ; vol 6 : 191-215

[19] Daemen M, Kurvers H, Bullens P, Barendse G, Van Kleef M, Van Den Wildenberg F, . Neurogenic inflammation and reflex sympathetic dystrophy (in vivo and in vitro assessment in an experimental model). *Acta Orthop Belg.* 1998 ; 64 : 441-447

[20] De Takats G. Sympathetic reflex dystrophy. *Med Clin North Am* 1965 ; 49 : 117-129

[21] Deuschl G, Blumberg H, Lücking CH. Tremor in reflex sympathetic dystrophy. *Arch Neurol* 1991 ; 48 : 1247-1252

[22] Didierjean A. Aspect psychologique de la dystrophie réflexe. In : Foucher G éd. L'algodystrophie de la main. Paris : Springer-Verlag, 1995 : 19-22

[23] Didierjean A. Psychological aspects of algodystrophy. *Hand Clin* 1997 ; 13 : 363-366

[24] Dielissen PW, Claassen AT, Veldman PH, Goris RJ. Amputation for reflex sympathetic dystrophy. *J Bone Joint Surg Br* 1995 ; 77 : 270-273

[25] Doury P. Algodystrophy, a spectrum of disease, historical perspectives, criteria of diagnosis, and principles of treatment. *Hand Clin* 1997 ; 13 : 327-337

[26] Doury P, Pattin S, Delahaye RP et al. La calcitonine dans l'algodystrophie sympathique réflexe. *Nouv Rev Méd* 1975 ; 7 : 3156

[27] Driessen JJ, Van Der Werken C, Nicolai JP, Crul JF. Clinical effects of regional intravenous Guanethidine (Ismelin) in reflex sympathetic dystrophy. *Acta Anaesthesiol Scand* 1983 ; 27 : 505-509

[28] Driessens M. Infrequent presentations of reflex sympathetic dystrophy and pseudodystrophy. *Hand Clin* 1997 ; 13 : 413-422

[29] Driessens M, Dijs H, Verheyen G, Blockx P. What is reflex sympathetic dystrophy? *Acta Orthop Belg* 1999 ; 65 : 202-217

[30] Drucker WR, Hubay CA, Holden WD, Bukovnic JA. Pathogenesis of post-traumatic sympathetic dystrophy. *Am J Surg* 1959 ; 97 : 454-465

[31] Dunningham TH. The treatment of Sudeck's atrophy in the upper limb by sympathetic blockade. *Injury* 1980 ; 12 : 139-144

[32] Farcot JM, Gautherie M, Foucher G. Regional intravenous sympathetic nerve blocks. *Hand Clin* 1997 ; 13 : 499-517

[33] Korpan MI, Dezu Y, Schneider B, Leitha T, Fialka-Moser V. Acupuncture in the treatment of posttraumatic pain syndrome. *Acta Orthop Belg* 1999 ; 65 : 197-201

[34] Flatt AE. Shoulder-hand syndrome. *Lancet* 1974 ; 1 : 1107-1108

[35] Foucher G. Aspects cliniques de la dystrophie réflexe. In : Foucher G éd. L'algodystrophie de la main. Paris : Springer-Verlag, 1995 : 1-12

[36] Gobelet C, Meier JL, Schaffner W, Bischof-Delaloye A, Gerster JC, Burckhardt P. Calcitonin and reflex sympathetic dystrophy syndrome. *Clin Rheumatol* 1986 ; 5 : 382-388

[37] Greipp ME, Thomas AF. New thoughts on reflex sympathetic dystrophy syndrome. *J Neurosci Nurs* 1990 ; 22 : 313-316

[38] Grundberg AB, Reagan DS. Compression syndromes in reflex sympathetic dystrophy. *J Hand Surg Am* 1991 ; 16 : 731-736

[39] Hannington-Kiff JG. Relief of Sudeck's atrophy by regional intravenous guanethidine. *Lancet* 1977 ; 1 : 1132-1133

[40] Hannington-Kiff JG. Reflex sympathetic dystrophy. *J R Soc Med* 1987 ; 80 : 605

[41] Hendler N. Depression caused by chronic pain. *J Clin Psychiatry* 1984 ; 45 : 30-36

[42] Hennart D, Leon M, Sylin P, Appelboom T. Sympathetic nerve blocks in refractory sympathetic dystrophy syndrome. *Acta Orthop Belg* 1999 ; 65 : 83-85

[43] Jänig W. The puzzle of (Reflex Sympathetic Dystrophy): mechanisms, hypothetic, open questions. In : Jänig W, Stanton-Hicks M eds. Reflex sympathetic dystrophy: a reappraisal. Progress in pain research and management. Seattle : IASP Press, 1996 ; vol 6 : 1-24

[44] Kozin F, Genant HK, Bekerman C, McCarty DJ. The reflex sympathetic dystrophy syndrome. II. Roentgenographic and scintigraphic evidence of bilaterality and of periarticular accentuation. *Am J Med* 1976 ; 60 : 332-338

[45] Kozin F, McCarty DJ, Sims J, Genant HK. The reflex sympathetic dystrophy syndrome. 1. Clinical and histologic studies: evidence for bilaterality, response to corticosteroids and articular involvement. *Am J Med* 1976 ; 60 : 321-331

[46] Kozin F, Ryan LM, Carerra GF, Soin JS, Wortmann RL. The reflex sympathetic dystrophy syndrome. III. Scintigraphic studies, further evidence for the therapeutic efficacity of systemic corticosteroids, and proposed diagnostic criteria. *Am J Med* 1981 ; 70 : 23-30

[47] Leriche R. De la causalgie envisagée comme une névrite du sympatique et de son traitement par la dénudation et l'excision des plexus nerveux péri-artériels. *Presse Méd* 1916 ; 23 : 148-180

[48] Mackinnon SE, Holder LE. The use of three-phase radionuclide bone scanning in the diagnosis of reflex sympathetic dystrophy. *J Hand Surg Am* 1984 ; 9 : 556-563

[49] Monsivais JJ, Baker J, Monsivais D. The association of peripheral nerve compression and reflex sympathetic dystrophy. *J Hand Surg Br* 1993 ; 18 : 337-338

[50] Müller LP, Rittmeister M, John J, Happ J, Kerschbaumer F. Frozen shoulder, an algoneurodystrophic process? *Acta Orthop Belg* 1998 ; 64 : 434-440

[51] Poplawski ZJ, Wiley AM, Murray JF. Post-traumatic dystrophy of the extremities. *J Bone Joint Surg Am* 1983 ; 65 : 642-655

[52] Price DD, Bennett GJ, Rafii A. Psychophysical observations on patients with neuropathic pain relieved by a sympathetic block. *Pain* 1989 ; 36 : 273-288

[53] Price DD, Gracely RH, Bennett GJ. The challenge and the problem of placebo in assessment of sympathetically maintained pain. In : Jänig W, Stanton-Hicks M eds. Reflex sympathetic dystrophy: a reappraisal. Progress in pain research and management. Seattle : IASP Press, 1996 ; vol 6 : 173-190

[54] Prough DS, McLeskey CH, Poehling GG, Koman LA, Weeks DB, Whitworth T et al. Efficacy of oral nifedipine in the treatment of reflex sympathetic dystrophy. *Anesthesiology* 1985 ; 62 : 796-799

[55] Ramamurthy S, Hoffman J and the Guanethidine study group. Intravenous regional guanethidine, in the treatment of reflex sympathetic dystrophy/causalgia. A randomised double blind study. *Anesth Analg* 1995 ; 81 : 718-723

[56] Rauïs A. Psychological aspects - a series of 104 posttraumatic cases of reflex sympathetic dystrophy. *Acta Orthop Belg* 1999 ; 65 : 86-90

[57] Roberts WJ. A hypothesis on the physiological basis for causalgia and related pains. *Pain* 1986 ; 24 : 297-311

[58] Schiepers C. Clinical value of dynamic bone and vascular scintigraphy in diagnosing reflex sympathetic dystrophy of the upper extremity. *Hand Clin* 1997 ; 13 : 423-429

[59] Schiepers C, Bormans I, DeRoo M. Three-phase bone scan and dynamic vascular scintigraphy in algoneurodystrophy of the upper extremity. *Acta Orthop Belg* 1998 ; 64 : 322-327

[60] Schott GD. Visceral afferents: their contribution to 'sympathetic dependent' pain. *Brain* 1994 ; 117 : 397-413

[61] Schuind A, Louvard A, Schoutens D, Itzkowitch D. The use of three-phase radionuclide bone scan after limb surgery. In : Arlet J, Mazières B eds. Bone circulation and bone necrosis. Berlin : Springer-Verlag, 1990 : 219-221

[62] Schuind F, Burny F. Radio-metacarpal external fixation. *Orthop Surg Tech* 1995 ; 9 : 7-19

[63] Schuind F, Burny F. Can algodystrophy be prevented after hand surgery? *Hand Clin* 1997 ; 13 : 455-476

[64] Schuind F, Burny F, Chao EY. Biomechanical properties and design considerations in upper extremity external fixation. *Hand Clin* 1993 ; 9 : 543-553

[65] Schuind F, Donkerwolcke M, Rasquin C, Burny F. External fixation of fractures of the distal radius : a study of 225 cases. *J Hand Surg Am* 1989 ; 14 : 404-407

[66] Schuind F, Nguyen T, Vancabeke M, Wautrecht JC. Modifications of arterial blood flow to the hand after carpal tunnel release. *Acta Orthop Belg* 1998 ; 64 : 296-300

[67] Schutzer SF, Gossling HR. The treatment of reflex sympathetic dystrophy syndrome. *J Bone Joint Surg Am* 1984 ; 66 : 625-629

[68] Schwartzman RJ, Kerrigan J. The movement disorder of reflex sympathetic dystrophy. *Neurology* 1990 ; 40 : 57-61

[69] Schwartzman RJ, McLellan TL. Reflex sympathetic dystrophy. A review. *Arch Neurol* 1987 ; 44 : 555-561

[70] Soucacos PN, Diznitsas LA, Beris AE, Xenakis TA, Malizos KN. Reflex sympathetic dystrophy of the upper extremity. *Hand Clin* 1997 ; 13 : 339-354

[71] Stilz RJ, Carron H, Sanders DB. Reflex sympathetic dystrophy in a 6-year-old: successful treatment by transcutaneous nerve stimulation. *Anesth Analg* 1977 ; 56 : 438-443

[72] Stolte BH, Stolte JB, Leyten JF. De pathofysiologie van het schouder-handsyndroom. *Ned T Geneesk* 1970 ; 114 : 1208-1029

[73] Van Der Laan L, Goris RJ. Reflex sympathetic dystrophy: an exaggerated regional inflammatory response? *Hand Clin* 1997 ; 13 : 373-385

[74] Van Der Laan L, Kapitein P, Verhofstad A, Hendriks T, Goris RJ. Clinical signs and symptoms of acute reflex sympathetic dystrophy in one hindlimb of the rat, induced by infusion of a free-radical donor. *Acta Orthop Belg* 1998 ; 64 : 210-217

[75] Van Houdenhove B, Vasquez G, Onghena P, Stans L, Vandeput C, Vermaut G et al. Etiopathogenesis of reflex sympathetic dystrophy: a review and biopsychosocial hypothesis. *Clin J Pain* 1992 ; 8 : 300-306

[76] Van Laere M, Claessens M. The treatment of reflex sympathetic dystrophy syndrome: current concepts. *Acta Orthop Belg* 1992 ; 58 (suppl I) : 259-261

[77] Veldman HJ, Reynen HM, Arntz IE, Goris RJ. Signs and symptoms of reflex sympathetic dystrophy: prospective study of 829 patients. *Lancet* 1993 ; 342 : 1012-1016

[78] Vikol J. L'algodystrophie dans son aspect psychologique. *Méd Hyg* 1986 ; 44 : 1237-1244

[79] Wang JK, Johnson KA, Ilstrup DM. Sympathetic blocks for reflex sympathetic dystrophy. *Pain* 1985 ; 23 : 13-17

[80] Watson HK, Carlson L. Treatment of reflex sympathetic dystrophy of the hand with an active "stress loading" program. *J Hand Surg Am* 1987 ; 12 : 779-785

[81] Wilhelm A. Stenosis of the subclavian vein, an unknown cause of resistant reflex sympathetic dystrophy. *Hand Clin* 1997 ; 13 : 387-411

[82] Wilson PR. Reflex? Sympathetic? Dystrophy? Paradigm shift ? *Clin J Pain* 1992 ; 8 : 281-284

[83] Zyluk A. Results of the treatment of posttraumatic reflex sympathetic dystrophy of the upper extremity with regional intravenous blocks of methylprednisolone and lidocaine. *Acta Orthop Belg* 1998 ; 64 : 452-456

Biopsy of bone tumours

R Capanna
P De Biase

Abstract. – The authors introduce current concepts of biopsy of bone lesions. The importance of an accurately placed biopsy together with obtaining a representative tissue for histology cannot be overstressed. Biopsy and definitive surgery should be preferably performed by the same centre. Clinical situations that do not necessarily need a initial biopsy are listed and the techniques of fine needle, tru-cut and incisional biopsy are detailed. Indications and pitfalls are discussed for each technique. For incisional biopsy, particular attention is paid to the type of incision, accurate haemostasis and closure. An explanation is provided on sample handling, preparation for freeze-dried section and definitive histology so that a secure diagnosis can be obtained.

Keywords: bone tumours, biopsy, fine needle biopsy, tru-cut biopsy, incisional biopsy, complications, frozen sections.

General requirements

Biopsy should not be considered a simple surgical procedure which can be performed by anyone as a preliminary investigation. The need to obtain representative and sufficient material for an accurate histological diagnosis should not compromise subsequent surgical treatment by spreading the tumour over its natural limits.

The biopsy should be performed by an experienced clinician (surgeon or radiologist) with knowledge of imaging techniques and pathology (to select representative areas) and surgical treatment of bone and soft tissue tumours (to select the appropriate approach). In a more modern approach, the biopsy strategy (modalities and techniques) for each individual patient should be preliminarily discussed and planned by a multidisciplinary team (surgeon, radiologist, pathologist, medical and radiation oncologist) after completion of all the necessary staging studies (X-rays, C.T., M.R.I., bone scan, angiogram) [11, 12].

Poorly performed biopsies, misplaced incisions and biopsy complications may compromise subsequent local management, expose the patient to unnecessary surgery, result in a higher local recurrence rate, worsen functional results or prevent limb salvage surgery [8].

The surgeon performing the biopsy should bear in mind all possible differential diagnoses and definitive surgical procedures. Because several different surgical approaches can be used to perform resection of a skeletal segment and several limb salvage reconstructive techniques can be applied, the biopsy should ideally be performed by the same surgeon who will carry out the definitive surgical treatment [6].

Indications

A biopsy can be omitted on rare occasions in certain benign lesions of bone and soft tissues (such as non-ossifying fibroma, fibrous dysplasia, unicameral bone cyst, exostosis, osteoma, osteoid osteoma, myositis ossificans, angioma, lipoma, pigmented villonodular synovitis, synovial chondromatosis). The clinical and radiographical picture is so typical that these lesions can often be excised without previous biopsy (so-called excision biopsy).

A biopsy can also be avoided in rare instances of malignant tumours, when all the following requirements are fulfilled:

– the diagnosis is quite clear from the clinical and radiographical appearance of the lesion;

– conservative surgery is indicated anyway;

– the histological report would neither modify the type of definitive surgical procedure nor the quality of anticipated surgical margins;

– no significant disability is expected from the surgical procedure.

On the contrary, a marginal or intralesional excision biopsy for a large, deep soft tissue mass should never be performed unless sophisticated imaging techniques (M.R.I. or C.T. scan) show an unequivocal lipoma.

General guidelines

The biopsy tract has to be widely excised from the skin to the tumour, together with all surrounding potentially contaminated tissues which should be included in the definitive surgical specimen.

In cases of conservative surgery, the biopsy skin incision has to be placed in line with the surgical approach for tumour removal (*fig 1*).

If an amputation is planned, the incision should be placed as distally as possible, or at least outside the flaps required for the amputation (*fig 2*).

With a needle (closed biopsy), or knife (incisional biopsy), the surgeon should avoid (*fig 3*):

Rodolfo Capanna, Dott, Director.
Pietro De Biase, Dott, Consultant, Oncological and Reconstructive Centre, II Divisione Ortopedia CTO, Largo P. Palagi, I-50139 Florence, Italy.

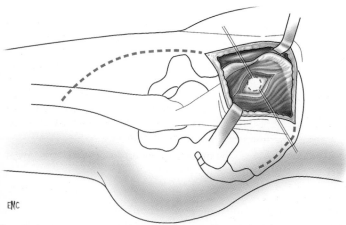

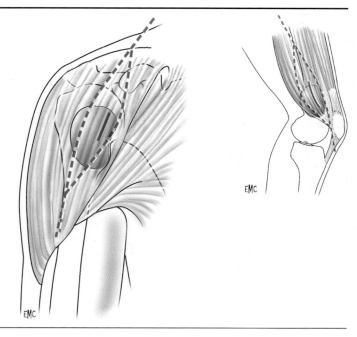

1   *The biopsy incision should be in line and excisable with the definitive surgical approach.*

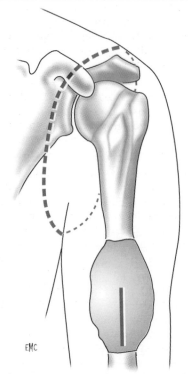

2   *In cases of amputation, the biopsy should be performed as distally as possible from the surgical flaps.*

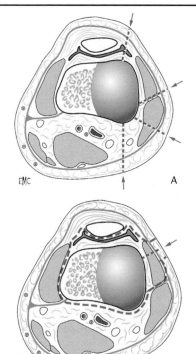

3   *A. A biopsy tract passing through a joint, extracompartmental spaces, fascial or muscles planes should be avoided.*
B. The correct approach should be direct through a muscle and excisable en bloc with the bone.

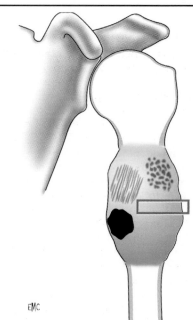

4   *The biopsy should be taken in normal tissue avoiding any calcified, sclerotic or cystic areas.*

– opening compartmental fascial barriers: at definitive surgery, this will mean removing two compartments instead of one;

– passing through extracompartmental spaces which will contaminate areolar tissue around neurovascular bundles or peridural spaces;

– dissecting along anatomical intermuscular planes;

– violating joint spaces.

Sample selection and handling

The biopsy should be taken in the most significant area of the tumour (i.e. the least differentiated part of the tumour), avoiding any liquid, necrotic, cystic, haemorrhagic, heavily ossified and calcified zones.

Areas of scar tissue and/or fibrosis are also not appropriate. The periphery of the tumour is usually more representative, viable and diagnostic than the centre which is often necrotic *(fig 4)* [4].

Useful information regarding growth modalities and invasiveness of the tumour can be obtained by histological examination of the pseudocapsule. However, a biopsy of the pseudocapsule should not performed alone.

The area of Codman's triangle must be avoided.

The tissue must not be crushed by surgical instruments.

To avoid excessive contamination, multiple samples of tissue must not be obtained.

The sample, if bulky, must be subdivided into smaller pieces (less than 0.5 cm.) to allow for quicker and better fixation. The separation should be done with sharp instruments (to prevent crushing the material). The tissue slices must be taken from the periphery (pseudocapsule) to the centre of the tumour.

The specimen should be immediately immersed in appropriate fixative solutions: if left to dry on the nurse's table it will fix inappropriately. Soft tumour and bone should be separated in different containers. Appropriate fixative solutions are required:

their volume should be at least 20 times the volume of the sample. Specific structures (such as eosinophilic granules in eosinophilic granuloma), special stains (histochemical and immuno-histochemical), and electron microscopy can be impaired if the sample has decalcified, or the fixative solution is not appropriate. A fresh piece of tumour should be sent to the pathology department for additional investigations.

If an infection is suspected, bacteriological tests should be carried out at the same time. The sample should never be deep frozen.

Biopsy techniques

Biopsies can be performed using different techniques: fine needle (aspiration) biopsy, tru-cut biopsy, and traditional open incisional biopsy (waiting for permanent sections and delayed diagnosis) or frozen section biopsy (for intraoperative assessment).

FINE NEEDLE BIOPSY

The biopsy is carried out with a thin needle (0.7 mm), aspirating the tumour with a vacuum lock syringe [1, 5, 7, 9]. The needle can be guided by echography, X-ray or C.T. scan. The material is smeared and stained and usually consists of scattered or small groups of cells interspersed with blood. Thus, it is more a cytological study than a histological examination and requires an expert cytologist. It has an accuracy level of 90% in assessing malignancy; however, accuracy is much lower (70-80%) for identifying histotype and malignancy grade, and this technique often does not provide sufficient material for more sophisticated studies (cytogenetics or flow cytometry) [10].

Being an atraumatic technique, performed on an outpatient basis, with a very limited risk of contaminating tissue plans, fine needle biopsy has become very popular for detection of soft tissue sarcomas, their local recurrence or to assess lymph node involvement.

This technique cannot be applied if a thick bony shell surrounds the lesion.

As the track of the needle biopsy has to be removed, the skin insertion should be marked with permanent Indian ink.

TRU-CUT BIOPSY

This is performed with a large needle (2-3 mm diameter) and allows not only a cytological but also a true histological examination. The rate of false negative results is usually low (5-10%). This method, guided by ultrasound or C.T. scan, has gained more and more popularity and now represents the method of choice in biopsies of deeply located tumours (spine, sacrum, pelvis) or of special anatomical regions (proximal tibia, elbow, wrist) in which minimal skin removal is mandatory [2].

The technique is apparently atraumatic and may be performed in an outpatient department under local anaesthesia. However, spillage of tumour (particularly if necrotic, liquid or myxoid) or contaminated blood (in case of hypervascular tumours) can sometimes be observed.

Because the biopsy track must be excised en bloc with the tumour later on, the skin overlying the needle insertion should be permanently marked. The direction of the needle must also follow the ideal line of the future surgical approach and it should be straight to the tumour, without performing several attempts in different directions. When carrying out a tru-cut closed biopsy, the inner needle must be inserted in a cannulated trocar to avoid losing the specimen in the muscles during needle retrieval. A gentle local compression is useful after biopsy. This method cannot be applied in sclerotic tumours or those encased in a thick layer of cortical bone.

INCISIONAL BIOPSY

It is the most traditional technique and should be considered in those "difficult cases" in which an accurate histological study on a relative large amount of tissue is desired, and previous attempts at biopsy (fine needle, tru-cut or frozen section) have been inconclusive. The retrieval of a large piece of tissue decreases the chances of a sampling error from an inexperienced surgeon, while the analysis of a large piece of tissue allows for a more confident diagnosis from a relatively inexperienced pathologist.

On the other hand, incisional biopsy is a more demanding procedure using several facilities (hospitalisation, operating room), with higher costs, morbidity and is more prone to complications (haematoma, tumour spillage, infection, fracture).

This technique should be avoided for deeply located tumours (vertebrae, pelvis for which trocar biopsy is preferred) or when a joint or an extracompartmental space has to be opened, with potential contamination of neurovascular bundles or the dural sac (in such cases a frozen section should be preferred).

■ *Tourniquet*

The use of a tourniquet is controversial. Venous stasis with tumour cell embolisation on tourniquet release is theoretically possible. However, the use of a tourniquet allows better tumour visualisation and reduces operative time, blood loss and blood contamination. If a tourniquet is used, two recommendations are made:

– to by-pass the tumour area when a compressive bandage is used to exsanguinate the limb, so as not to squeeze tumoral cells;

– to release the tourniquet before (and not after) wound closure, to allow for meticulous haemostasis.

■ *Skin incision and approach*

The skin incision should be as short as possible and should be a segment of the incision line used for the definitive surgery. The approach should be through muscle, straight to the tumour. Any dissection (subcutaneous tissue from fascia, fascia from muscle, muscle from periosteum and periosteum from bone) should be avoided or be kept to a minimum.

The most frequent errors observed in clinical practice are (*fig 5*):

1) Misplaced incision due to a tendency to use standard orthopaedic surgical approaches:

In the shoulder, an approach to the proximal humerus that follows the conventional deltopectoral interval may disseminate the tumour along normal neurovascular planes. In these circumstances, a direct anterior transdeltoid approach is indicated.

In the pelvis, a biopsy using an direct approach through the gluteus major is another common error: in fact an intact gluteus major muscle flap is required both for conservative (pelvic resection) and ablative (hemipelvectomy) surgery.

In the knee, tumours which often protrude into the popliteal fossa are reached by a Trickey approach, and tumours bulging under the synovial pouch are approached arthroscopically, causing contamination of the neurovascular bundle or joint space.

2) Approaching the tumour through the central full-thickness part of a muscle surrounding a bone tumour (for instance, a biopsy of the femoral diaphysis performed through an anterior approach), will later require a partial removal of the quadriceps muscle with possible denervation of the residual muscle. In such cases, a biopsy performed by a lateral approach will only require removal of the vastus lateralis, with an anticipated excellent function.

3) Using transverse incisions in extremities. Such incisions cannot be excised en bloc with the underlying longitudinally directed muscles or bone segments, without excessive skin removal. In definitive surgery, exposure to complications of the wound healing process or requiring otherwise unnecessary skin flaps will result.

4) Using different incisions in cases of repeated biopsies. In particular, if they are parallel, they will require wide skin removal and complex reconstructive surgery (free flaps).

5) "Over the top" incision through distended, discoloured and altered skin in cases of bulging tumours. The skin closure is very tight with possible complications (wound sloughs or superficial infections). In these cases, a peripheral biopsy through more normal skin, or a different technique (closed biopsy, frozen section) should be considered.

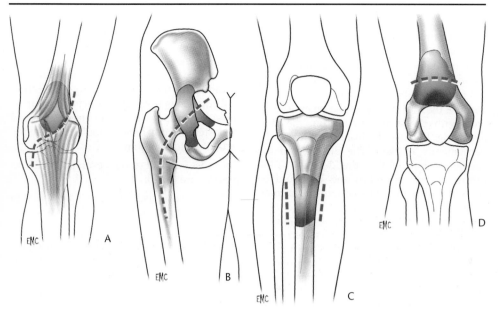

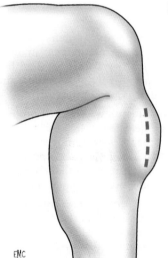

5 *The most frequent errors in incisional biopsy.*
A. Popliteal approach for tumours of the posterior distal femur.
B. Transgluteal approach for acetabular tumours.
C. Multiple parallel incisions.
D. Transverse incision.
E. Incision over distended skin.

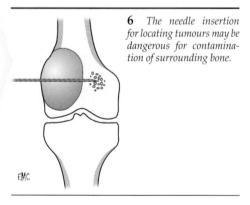

6 *The needle insertion for locating tumours may be dangerous for contamination of surrounding bone.*

■ Sampling

Close to the tumour, the colour of muscles around the pseudocapsule changes from red to pale because of reactive oedema. The tumour surface must be exposed over 2-3 cm².

Do not insert Kirschner wires transfixing the tumour to localise it; these may act as potential tracts for tumour contamination of the surrounding bone *(fig 6)*.

Any large dilated vessels surrounding the pseudocapsule and running on its surface should be coagulated or ligated. In cases of osteolytic and hypervascular tumours, a preliminary puncture of the cavity is recommended *(fig 7A)*. In cases of intensive bleeding, a trocar biopsy or a very small and cautious incision must be made. A H-shape incision is made on the tumour surface and two flaps of the reactive pseudocapsule can be elevated, then repositioned and sutured at the end of the biopsy.

A full thickness sample of 0.5-1 cm³ using a knife (soft tissue mass) or a sharp osteotome (bone) is retrieved. This should be handled gently so as not to crush it *(fig 7B, C)*.

Avoid violating the bone cortex, taking the samples in the soft tissue extension of the tumoral mass. If a biopsy of the intramedullary cavity is required, the bone should be opened, making a small hole with a circular saw to avoid stress risers which can cause subsequent pathological fractures [3]. If a large window is necessary, two circular holes with a power saw, connected by two parallel sections should

be made, instead of using several drill holes connected to an osteotome *(fig 7D)*.

An indirect approach through a bone tunnel is recommended in special situations, such as for the vertebral body (reached along the vertebral pedicle), the femoral neck (through the trochanter), the supracetabular area (through the antero inferior iliac spine) *(fig 8)*. In these situations, a direct approach to the tumour would contaminate the peridural space, the hip joint and the gluteal muscles respectively. Obviously, such a technique is indicated when en bloc resection is anticipated, removing the involved bone en bloc with the bone tunnel. On the contrary if a curettage is foreseen, the direct approach is preferred otherwise the bone tunnel must also be curetted.

The macroscopic appearance of the retrieved specimen should be of a viable tumour. If it contains reactive tissue, necrosis, calcification etc. more material should be obtained through the same window. It is recommended performing a frozen section for any incisional biopsy of which the macroscopic aspect of the specimen is not clearly pathological. This is to confirm the representativeness of the material and avoid repetitive surgical biopsies.

■ *Haemostasis and skin closure*

At the end of the procedure, the surgical bed and borders have to be meticulously electrocauterised and argon coagulation is particularly useful in these cases. Haemostasis may be obtained with compression and/or lavage with hydrogen peroxide *(fig 7E)*.

In soft tissue, the biopsy cavity may be obliterated with sponge collagen. In bone, bleeding can be prevented using bone wax or methylmethacrylate. Cement should only be used to seal the bone surface and should not be injected inside the medullary canal so as not to increase medullary pressure or push the tumour up and down *(fig 7F)*.

The suture must be tight and, possibly, in multiple layers. The stitches (both deep and superficial) must be performed very close to the incision to minimise the width of skin and muscle removal.

Suction drainage should be avoided as it acts as a tract for tumour spread. If used, its exit should be in line with and near the biopsy tract *(fig 7G, H)*.

FROZEN SECTION

Frozen sections may be performed from samples taken either by trocar or incisional biopsy. Compared to conventional histology (which necessitates at least 1 day for embedding, cutting and staining), this technique requires only a few minutes: it therefore allows intraoperative diagnosis and immediate therapeutic action.

However, it has two major disadvantages:

– It can only be performed by taking samples from a soft (cellular) component of

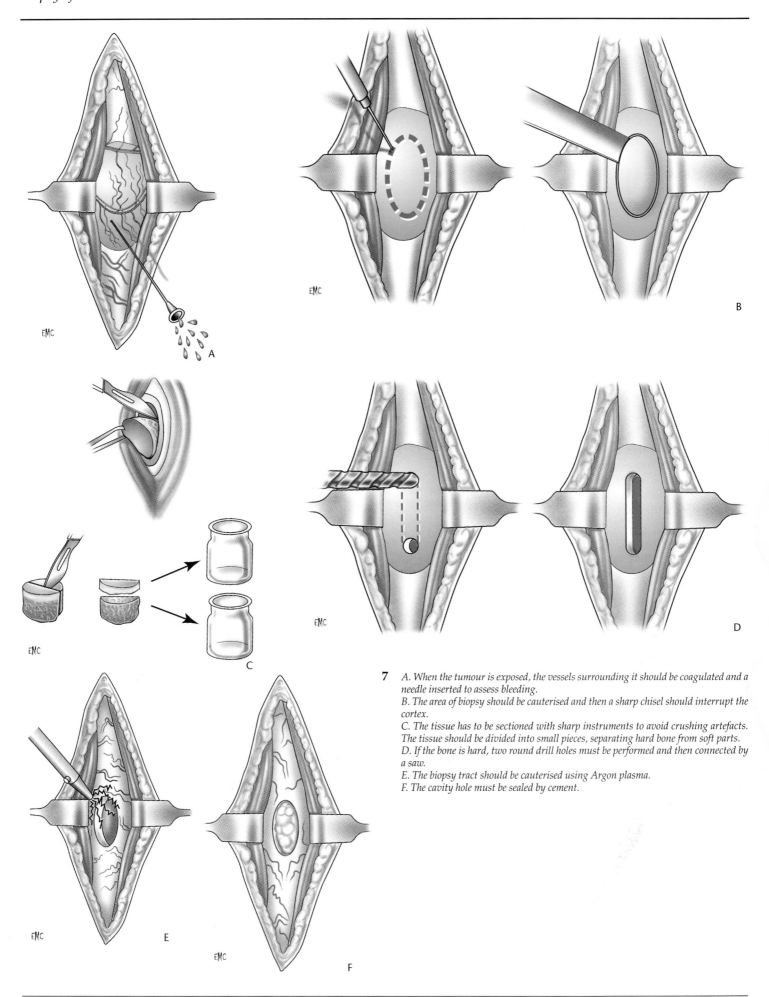

7 A. When the tumour is exposed, the vessels surrounding it should be coagulated and a needle inserted to assess bleeding.

B. The area of biopsy should be cauterised and then a sharp chisel should interrupt the cortex.

C. The tissue has to be sectioned with sharp instruments to avoid crushing artefacts. The tissue should be divided into small pieces, separating hard bone from soft parts.

D. If the bone is hard, two round drill holes must be performed and then connected by a saw.

E. The biopsy tract should be cauterised using Argon plasma.

F. The cavity hole must be sealed by cement.

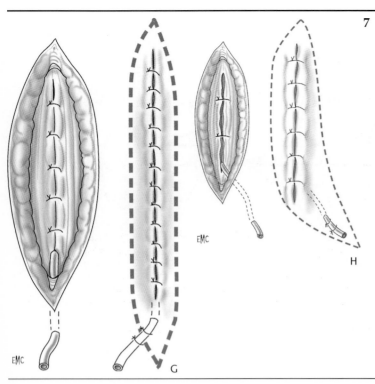

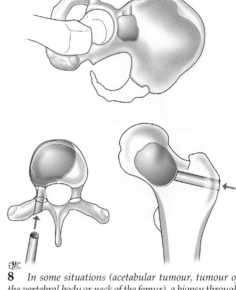

7 *G. The overlying planes (muscle and skin layer) should be meticulously closed and drainage should exit in line with the incision. This allows excision of only a small amount of skin.*
H. A wide skin suture and a drainage exit far from the wound require wide skin removal.

8 *In some situations (acetabular tumour, tumour of the vertebral body or neck of the femur), a biopsy through a bone tunnel may be considered.*

the tumour. In fact any hard (calcified or ossified) part cannot be processed and cut.

– An expert pathologist with great experience in this field must be available: the histological details are often not so clear as to allow for a confident diagnosis in difficult cases.

This method is particularly useful:

– in cases in which an intraoperative confirmation of an already clear diagnosis, based on pre-operative imaging studies, is sufficient;

– in cases of deeply located intra-articular or extracompartmental tumours (with a "typical" radiological aspect), to avoid contamination of joint or neurovascular structures;

– to confirm intraoperatively the adequacy of surgical margins achieved;

– to confirm the representativeness of the specimen and to determine if complementary studies are required, in cases of doubtful incisional biopsy.

In frozen sections, all principles and rules as illustrated for an incisional biopsy must also be satisfied.

If a definitive surgical procedure (resection) is performed immediately after a frozen section:

– the biopsy track must be closed and sealed, as previously described;

– the limb must be redraped;

– all sterile instruments (gloves, gowns etc.) must be changed.

Obviously this is not necessary, if curettage is selected as the definitive treatment.

References

[1] Akerman M, Rydholm A, Persson BM. Aspiration cytology of soft tissue tumors: the 10-year experience at an orthopaedic oncology center. *Acta Orthop Scand* 1985 ; 56 : 407-412

[2] Ball AB, Fisher C, Pittam M, Watkins RM, Westbury G. Diagnosis of soft tissue tumours by Tru-cut biopsy. *Br J Surg* 1990 ; 77 : 756-758

[3] Clark CR, Morgan C, Sonstegard DA, Matthews LS. The effect of biopsy-hole shape and size on bone strength. *J Bone Joint Surg Am* 1977 ; 59 : 213-217

[4] Den Heeten GJ, Oldhoff J, Oosterhuis JW, Schraffordt Koops H. Biopsy of bone tumors. *J Surg Oncol* 1985 ; 28 : 247-251

[5] Desantos LA, Murry JA, Ayala AG. The value of percutaneous needle biopsy in the management of primary bone tumors. *Cancer* 1979 ; 43 : 735-744

[6] Enneking WR. Editorial: the issue of biopsy. *J Bone Joint Surg Am* 1982 ; 64 : 1119

[7] Haidu SI, Meramed MR. Needle biopsy of primary malignant bone tumors. *Surg Gynecol Obstet* 1971 ; 133 : 829

[8] Mankin HJ, Lange TA, Spanier SS. The hazard of biopsy in patients with malignant primary bone and soft tissue tumors. *J Bone Joint Surg Am* 1982 ; 64 : 1121-1127

[9] Moore TM, Meyers MH, Patzakis MJ, Terry R, Harvey JP Jr. Closed biopsy of musculoskeletal lesions. *J Bone Joint Surg Am* 1979 ; 61 : 375-380

[10] Schajowicz F, Derqui JC. Puncture biopsy in lesions of the locomotor system: review of results in 4050 cases, including 941 vertebral punctures. *Cancer* 1968 ; 21 : 531-548

[11] Simon MA. Current concepts review: biopsy of musculoskeletal tumors. *J Bone Joint Surg Am* 1982 ; 64 : 1253-1257

[12] Simon MA, Biermann JS. Biopsy of bone and soft-tissue lesions. *J Bone Joint Surg Am* 1993 ; 75 : 616-621

Excision of bone tumours

R Capanna
P De Biase

Abstract. – The authors discuss general principles of tumour growth, the definition of anatomical compartments in bone, and the anatomical barrier to enlargement of tumours which characterise the surgical staging as proposed by Enneking. They also explain the concept of surgical margins (intralesional, marginal, wide and radical) and its importance in surgery. On the basis of these concepts, general guidelines for excision of bone tumours and a comprehensive explanation of surgical procedures for bone tumour excision are provided; the muscles, vessels and nerves encountered during surgery are described. Various indications and techniques to be used in benign and malignant bone tumours are given. The technique of curettage is highlighted, with particular accent on the use of local adjuvants (phenol, hydrogen peroxidase, liquid nitrogen) to lower recurrence.

Keywords: bone tumours, excision, resection, curettage, surgical staging, surgical, margins, Enneking's classification.

Introduction

It is a common observation that tumours with the same histological appearance may have a different clinical course in different patients, ranging from an indolent, static lesion to an aggressive malignant or even a metastasising tumour.

It is fundamental to adopt a staging system, in order to:

– classify tumours into groups having similar behaviour and prognosis;

– produce general guidelines for treatment;

– introduce a common language for a more uniform and comparable evaluation of the oncological results.

General concepts on tumour growth

Tumour growth depends on the following factors:

– the tumour type (well represented by its histogenesis and histological grade). This factor influences growth and rate modalities;

Rodolfo Capanna, Dott., Director.
Pietro De Biase, Dott., Consultant, Oncological and Reconstructive Centre, II Divisione Ortopedia CTO, Largo P. Palagi, I-50139 Florence, Italy.

– the local reaction of the host to the tumour;

– the anatomical setting of the lesion.

LOCAL GROWTH

Two different behaviours of local growth are observed: "pushing" or "permeative" mechanism. The pushing mechanism is typical of benign tumours, but is sometimes also observed in very low-grade, malignant lesions. It causes atrophy by compression of the surrounding soft tissue and resorption of bone because of osteoclastic activation. When this "stimulated" bone resorption is very slow, contemporary activation of osteoblasts on the outer side of the resorbed cortex may produce new bone apposition. In this case, the bone may be expanded, but it retains a cortical shell. The pushing mechanism may therefore produce a true "capsule" around the tumour, due to a thin layer of normal, mature, fibrous or bone tissue. The permeative mechanism is more often seen in malignant tumours. Malignant cells may play a direct part in destroying surrounding bone and soft tissues, and may grow in the surrounding area, forming tumour digitations and satellites. These tumoural foci (satellites) propagate via the veins and may be found far from the original mass (skip metastases), but are more often proximal to the tumour, in the same or in an adjacent compartment. Sometimes skip

metastases may be transarticular involving the adjacent bone. The preferred directions of growth are: cancellous bone, the medullary canal, the thin metaphyseal cortex (particularly where it is perforated by capsular and tendinous insertions), the areolar fat present in fascial planes and along the neurovascular bundles, muscle, the peridural space, and in all areas where natural barriers are perforated by vessels.

LOCAL REACTION

Around a tumour, a local reaction is elicited which is very similar to the inflammatory phase of reparative tissue, observed in the wound healing process or callus formation. This reactive zone consists of:

– oedema, fibrin and infiltration by inflammatory cells;

– proliferation of mesenchymal cells (histiofibroblasts, osteoblasts) and blood vessels;

– areas of pre-existing degenerated (muscle, fat) or resorbed (bone, cartilage) tissues;

– tumoral digitations and satellites in malignant tumours.

The local reaction is related to several factors:

– mode and rate of tumour growth (permeative and rapid growth allow less "reaction" from the host);

Table I. – *Effectiveness of natural barriers to tumour growth.*

Strong barrier	Relative (thin) barrier	Ineffective barrier
Articular cartilage	Periosteum	Bone marrow
Growth plate	Synovial membrane	Fat and peridural space
Cortical bone	Sheath of major nerves	Muscle
Fascia and fascial septa	(perineurium)	Fat and interstitial areolar tissue around neurovascular bundles
Joint capsule	Tendon sheath	Tendons and capsular insertions into epiphysis, apophysis or metaphysis
Tendons		Areas of vascular perforations of strong natural barriers (growth plate, cortex, fascia)

Table II. – *Anatomical compartments according to Enneking's classification* [3]

Intracompartmental (T1)	Extracompartmental (T2)
Intraosseous	Soft tissue extension
Intra-articular	Deep extension to fascia
Superficial to fascia	Intraosseous or extrafascial extension
Paraosseous	Extrafascial planes or spaces
Intrafascial compartments	Midfoot and hindfoot
Ray of hand or foot	Popliteal space
Calf	Inguinofemoral triangle
Anterolateral leg	Intrapelvic
Anterior thigh	Midhand
Medial thigh	Antecubital fossa
Posterior thigh	Axilla
Buttock	Periclavicular
Anterior forearm	Paraspinal
Posterior forearm	Head and neck
Anterior arm	
Posterior arm	
Periscapular	

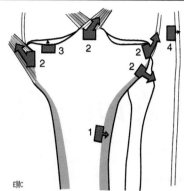

1 *Anatomical barriers: strong barrier (cartilage), medium barrier (diaphyseal cortex, periosteum, fascia), ineffective barrier (thin meta-epiphyseal cortex with capsular and ligament attachments).*

Anatomical compartments

Enneking [2, 3] defined a compartment as an anatomical structure bounded by natural barriers to tumour growth. Natural barriers may be subdivided into strong, relative (because too thin) and ineffective (or at risk) (*table I*). The only real and effective barrier is the articular cartilage, because it has no vascular perforations and probably presents an intrinsic resistance to tumours (*fig 1*). The tumour may, however, involve the joint because of a fracture, or by extension through epiphyseal attachments of the capsule, ligaments, or synovial membrane. These areas are at risk because only a thin cortex with vascular perforation is present, and the tumour may easily extend from the cancellous bone to such structures and vice versa. Ulceration and bleeding of the synovial membrane may also produce a haemarthrosis containing tumoral cells and consequent joint contamination. Several strong natural barriers such as cortical bone, fascia and fascial septa may also be passed through their vascular perforations. The growth plate may act as a natural barrier to joint invasion, except in cases where it is intra-articular (as in the hip), or in early infancy or after puberty (when it is perforated by vessels). According to Enneking [2, 3] and on the basis of their anatomical location and extension, tumours may be subdivided into intracompartmental (T1) and extracompartmental (T2) (*table II*).

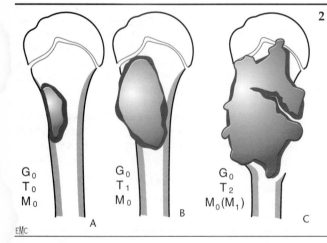

2 *Stages of benign tumours.*
A. Stage 1: the tumour is well defined and marginated by a rim of sclerotic bone.
B. Stage 2: the tumour may expand the bone but is surrounded by a thin ring of reactive bone and periosteum; its margins are still defined but discontinuous.
C. Stage 3: the tumour has aggressive behavior with indistinct margins and may destroy the cortex and expand into soft tissue, limited only by the periosteum.

G_0 T_0 M_0 A

G_0 T_1 M_0 B

G_0 T_2 $M_0(M_1)$ C

– existence of spontaneous tumour necrosis and internal haemorrhage;

– production of tumoral substances (tumour angiogenetic factors);

– immunological cellular response of the host to tumour associated antigens. This "reactive" zone spontaneously regresses in benign lesions when the tumour is removed, whereas in malignant lesions, it may become thicker and mature when the tumour is devitalised by preoperative treatments.

ENCAPSULATION

The tumour may be encapsulated by: 1) a thin layer of normal tissue, caused by the pushing growth mechanism (true capsule) and/or 2) a variable amount of reactive

tissue. In malignant tumours, this reactive tissue is filled by tumoral digitations and satellites, and is considered a pseudocapsule representing an unsafe surgical margin.

METASTASES

Metastases are usually found in the lung because bone sarcomas usually metastasise via the venous blood stream. Moreover, lymph node involvement is rare, because bone lacks lymphatic vessels. Lymph node metastases are more often observed when the tumour has a large soft tissue component or involves the skin (which, on the contrary, is rich in lymphatic vessels). However, this is more common in soft tissue sarcoma, particularly in epitelioid sarcoma, synovial sarcoma and rhabdomyosarcoma.

Surgical staging system (Enneking's classification)

Tumours are classically staged according to their histological grade (G), anatomical extension (T) and presence of regional or distant metastases (M). The staging also takes into account all data regarding clinical, imaging, and histological studies.

Benign lesions (*fig 2*) are subdivided into:

– Stage 1 or "latent", "inactive" lesions that remain static or heal spontaneously (such as most non-ossifing fibromas).

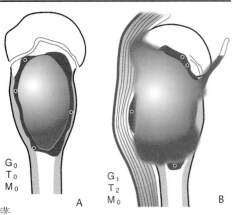

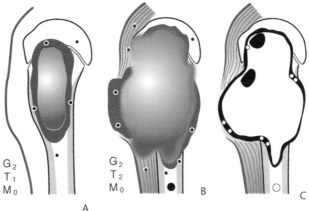

4 *Stages of high-grade malignant tumours.*
A. Intracompartmental (IIA).
B. Extracompartmental (IIB).
These tumours do not usually have well defined margins, but several areas of permeative growth. Satellites are numerous both inside and outside the pseudocapsule. Skip metastases may be found at a distance.
C. After chemo- or radiation therapy the tumour may become largely necrotic, the pseudocapsule matures with better margination with reactive bone or fibrous tissue, while satellites may be destroyed.

3 *Stages of low-grade malignant tumours.*
A. Intracompartmental (IA).
B. Extracompartmental (IB). These lesions are usually well circumscribed by a pseudocapsule, and permeative growth is limited to restricted areas. Satellites are few and usually present inside the reactive pseudocapsule.

– Stage 2 or "active" lesions that show progressive growth but are limited by a natural barrier (such as most giant cell tumours).

– Stage 3 or "aggressive" lesions that present progressive growth which is not limited by natural barriers (such as some pseudo-malignant giant cell tumours, aneurismal bone cysts, or osteoblastomas).

Malignant tumours (*fig 3, 4*) are subdivided into:

– Stage I (low grade),

– Stage II (high grade),

– or Stage III (presence of metastases) (*table III*).

Moreover, each stage is subdivided into A or B, according to the intra- or extracompartmental extension of the tumour.

After extensive study of the entire surgical specimen, the preoperative stage (based on biopsy) must sometimes be reviewed, because of the presence of areas of dedifferentiation, or malignant progression.

Surgical margins

Surgical margins should be assessed in the operating theatre, both by the surgeon and the pathologist. Any doubtful areas in the surgical field or in the resected specimen must be controlled by frozen section. The obtained margins are easily determined in the surgical specimen if any area of suspicion is marked with permanent ink. Several samples for histology are taken perpendicularly to the marked surface, to assess quantity and quality of the tissues surrounding the tumour. According to Enneking [3], surgical margins can be classified in 4 categories (*fig 5*):

– *Intralesional:* the tumour is entered, leaving macroscopic residual areas of disease.

– *Marginal:* the tumour is removed en bloc, but following a dissection plane through its capsule or pseudocapsule ("shell out" technique). Such procedures can be adequate for benign lesions but, in malignancies, they leave microscopic residual areas of tumour in the surgical field. These are represented by isolated cells or neoplastic digitations present in the thickness of the pseudocapsule, plus possible satellites and distant skip lesions, often observed in high-grade lesions;

– *Wide:* the tumour is resected en bloc, wrapped by a cuff of normal tissue. This procedure enables the removal of satellites around the pseudocapsule but it may leave distant or transarticular skip lesions in situ. The safety of this cuff is related more to the type of tissue than to its amount: a 1 mm fascial plane is a more effective barrier than 2 cm of muscle. The effectiveness of these barriers is reported in table I;

– *Radical:* the tumour is removed with the entire compartment (for instance a total femur resection for an intraosseous tumour of the distal femur; total quadriceps resection for a soft tissue sarcoma of the vastus medialis; a forequarter amputation

Table III. – Surgical staging system according to Enneking [3] and related surgical procedures.

Stage	Grade	Site	Metastases	Type of surgery	Surgical margins
1 latent - inactive	G0	T0	M0	None or excision	Intralesional or marginal
2 or active	G0	T1	M0	Excision	Intralesional plus adjuvant or marginal
3 or aggressive	G0	T2	M0	Excision rarely amputation	Marginal or intra plus adjuvants Wide
I A	Low (G1)	Intracompart (T1)	M0	Excision	Wide
I B	Low (G1)	Extracompart (T2)	M0	Excision rarely amputation	Wide
II A	High (G2)	Intracompart (T1)	M0	Excision +/- chemo & rx th.	Wide
II B	High (G2)	Extracompart (T2)	M0	Excision +/- chemo & rx th. Rarely amputation	Wide Radical
III A	Low (G1)	Intra or Extra comp. (T1 T2)	Regional or Distant (M1)	Individually selected	Wide
III B	High (G2)	Intra or Extra comp. (T1 T2)	Regional or Distant (M1)	Individually selected	Wide Radical

The grade of tumour is subdivided into: G0 (benign); G1 (low grade or grade 1-2 of Broder's classification), G2 (high grade, or grade 3-4 of Broder's classification).
The anatomical extension (T) is subdivided into: T0 - benign tumour surrounded by a true capsule; T1 - benign or malignant tumour surrounded by a pseudocapsule but confined inside an anatomical compartment; T2 - benign or malignant tumour surrounded by a pseudocapsule (with extracompartmental origin or extension).
The presence of metastases, either regional (skip, lymph nodes) or distant, are subdivided into: M0 - absence of metastases; M1 - presence of metastases.

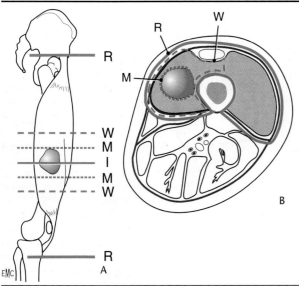

5 *Surgical margins according to Enneking's classification.*
A. In bone.
B. In soft tissue tumours (R = radical, W = wide, M = marginal, I = intralesional).

Table IV. – Recommended surgical procedures according to Simon [6].

Intralesional	Stage 1 and 2 benign bone tumours (simple curettage)
	Stage 3 bone tumours and adjuvants (extended curettage)
Marginal	Benign capsulated soft tissue tumours
	Stage 3 bone tumours and adjuvants
	Recurrent stage 2 and 3 benign bone tumours
	Selected low and high grade sarcomas (good responders to preoperative treatment)
Wide	Stage 3 benign recurrent lesions
	Most low and high grade sarcomas with or without adjuvant treatment
Radical	Recurrent sarcomas
	Displaced pathological fracture of bone sarcomas
	Sarcomas that could not be adequately imaged

for a tumour of the arm, etc.). This procedure can even remove skip lesions, except transarticular ones.

The procedure is finally characterised by its closest margin (for instance, a wide resection that in a limited area shows an exposed pseudocapsule will be defined as marginal).

Any of the previous procedures must also be called "contaminated" if the surgeon inadvertently enters the lesion, even in a limited zone and even if, subsequently, he is able to widen the margins in normal tissue.

Such classification is used both in limb salvage and ablative surgery. The suggested margins in relation to the stage of the tumour are reported *(tables III, IV)*, according to Simon [6].

General guidelines on resection

A tumour resection usually aims at achieving wide surgical margins. Focal areas of marginal margins are acceptable only in benign tumours, or in cases of malignancies showing good response to neoadjuvant treatment, and with the purpose of saving important functional structures. Exceptionally, resection may achieve radical margins (scapulectomy, compartmental myectomy, and en bloc removal of an entire bone from joint to joint).

The following guidelines are given to the surgeon with the aim of achieving wide margins and avoiding contaminated procedures:

– Mentally define the tri-dimensional configuration of the tumour on the basis of preoperative imaging studies, and select the most appropriate plane of dissection.

– Feel tumoral edges only by gentle palpation during surgery, without exposing the tumoral pseudocapsule.

– Promptly change the plane of dissection and increase the surgical margins, if the reactive or degenerated oedematous area around the tumour is visualised or entered.

– Improve the effectiveness of the surgical margins by including intact anatomical barriers (bone cortex, periosteum, fascia, growth plate, articular cartilage, capsule joint, tendons and ligaments, tendon sheath, perineurium) in the specimen.

– When dealing with tissues that do not include any compartmental barrier (muscle, cancellous bone, extracompartmental fat, medullary canal), try to maximise the amount of healthy tissue removed around the tumour. This does not prevent selected reconstructive procedures and desired functional results.

– Be prepared to modify or switch intraoperatively to different reconstructive methods, if the adequacy of surgical margins

requires a more extensive resection than was originally planned with changes in the feasibility of the reconstruction.

These rules are fundamental when:

– the tumour is of high-grade malignancy;

– the tumour shows a permeative growth pattern;

– the tumour is known to have frequent occult and extracapsular extensions (Ewing's sarcoma, osteosarcoma, malignant fibrous hystiocytoma, leiomyosarcoma);

– a poor response to preoperative treatment is observed.

BIOPSY TRACT AND SCAR FROM PREVIOUS SURGERY

The surgical approach should include the biopsy tract and scar of any previous surgery, removing a wide elliptical area of normal tissue around it. The removal of a large skin area because of previous, displaced biopsies (multiple parallel or transverse incisions), or as treatment of superficial, soft tissue tumours sometimes requires the use of a pedicled or free flap for coverage. The subcutaneous tissue is split outwards in oblique directions and removed more widely than the skin. The underlying fascia is widely excised and left as an anatomical barrier that covers the tumour *(fig 6)*. In some instances, dissection can be carried out between the subcutis and fascia, partially or totally removing the fascia. This technique, although oncologically correct, may create wound healing complications due to damage to the blood supply of the cutaneous flap: it is thus only recommended for pushing tumours and those extensively protruding under superficial planes.

MUSCLE

If the bone tumour is intraosseous (intracompartmental), the surrounding muscles can be saved, and it is sufficient to resect the bone en bloc with its periosteum, cutting all septa, tendons and ligaments 0.5 cm from their insertions, and leaving a small amount of insertional muscle fibre attached to the bone.

However, the muscle must be widely resected on both sides of the biopsy tract, over all the extraosseous extension of a bone sarcoma, and all around a soft tissue tumour *(fig 5)*. This cuff of freely movable, normal looking muscular tissue should be at least 2-3 cm in size. A muscle covering the extra-osseous extension of a high-grade bone sarcoma which has its insertion fibres in the same area as the tumour should be removed en bloc (i.e., the vastus intermedius or vastus lateralis for tumours of the distal femur). Splitting the muscle, saving half while leaving the remaining half as tumour coverage, may be done only by an expert surgeon and only in cases of high-grade malignancy with good response to preoperative treatments. A more

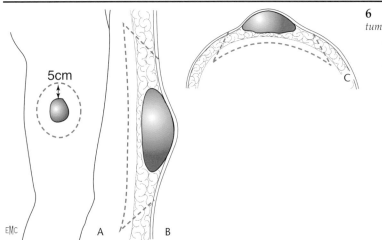

6 *In superficial soft tissue tumours:*
A. A large removal of skin is required to achieve radical margins.
B. The subcutaneous tissue must be resected in an oblique fashion, maximising surgical margins.
C. The underlying fascia is used as a natural barrier.

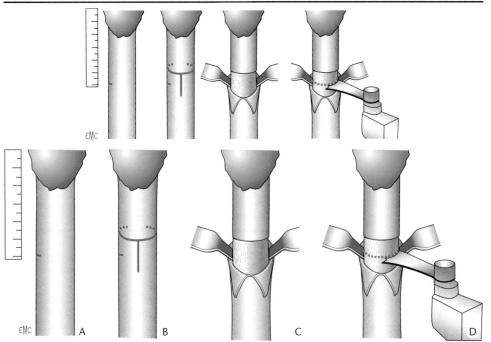

7 *Bone resection.*
A. The diaphysis is marked at the level of the desired osteotomy.
B. The periosteum is cut using a T section.
C. The periosteum is elevated and two Hohmann retractors are inserted for protection.
D. The bone is sectioned with an oscillating saw. A bone marrow sample is taken for frozen section. The osteotomy is then opened gently and the periosteum is immediately cut on the other side. The muscle and septa are finally divided at a distance from their bone insertion. Immediate forceful traction is dangerous, causing stripping of the periosteum with tumour exposition.

conservative attitude can be used for those muscles crossing the tumoral area with no attachments over the involved bone (i.e., the vastus medialis or rectus femoris for tumours of the lateral metaphysis or the distal femur).

BONE

The extension of the tumour and the presence of possible skip lesions within the medullary canal must be carefully evaluated before surgery, using M.R.I., bone scan and P.E.T. examination. The presence of a reactive zone (and its changes before and after preoperative chemo- or radiation therapy) should also be recorded. The radiologist should provide this information, taking measurements from objective landmarks which can be easily recognised intraoperatively. A supplementary biopsy may be justified in areas of suspected, but doubtful, tumoural extension. It has always been stressed that an osteotomy must be performed in normal bone, but the ideal distance from the top of the tumour (or oedematous-reactive zone if present) has not always been well defined. Some authors suggest a safety zone of up to 7 cm. Our personal preference is to obtain 1 cm in benign, 2 cm in low, and 3 cm in high-grade lesions. However, these safety margins can be increased (if no changes in reconstruction or functional results are expected) or decreased to save important anatomical structures (growth plate or articular surface) and/or in the presence of a good response to preoperative treatment.

During surgery, the periosteum is exposed at the level of the planned osteotomy; it is marked, cut and elevated just enough to insert two Hohmann retractors for protection while performing the osteotomy with an oscillating saw. After osteotomy, the medullary canal should be immediately inspected to check for the presence of normal bone marrow, and a sample of this must be taken from the remaining bone and sent for frozen section. It is crucial to section the periosteum circumferentially, immediately after the osteotomy and before applying any traction. This avoids stripping the periosteum from the shaft of the bone segment to be resected, which may expose the tumour and contaminate the surgical field. After osteotomy, a bone forceps has to be applied around the stump of the segment to be removed, gripping the sectioned periosteum over the cortex: the space at the osteotomy level is then opened by gradual mobilisation, so that the muscles, tendons and septa insertions can be divided *(fig 7)*.

A trick may be used to avoid an incidental break through the tumour while performing a close osteotomy, particularly in cases of transepiphyseal resections. A Kirschner wire is introduced at the level of the planned osteotomy and its direction is controlled by radiographic control. Several wires are then inserted under radiographic guidance, to define the line of the osteotomy. These wires act as a path, directing an osteotome or oscillating saw to slide over them. They also represent a barrier by preventing taking a wrong direction towards the tumour and minimising the risks of an incidental fracture of the posterior cortex that can produce a bone spike involving the tumour *(fig 8)*.

JOINTS

Joint invasion may be suspected in the presence of clinical symptoms such as effusion, stiffness or pain. Imaging techniques (particularly M.R.I.) are able to detect tumour growth into capsular attachments and ligaments preoperatively, as well as to demonstrate effusion or haemarthrosis. If the bulging of the lesion inside the joint is minimal, the tumour is covered by a shell of bone or at least by an intact synovial membrane, and the capsule or ligament are only partially invaded, an intra-articular resection can be carried out *(fig 9)*. Usually, the capsule and ligaments have to be sectioned in their middle substance to allow reconstruction with an osteoarticular allograft. These structures can be totally removed if a constrained prosthesis is selected as the reconstructive method. However, if joint contamination is secondary to a pathological fracture, ulceration of the synovial membrane with macroscopic bulging of the tumour inside the joint, or into ligaments, massive haemarthrosis, transarticular biopsy, or an intra-articular origin of the tumour (synovial sarcoma), an extra-articular resection is more appropriate *(fig 10)*.

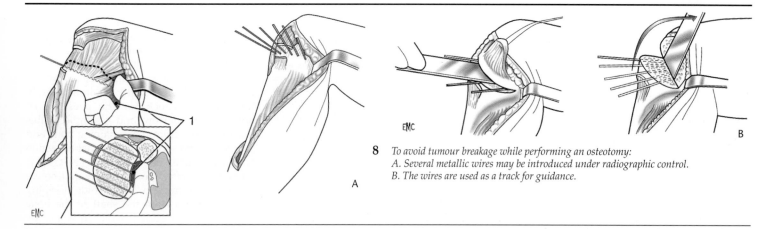

8 To avoid tumour breakage while performing an osteotomy:
A. Several metallic wires may be introduced under radiographic control.
B. The wires are used as a track for guidance.

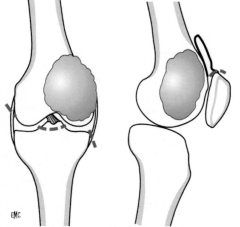

9 Minimal joint invasion is treated by intra-articular resection.

10 A. Pathological fracture.
B. Massive haemarthrosis.
C. Massive joint invasion or intra-articular tumour requiring extra-articular resection.

VESSELS

Involvement of major vessels is easily detected preoperatively, using echo-Doppler, C.T. scan with contrast medium, or angio-M.R.I. Nowadays, the more invasive classical angiography is still indicated preoperatively, but only when a by-pass is already scheduled and information is required on size of vessels and site of anastomosis.

During surgery, if the vessels are compressed by the tumour, these are identified proximally, prepared and gently retracted using a vaseloop. If a "blunt dissection" is feasible using only a tampon, and retracting the vessels and ligating collateral branches, the vessels may be retained and isolated from proximal to distal (fig 11). If the artery is not involved, but difficulties are encountered in dissecting the major vein (or tumoural clots are observed within collateral vein branches), the latter can be sacrificed (without reconstruction), if the superficial circle is preserved.

However, if a "sharp dissection" using scissors is required because the vascular adventitia has become part of the tumoural pseudocapsule, the vessels have to be resected en bloc, so that adequate margins can be achieved (fig 12). In this case, several authors suggest reconstructing only the

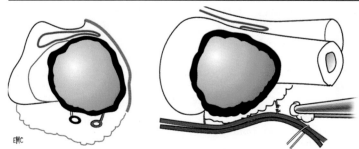

11 The vessels may be spared if they can be isolated by blunt dissection.

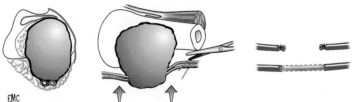

12 If the vascular adventitia is part of a tumoral pseudocapsule, a sharp dissection with scissors is required and the vessels should be resected en bloc, performing a by-pass.

artery, because the vein by-pass will be rapidly obstructed by a thrombus. However, we generally prefer to reconstruct both artery and vein for the beneficial effects on blood circulation, at least in the immediate, and during the more critical postoperative period. In any case, if a deep vessel by-pass is scheduled, particular care has to be taken in preserving the superficial circle while performing skin incision and tumour approach. Usually, we prefer biological reconstruction (saphenous vein autograft) instead of artificial prostheses, except in cases where postoperative radiation therapy

is required. In the past, the success rate of a conventional by-pass on peripheral vessels (distally to the elbow or knee) was discouraging. Recently, however, this limitation has been solved by performing these by-passes using more advanced microsurgical techniques.

The same criteria ("blunt" versus "sharp" dissection) are used to decide whether or not to remove, en bloc with the tumour, a part of the adjacent and adherent viscera (for instance, bladder or bowel in pelvic tumours).

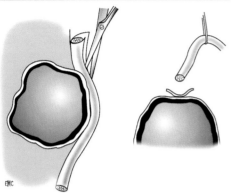

13 *If the nerve is compressed, the perineurium may be opened and left in situ as a barrier.*

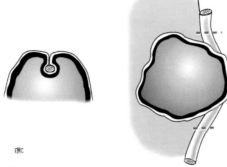

14 *If the nerve is entrapped in the tumour, it should be resected and repaired with nerve grafts.*

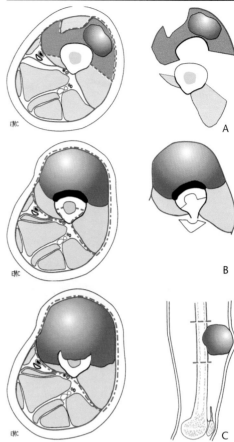

15 *In soft tissues sarcomas:*
A. If the tumour is mobile over the bone, removing the periosteum is sufficient.
B. If the pseudocapsule involves the periosteum, a partial diaphysectomy is required.
C. If the cortex is eroded or the tumour surrounds the bone, an en bloc resection is mandatory.

NEOPLASTIC THROMBI IN THE VENOUS BRANCHES

This is a rare event, usually observed in large tumours pushing or compressing the main vascular bundle. The surgeon finds some venous branches, running from the tumour area and confluent into the major vessels, clotted by neoplastic thrombi: occasionally, the obstruction extends far into the principal vein. Unfortunately, such occurrence is rarely detected preoperatively, even using the most advanced imaging techniques (C.T., M.R.I., angiographies), particularly if major vessels are not involved and the phenomenon is limited to the peripheral branches. The suspicion of clotted vessels (hard in consistency while ligating or cutting) should warn the surgeon and a frozen section is mandatory. If neoplastic thrombi are confirmed, a wider dissection (possibly with major vessel removal) or an amputation should be considered, instead of relying on postoperative radiation therapy.

NERVES

Rarely, nerves will show strong adherences with the pseudocapsule of a sarcoma. Paradoxically, this is more often observed in dysplastic lesions (fibromatosis, myositis ossificans). The epineurium, although thin, represents a strong anatomical barrier to tumour infiltration. For this reason, the nerve is approached and exposed on its side opposite to the lesion, the epineurium is longitudinally split, the nerve is peeled off and extracted: the epineurium remains attached to the tumour and is removed en bloc with the lesion *(fig 13)*. This technique is usually feasible in new tumours, but often cannot be applied to recurrent tumours in which a previous neurolysis has already been performed and/or the nerve is included in scar tissue and fibrosis. If the nerve, instead of being pushed, is surrounded by the tumour, a nerve resection should be considered *(fig 14)*. Functional restoration may be achieved by nerve grafts, motor unit transplantation, or tendon transfers [1]. If nerve grafts are chosen as a reconstructive method, it is useful, before cutting, to map the nerve by electrical stimulation at the level of the proximal and distal transsection, in order to recognise motor and sensitive fibres. This will help in selecting priorities in grafting (often the availability of nerve grafts allows only partial anatomical restoration after extensive resection of major nerves) and greatly improves accuracy and quality of reconstruction. In cases of major nerve resection (sciatic trunk, brachial plexus, multiple removals), the expected functional results should be considered and compared to function obtainable by amputation, also taking into account the oncological adequacy of the surgical procedure.

ADJACENT BONE (IN SOFT TISSUE TUMOURS)

If a soft tissue tumour is adjacent to a bone, a decision should be taken as to whether the latter must be removed en bloc with the lesion. The following criteria are usually selected *(fig 15)*:

– If the tumour is clinically, freely movable, and the imaging studies are negative, no removal of bone is required.

– If the tumour is clinically not movable, with a negative bone scan and negative imaging studies, en bloc removal of the adjacent periosteum is recommended.

– If an increased isotope uptake of the adjacent bone is observed, partial removal of the bony shaft is required, the periosteum being involved in the tumoral pseudocapsule.

– If the bone scan uptake is associated with a periosteal reaction or superficial cortical erosion or oedema inside the medullary canal, a complete en bloc removal of the bone is recommended. Periosteal reaction and cortical erosion are best assessed by C.T. scan, while oedema or intramedullary skip lesions are only detected by M.R.I.

– If the bone scan is positive, even if all other studies (X-rays, C.T., M.R.I.) are negative, an en bloc removal of the entire bone is also recommended when the tumour completely surrounds the shaft.

If extensive stripping of the periosteum or partial bone resection is performed, there is an increasing risk of pathological fracture, particularly if adjuvant radiation therapy is included in the treatment. In this case, a prophylactic osteosynthesis and/or grafting procedures should be considered.

General guidelines on curettage

Curettage or intracapsular excision is a technique recommended for benign tumours (stage 1 or 2, rarely 3). Exceptionally, this procedure is used for low-grade malignant tumours (grade 1 chondrosarcoma, desmoplastic fibrosarcoma). We follow the same guidelines suggested by Gitelis and Mc Donald [4], and we recommend the following steps in particular *(fig 16)*:

1. Approach the lesion by dissecting in normal tissue (wide) or at least between normal tissue and the reactive capsule (marginal), and expose a large surface on the side where the cortex is more attenuated and expanded. The exposure should be 1 or 2 cm larger than the diameter of the surface involved by the tumour.

2. If muscles, aponeuroses, tendons or joint capsule insertions are to be sectioned, these structures can be divided at a short distance from the bone so they can be easily reinserted at the end of the procedure.

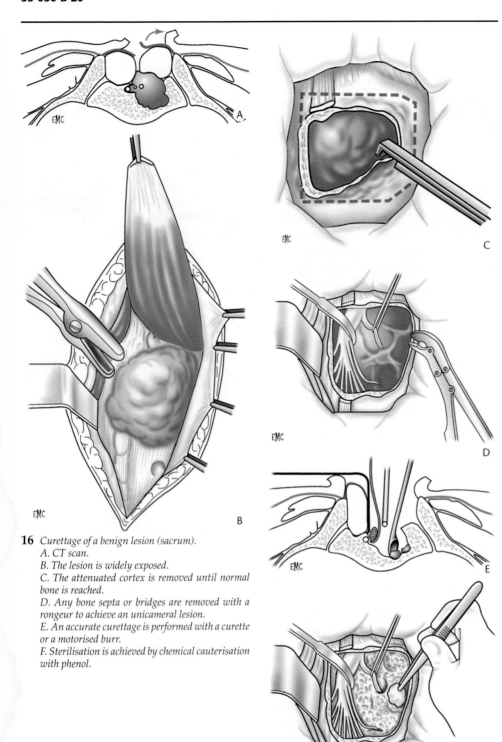

16 *Curettage of a benign lesion (sacrum).*
A. CT scan.
B. The lesion is widely exposed.
C. The attenuated cortex is removed until normal bone is reached.
D. Any bone septa or bridges are removed with a rongeur to achieve an unicameral lesion.
E. An accurate curettage is performed with a curette or a motorised burr.
F. Sterilisation is achieved by chemical cauterisation with phenol.

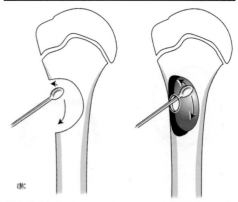

17 *Curettage must be performed through a large window; a limited approach is practically blind, leaving some areas unreached by the curette.*

from the normal bone to the tumour and not vice versa.

7. Perform an accurate curettage of the tumour through a large window to achieve direct visualisation of the internal walls of the cavity. Any attempt to perform a curettage through a small window (or through "the neck of a bottle" such as a curettage of the femoral head by a transtrochanteric approach) leaves some dark areas not reached by the curette, and is a risk for local recurrence *(fig 17)*.

8. The cavity having been widely saucerised, the remaining deep wall must be generously freshened to the normal bone using a curette, gouges and a motorised burr. Any abnormal areas of cancellous bone, as well as any bony ridges, should be removed, and the cavity must appear unicameral with smooth walls.

9. A pressurised lavage with saline solution must be used to wash out curettage detritus, repeatedly and abundantly.

10. While performing the surgical procedure, the medullary canal of the diaphysis should not be opened until the very end, to avoid inadvertently pushing the tumour distally.

II. Improve margins using a local adjuvant, particularly if it is not possible to remove the thinned wall of the cavity completely. This prevents a substantial mechanical loss, or avoids opening the bone in a dangerous area (popliteal fossa), or because the wall itself is represented by the joint cartilage or the growth plate.

12. The following local adjuvants have been demonstrated to be effective either alone or in combination [5]:

a) Soak the surface three times with highly concentrated phenol (80%), followed first by lavage with alcohol, and then with saline solution. This technique is only effective in contact and thus, only sterilises the surfaces.

b) electrocauterise extensively the bony walls and the tissue layer around the rim of the cavity. This procedure, particularly if performed with argon, has a haemostatic effect and a sterilising property of 1 mm.

c) Use the thermal and toxic effect of methylmethacrylate during polymerisation.

3. Using electrocautery, section the periosteum all around and lift it from its circumference towards the centre, until the edges of the lesion are exposed.

4. Before opening the tumour, protect the surrounding soft tissues with moistened sponges to avoid contamination by tumour cells. For the same reason, in approaching the tumour, avoid opening the joint cavity or exposing the neurovascular bundle.

5. Through a small opening, take a tumour sample to confirm the diagnosis by frozen section.

6. Then with rongeurs enlarge the access, removing all the eroded cortex and the overlaying periosteum until normal bone is reached. The tumour often clings to the walls and fills in little out-pockets of the walls. Therefore, whenever possible, removal of all attenuated cortex is recommended. Instead of progressively enlarging an initial small access, some authors prefer to cut the periphery of the lesion directly with osteotomes and gouges, mobilising and elevating in one block a large cover made of the outer wall of the lesion and a major portion of the tumour. This procedure requires more skill and, to avoid contamination, the surgeon should make sure he orients the osteotome continuously

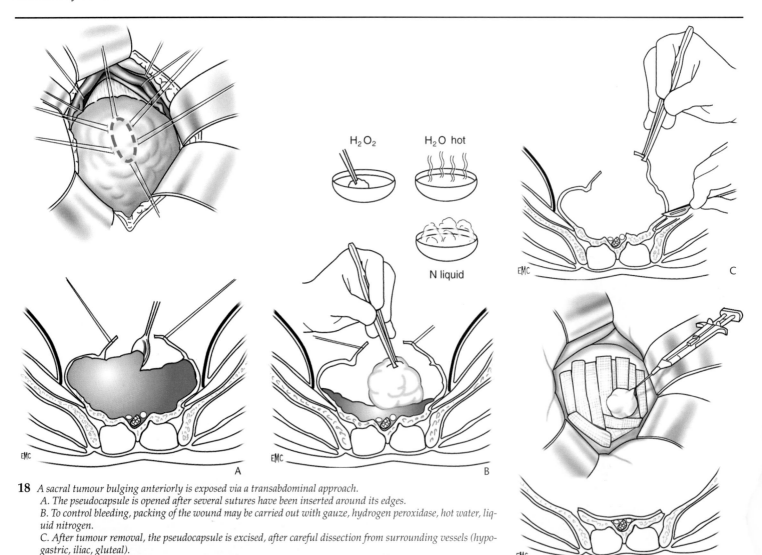

18 *A sacral tumour bulging anteriorly is exposed via a transabdominal approach.*
A. The pseudocapsule is opened after several sutures have been inserted around its edges.
B. To control bleeding, packing of the wound may be carried out with gauze, hydrogen peroxidase, hot water, liquid nitrogen.
C. After tumour removal, the pseudocapsule is excised, after careful dissection from surrounding vessels (hypogastric, iliac, gluteal).
D. Haemostasis of the deep exposed surface is obtained by fibrin glue and gauze, or by a rotated omentum flap.

This thermal effect is dependent on several parameters: the amount of cement used (very little in filling small cavities of less than 1cm in diameter, more important in cavities larger than 3 cm); the conductivity of bone (the effect being greater in cancellous bone of 2-3 mm, less in cortical bone of 0.5 mm); the pressurisation inside the trabeculae; the rate of heat dissipation (better if the vascular supply of the bone is diminished by tourniquet application). The toxic effect depends on monomer release: thus it is more pronounced if the cement is prepared using unsophisticated older generation technology. The overall effect is a ring of necrosis of about 1-2 mm.

d) Deep freeze and thaw the cavity using liquid nitrogen or more advanced techniques (filling the cavity with a sterile gel and using a probe connected to a machine that controls temperature and rate of freezing). The procedure (freeze and thaw) should be repeated at least three times. This technique produces a ring of necrotic bone of 1-2 cm and therefore represents the most effective local adjuvant. The surgeon must be aware of bone fragility and damage to soft tissues. (*fig 18*).

13. Once the curettage has been completed, all sponges are removed, the wound is abundantly and repeatedly irrigated, the surgeon changes gloves and instruments.

14. The cavity is filled with autogenous or homologous grafts, bone substitutes or derivatives according to the surgeon's personal preferences. Cement is useful, not only for its adjuvant effect, but also for its filling capacity (strengthening the osteosynthesis and affording better screw grip), its ability to support immediate weight-bearing and allow early detection of local recurrence. Filling with methylmethacrylate is recommended in cases of very aggressive lesions (at risk of local recurrence) or to prevent fractures when local adjuvants with a cracking effect are used. Because the cement increases the subchondral stiffness and may create the risk of a degenerative change of the joint, a subchondral layer of bone graft in association with cement is recommended to reconstitute subchondral bone (*fig 18, 19*).

References

[1] Capanna R. Le traitement des sarcomes des tissus mous. In : Cahiers d'enseignement de la SOFCOT. Paris : Expansion scientifique française, 1998 : 175-189

[2] Enneking WF. A system of staging musculoskeletal neoplasms. *Clin Orthop* 1986 ; 204 : 9-24

[3] Enneking WF, Spanier SS, Goodman MA. A system for the surgical staging of muscoloskeletal sarcomas. *Clin Orthop* 1983 ; 153 : 106-120

[4] Gitelis S, McDonald DJ. Curettage. In : Simon MA ed. Surgery for bone and soft tissue tumours. Springfield : Lippincott-Raven, 1998 : 133-157

[5] Gitelis S, McDonald DJ. Adjuvant agents and filling materials. In : Simon MA ed. Surgery for bone and soft tissue tumours. Springfield : Lippincott-Raven, 1998 : 133-157

[6] Simon MA. Surgical margins. In : Simon MA ed. Surgery for bone and soft tissue tumours. Springfield : Lippincott-Raven, 1998 : 77-92

Figures 19 and 20 ▶

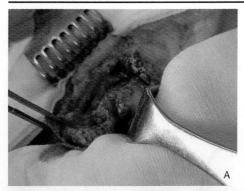

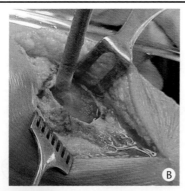

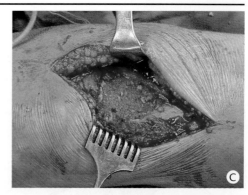

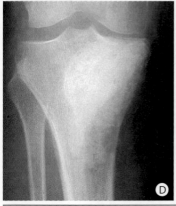

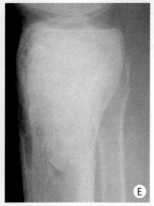

19 *A 14-year old girl with a giant cell tumour of the proximal tibia. After the initial biopsy the girl was operated with curettage and filling of the cavity with bone autografts from the iliac crest.*

A. The bone is opened through a large window and the tumour is exposed presenting the typical aspect of a giant cell tumour. After adequate curettage the cavity presents without bony bridges or recesses. A mechanical burr is used to complete manual curettage and improve thermal effects. The use of local adjuvants is recommended to lower the recurrence of disease. Phenol is used to "clean" the walls of the cavity three times and is inactivated with alcohol solution after every use.

B. Deep freezing is another local adjuvant; it can be used through liquid nitrogen or with devices as seen in the image. This uses liquid nitrogen to release freezing through local applicators such as this stick.

C. The autograft bone is divided into small chips and packed into the cavity.

D, E. X-ray appearance of the tibia after operation. The cavity has been completely filled with well-packed bone chips to achieve rapid healing.

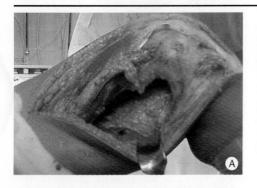

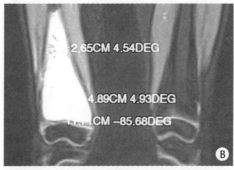

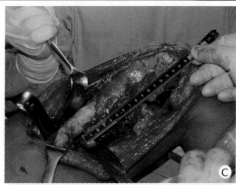

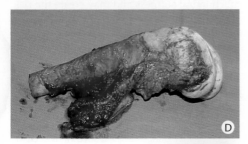

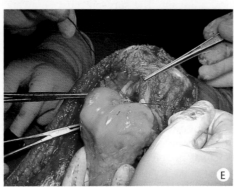

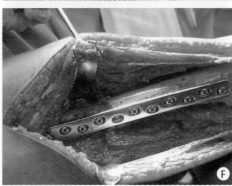

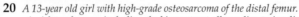

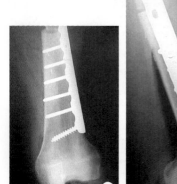

20 *A 13-year old girl with high-grade osteosarcoma of the distal femur.*

A. A lateral access including the biopsy tract allows direct visualisation of the distal femur. The tumour is exposed with a surrounding cuff of normal muscle.

B. Preoperative MRI shows the intracompartimental extension of the tumour, and its length in the medullary canal.

C. Using instrumental measurements, an adequate length of bone is resected. The excised bone with the biopsy tract is left in situ.

D. The bone excised with normal tissue coverage.

E. The osteo-articular graft is fixed to the tibial ligament stumps with multiple non-reabsorbable stitches. It is important to try to achieve the right tension of the cruciate ligaments and of the posterior capsule.

F. After joint reconstruction, the allograft is fixed to the host bone with the longest 4.5 mm plate available.

G, H. X-ray appearance of the osteo-articular allograft.

Surgical management of long bone and pelvis metastases

J Keller

Abstract. – *Bone metastasis is a serious complication of cancer. The most frequent locations are the spine, pelvis and proximal femur, with pain as the dominant symptom. Cure is seldom possible and the aim of treatment is palliation. It is controversial if radical surgery is carried out in solitary bone metastasis. In general, the role of surgical treatment is to treat or prevent fracture and maintain function. The guidelines for predicting the risk of fracture are of limited value. Osteosynthesis may provide initial stability. In combination with PMMA (polymethylmethacrylate), a better and more long standing stability can be obtained. Moreover, the tumour mass is reduced making radiation more effective. The use of prostheses has been increasing after development of calcar bearing prostheses, but the indications for their use is controversial. In selected patients there is a need for radical tumour resection and reconstruction with a megaprosthesis.*

Keywords: bone metastasis, pelvis, long bone, osteosynthesis, prosthesis.

Introduction

Bone metastasis is a serious complication of cancer. Most patients will present multiple metastatic bone lesions. The spine is involved in 70% of patients, the pelvis in 40% and the femur in 25%. Cure is seldom possible at this stage of the disease and treatment can only be palliative. The strategy of treatment of bone metastasis will focus primarily on minimising pain and maintaining function in order to improve quality of life. Only in solitary bone metastasis may radical tumour removal be indicated. In more than 75% of the patients, pain is the dominant symptom. In some cases mild analgesics may be sufficient, but often these patients need narcotics. Radiation has shown good effects on pain whereas its effect on bone healing is questionable. Previously, radiation was given in multiple fractions (4 x 5 Gy), but recent evidence demonstrates good pain relief after a single dose (8 Gy) [12]. Responding patients with recurrent pain can be retreated with radiation. Patients with multiple lesions may be treated with half body therapy (7 Gy) with similar efficacy as after local radiotherapy. Pain relief occurs in half of the patients within 2 days, but in other patients the effects may occur within the first 2 weeks [13].

Johnny Keller, M.D., DMSc, Associate Professor, Consultant in Orthopaedic Surgery, Department of Orthopaedic Surgery, University Hospital of Aarhus Norrebrogade, Denmark.

In long bones with metastasis, the fracture risk is difficult to predict. Many factors influence strength reduction: type of lesion, geometry of the defect, size and anatomical site [3]. The classical guidelines for prophylactic surgery are: bone lesions of more than 25 mm in long bones or destruction of more than 50% of the cortical bone [4]. However, fracture may easily occur in even smaller lesions. Pain may be a sign of impending fracture, especially if it persists after radiation therapy. Mirel [11] proposed a scoring system for prophylactic surgery taking additional aspects into account, such as site, pain and blastic response in the metastasis.

In a few patients with myeloma or breast cancer, bone healing is possible after adjuvant chemotherapy, hormonal therapy or radiation. However, in most patients bone healing is not possible. The surgical procedure must be simple, provide immediate stability and aim to last for the lifetime of the patient. The procedures can be divided into the following options:

– Osteosynthesis.

– Curettage of the tumour followed by osteosynthesis reinforced with polymethyl-methacrylate (PMMA).

– Prosthesis.

Osteosynthesis is a simple procedure which can be performed even in very sick patients. The aim is to obtain immediate stability and a short rehabilitation period. The method of choice, when possible, is nailing which will maintain stability despite progression of the metastasis. On the other hand, the procedure itself may cause a local progression of the disease due to implantation of metastatic tissue into the medullary canal. Plate fixation has very few indications as an isolated procedure. Stability can be improved if osteosynthesis is combined with curettage of the tumour and filling in with PMMA [3, 7, 19]. Furthermore, the tumour mass reduction improves the effects of adjuvant radiation therapy. The use of prostheses has increased after development of calcar replacement implants. In some cases, the intact bone stock is not sufficient for reconstruction and the only possibility may be resection of the tumour area. Reconstruction with a megaprosthesis often requires major operations and longer rehabilitation compared to osteosynthesis. Amputation is seldom indicated as a palliative procedure.

Surgical techniques

PELVIS

The pelvis is a common region for bone metastases. Most of these can be treated conservatively, but if the acetabular region is involved, patients often need surgery. The main goal is to maintain walking ability and avoid protrusion of the femoral head into the weakened acetabular bone. The most common classification of the lesions in the periacetabular region has been described by Harrington [6].

– Class I: The lateral, superior and medial parts of the wall are intact.

– Class II: The medial part of the wall is deficient.

– Class III: The lateral, medial and superior parts are deficient.

■ *Class I*

Patients in this class have enough unaffected periacetabular bone to make conventional fixation of a prosthesis sufficient.

■ *Class II*

In these patients a protrusio shell is needed in order to transfer the stress from the deficient wall to the intact acetabular rim.

■ *Class III*

The reconstruction must transmit the load from the deficient acetabulum onto the upper part of the ilium and sacroiliac joint. Harrington [6] has described a simple procedure whereby load is transferred to the pelvis via multiple Steinmann pins *(fig 1)*.

In a few special cases, the defect can be reconstructed with a saddle prosthesis [1].

■ *Operative techniques*

A posterior approach or lateral approach is used for class I and II lesions. For class III lesions, a lateral or anterior approach can be used depending on the extension of the lesions. The anterior approach is used for larger lesions requiring possible access to both the inner and outer aspects of the pelvis. Groups of large Steinmann pins are drilled across the pelvis proximally from the acetabular bed and distally through the acetabular bed. The first group of pins is drilled into the sacroiliac joint. It is essential to put a finger in the foramen ischiaticum to be sure not to drill into the ischiatic nerve. The second group of pins is drilled from the anterior superior iliac spine through the acetabular bed and into the ischium. Intra-operative radiographs are necessary to check the position of the pins. The pins in combination with a protrusio shell provide support for the cemented acetabular component [6]. In patients with lesions in the femoral bone, a long femoral stem is used to prevent fracture in this area. A sufficient soft tissue coverage over the implants is mandatory in order to avoid infection and allow early mobilisation. In classes I and II, full weight-bearing is allowed after surgery. In class III, full or partial weight-bearing is allowed, but the patient must wear an abduction orthosis for 1-3 months.

LOWER EXTREMITY

In the femur, stress on the bone is extremely high in the proximal part, making prophylactic osteosynthesis necessary even in minor lesions which do not strictly fulfil the criteria of impending fracture.

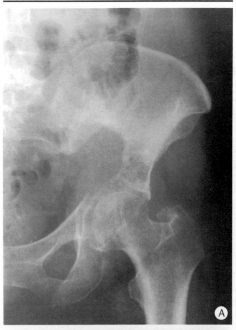

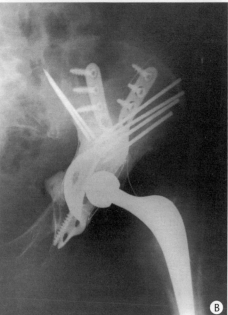

1 *A. Anteroposterior radiograph of the pelvis in a 50-year-old woman with metastatic breast carcinoma. The destruction involves the medial and lateral wall (class III).*
B. After excision of the tumor and reconstruction with multiple Steinmann pins and an antiprotusio shell.

■ *Femoral head and neck*

Hemiarthroplasty is the preferred method if the acetabulum is not involved; otherwise a total hip arthroplasty must be performed [10].

Surgical techniques

A posterior lateral approach without trochanteric osteotomy is used. For simple cases a standard hip replacement prosthesis can be used. If the intertrochanteric bone is involved, additional support is needed and consequently a prosthesis for calcar replacement must be used. In case of further metastases in the femoral bone, a long stem must be used in order to include these metastases in the stabilisation. The stem

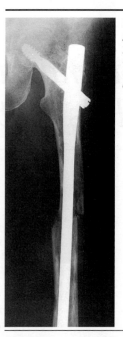

2 *Anteroposterior radiograph of the femur in a 75-year-old woman with metastatic myeloma. Stabilisation was performed with a long gamma nail.*

should be cemented for immediate weight-bearing. Rehabilitation follows the procedures for standard hip replacements.

■ *Intertrochanteric and subtrochanteric region*

Surgical treatment in this region is controversial, with a choice between internal fixation and prosthetic replacement. Internal fixation has been widely used with or without bone cement. Cementation can be performed under direct vision and improves stabilisation. If the bone does not heal, the bone cement will avoid fatigue fracture of the metal.

The compression hip screw fixed with a plate and reinforced with PMMA may be sufficient for an intertrochanteric lesion, but is insufficient for a subtrochanteric lesion. For this latter lesion, a locking intramedullary nail should be preferred due to the strong forces on this area *(fig 2)*. With the development of calcar replacement implants, arthroplasty has become more widely used. Resection of the proximal femur and use of a massive prosthesis may be indicated in patients with large destructions and insufficient bone stock for implant fixation *(fig 3)*. Due to increased risk of dislocation and longer rehabilitation, this procedure should be limited to selected patients [15].

Surgical techniques

Osteosynthesis is performed through a lateral approach. Rehabilitation is short and the patient is usually allowed weight-bearing immediately after operation.

Arthroplasty without intertrochanteric resection can be performed through a posterior approach. An anterior approach is preferred for proximal resections. Sufficient soft tissue coverage of the prosthesis is mandatory in all cases. After intertrochanteric resections, the abductor muscles must

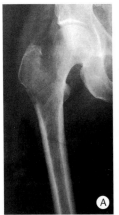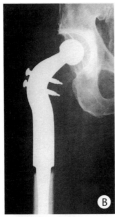

3 *A. Anteroposterior radiograph of the femur in a 46-year-old man with a solitary metastasis from a renal cell carcinoma. The destruction involved the neck and the intertrochanteric region.*
B. The patient was treated by kidney removal and resection of the proximal femur. The reconstruction was performed with a megaprosthesis (Müller).

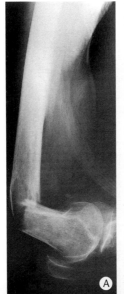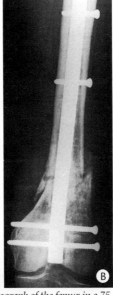

4 *A. Anteroposterior radiograph of the femur in a 75-year-old woman with a metastatic myeloma. The destruction occurred in the supracondylar region.*
B. Stabilisation was performed with a retrograde nail (Smith and Nephew). PMMA would have improved stability.

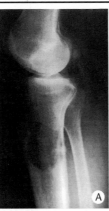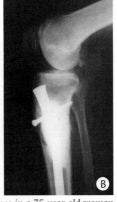

5 *A. Radiograph of the knee in a 75-year old woman with a metastatic renal cell carcinoma (same patient as Fig. 4).*
B. She had kidney removal and the bone destruction was curetted. Stabilisation was achieved with a locked nail and PMMA. She survived more than 3 years without progression of the disease.

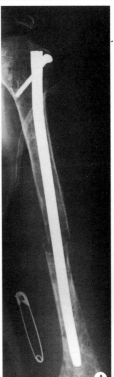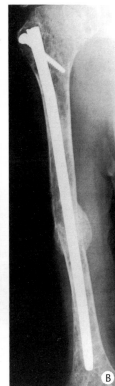

6 *A. Radiograph of the arm in a 75-year-old woman with metastatic myeloma (same patient as Fig. 4, 5). The humerus was stabilised with a nail locked proximally and distally.*
B. The fracture healed after 3 months.

be sutured to the lateral aspect of the vastus lateralis muscle. The iliopsoas muscle is placed anteriorly to the prosthesis and sutured to the abductor muscles and the quadriceps muscle. The fixation of the soft tissue to the prosthesis is the main problem. A recent study showed that porous coating will facilitate soft tissue ingrowth [17].

In patients without intertrochanteric resection, rehabilitation can follow the regimens used after standard total hip replacement. After intertrochanteric resection, full or partial weight-bearing is allowed, but the patient must use an abduction brace for 1-3 months. We use a custom-made plastic brace. For the first 5 weeks, we allow flexion from 5-70°, and from the 6th to the 12th week we allow flexion from 5-80°.

■ *Femoral and tibial diaphysis*

The treatment of choice at present is intramedullary nailing. The use of additional bone cement is questionable. It is obvious that local curettage of the tumour followed by nailing and cementing gives optimal local tumour control and probably better stability. On the other hand, the open technique increases operation time and risk of infection compared with the closed technique.

For selected cases, en bloc resection may be needed. Reconstruction can be performed using a prosthesis for replacement of the diaphyseal bone.

Surgical techniques

Operation is most convenient on the extension table in a supine position. Care should be taken since the bone is weakened with impending fractures. If bone cement is used the open technique is preferred. For the femoral diaphysis, the incision is placed laterally. The tumour is carefully removed with curettage as the first step. After reaming, the nail is introduced and locked at both ends. Finally, bone cement is pressed proximally and distally through the cortical defect. Full weight-bearing is allowed after operation.

■ *Knee*

In this region, alternative procedures are possible. The lesion is often underestimated and MRI scanning may be necessary to evaluate the extension of the lesion. Many authors prefer plating or retrograde nailing with additional bone cement (*fig 4, 5*). In extensive lesions, the treatment is resection and a tumour reconstruction prosthesis.

Surgical techniques

The operation is performed using a tourniquet. The patient is placed in a supine position. Osteosynthesis is performed through a lateral approach and may be combined with an additional anteromedial approach. Arthroplasty is performed through a medial parapatellar approach. Rehabilitation is with partial or full weight-bearing after operation.

UPPER EXTREMITY

■ *Humeral head and neck*

Evaluation of the lesion may be difficult in this region without additional MRI scanning. In most cases, the bone stock is insufficient for osteosynthesis and a prosthesis is recommended.

Surgical techniques

An anterior approach is used with the patient in a supine sitting position. The approach can be extended distally for further resection. If the major tuberosity is not destroyed, it should not be resected, so that fixation of the rotator cuff to the prosthesis can be secured. After operation the patient must use a sling for 6 weeks, in which only passive motion is allowed.

■ *Diaphyseal bone in upper extremity*

The load on the humerus is relatively much smaller than on the femur. The preferable method is probably nailing with or without curettage and PMMA (*fig 6*). Some authors advocate curettage and fixation with two metal plates combined with PMMA. In selected cases a tumour resection prosthesis is needed (*fig 7*).

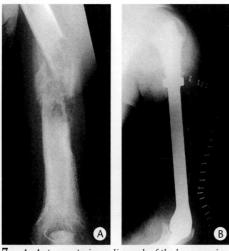

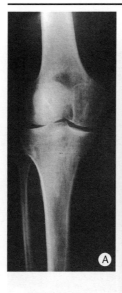

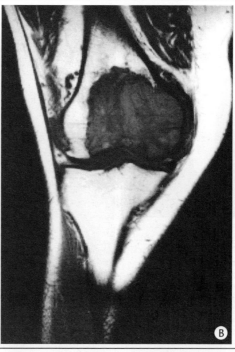

8 *A. The extension of a bone metastasis is difficult to evaluate from a plain radiograph.*
B. MRI scanning or CT scanning is needed to visualise the destruction.

7 *A. Anteroposterior radiograph of the humerus in a 25-year-old man with a metastatic Ewing sarcoma.*
B. After preoperative chemotherapy a marginal excision was performed and reconstruction was carried out with a custom made prosthesis (Link).

Surgical techniques

A posterior approach is widely used.

■ *Elbow*

If the bone stock is sufficient, osteosynthesis in combination with PMMA is preferred. In other cases, an elbow prosthesis is the method of choice.

Surgical techniques

A posterior approach with splitting of the triceps aponeurosis gives an excellent approach.

Indications

PREOPERATIVE EVALUATION

In patients with a history of malignancy, a bone lesion is probably a metastatic lesion. In solitary bone lesions, other malignancies should be suspected. This is especially true if the area has had high dose radiation previously. In such a case the patient should be referred to a tumour centre before biopsy [14].

The preoperative examination of a patient with a suspected metastasis must include evaluation of the general condition and a search for the most frequent primary cancers:

– lung (radiograph, CT scan).

– breast (palpation, mammography).

– prostate (exploration, prostate-specific antigen).

– kidney (abdominal ultrasound or CT scan).

– thyroid (palpation, scanning).

– myeloma (immune electrophoresis).

– lymphoma (lymph nodes, abdominal ultrasound or CT scan).

The body should be examined for multiple metastases (whole body bone scintigraphy). The scan is positive for most metastases except those with an osteoblastic response, such as myelomas and some lymphomas. Each metastatic lesion should be radiographed. In trabecular bone, the lesion may be underestimated and a CT scan or an MRI scan should be performed (fig 8). In most cases the diagnosis should be verified with a needle biopsy before surgery. Embolisation should be considered before operation, especially in renal cell carcinoma [5].

SURGICAL STRATEGY

Surgical treatment should be individualised for each patient. Fracture of the long bones in the lower extremity is usually a major criterion for surgery, whereas fracture in the upper extremity can be alternatively treated with a brace. Impending fracture is another major criterion for surgery. However, the guidelines for predicting fracture are of limited value [3, 11]. In some patients, several bone metastases need operation. A simple procedure may not be the most stable in the long run, but for a patient with a short survival it may be sufficient for the rest of his life. Tokuhashi et al [16] proposed a scoring system for survival based on the general condition of the patient, number of metastases, metastases to major internal organs, site of the primary cancer and presence of fracture. Except for the factor for general condition, they were all found to be true prognostic factors for survival in a later study [2]. Survival was correlated to the number of factors with positive effect on survival.

ADJUVANT THERAPY

It is important to have a multidisciplinary approach in these patients for optimal treatment. The effect of postoperative systemic treatment depends on the primary malignancy (endocrine therapy, chemotherapy and radiotherapy). At present the most important effect of chemotherapy, endocrine therapy and radiation have been noted in breast cancer, of endocrine therapy in prostatic cancer, of radiation and of chemotherapy in myeloma, and chemotherapy in lymphoma.

Postoperative radiation has a well documented effect on pain [12]. Furthermore, radiation may help to control tumour growth. Radiation is usually given in doses up to 20 Gy, although high dose radiation may be considered in solitary bone metastasis. Recently, biphosphonates seem promising, but their role has not been clarified [9].

COMPLICATIONS

The patients are often in a poor condition, increasing the risk of infection and thromboembolic complications. In highly vascularised tumours (renal cell carcinoma), there is a risk of excessive peroperative blood loss. This can be reduced with preoperative embolisation of the tumour. The use of PMMA and intramedulary nailing have been sporadically associated with cardiovascular collapse and intraoperative death. The risk of nailing seems to be associated with reaming. Probably use of unreamed nailing reduces the risk of cardiovascular collapse. Other complications may be the local and systemic spread of the tumour cells, secondary to the surgical trauma (the risk is high in renal cell carcinoma). Failure of the fixation may occur due to improper initial fixation, fatigue fracture (fig 9, 10) of the metal or local progression of the bone lesion (fig 11) [18].

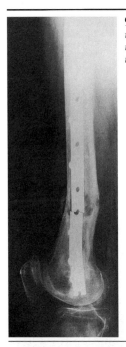

9 *Fatigue fracture in a retrograde nail due to an ununited pathological fracture.*

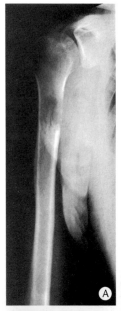 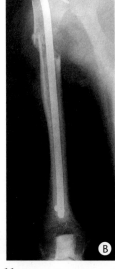

11 *Progression of renal cell carcinoma in a nailed renal cell carcinoma metastasis.*

A. Preoperatively.
B. One month after operation.
C. Four months after operation. The patient died 2 months later.

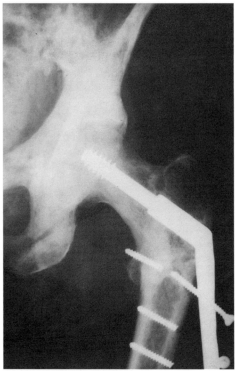

10 *Fatigue fracture of the diaphyseal screws of a hip screw due to an ununited pathological fracture.*

References

[1] Aboulafia AJ, Buch RB, Mathews J, Li W, Malawer MM. Reconstruction using the saddle prosthesis following excision of primary and metastatic periacetabular tumors. *Clin Orthop* 1995 ; 314 : 203-213

[2] Bauer HC, Wedin R. Survival after surgery for spinal and extremity metastases. Prognostication in 241 patients. *Acta Orthop Scand* 1995 ; 66 : 143-146

[3] Damron TA, Heiner JP, Freund EM, Damron LA, McCabe R, Vanderby R. A biomechanical analysis of prophylactic fixation for pathological fractures of the distal third of the humerus. *J Bone Joint Surg Am* 1994 ; 76 : 839-847

[4] Fidler M. Incidence of fracture through metastases in long bones. *Acta Orthop Scand* 1981 ; 52 : 623-627

[5] Galasco CS. Diagnosis of skeletal metastases and assessment of response to treatment. *Clin Orthop* 1995 ; 312 : 64-75

[6] Harrington KD. Orthopaedic management of extremity and pelvic lesions. *Clin Orthop* 1995 ; 312 : 136-147

[7] Harrington KD, Sim FH, Enis JE, Johnston JO, Dick HM, Gristina AG. Methylmethacrylate as an adjunct in internal fixation of pathological fractures. experience with three hundred and seventy-five cases. *J Bone Joint Surg Am* 1976 ; 58 : 1047-1055

[8] Hipp JA, Springfield DS, Hayes WC. Predicting pathologic fracture risk in the management of metastatic bone defects. *Clin Orthop* 1995 ; 312 : 120-135

[9] Houston SJ, Rubens RD. The systemic treatment of bone metastases. *Clin Orthop* 1995 ; 312 : 93-104

[10] Lane JM, Sculco TP, Zolan S. Treatment of pathological fractures of the hip by endoprosthetic replacement. *J Bone Joint Surg Am* 1980 ; 62 : 954-954

[11] Mirel H. Metastatic Disease In Long Bones. A proposed scoring system for diagnosing impending pathologic fractures. *Clin Orthop* 1989 ; 249 : 256-264

[12] Nielsen OS, Bentzen SM, Sandberg E, Gadeberg CC, Timothy AR. Randomized trial of single versus fractionated palliative radiotherapy of bone metastases. *Radiother Oncol* 1998 ; 47 : 233-240

[13] Nielsen OS, Munro AJ, Tannock IF. Bone metastases. Pathophysiology and management policy. *J Clin Oncol* 1991 ; 9 : 509-524

[14] Rougraff BT, Kneisl JS, Simon MA. Skeletal metastases of unknown origin. *J Bone Joint Surg Am* 1993 ; 75 : 1276-1281

[15] Sim FH, Frassica FJ, Chao EY. Orthopaedic management using new devices and prostheses. *Clin Orthop* 1995 ; 312 : 160-172

[16] Tokuhashi Y, Kawano H, Toriyama S. Score assessment of metastatic bone tumor for operative treatment. In : Langlais F, Tomeno B eds. Limb Salvage - Major reconstructions in oncologic and nontumoral conditions. Berlin : Springer-Verlag, 1991 : 725-732

[17] Ward WG, Freels DV, Kilpatrick S, Gordon S. Soft tissue in growth into various tumour endoprothesis surface coatings. In : Choong P ed. 10th International Conference Proceedings Symposium on Limb Salvage. Cairns, Australia, 1999 : 14-15

[18] Wedin R, Bauer CF, Wersäll P. Failures after operation for skeletal metastatic lesions of long bones. *Clin Orthop* 1999 ; 358 : 128-139

[19] Yazawa Y, Frassica FJ, Chao E, Pritchard DJ, Sim FH, Shives TC. Metastatic bone disease. A study of surgical treatment of 166 pathologic humeral and femoral fractures. *Clin Orthop* 1990 ; 251 : 213-219

Spinal metastases

H Bauer
C Olerud

Abstract. – The aim in treating spinal metastases is palliation. The treatment should allow the patient to gain an improved quality of life. A thorough analysis of symptoms, extent, anticipated outcome of the operation, as well as the expected survival of the patient, all have to be considered. The most frequent indication for surgery in cervical metastases is pain, whereas neurological dysfunction is more common in the thoracic and lumbar spine. Strategic decisions, based on pre-operative investigations, must be made concerning how the spine is best decompressed (if necessary), and how it is best reconstructed. Application of the above principles of treatment should allow good and lasting pain relief. In patients with mild to moderate neurological damage, a good recovery can be anticipated. Treating patients with spinal metastases is a multidisciplinary team undertaking. An oncologist should be involved both in the pre-operative planning and in the postoperative care.

Keywords: spine, bone metastases, spinal instability, spinal cord compression, pathological fracture, palliative care.

Introduction

The vast majority of metastases to the spine are metastases to the bone marrow of the vertebrae. The metastasis undermines the mechanical integrity of the bone tissue and can cause a pathological fracture with pain and/or neurological deficit through epidural compression. This compression can be caused by a bulging tumour and bone fragments or by tumour growth in the spinal canal (fig 1). The neurological symptoms come from the spinal cord, cauda equina, or nerve root, depending on the location of the compression. Slow progression of neurological dysfunction, usually without pain, indicates a slow tumour expansion whereas a sudden, painful onset of neurological deficit is often due to pathological fracture. In these cases, radiotherapy will not be sufficient. Instead, surgical decompression of the dural sac and stabilisation of the spine can lead to both neurological restitution and long-standing pain relief [5]. On the other hand, a very rapid, total loss of neurological function may

Henrik CF Bauer, M.D., Ph.D., Orthopedic Oncology Service, Department of Orthopedics, Karolinska Hospital, SE-171 76 Stockholm, Sweden.
Claes Olerud, M.D., Ph.D.
Section for Spine Surgery, Department of Orthopedics, Uppsala University Hospital, SE-751 85 Uppsala, Sweden.

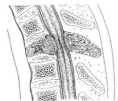

1 *The drawing shows how the spinal cord is compressed by a pathological fracture of the vertebral body and by a tumour in the posterior elements of the vertebra.*

indicate a vascular catastrophe with poor prognosis for recovery whatever the treatment modalities. Intradural metastases also exist, but they are uncommon and will not be dealt with here.

Treatment aims

The overall aim for treating patients with epidural metastases is palliation, i.e. to relieve pain and restore function. The malignant disease is disseminated and surgical treatment will only marginally affect the patient's survival. A severe neurological complication (tetraplegia or paraplegia) shortens life [3, 14], but other factors such as the general condition of the patient, the degree of tumour dissemination, and the inherited biology of the primary tumour are decisive for life expectancy.

Cost-benefit

Surgical treatment always carries a cost to the patient. There are risks of complications, and the chance of relief varies. Pain, even severe, carries a good prognosis. A mild neurological injury will probably recover, whilst a severe one, e.g. tetraplegia, will probably not [2, 3, 9, 13]. There is also always a convalescent time after a surgical procedure, during which the patient is worse off than before. Post-operative infection causes increased morbidity and may delay or prevent other palliative treatments, such as radiotherapy or chemotherapy. The length of the convalescent time depends on the general condition of the patient and the extent of the surgical intervention. Anterior decompression and stabilisation of the cervical spine are easily overcome by the patient while a similar procedure in the thoracic or lumbar spine is associated with considerable morbidity. Most patients' expected survival is short, so the time during which they may benefit from an operation is limited [4].

As the treatment aim is palliation, the surgeon will have to decide if the benefit for the patient outweighs the cost. Several factors have to be included in this analysis. First of all, the level of symptoms and the chances of alleviation are primordial, as these decide the maximal relief the patient might experience. Another important issue is the expected survival of the patient. The tumour type has a great impact on survival, e. g. patients with lung cancer have a much poorer chance of surviving 6 months than do kidney cancer patients. Furthermore, the degree of dissemination is important. Patients with solitary metastases have the best prognosis, whereas those with non-skeletal metastases have the worst. The general condition of the patient and the degree of neurological deficit play important roles. Tokuhashi et al [21] and others have developed scoring scales for estimating prognosis. However, these scales are coarse tools, and consultation with an experienced oncologist to assess prognosis and possible benefits of chemotherapy or radiotherapy is crucial in the decision-making process.

Symptoms

The most common initial symptom of an epidural metastasis is severe pain locally in the spine. This can be combined with radiating pain and neural dysfunction, if nervous tissue is compressed as well. In the cervical region, in contrast to other areas of the spine, pain is usually the dominating symptom whereas neurological symptoms are rare and develop late in the course of the disease [9, 18]. Pain may radiate into the upper extremities. The prognosis for survival is poor once tetraplegia has developed.

In the thoracic spine, neural compression will cause radiating pain across the thoracic or abdominal wall. Severe compression of the spinal cord will lead to paraplegia including paresis of the abdominal muscles. Compression of the cauda equina causes radiating pain to the lower extremities and sometimes paresis. Urinary bladder and anal sphincter paresis are uncommon as initial symptoms, but unfortunately are often already present when the patient comes for treatment.

Differential diagnoses

There are several differential diagnoses to be considered in the assessment of a cancer patient suspected of having spinal cord compression due to vertebral metastases. Among these are cerebral disorders such as brain metastases and cerebral vascular insults. Local tumour growth involving peripheral nerve plexus can lead to radiating pain and paralysis. For example, lung cancer involvement of the cervical plexus or prostate cancer involvement of the presacral plexus are not uncommon. Spontaneous compression fractures of vertebral bodies with neurological symptoms due to osteopenia (Kümmell's disease) are rare and offer diagnostic difficulties. A chronic low-grade infection may also be mistaken for a malignancy, usually requiring biopsy with

both histology and culture for definite diagnosis. Pathological fractures of the pelvis or hip lead to pain and loss of function which can be mistaken for symptoms of spinal involvement.

Acute investigations and treatment

- Patient history and assessment of neurological deficit.

- High dose steroids.

- Adequate analgesia to permit adequate radiological examinations.

- Bladder catheter.

- Plain radiographs.

- MRI of the entire spinal column. CT myelography if MRI is contraindicated.

- Needle biopsy of the most accessible lesion, if there is no known primary lesion.

- Pre-operative embolisation if there are kidney or thyroid cancer metastases.

- Decision on surgical treatment with an oncologist.

Pre-operative assessment

Patients suspected of having epidural compression should be seen urgently by the oncologist and the surgeon conjointly, even if the neurological deficit is not alarming. It is important to assess how long the neurological symptoms have been present and whether they are progressing or stable. The clinical level and extent of paresis is determined, as well as possible bladder or anal sphincter dysfunction. Radiological examinations include MRI of the entire vertebral column and plain radiographs of all involved areas of the spine. MRI reveals the extent of bone involvement and compression of neural structures. Spiral CT with sagittal and frontal plane reconstruction contributes to assessing skeletal integrity and is sometimes useful for planning the operative stabilisation.

Indications for treatment

Decision as to surgical treatment is made together with the responsible oncologist after complete clinical and radiological examinations. Factors of relevance when choosing between surgery and other treatment modalities include: the extent of pain, the neurological deficit, and the speed with which these have developed; type of primary tumour, and its sensitivity to radio-, hormone, or chemotherapy; the dissemination of the disease in terms of other skeletal and non-skeletal metastases; the general condition of the patient and, finally, the technical possibility of performing surgical decompression and stabilisation.

INDICATIONS FOR RADIOTHERAPY

- Slow onset of symptoms.

- No or only slight neurological symptoms.

- Non-skeletal metastases.

- Extensive spine metastases.

- Radiosensitive tumour, e.g. lymphoma.

- Complete paraplegia.

INDICATIONS FOR SURGICAL TREATMENT

- Progression of neurological deficit.

- Inability to walk.

- Severe pain.

- Spinal instability.

- Solitary metastases.

- Continued pain after radiotherapy.

Strategy for choice of operative approach

The primary concern is to choose the surgical procedure which fits the patient's symptoms and radiological findings. If the patient has neurological symptoms, decompression of the spinal cord is paramount. If the main problem is pain, decompression is seldom needed and restoration of spinal stability is the primary goal.

There are several different mechanisms of neural compression due to metastases in the spine, but more than one mechanism may be present at the same time. Sometimes a lytic metastasis has destroyed a vertebral body causing collapse of the anterior column with kyphosis, and the tumour infested bone will bulge into the spinal canal without any actual epidural growth. Decompression may be achieved merely by reduction of the fracture [16], or by anterior resection of the vertebral body [10]. Bone destruction, especially of the posterior structures of the cervical spine, can cause a translational deformity, as the mechanism for neural compression is secondary to the slip. In this situation, reduction of the deformity will result in an effective decompression. Finally, the neural compression may be due to tumour epidural growth, either as a tumour cuff strangulating the dural sac, or more often compressing the sac from one direction. In these patients, decompressive resection of the bone must be part of the operation. A thorough analysis of the best way to decompress and reconstruct will be needed to decide on the operative approach. As a general rule, the decompression should be performed from the side of maximal compression. However, it is also important to consider how spine realignment will contribute to the decompression.

A different mechanism of neural compression is commonly seen in prostate cancer metastases [6]. The tumour infiltration leads to bony hypertrophy, causing spinal stenosis, often at several adjacent levels. If the area of stenosis is lordotic, a laminectomy will suffice. If the area is kyphotic, however, a laminectomy will not result in effective decompression but will lead to instability instead. In such situations, other strategies have to be considered, such as combined anterior and posterior approaches to decompress the spinal cord and restore stability.

Restoration of spinal stability

The means of achieving stability is a key issue in the surgical approach to spinal metastases. If the instability is secondary to compression of one or two adjacent vertebral bodies, an anterior approach with resection of the metastasis and reconstruction with some form of spacer and a plate or rods will be sufficient [7, 19]. If more than two vertebral bodies are affected, the anterior reconstruction alone may not be strong enough and a posterior stabilisation will have to be considered instead. In this situation, the posterior reconstruction aims to stabilise (bypass) the unstable segments indirectly and no anterior pillar reconstruction is performed (*fig 2*). To avoid failure leading to kyphosis, it is recommended that a bypass stabilisation be fixed to at least two vertebrae on each side of the destruction. The internal fixation device will be load-bearing and not load-sharing, and the construct may fail if the patient lives long enough. Therefore, if the patient has a long survival expectancy, a combined approach of posterior stabilisation and anterior pillar reconstruction is recommended. In cases of pure posterior element insufficiency, the best way to reconstruct is from behind. Most patients with neurological symptoms due to metastases in the thoracic or lumbar spine have a short life expectancy, and posterior decompression and stabilisation will be sufficient to maintain stability and restore neurological function [3].

Surgical treatment

ANTERIOR APPROACH TO THE CERVICAL SPINE

Under general anaesthesia, the patient is placed supine on the operating table. The head rests on an adjustable head support and skull traction of 3-4 kg is applied. In lateral projection fluoroscopy, the spinal misalignment is reduced. To avoid injury to the recurrent laryngeal nerve, the spine is exposed through a left-sided anterolateral approach. The vertebral body is excised down to the posterior longitudinal ligament. If the pre-operative MRI showed intraspinal

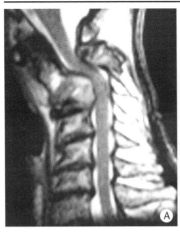
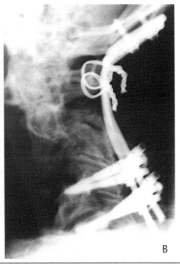

2 *A. A patient with cancer of the oesophagus who had severe pain and paraparesis due to destruction of C3, causing epidural compression of the spinal cord. An anterior approach was not feasible due to the poor quality of the soft tissues secondary to previous radiotherapy. B. Treated with reduction and posterior stabilisation from the occiput to C5 with the Olerud cervical fixation instrument.*

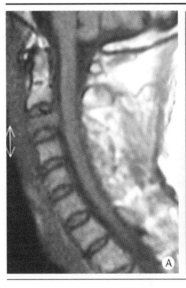
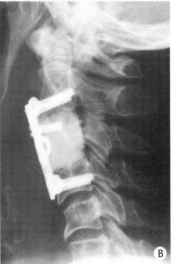

3 *A. This patient with lung cancer had pain due to a pathological fracture of the body of C3 but no neurological symptoms. B. Treated with anterior decompression and reconstruction with cement and AO/ASIF O'Roscoe plate.*

tumour growth, the ligament is resected to allow decompression of the epidural space. If, on the other hand, no tumour growth was seen deep to the ligament, the spinal canal is not opened. The spine is stabilised with a plate and the defect is filled with bone cement (*fig 3*). Most patients will require postoperative radiotherapy [12] which may cause problems in healing if a bone graft is used.

The standard exposure can be extended upwards into the upper cervical spine. By using nasal intubation, which allows the mouth to close, and by rotating the head slightly away from the exposure, it is usually possible, through this exposure, to reach the C1 arch from below.

POSTERIOR APPROACH TO THE CERVICAL SPINE

Just as in anterior surgery, the head is resting on a head support, skull traction is applied, and the spine is reduced to a correct position. A midline exposure is made. To use pedicle screws, the lateral border of the facet joints must be exposed (*fig 4*). If transarticular C1-C2 screws are planned, the upper and inner surfaces of the C2 pedicles should be exposed to the posterior capsule

of the C1-C2 facet joint. By doing so, both the entrance point and the direction of the screws can easily be decided. Pedicle screws are very useful in metastatic disease because of their superior biomechanical properties [8]. Probably the safest technique for inserting these screws is that described by Abumi [1]. The procedure is carried out under lateral projection fluoroscopy (*fig 5*). The insertion point is identified by anatomical landmarks and a large hole is prepared in the posterior cortex. With the aid of "tactile feedback", the pedicle is gently probed with a blunt instrument in the direction of the anticipated screw trajectory. The screw is inserted after tapping of the screw canal and the longitudinal members of the construct are assembled. The exact extent of fixation depends on the current mechanism of instability.

CRANIOCERVICAL JUNCTION

The special anatomical features and biomechanical properties of the craniocervical junction must be taken into consideration for the analysis of metastases in the upper cervical spine. The vertebrae in this region are very mobile. The occiput - C1

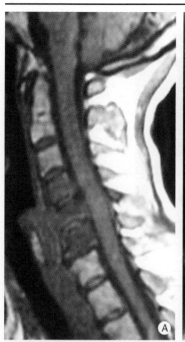
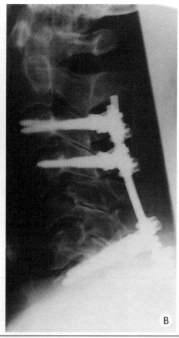

4 *A. Patient with breast cancer and pathological fractures of C4, C5 and C6 causing pain.*
B. Treated with laminectomy and posterior fusion from C3 to T2 with the Olerud cervical fixation instrument.

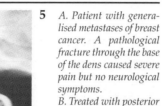

5 *A. Patient with generalised metastases of breast cancer. A pathological fracture through the base of the dens caused severe pain but no neurological symptoms.*
B. Treated with posterior fusion C1-C2 with the Olerud cervical fixation instrument.

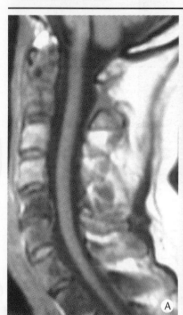
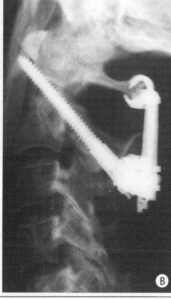

CERVICOTHORACIC JUNCTION

The principles of anterior cervical spine decompression and reconstruction can be applied down to the upper thoracic spine. It is usually possible to reach down to decompress T1 and to put screws in T2 above the jugulum (*fig 6*). To reach more distal vertebrae, the sternum has to be split. For reconstruction after a posterior approach to the cervicothoracic junction, a pedicle screw technique is recommended both for the thoracic and cervical vertebrae. If the fixation has to be extended down into the thoracic spine there are connection devices available which adjust cervical spine fixation instruments to traditional spine fixation instruments used in that region.

ANTERIOR APPROACH TO THE THORACIC AND LUMBAR SPINE

In most cases of pathological fracture of the spine, the whole vertebral body is collapsed, pressing the spinal cord or cauda equina backwards. To restore the integrity of the anterior and medial columns, and reduce the kyphotic deformity, full access to the vertebral bodies is required. A costotransversectomy approach will not be sufficient in most cases. Therefore, an anterior thoracotomy approach is recommended to reach tumours from the upper thoracic spine to the upper lumbar spine. Access to L1 and occasionally L2 is achieved by resection of the 10th rib and incision of the diaphragm (*fig 7*). To reach L2, L3 and L4, a retroperitoneal approach is needed.

The patient is placed in the lateral decubitus position with the arm over the head. The curved incision follows the rib to be resected, which should be the same as the involved vertebra or the one above. For mid- or upper thoracic approaches, either a right or left thoracotomy may be chosen, but for lower thoracic and upper lumbar lesions, the left side is preferable to avoid the liver. The incision stretches from the anterior axillary line towards the paraspinal muscles. The latissimus dorsi muscle is mobilised posteriorly and the serratus anterior muscle anteriorly. For the thoracotomy, the same rib or the one above the vertebra involved is resected. It is easy to count the ribs by moving the hand under the scapula to the second rib. After resection of the rib, the parietal pleura is incised and the lung is either deflated or just retracted. The segmental vessels running across the midline of each vertebra are identified and ligated. Using blunt dissection anteriorly, a finger should reach around the vertebra so that a malleable retractor can be placed to protect the great vessels.

If the involved vertebra is not obviously macroscopically abnormal, the vertebra should be identified with an image intensifier. A complete vertebrectomy is performed by curettage using curettes or a bone nibbler. If the bone is very hard, a high speed burr may be used. The intervertebral

joint has a large range of motion in extension and flexion whereas the C1 - C2 joint contributes to half the cervical spine's axial rotation [17]. Biomechanically, the spine starts as a two pillar structure at the craniocervical junction and transforms into a three pillar structure at the isthmus of C2 [11]. Thus, metastatic destruction above this area will behave differently biomechanically than it will below. If a lesion involves an occipital condyle or the lateral mass of C1, an insufficiency of axial stability will occur resulting in a lateral tilt of the head. The patient is likely to experience severe mechanical pain, whereas neurological symptoms will be absent or slight. A reconstruction will have to breach the insufficient area and basically extend from the occiput to the intact cervical spine below the lesion. The further down the

fixation is extended, the more mobility will be lost. In such cases, it is necessary to pay attention to the craniocervical alignment as an incorrect position will result in discomfort for the patient.

With a pathological dens fracture, if the lateral masses of C2 are intact, a special reconstruction can be considered to preserve craniocervical motion. Intramedullary screws are placed inside the dens and incorporated in a bone cement replacement of the C2 vertebral body. The bone cement is fixed with a plate to C3 [19, 20]. If the destruction involves the lateral masses of C2, the axial rotation cannot be preserved. The spine can be stabilised by placing screws in the anterior arch and lateral masses of C1 and then imbedded in bone cement, fixed to the lower cervical spine with a plate, thus preserving some craniocervical motion [15].

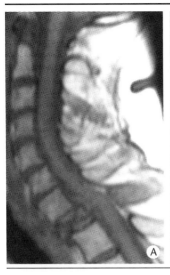
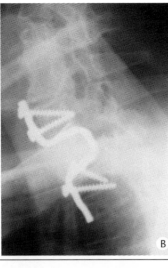

6 *A. Metastasis of thyroid cancer in T1 causing local pain and radiculopathy in both arms.*
B. Treated with anterior decompression and stabilised with a U-bent AO/ASIF reconstruction plate and cement. The configuration of the plate permits screw insertion into the body of C2 from above, as the jugulum prohibits horizontal insertion.

discs above and below the vertebra are also removed without damaging the endplates of the adjacent vertebrae. The intervertebral foramen is identified so as to appreciate the posterior margin of the vertebral body. The posterior wall of the vertebral body is removed to provide decompression of the spinal cord if the pre-operative MRI shows the posterior longitudinal ligament is intact and there is no tumour tissue in the spinal canal. If there is tumour in the canal, this must be gently removed from the spinal cord to achieve decompression.

Mechanical stability is restored by a plate or rods fixed with screws into the body of the adjacent vertebrae. The instrumentation can be used to reduce the kyphotic deformity, and the space created by the vertebral and intervertebral disc removal is filled with acrylic bone cement. There is seldom an indication for bone grafts in metastatic bone disease. Studies have not shown that the heat of the cement will injure the spinal cord but care must be taken that the cement itself does not cause epidural compression. After the cement has set, the rods or plate can be loosened to allow compression of the cement against the adjacent vertebral endplates and then tightened again.

The mid-lumbar spine is approached through an anterolateral incision running between the twelfth rib and the iliac crest. The retroperitoneal space is accessed by dividing the abdominal wall muscles and, by blunt dissection, the peritoneum and fat are moved anteriorly exposing the sympathetic trunk, the psoas muscle and the vertebral bodies. The segmental vessels are identified and ligated, and corporectomy and stabilisation are similar to that for thoracic and upper lumbar vertebrae.

POSTERIOR APPROACH TO THE THORACIC AND LUMBAR SPINE

For posterior decompression and stabilisation, the patient is placed prone and

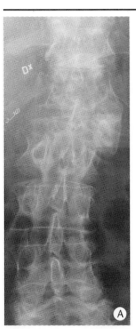
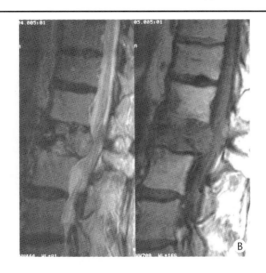
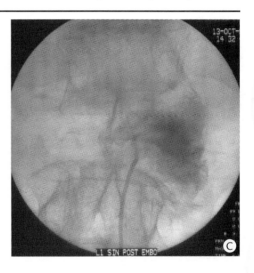

7 *A. Patient with metastasis of kidney cancer in the body of L1 causing pain and weakness in lower extremities. Note translational deformity.*
B. MRI shows epidural compression due to pathological fracture and tumour.
C. Pre-operative embolisation was performed. Note the hypervascular tumour before embolisation.
D. Treated with anterior decompression and reconstruction with cement and a Z-plate.

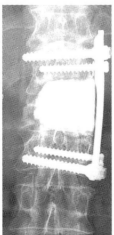
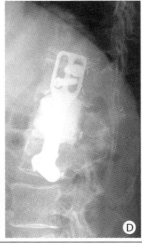

the appropriate level is identified using fluoroscopy. The involved vertebra can also be marked with charcoal by the radiologist pre-operatively. A longitudinal incision in the midline is extended on both sides of the spinous process and the subperiosteal dissection is extended laterally to the transverse processes in the thoracic spine and to the facets in the lumbar spine. Decompression of the spinal cord or cauda equina is achieved by removing the spinous process of the involved vertebra and removing tumour tissue that often grows as a cuff around the dural sac. The pedicles are often destroyed by tumour and with a curette, tumour tissue compressing the dural sac can be removed. Stabilisation is performed with rods based on pedicle screw and/or hook fixation (*fig 8*). Bone grafts are seldom indicated.

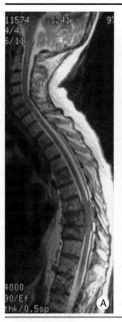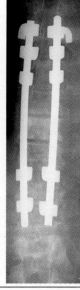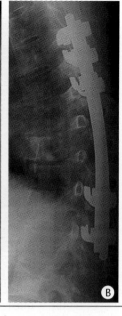

8 *A. Patient with metastases of prostate cancer in the mid-thoracic spine. Epidural compression caused severe neurological symptoms with inability to walk.*
B. Treated with posterior decompression and stabilisation with Isola rods and hooks from T5 to T10.

References

[1] Abumi K, Kaneda K. Pedicle screw fixation for nontraumatic lesions of the cervical spine. *Spine* 1997 ; 22 (16) : 1853-1863

[2] Atanasiu JP, Badatcheff F, Pidhorz L. Metastatic lesions of the cervical spine. A retrospective analysis of 20 cases. *Spine* 1993 ; 18 (10) : 1279-1284

[3] Bauer HCF. Posterior decompression and stabilization for spinal metastases. Analysis of 67 consecutive patients. *J Bone J Surg* 1997 ; 79 : 514-522

[4] Bauer HCF, Wedin R. Survival after surgery for spinal and extremity metastases. Prognostication in 241 patients. *Acta Orthop Scand* 1995 ; 66 (2) : 143-146

[5] Byrne TN. Spinal cord compression from epidural metastases. *N Engl J Med* 1992 ; 327 (9) : 614-619

[6] Galasko CS. Mechanism of lytic and blastic metastatic disease of bone. *Clin Orthop* 1982 ; 169 : 20-27

[7] Harrington KD. Anterior decompression and stabilization of the spine as a treatment for vertebral collapse and spinal cord compression from metastatic malignancy. *Clin Orthop* 1988 ; 233 : 177-1797

[8] Jones EL, Heller JG, Silcox DH, Hutton WC. Cervical pedicle screws versus lateral mass screws. Anatomic feasibility and biomechanical comparison. *Spine* 1997 ; 22 (9) : 977-982

[9] Jonsson B, Jonsson H, Karlstrom G, Sjostrom L. Surgery of cervical spine metastases: a retrospective study. *Eur Spine J* 1994 ; 3 (2) : 76-83

[10] Jonsson H, Sjostrom L, Karlstrom G, Olerud S. Internal stabilization of pathological fractures in the cervical spine. *Acta Orthop Scand* 1988 ; 59 : 91-92

[11] Louis R. Spinal stability as defined by the three-column spine concept. *Anat Clin* 1985 ; 7 (1) : 33-42

[12] Missenard G, Lapresle P, Cote D. Local control after surgical treatment of spinal metastatic disease. *Eur Spine J* 1996 ; 5 (1) : 45-50

[13] Nakamura M, Toyama Y, Suzuki N, Fujimura Y. Metastases of the upper cervical spine. *J Spinal Disord* 1996 ; 9 (3) : 195-201

[14] Olerud C, Andersson S, Svensson B, Bring J. Cervical spine fractures in the elderly: factors influencing survival in 65 cases. *Acta Orthop Scand* 1999 ; 70 (5) : 509-513

[15] Olerud C, Jonsson B. Surgical palliation of symptomatic spinal metastases. *Acta Orthop Scand* 1996 ; 67 (5) : 513-522

[16] Olerud C, Sjostrom L, Jonsson JRH, Karlstrom G. Posterior reduction of a pathologic spinal fracture. A case of indirect anterior dural decompression. *Acta Orthop Scand* 1992 ; 63 (3) : 345-346

[17] Panjabi M, Dvorak J, Duranceau J, Yamamoto I, Gerber M, Rauschning W, Bueff HU. Three-dimensional movements of the upper cervical spine. *Spine* 1988 ; 13 (7) : 726-730

[18] Rao S, Badani K, Schildhauer T, Borges M. Metastatic malignancy of the cervical spine. A nonoperative history. *Spine* 1992 ; 17 (10 Suppl) : 407-412

[19] Siegal T, Tiqva P, Siegal T. Vertebral body resection for epidural compression by malignant tumors. Results of 47 consecutive operative procedures. *J Bone Joint Surg* 1985 ; 67 (3) : 375-382

[20] Sjostrom L, Olerud S, Karlstrom G, Hamberg H, Jonsson H. Anterior stabilization of pathologic dens fractures. *Acta Orthop Scand* 1990 ; 61 (5) : 391-393

[21] Tokuhashi Y, Matsuzaki H, Toriyama S, Kawano H, Ohsaka S. Scoring system for the preoperative evaluation of metastatic spine tumor prognosis. *Spine* 1990 ; 11 (15) : 1110-1113

Systems of external contention

I Kempf
LE Pidhorz

Abstract. – Casts ensure good immobilisation for the conservative treatment of fractures or the progressive correction of deformity.

Plaster is the reference material for casts and has been in use since the19[th] century. There are codified rules concerning such immobilisation, allowing preparation of a "comfortable" cast which is well accepted by the patient. A plaster cast can be prepared by a technician, but always under the control of a medical doctor. One must explain to the patient why this type of treatment was selected and inform him about the need for monitoring by a general physician and the patient himself to avoid complications, in particular compartment syndrome and thromboembolism.

Since the 1970s, new synthetic materials have been used for external contention, for specific indications or following a plaster cast. In comparison with plaster, the new materials are lighter, stiffer and radiolucent; however, they are more difficult to prepare and more expensive.

Immobilisation by external contention is a therapeutic method which can be used alone in conservative treatment or after a surgical operation.

Keywords: external contention, conservative treatment, plaster cast, synthetic resins.

Introduction

Casts maintain immobilisation for conservative treatment of a fracture or progressive correction of a deformity. Various types of immobilisation have been used since prehistoric times. From antiquity, the materials used have had two major disadvantages: sensitivity to humidity and insufficient solidity over time. It appears that the plaster cast was introduced by the Persians around the 10th century. The use of bands sprinkled with dry plaster and the method of making the cast are attributed to Mathijsen, a 19th century Dutch physician. Modern chemistry has allowed improvement of the plaster bands and today, plaster casts are made within a short time, have good mechanical resistance and pose no risk of secondary deformation.

Plaster is still the most widely used material, although new materials have appeared which are lighter, easier to use and more comfortable for the patient. These materials may be considered as additions to – and not replacements of – plaster.

Ivan Kempf, M.D., Professeur honoraire de chirurgie orthopédique et traumatologique à la Faculté de Médecine de Strasbourg, Laboratoire de Biomécanique, 4, rue Kirschleger, 67000 Strasbourg, France.
Laurent E Pidhorz, M.D., Praticien hospitalier, Chirurgien orthopédiste et traumatologique, Centre Hospitalier du Mans, 194, avenue Rubillard, 72000 Le Mans, France.

Plaster casts [7]

MATERIALS

The plaster used is based on a natural product, gypsum (hydrated calcium sulphate). Associated with organic solvents, this crushed sulphate is placed on gauze bands and heated to 150 °C. When wet, the plaster is transformed into gypsum, which is characterised by long thin crystals which are tightly interwoven. After the water has evaporated, it becomes a solid mass. The drying process gives a thin porosity to the plaster, which favours skin ventilation. The plaster begins to set within 100 seconds to 5 minutes. The drying time varies from 30 to 48 hours, depending of the thickness of the cast, the humidity of the air, the ambient temperature and the air circulating around the cast.

MAKING THE CAST [2, 7]

The basic rules for making a cast are the same whatever the materials used. We will describe the procedure for a plaster cast. It is important to adhere to these rules; otherwise there is a risk of malunion or skin ulceration. Making the cast must be considered a medical act, to be performed by a medical doctor or by well-trained auxiliary personnel under the supervision of a doctor.

– The cast must be as solid and as light as possible.

– The skin should be protected with a tubular stockinet.

– The cast should be moulded onto the limb and smoothed before drying.

– The cast should never extend beyond the metacarpophalangeal joints of the upper limbs. For the lower extremities, it must sustain the plantar side of the toes or stop at the roots of the toes. It must never cover the extremities of the limbs, unless there is a specific indication.

– All circular casts ensuring contention of a recent injury must be split longitudinally, end to end and "to the last thread" after hardening, in order to avoid compression due to oedema.

■ Preparation

The cast should be prepared in one session, without interruption. The limb is covered with a cotton tubular stockinet of the appropriate diameter, which is first rolled up. After skin preparation, it is then applied by unrolling; creases or wrinkles are to be avoided as they may be a source of local irritation or skin ulceration. Padding is used to protect bony projections and the various pressure zones; it is usually made of orthopaedic cotton wool. The padding also makes it easier to open and remove the cast.

A double stockinet without cotton wool can be used in cases of conservative reduction to allow better modelling of the plaster, but in this case it is imperative that it be split. Some surgeons protect the pressure zones with felt.

The plaster bands are prepared, according to their size and their characteristics, as well as the splints which reinforce the cast. The water should be cold or slightly lukewarm (20-25° C) and changed between each cast. Increasing the temperature of the water will shorten the time until the plaster sets.

The position of the limb is defined before making the cast. This position can be maintained by the patient, who is comfortably installed, or by an assistant who supports the limb with his hands held flat, without gripping it with his fingers. The criteria for positioning are discussed in the following pages. The position must not be modified during drying of the plaster; otherwise, there is the risk of excessive compression occurring at the flexion creases of the joints, which can cause ulceration or vascular or nerve compression.

■ *Immersion and application*

The plaster bands are kept in the water until there are no more bubbles. They are then lightly pressed to eliminate the water, but without real wringing which would eliminate too much plaster. They are applied on the stockinet following the anatomical shape of the limb. The band is unrolled with one hand, avoiding wrinkles; at the same time, the other hand spreads and smoothes the unrolled band. This smoothing avoids layering of the cast, ensures homogeneity of the plaster and eliminates air bubbles. At the flexion creases of the joints, the bands must not be applied transversally, otherwise a source of constriction may be created. As each band is unrolled, it covers half of the width of the previous band. The stockinet is turned inside out at the extremities of the cast before the last bands are applied to avoid direct contact between the plaster and the skin. The plaster is modelled with the hand flat to avoid leaving fingerprints. The cast should be smoothed with the ulnar side of the hand, the first web or a humidified piece of plastic or latex. The solidity of the cast does not depend of the number of bands used, but rather on the distribution of the bands.

A note should be made on the cast indicating the date it was applied, the estimated dates for changing and removal, the names of the prescribing physician and the person who prepared the cast, and, if applicable, a sketch of the fracture. The cast will dry within 36 to 48 hours. Weight-bearing is allowed after 48 hours. Casts should never be dried by artificial means, nor placed on a hard surface, in order to avoid deformation.

Two other classical rules must be emphasised:

– For fracture immobilisation, the joints above and below the fracture must be included in the cast.

– The bands must not be too tight to avoid constriction after drying.

Sarmiento [6] has proposed changes to the above rules, and these will be discussed later.

Once the cast is finished, if the injury is recent, the cast must be split from one end to the other; this will avoid compression and allow spreading the two edges of the cast, should this be necessary due to oedema. This split is guided by a cord placed on the stockinet before preparing the cast. It is necessary to check that there is no compression and that the functional possibilities of the joints above and below the fracture are preserved. After the oedema has subsided, the cast is closed with a plaster band. The patient must be informed about care of the cast and monitoring of symptoms.

■ *Removal*

For plaster casts, removal is carried out with an oscillating saw. The cast is split longitudinally and removed with pliers or scissors. Care must be taken not to cut the cast near bony projections to avoid wounding the skin.

ADVANTAGES OF PLASTER CASTS

The general advantages of plaster casts include:

– Relative ease of preparation.

– Low cost compared to that of the more recent materials.

– Plaster is well tolerated by most patients, with few allergic reactions.

– The porosity of the plaster allows ventilation of the skin.

The specific advantages of plaster casts for the treatment of fractures include:

– The cast is innocuous.

– The risk of infection is reduced.

– Good mechanical quality of the callus.

– In case of imperfect reduction, alterations can be made by cast wedging.

– Better cosmetic results (absence of scars).

DISADVANTAGES OF PLASTER CASTS

The general disadvantages of plaster casts include:

– Discomfort due to immobilisation of the joints above and below the fracture, especially in elderly patients.

– Risk of thromboembolism and other complications.

The specific disadvantages of plaster casts in the treatment of fractures are:

– Imprecision of reduction.

– Heterogeneous radio-transparency which makes it difficult to monitor fractures by X-ray (for joint fractures, carpal or tarsal fractures, and in the case of osteoporosis).

COMPLICATIONS

Complications are frequent and have been called by some "the plaster disease". Combined with the inescapable discomfort of wearing a cast, these complications explain the relative unpopularity of casts with patients. In addition, due to the risk of complications, the surgeon must ensure that the patient is monitored during healing, an important task which some wrongly consider to be fastidious.

■ *Orthopaedic complications*

Secondary fracture displacement

This is due to several factors, which may be associated:

– The limits of this method: the cast provides an imperfect immobilisation of the fragments, especially in the case of unstable fractures, and more so in some locations (arm, thigh).

– Subsidence of oedema, resorption of the haematoma surrounding the fracture and amyotrophy, which can be detected by a radiolucent line between the cast and the outline of the limb.

– Weakening of the cast.

This displacement can be avoided by clinical and radiological follow-up, by early closing of the split cast after subsidence of the oedema, by reinforcement of the cast or even better by changing it in case of damage, by regular muscular contractions under the plaster and by early weight-bearing. If secondary fracture displacement occurs, reduction can be performed again under general anaesthesia.

Stiffness after cast removal

Walking and appropriate exercises while in the cast can attenuate stiffness. Stiffness occurs during the treatment of diaphyseal fractures but disappears more or less after physiotherapy. Sarmiento has made a significant contribution to the prevention of this complication by recommending the release after 10 days of the joints above and below the fracture, early joint mobilisation and early weight-bearing, The stiffness occurring after joint fractures is much more stubborn and frequently leaves permanent sequelae. Therefore, treatment of such fractures is almost always surgical.

Reflex sympathetic dystrophy (Sudeck-Leriche syndrome)

This is a fearsome and unpredictable complication. Its symptoms are well known. The outcome is not always reversible and can lead to definitive anatomical and functional sequelae.

■ Cutaneous complications

Cutaneous complications are frequent with circular casts.

Some minor complications are common after cast removal: desquamation, dry skin, increased pilosity, cyanosis of the extremities. These will disappear with appropriate care.

On the other hand, cutaneous ulcerations can occur at any time during cast immobilisation, especially at the level of the bony projections. Ranging from simple skin irritations to deep sores, these lesions can be revealed by suspicious spotting on the cast surface or by signs of infection. Such complications are avoidable if the cast is carefully prepared and regularly monitored. If ulceration is suspected, a window should be made in the cast or it should be removed.

■ Serious complications

These are exceptional and can be avoided by good supervision of the patient.

Thrombophlebitis and thromboembolic disease

These are a frequent and serious complication of immobilisation of the lower limbs. Early diagnosis is made difficult due to the presence of the cast. The patient may present symptoms such as pain or constriction under the cast, rapid pulse, high temperature, oedema of the toes, or anguish, but often this complication is first recognised due to the more or less obvious symptoms of embolism. After cast removal, the diagnosis must be confirmed by clinical examination, phlebography or echo-Doppler, to be followed by appropriate treatment. Systematic prophylaxis is imperative. The surgeon should prescribe the appropriate medication, and the patient's general practitioner must ensure that it is taken until the end of immobilisation.

Complications involving the nervous system

Rare at the upper limbs, these complications usually concern the lateral popliteal nerve of the lower limb.

Vascular complications

Vascular complications are the most dangerous, especially in upper limb immobilisation for fractures in children and in leg fractures. Symptoms such as pain, cyanosis or livid extremities, dysaesthesia or anaesthesia, immobility of fingers or toes require that the cast be removed.

Two situations can exist:

– The most frequent is absence of pulse due to an arterial lesion, which must be confirmed by arteriography and followed by emergency vascular restoration.

– The existence of a compartment syndrome with excess pressure in the muscle

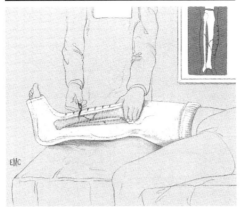

1 *Cast wedging: the exact level is located on the X-ray by metallic marks.*

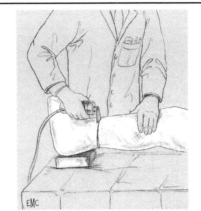

2 *Cast wedging: An almost complete circumferential section of the cast with an oscillating saw.*

compartments, the presence of pulse, some dysaesthesia. Unless there is immediate decompression, this very dangerous complication can lead to definitive sequelae in the form of Volkmann's Syndrome.

In conclusion, for all circular plaster casts:

– when treating fresh fractures, the cast must be split along its entire length to avoid compression;

– careful clinical monitoring is mandatory;

– when there is suspected ischaemia, the cast must be removed and emergency treatment instituted for a muscular lesion or compartment syndrome.

Cast wedging ("gypsotomy")

In some cases of reduction of fractures of the long bones, it may be necessary to correct the axis after the cast has been applied (*fig 1, 2, 3, 4*). Cast wedging allows angular correction by means of an almost circumferential section made on the dry cast, leaving only a small hinge of plaster. This is carried out without general anaesthesia. The cast is opened and fixed at the correct position by a wooden or cork wedge of the appropriate size, reinforced by a few plaster bands.

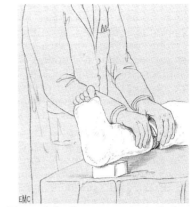

3 *The cast is fixed by an appropriately sized wooden or cork wedge.*

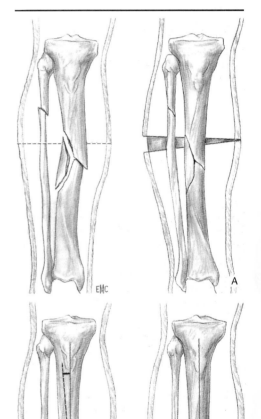

4 *Cast wedging: correction in varus (A) or valgus (B).*

Monitoring the cast-immobilised patient

The rules for supervision must be rigorously followed for the duration of the immobilisation. If the patient is discharged immediately after the cast is applied, he must be given precise instructions concerning the cast itself (condition, suspicious spots on the cast surface) and possible symptoms – pain under the cast (sleep-preventing, shooting, not influenced by the limb position) or sensations of irritation, dysaesthaesia or burning. During immobilisation, the patient should undergo regular clinical examination at the extremities of the cast (motion, trophicity, colour, cyanosis, sensitivity, oedema, smell) and regular X-ray controls.

The discovery of any of these signs, even if the pulp or peripheral pulse rates are normal, requires immediate consultation, opening of the cast (stockinet included), raising the limb, measuring compartmental pressure and, if necessary, a fasciotomy in the case of compartment syndrome.

Golden rules:

– Always take the patient's complaints seriously.

– If the patient has symptoms, make a window in the cast, split it or change it; this is better than committing the sin of omission.

Cast immobilisation according to location

The types of casts currently in use will be described, with the appropriate material and preparation for each location. The cast is always prepared beginning at the proximal part of the limb and continuing to the extremity. The goals of treatment should be explained to the patient, as well as the duration of immobilisation and the different sequences of the treatment.

CAST IMMOBILISATION OF THE UPPER LIMB [2, 3, 6]

Rings and bracelets should be removed. The functional position is with the elbow in 90° flexion, the forearm in neutral pronation, the wrist in 20° dorsiflexion and the fingers in the intrinsic plus position (metacarpophalangeal joints in flexion and interphalangeal joints in extension). The patient is placed in a sitting position or in decubitus, the upper limb sustained by an assistant or by traction.

■ *The shoulder spica* (fig 5)

This immobilisation is now rarely used; most indications are surgical or orthopaedic with the use of manufactured abduction apparatuses or a simple elbow bandage. The shoulder spica immobilises the shoulder, arm, elbow and forearm. The patient is positioned sitting or in decubitus; the cast has two parts: thoracic and brachial.

– The thoraco-abdominal brace with 2 straps is prepared first.

– The limb is immobilised with 2 splints attached to the brace with the straps; the armpit is protected.

– The position of the limb in relation to the brace is generally with the shoulder in 45°

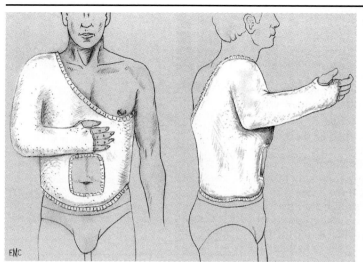

5   *The shoulder spica.*

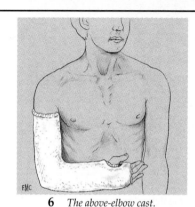

6   *The above-elbow cast.*

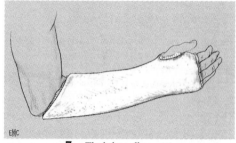

7   *The below-elbow cast.*

abduction, 45° antepulsion and neutral rotation. The position of the upper limb is the same as for an above-elbow cast.

– The two splints are jointed with circular bands and the contralateral strap is cut and removed.

– The cast can be reinforced with a wooden splint placed between the arm and the lower part of the brace; the splint is surrounded with plaster.

■ *The above-elbow cast* (fig 6)

The elbow, forearm and wrist are immobilised (elbow in 90° flexion, the forearm in neutral pronation, the wrist in 20° dorsiflexion), unless there is an indication to do otherwise.

– The stockinet and the cotton wool are placed on the limb, making a hole for the thumb. The cast is begun proximally, under the armpit and over the greater tubercle of the humerus, taking care not to compress the radial nerve at the posterior aspect of the arm.

– At the level of the elbow crease, the bands should not be placed transversally, unless an anterior chamber is first made. It is preferable to apply the bands in a figure-of-eight fashion. At this point, it is imperative not to modify the angle of the cast.

– At the dorsal aspect of the hand, the cast is stopped at the level of the metacarpal heads to allow effective drainage of the

dorsal veins. At its volar aspect, the cast is stopped at the proximal flexion crease to allow flexion of the metacarpophalangeal joints. The base of the thumb must be kept free to permit adduction.

– The wrist is maintained higher than the elbow with a sling.

This immobilisation is used in the conservative treatment of elbow, forearm or wrist injuries, in the postoperative period after operations on the upper limb, or for treatment of fractures of the humerus by a hanging cast (with a weight fixed to the forearm part of the apparatus).

■ *The below-elbow cast* (fig 7)

This cast immobilises the forearm and the wrist; the elbow is left free.

– The cast is placed two finger-breadths below the elbow flexion crease, the freedom of which is checked again after the cast is finished.

– The distal limits are the same as for the above-elbow cast.

– The cast has to be very well moulded to avoid its sliding and losing its contention action.

This cast is used for forearm and wrist injuries, most of the time 3 or 4 weeks after an above-elbow cast immobilisation or after wrist surgery.

Alternatives

● *The carpal scaphoid below-elbow cast* (fig 8)

The limits are the same as for the below-elbow cast with the addition of a band

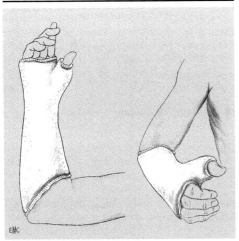

8   *The carpal scaphoid below-elbow cast. The thumb is immobilised in abduction and opposition; the interphalangeal joint is not included.*

which immobilises the thumb, metacarpophalangeal joint included, with maximal abduction and anteflexion. This cast is used for carpal scaphoid injuries or ligament ruptures of the first metacarpophalangeal joint. For scaphoid fractures, some surgeons recommended an above-elbow plaster cast during the first weeks.

- *The gauntlet cast*

This is a carpal scaphoid below-elbow cast which stops at the wrist level. It is sometimes used for sprains of the metacarpophalangeal joint of the thumb.

CAST IMMOBILISATION OF THE PELVIC RING AND LOWER LIMB

All of these casts allow standing, with the inclusion of a heel piece or a walking sole, or with the foot free. This avoids long immobilisation in bed and allows mechanical prompting of the skeleton and muscles (dynamisation) which is beneficial for healing. Preparation of such casts often requires an assistant. The patient is positioned in decubitus or with the leg hanging. The functional position for the lower limb is with the knee in 10° of flexion and the ankle in 90° of flexion, maintaining the axis of the hind foot. Systematic anti-thrombosis prophylaxis must be administered.

■ **The simple hip plaster spica** *(fig 9)*

This immobilises the pelvis and the entire lower limb. It is still used for young children, but only exceptionally for adults.

Place the stockinet from the base of the thorax to the proximal part of the thigh and a ball of padding at the pit of the stomach to allow expansion after food intake (epigastric window). The stockinet from the lower limb overlaps it.

The patient must be positioned on the table with a pelvic support.

Mould the iliac crests, the pubis, the greater trochanters, the protrusions of the knee and the malleoli.

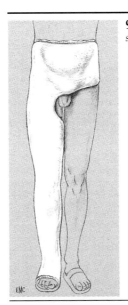

9   *The simple hip plaster spica.*

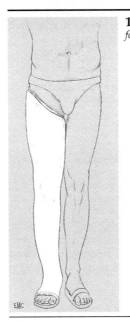

10   *The KAF (knee, ankle, foot) cast.*

Reinforce the cast with splints, especially at the junction between the two parts of the cast; a splint is placed around the top of the thigh.

Alternative: the double hip plaster spica

This very heavy apparatus, which should be applied in decubitus, is necessary for young children to block the pelvis in cases of congenital dislocation of the hip.

■ **The KAF (knee-ankle-foot) cast** *(fig 10)*

This is one of the most frequently used casts. The limb is immobilised in the functional position (if necessary, this cast is made with a knee support under the popliteal fossa and with an assistant who maintains knee flexion). The patient is in decubitus, with the homolateral buttock heightened by padding (to allow correction of the automatic external rotation of the limb).

- Begin the cast by making a good trochanteric support.

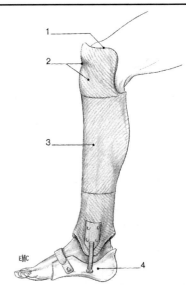

11   *Sarmiento's apparatus (functional below-knee brace). 1. Lateral anti-rotation fins applied on the lateral part of the condyles; 2. anterior shield moulded on the patellar tendon. 3. cast muff; 4. sole with an articulated heel.*

- Reinforce the posterior part with a long splint and the anterior part with a short one.

- Stop the cast under the metatarsal heads or make a sole under the toes.

- Remove the knee support and place a band around the knee.

- If the patient is to walk, place a heel piece or a walking sole.

The indications for this cast are numerous and concern all age groups: postoperative immobilisation after bone, tendon or joint surgery, orthopaedic treatment of tibial or ankle fractures, and sometimes hind foot fractures. This long cast is unquestionably awkward, especially in older patients. It may also lead to stiffness, amyotrophy and cutaneous lesions.

■ **The Sarmiento apparatus** [4, 5, 6] *(fig 11)*

In 1967, Sarmiento introduced a new concept in the treatment of leg fractures based on three principles:

- Immobilisation of the joints above and below a fracture is not essential for consolidation.

- The early resumption of function furthers osteogenesis.

- The strict immobilisation of a fracture is not a preliminary condition for healing.

His cast is placed between the 12th and the 15th day after the injury. It is composed of:

1) An upper part inspired by the patellar tendon bearing prosthesis used in leg amputations. This is composed of an anterior shield which goes up three finger-breadths above the superior limit of the patella. It is moulded on the patellar tendon and extended by lateral anti-rotation fins applied on the lateral part of the condyles

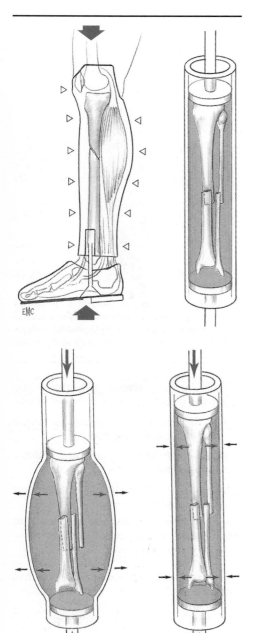

12 *Hydraulic principle of Sarmiento's method: unstretchable and incompressible system which puts a cap around the fracture.*

which leave the popliteal fossa completely free. In this way, full articular freedom is obtained, with preservation of rotational stability.

2) The muff cast itself is applied with tight contact on the leg and moulded onto the tibial tuberosities and on the medial aspect of the tibia. Because the aponeuroses around the muscles of the leg cannot be stretched, this "total" contact converts the leg segment into a incompressible system that maintains its shape, stabilises and "puts a cap around" the leg, and prevents angulation and shortening *(fig 12)*.

3) A distal part, which may be made in two ways:

– either it stops at the ankle, bearing on the malleoli, with the anterior and posterior edges trimmed to allow ankle movements.

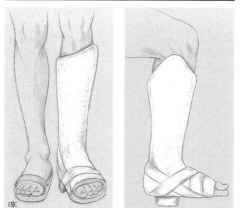

13 *The below-knee cast: the heel is in the tibial axis.*

A plastic articulation with a heel is fixed to its extremity to allow wearing a shoe. This is the true functional brace.

– or the foot is moulded in the cast and the entire apparatus is fitted with a sole or a heel. This is the Sarmiento boot.

This apparatus can also be made with thermoplastic. Sarmiento extended these same principles to diaphyseal fractures of the humerus. On the other hand, for fractures of the femur and the forearm, Sarmiento has found few adepts.

■ *The knee and ankle cast or plaster girdle*

Its preparation is identical to that of the KAF cast; it ends at the level of the malleoli. It immobilises the knee and allows tibiotalar mobility. It is used for bony or ligament lesions of the knee. It is frequently replaced by a posterior plaster splint or by removable splints.

■ *The below-knee cast* (fig 13)

This immobilises the ankle and the foot. It is made with the leg hanging, the foot at 90°, or with the patient in decubitus, the knee on a support, and the foot maintained at 90° by an assistant.

The cast is begun at the tibial tuberosity level. The popliteal fossa must be cleared to allow 90° of knee flexion. Laterally, the fibular head should be covered. The bands should not be placed just at the level of the fibula neck to avoid compression of the lateral popliteal nerve.

The below-knee cast should be reinforced with a posterior splint.

The cast should end at the level where the toes begin, or still better, a plantar sole should be made on which the toes rest.

In some cases, a heel may be placed in the continuation of the tibial axis.

The below-knee cast is widely used for injuries and after surgery of the ankle and foot. It can include a heel chamber, as proposed by Graffin, for fractures of the calcaneus.

CAST IMMOBILISATION OF THE SPINE [2, 3]

Reduction casts for scoliosis, such as the EDF cast, are discussed in another chapter and will not be presented here, nor will scoliosis contention systems made of synthetic materials.

■ *The collar brace*

This immobilises the cervical spine. The chin, ear lobes and occipital tuberosities are the upper limits of the cast, and it extends to the lowest ribs, or preferably to the iliac crests. The head is the neutral position for tilt and rotation and in slight anteflexion (10° to 20°). The cast is prepared with the patient sitting on a stool. The head is maintained with slight traction by a Gardner calliper hung from a pulley or held by an assistant who corrects its tilt and rotation.

Care must be taken to check for orthostatic low blood pressure or the frequent vagal faintness which may occur in these patients who have been bedridden some days before the collar is made.

Place a stockinet around the head and the neck, and link it with the stockinet of the brace. Make holes for the nose and the eyes. The various compression points are padded with felt, especially at the tracheal axis.

Begin the cast with a band put around the cervical spine, then make the thoracic part. Anterior and posterior splints must be crossed around the neck and lateral splints cover the shoulders.

Mould the neck, mandible, interscapular area and the sternal manubrium.

Release the ears and make an opening for the mouth. Release the armpits and the acromioclavicular joints to allow shoulder abduction.

This collar is indicated in orthopaedic treatment of undisplaced fractures of the spine. For fractures of the upper cervical spine, a frontal support (or headband) is added.

■ *The Böhler-type plaster brace* [1]

This apparatus allows contention of the thoracolumbar and lumbar spine. It is based on three-point support (manubrium, pubis and thoracolumbar spine *(fig 14)*). The upper limits of the brace are the top the manubrium and the 5th or 6th thoracic vertebra, and the lower limit the pubis and the sacrum. Classically, it is made in the decubitus position, with the sacral area and the top of the shoulders lying on two tables; a strap is placed at the level of the lesion and linked to a pulley fixed to the ceiling (a Cotrel table can be used). If reduction is not required, the cast is made on a standing patient with a lumbar lordosis; the patient is maintained by two assistants or by crutches. In the case of a recent fracture, the cast is made after the return of intestinal movements.

Dress the patient with a double stockinet before he is placed on the table. Protect the

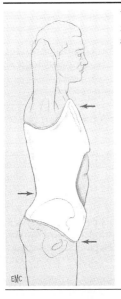

14 *The Böhler-type plaster brace with three-point support.*

iliac crests. Place a ball of padding at the pit of the stomach to facilitate cutting the epigastric window.

After the first bands have been applied, place splints along the entire height of the brace: anterior at the nipple lines, posterior on the spinous line, crossed in the lumbar area and at the armpits.

Mould the crests, and the superior and inferior supports. Release the armpits and the inguinal creases to allow hip flexion to 90°.

Remove the strap and finish the cast. Cut the epigastric window.

The patient must be instructed to avoid large food intake, but rather to eat small but frequent meals. In case of vomiting or stomach pain, the apparatus must be removed without hesitation. This brace is indicated for the reduction of some fractures of the inferior thoracic spine and the lumbar spine. After 6 weeks, this brace can be changed and replaced by a removable resin brace.

The new synthetic materials

In the 1970s, synthetic materials became available for orthopaedic immobilisation. Their preparation differs in some ways from that of plaster casts, and they are used for specific indications.

RESIN BANDS [3]

Used for immobilisation and contention, these bands are composed of a synthetic support made of woven fibres (glass, polyester and/or nylon) impregnated with a polyurethane resin which polymerises in the water. For the majority of indications, we prefer plaster bands for emergency immobilisation of injuries. Casts made of resin bands are often used after the plaster immobilisation.

■ *Preparation*

Preliminary preparation resembles that of a plaster cast. The stockinet is made of cotton or fire-resistant polypropylene (this material may lead to heavy perspiration). It is applied in the same manner as for a plaster cast and covered with synthetic orthopaedic wool. The resin bands are then prepared. They should be removed from their protective bag just before use; otherwise, they will polymerise on contact with the humidity in the air. The hands of the technician must be protected by latex gloves.

Before the cast is begun, the limb position is defined using the same criteria as for a plaster cast. This position must not be modified, due to the risk of inducing a flexion crease which could lead to skin ulceration.

■ *Immersion and application*

The resin bands are immersed in water until the bubbles disappear, taking care to note the location of the beginning of the band. The water should be at room temperature or lukewarm; hot water speeds up the polymerisation. After the bands are removed from the water, with only slight or no wringing, they are applied following the anatomy, without tightening and taking care not to create creases. Each band is unrolled, covering half of the width of the previous band (or two-thirds if greater stiffness is required). At the extremities of the cast, the stockinet is turned inside out after the first band is applied to avoid contact between the blunt edge of the resin and the skin. The bands polymerise quickly after wetting and must be applied within five minutes. The resin acquires its maximal hardness within 30 to 60 minutes. The manufacturers recommend 4 to 5 layers of resin (once back and forth, if the application technique is correct). The bands can also be applied without preliminary immersion in water, by wetting them with a spray or wrapping the cast with a wet cloth.

■ *Removal*

Removal is performed using an oscillating plaster saw with a special blade made of tempered steel or carbide tungsten, or with special shears. The apparatus is cut into two parts and taken off. Care should be taken that the heat of the blade does not lead to burns (cut the resin with small touches) and to avoid projections of fibre glass particles, especially into the eyes.

■ *Advantages of these materials*

– Lighter weight and greater stiffness of the cast.

– Radiolucency allowing better X-ray follow-up.

– The possibility of drying the cast with a hair-drier (set at the minimum position) in case of accidental contact with water. It is recommended not to wet the cast in a regular or prolonged fashion.

– Patients frequently request this kind of modern, water-resistant and coloured material.

■ *Disadvantages and specific complications*

– The cast requires more meticulous preparation than does a plaster cast. The synthetic bands are less malleable, which makes their application more difficult.

– Higher cost of a resin cast (5 to 10 times that of a plaster cast).

– The specific complications are mainly cutaneous. The vascular, neurological or orthopaedic complications are the same as for a plaster cast. However, the water-resistant nature of these resins does not allow normal ventilation of the skin, which can cause maceration, itching or smells. The exothermic reaction during drying can cause some burning, especially in the child.

– The impossibility of altering the set resin, requiring a complete change of cast in case of compression or creases.

– Emanation of isocyanate vapours during the polymerisation which can induce some allergies (asthmatic or cutaneous reactions) even up to 15 years afterwards.

■ *Indications*

Resin bands may be used in the following cases:

– In place of a postoperative plaster cast.

– In the immediate postoperative period after neurological surgery.

– To change a reduction brace for a spinal fracture (a removable apparatus can be made).

– For some fragile patients (paraplegia, arteritis, neuropathology).

Although it is possible to wet these casts, we advise against immersion in a swimming pool or in salt water to avoid maceration of the skin or cutaneous "salting". We do not feel that this sales argument for resin casts is appropriate, unless the apparatus is removable, because of the potential skin complications.

Thermoplastics

Other materials are available on the market which have the lightness of resin and the additional advantage of allowing alteration.

LOW TEMPERATURE THERMOPLASTICS

The advantage of these materials is that the cast can be made directly on the patient without preliminary moulding. They are used especially for small apparatuses. Light, radiolucent and well tolerated by the skin, these materials become stiff below 40° C and can be worked above this temperature. They soften in hot water between 55 and 80° C (according to the material) or with steam. Some local alterations can be made with a hair dryer, a steam boiler or by local wetting with hot water. Several groups of these materials exist: polyisoprenes, polyester copolymers, polycaprolactum and polyvinyl alcohol. Each product has its specific characteristics: elasticity, self-adherence, colour and texture changes during heating, malleability during cast making, speed of softening and cooling, resistance and upkeep of the apparatus.

■ *High and medium temperature thermoplastics*

Used for large apparatuses, they require preliminary moulding. Supple, semi-stiff or stiff, these materials are worked between 130° and 240° C. These materials may be made of polyethylene, polypropylene, copolymers (methacrylate, cellulose acetate), polymethyl methacrylate (PMMA), acrylic fibre glass, etc.

■ *Expanded foam materials*

Neofrakt® (expanded polyurethane foam) may be used for immobilisation of numerous parts of the body. Two liquids must be mixed and poured into the stockinet. This is then placed around the part to be immobilised and closed with a tab. These casts are easy and quick to make; however, this type of immobilisation is costly, does not allow alterations and the skin is poorly ventilated.

ORTHOSES

Orthoses made of thermoplastics are used in particular at the level of the limb extremities, especially the hand and wrist. They are removable. They can have various functions: simple immobilisation, or "static" or "dynamic" (active or passive) immobilisation. They can be custom-made (moulded on the patient) or manufactured (which makes them convenient, as they are always available ready to use).

The main orthoses available and their main indications are:

■ *For the upper limb*

Immobilisation of the:

– fingers (sprains of the interphalangeal joints, fractures of the phalanges);

– thumb (sprains of the metacarpophalangeal joint, root arthrosis);

– wrist, with more or less integration of one of the fingers (sprain or fracture of the wrist or carpus, De Quervain's tendinitis);

– hand (tendon suture, arthritis or neurological pathology).

In addition, passive and dynamic orthoses may be used for extension of the joints of the finger (post-traumatic stiffness or radial or ulnar paralysis) or for flexion of the joints (articular stiffness).

Active and dynamic orthoses, such as the Kleinert orthosis, may be used for section of the finger flexors or for active extension of the fingers in radial paralysis.

■ *For the lower limb*

Immobilisation:

– foot (paralysis of the lateral popliteal nerve, reducible equinus in neurological pathology);

– leg orthoses, such as a simple hip spica or KAF cast, are especially indicated for cerebral palsy patients or in degenerative neurological pathologies;

– Sarmiento's leg orthosis (in place of a cast for orthopaedic treatment of a leg fracture).

■ *For the spine*

An orthosis can be used in place of a brace for the treatment of a spinal fracture, in the treatment of scoliosis or kyphosis, for some cases of low back pain, in some rheumatological pathologies, after spinal surgery or in some neurological troubles of the spine.

References

[1] Böhler L. Die Technik der Knochenbruchbehandlung. Wien : W Mandrich, 1953

[2] Borgi R, Butel J. Manuel du traitement orthopédique des fractures des membres et des ceintures. Paris : Masson, 1981

[3] Fiches techniques d'immobilisations plâtrées. Vibraye : Laboratoires FISH - SMITH + NEPHEW, 2000

[4] Kempf I, Graf H, Lafforgue D, Francois JM, Anceau H. Traitement orthopédique des fractures de jambe selon la méthode de Sarmiento. *Rev Chir Orthop* 1980 ; 66 : 373-381

[5] Sarmiento A. A functional bracing of tibial and femoral shaft fractures. *Clin Orthop* 1972 ; 82 : 2-13

[6] Sarmiento A, Latta LL. Closed functional treatment of fractures. Berlin : Springer-Verlag, 1981

[7] Watson-Jones R. Fractures and joint injuries. Edinburgh : Churchill Livingstone, 1955

Traction treatment of fractures

F Langlais
JC Lambotte

Abstract. – The reliability of current internal fixation techniques and low morbidity of modern anaesthesia have limited the use of traction as a means of obtaining and maintaining fracture reduction. However, traction is still used for this purpose in acetabular fractures in adults. In some diaphyseal fractures of the femur or tibia, skeletal traction is useful while awaiting further treatment. Skin traction is an atraumatic technique that is used before surgery to relieve pain in some forms of trochanteric fracture. Combined traction and continuous passive motion can be used in some inoperable articular fractures of the knee. Finally, suspension in a splint can allow painless rehabilitation therapy in some complex fractures treated by internal fixation. We will describe six traction techniques, after indicating which technique is in our view most appropriate for each type of fracture. These techniques are:
– skin traction;
– skeletal traction using a proximal tibial Kirschner wire (acetabular fracture);
– skeletal traction using a calcaneal Kirschner wire (tibial traction);
– skeletal traction using a tibial Steinmann pin (acetabular fracture);
– traction combined with continuous passive motion (tibial plateau fracture);
– suspension (rehabilitation of operated articular fractures of the knee).

© 2001, Editions Scientifiques et Médicales Elsevier SAS. All rights reserved.

Keywords: skin traction, skeletal traction, continuous passive motion, suspension, Kirschner wire, Steinmann pin.

Traction techniques and their indications

The system used to provide traction varies with the desired traction weight and duration. For weights of no more than 3 kg applied for less than 3 days, skin traction is usually adequate and has the advantage of being simple. If a heavier weight (3 to 8 kg) is to be applied for up to four weeks, a Kirschner wire is usually well tolerated and effective. A Steinmann pin is recommended for longer traction treatment (up to two months), as tolerance is usually better than with a wire [1, 2].

The best indications for traction treatment are reviewed below.

SKIN TRACTION

Skin traction is used primarily to provide pain relief to a patient who is awaiting internal fixation of a fracture. The skin must

Frantz Langlais, Professor, Chef de service.
JC Lambotte, M.D., Praticien hospitalier.
Service de Chirurgie Orthopédique, traumatologie et réparatrice,
Hôpital Sud, 16, boulevard de Bulgarie, 35056 Rennes, France.

be unbroken. Non-adhesive foam strapping is usually preferred over adhesive strapping which can cause blistering and other complications. Skin traction is often used to achieve lower limb immobilisation in elderly patients with trochanteric fractures whose surgical treatment must be deferred for a few days to allow clearance from the body of drugs that contraindicate immediate anaesthesia.

SKELETAL TRACTION WITH A KIRSCHNER WIRE

A Kirschner wire driven through the proximal tibia is often used to apply a traction weight of more than 3 kg to avoid pain due to overlapping of bony fragments, for instance, in some fractures of the femoral or tibial shaft for which immediate surgical treatment is not possible or not desirable. Skeletal traction is indispensable to counteract the effects of muscle contracture. Furthermore, by pulling the wire through a double horizontal and vertical stirrup, the traction can be used to control rotation. Tolerance is usually good if the duration of the traction does not exceed four weeks. This technique is used mainly in femoral shaft fractures and acetabular fractures scheduled

for surgical therapy. Another indication is prevention of secondary displacement after internal fixation of comminuted acetabular fractures with very small fragments. Traction for three weeks ensures bonding of the fragments and is compatible with gentle passive rehabilitation therapy.

Traction with a Kirschner wire driven through the calcaneus can be used in some leg fractures with skin lesions which preclude direct internal fixation and where external fixation is not possible or not desirable. The wire driven through the calcaneus ensures reduction of the fracture and gives the skin lesions time to heal, so that surgery or orthopaedic treatment (cast or Sarmiento splint) can be used later.

SKELETAL TRACTION WITH A STEINMANN PIN THROUGH THE PROXIMAL TIBIA

This technique is used to obtain and to maintain reduction of acetabular fractures. A heavy weight is often applied initially to obtain reduction of the fracture. The traction is applied for about two months to allow bonding of the fragments. This eliminates the risk of secondary displacement. A Steinmann pin, 4 mm in diameter, usually

Table I. – Indications for different types of traction or suspension.

Type of fracture	Skin Traction	Skeletal Traction K-wire	Skeletal Traction S-Pin	Traction-Motion Mobilisation	Suspension
Trochanteric fracture (pre op)	+				
Acetabular fracture • Full orthopaedic treatment • Pre op • Post op (ORIF)		+ +	+		
Femoral head fracture Hip dislocation	+	+			
Femoral diaphysis fracture (pre op)		+			
Tibial fracture (pre op, or pre-orthop)		+			
Complex tibial plateau fracture (operation not recommended)				+	
Articular knee fracture (post op)					+

provides an excellent purchase on the bone and consequently is well tolerated during prolonged traction.

TRACTION WITH CONTINUOUS PASSIVE MOTION

Some articular fractures of the knee are inoperable, for instance, because there is contusion or a skin lesion in the area of the incision or because the fragments are so small as to compromise the chances of successful internal fixation. In this situation, traction is applied along the axis of the leg to ensure reduction by osteotaxis of the articular fragments (particularly in separation fractures of the tibial plateaux). A motorised system provides continuous passive flexion and extension of the knee to maintain range of motion.

SUSPENSION

Operated articular fractures of the knee require early mobilisation. In some comminuted fractures, the internal fixation is not strong enough to allow active mobilisation. Continuous passive motion provided by a motorised system is widely used in this situation. Alternatively, the leg

can be suspended in a splint to reduce the pull of gravity, thus facilitating rehabilitation therapy and nursing.

A recapitulation of the main indications for traction in lower limb fractures is provided (*table I*).

Skin traction *(fig 1)*

DESCRIPTION

Traction on the leg to obtain temporary immobilisation of a trochanteric fracture in an elderly patient, the goal being to relieve pain.

TECHNIQUE

Non-adhesive foam-rubber strapping is used. An assistant lifts the foot above the bed, pulling gently and keeping the medial edge of the foot perpendicular to the plane of the bed. A strip of foam rubber is applied to protect the malleoli. Foam rubber strapping, 5 to 6 cm in width, is then applied to both sides of the leg up to the knee and down to about 10 cm below the heel. To ensure adhesion of the foam rubber, an

elastic bandage is wrapped loosely around the leg over the strapping. Axial traction is applied to check that the system is effective. A spreader bar is placed in the loop and attached to a pulley with a weight of 2 to 3 kg. A springy cushion is placed under the calf or Achilles tendon to prevent development of a pressure sore where the heel rests on the bed. Care is taken to make sure that neither the strapping nor the bandage is applied too tightly, particularly at the proximal end of the fibula where excessive compression can cause palsy of the common peroneal nerve. A foam rubber cushion placed against the lateral edge of the foot can be useful if there is a marked tendency toward external rotation. Finally, a hoop should be placed under the bedclothes to lift these off the tips of the toes. The foot of the bed should be raised by about 10 cm so that the weight of the body provides counter-traction (a tilting bed is convenient). The absence of pain in the strapped area and the presence of signs of adequate blood circulation in the foot should be checked daily.

OTHER INDICATIONS

Skin traction can be used after reduction of a trauma-related dislocation of the hip or of a dislocated hip prosthesis and to maintain the hip in the desired position after a surgical procedure (abduction after adductor tenotomy, prevention of dislocation after surgery for cancer with extensive resection of the soft tissues that stabilise the hip).

Skeletal traction with a proximal tibial Kirschner wire

GENERAL REQUIREMENTS FOR SKELETAL TRACTION

■ *Kirschner wire or Steinmann pin?*

A wire is well tolerated as long as there is no infection. Consequently, the wire should

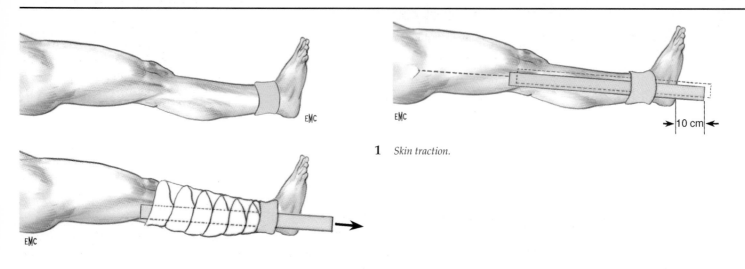

1   *Skin traction.*

be inserted aseptically and there should be no pull whatsoever of the wire on the soft tissues, particularly the skin. Necrosis of the skin due to pull from the wire creates an entry portal for micro-organisms. Necrosis of the skin or even of the bone can occur if heavy traction is applied: if heavy traction is needed, a Steinmann pin is preferable. To avoid thermal necrosis, the rotation of the wire during motorised insertion must be extremely slow to minimise the increase in temperature. At the femur and tibia, the wire is driven through the metaphysis at a sufficient distance from the joint to eliminate all risk of arthritis, yet in a zone that offers high resistance. Insertion of a Steinmann pin into the diaphyseal cortex should be avoided because there is a non-negligible risk of fissuring the bone. The wire is inserted on the side that contains structures susceptible to injury, as these are then more easily avoided: the medial aspect of the limb at the femoral condyles (femoral artery), the lateral aspect of the leg at the proximal tibia (common peroneal nerve), and the medial aspect of the foot at the calcaneus (posterior tibial pedicle).

▪ *Controlling rotation and equinus*

Axial rotation must be controlled, particularly when traction is used both to obtain and to maintain reduction of a fracture. Two stirrups perpendicular to one another are used: one provides the traction and controls varus-valgus motions and the other controls rotation. The foot tends to drop into equinus, which rapidly becomes fixed as a result of contracture of the gastrocnemius muscle and talocrural capsule. Use of a board to prevent equinus can be ineffective and can cause insidious development of pressure sores over the metatarsophalangeal joints. A better method is extremely gentle (500 g) but permanent traction by an adhesive sock to keep the ankle in dorsal flexion.

▪ *Checking the efficacy of traction treatment* (fig 2)

Counter-traction must be applied. For the weight of the body to serve as counter-traction, the upper body must tend to slide toward the head of the bed and the suspension system must be designed in such a way that it does not reduce the force of the traction. Care should also be taken to check that the traction weight falls freely, i.e. that the ropes glide freely in the pulley and that the weight does not rest on the bed or floor.

▪ *Checking patient comfort* (fig 3)

At a given level of efficacy, some systems are better than others in terms of patient comfort. Traction-suspension in a U-shaped splint (leaving the posterior aspect of the knee and thigh free) is far more comfortable than traction on a Boppe-Braun frame which has lateral posts that press against the thighs

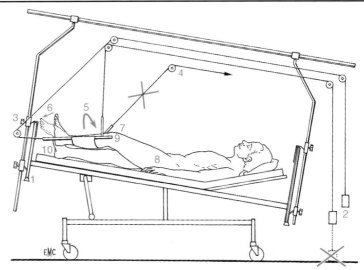

2 *The ten points used to monitor transtibial traction:*
To be effective: 1. Foot of the bed raised or bed tilted; 2. no contact between the weights and the floor; 3. no impediment to free sliding of the ropes in the pulleys; 4. no divergent tractions.
To be properly oriented: 5. control of leg rotation; 6. control of equinus of the foot; 7. slight flexion of the knee; 8. minimal flexion of the hip.
To be well tolerated: 9. at the wire (no pain or mobility); 10. at the heel and foot.

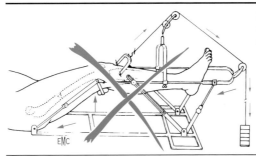

3 *The Boppe splint is not recommended because the counter-supports at the popliteal fossa and thigh can cause pain.*

and is so cumbersome that it prevents all motion, thus increasing the risk of pressure sores.

DESCRIPTION OF SKELETAL TRACTION WITH A KIRSCHNER WIRE

▪ *Indication*

Temporary traction-suspension with a wire after internal fixation of a comminuted acetabular fracture (fig 4).

▪ *Material needed*

– Kirschner wire.

– Kirschner stirrup.

– U-shaped splint.

– Two wire tighteners that can slide over the wire.

– Sterile gloves.

– Material for local anaesthesia.

– Pointed knife.

– Slowly rotating motor and wire-guide.

▪ *Insertion of a transtibial wire* (fig 4A)

The lower limb is stretched out. An assistant holds the medial edge of the foot

perpendicular to the plane of the bed (or in slight external rotation at the same degree as on the normal side). The other limb is in abduction.

The entry site, located 2 to 3 cm behind the bulge of the anterior tibial tuberosity and 5 to 6 cm under the joint space (which is at the level of the tip of the patella), is disinfected. Lidocaine is injected successively into the lateral skin, the anterior tibialis muscle, the lateral and medial periosteum, and the medial soft tissues.

The skin is punctured with the knife. The wire is inserted down to the periosteum by hand, then driven through the bone using a slowly rotating motor (the wire is held in the right hand and a guide in the left hand to ensure that the wire stays on track despite its relative flexibility).

When the tip of the wire bulges under the skin on the medial aspect of the limb, lidocaine is injected into the area and the skin is punctured with the knife. There should be no tension of the skin; if tension occurs, an incision must be made in the skin (or even the underlying soft tissues) by cutting with the knife against the wire.

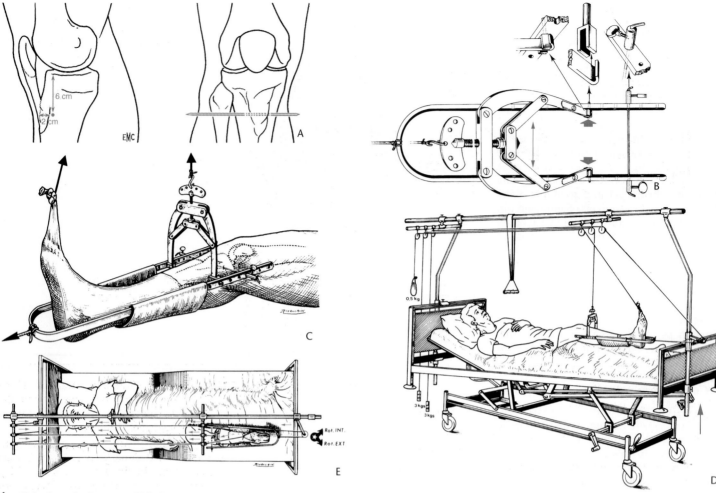

4 *Skeletal traction by a transtibial wire.*
A. The wire is inserted at the lateral aspect of the leg.
B. The U-shaped splint and Kirschner stirrup are put in place.
C. The leg sling and anti-equinus sock are put in place.

D. The position of the bed is adjusted.
E. Rotation of the limb can be adjusted by changing the position of the traction pulley
on the stirrup: moving the pulley medially induces internal rotation of the leg.

■ **Setting up the traction system**
(fig 4B, C)

The traction system has two main components:

– a U-shaped splint (on which the leg rests maintained in a knitted sling) to which the axial traction is applied;

– a Kirschner stirrup that maintains the wire taut, allows suspension, and controls rotation of the limb.

The system is set up as follows:

– The wire is threaded through the holes in the splint so that the axis of the splint matches that of the leg and the base of the U is at least 5 cm beyond the heel.

– The two wire-tighteners are threaded over the wire.

– The two tabs are placed on the bits of the Kirschner stirrup, and the lugs are pushed into the holes of the splint, usually two holes beneath the wire.

– The opening of the stirrup is adjusted so that the smallest distance between the stirrup and the skin of the leg is 1 to 2 cm.

– The wire-tighteners are screwed on, and the tip of the wire is twisted and cut 2 cm beyond its point of exit from the butterfly nut.

– The Kirschner stirrup is pulled to maximum tautness.

■ **Position of the bed** *(fig 4D, E)*

Counter-traction

Traction is effective only if counter-traction is applied to ensure that the patient is not pulled gradually to the foot of the bed by the weights. One means of providing counter-traction is to raise the foot of the bed by about 10 cm. Alternatively, the bed can be tilted around its axis to obtain a similar degree of elevation (this is the simplest and most effective method).

Care should be taken that the lower part of the splint does not come into contact with the traction pulleys and that the suspension is applied exactly along a vertical line and not in the direction opposite to the traction, since this would reduce the efficacy of the treatment.

■ **Setting up the pulleys and weights**

Three bars are placed on the traction frame:

– one at the foot of the bed with one pulley (traction);

– one exactly above the stirrup, with three pulleys, i.e. from the inside to the outside:

– reflection of the axial traction;

– suspension;

– and anti-equinus traction;

– the third bar is placed at the head of the bed: this bar keeps the weights away from the bed frame.

A knitted sling is slipped over the U-shaped splint, and the leg is positioned so that the calf above the Achilles tendon rests in the sling. A knitted sock with a 500 g weight maintains dorsal flexion of the foot. The sock is attached to the splint. Usually, 3 kg of traction and 3 kg of suspension are adequate. The suspension weight should be increased until the hand can be slipped under the popliteal fossa.

■ **Monitoring traction treatment**
(fig 2)

An advantage of these set-ups is that the patient can move (for rehabilitation therapy, eating, using the bedpan, and while the sheets are changed). However, this requires that the set-up be checked daily: the physicians and other health care providers should check the ten points listed below.

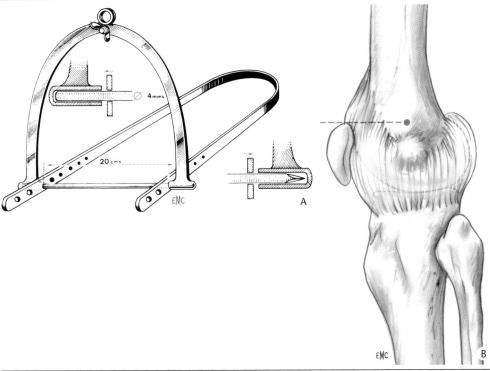

5 *Traction by a Steinmann pin.*
A. The pin turns freely in the stirrup, which also maintains the U-shaped splint.
B. Application of the pin for transcondylar traction.

The traction is effective if:

1. The foot of the bed is raised (to provide counter-traction).

2. The weights are not in contact with the floor or bed.

3. The traction is not impeded by the stirrup or a knot caught in a pulley.

4. The suspension does not impede the traction (divergent forces).

The direction of traction is satisfactory if:

5. There is no abnormal rotation of the distal extremity of the foot (change the position of the suspension pulley as needed).

6. The foot has not dropped into equinus.

7. The knee is in slight flexion (a hand can be slipped under the popliteal fossa).

8. The hip is not in marked flexion (i.e. the upper body is not too vertical).

The traction is well tolerated if:

9. There is no necrosis of the skin or infection at the wire entry and exit sites. The wire is fixed and does not cause pain. A wire that moves or causes pain must be removed and replaced by another wire inserted 1 to 2 cm from the first wire.

10. There are no skin lesions at the foot or the Achilles tendon.

Traction-suspension with a proximal tibial Steinmann pin

INDICATIONS

This method is used to obtain and to maintain reduction of comminuted acetabular fractures that are not treated surgically.

TECHNIQUE

■ ***Material***

– Steinmann pin 4 mm in diameter and 20 cm in length.

– Boehler-type stirrup (allowing axial rotation of the pin).

– U-shaped splint with 6 mm holes.

– Material for local anaesthesia.

– Pointed knife.

– "American-nose" pin holder.

■ ***Insertion of the transtibial Steinmann pin***

This is done at the same level as the Kirschner wire. After anaesthesia, the pin is pushed down to the lateral periosteum, then driven through the bone using a handle; a rapidly rotating motor should not be used. The skin must be debrided if the pin causes tension.

■ ***Setting up the traction system***
(fig 5A)

It is usually easier to set up the U-shaped splint first and then the stirrup. As the splint is elastic, it usually rests against the internal aspect of the bits of the stirrup.

The leg suspension sling and anti-equinus sock are put in place.

■ ***Position of the bed***

To ensure that the traction force is applied in the plane of opening of the acetabulum, the hip should be abducted 10 to 15°. This can be achieved by a traction force that pulls the leg laterally with reference to the axis of the bed (by using longer transversal bars).

However, unilateral axial traction alone often causes the pelvis to tilt around the lumbosacral junction, thus producing a sufficient degree of abduction.

Heavy traction (1/10th of the body weight) is often needed initially. The weight is then decreased gradually down to about 3 kg, according to findings on follow-up radiographs. The heavier the weight, the higher the foot of the bed must be raised.

Rotation of the limb is corrected by adjusting the position of the suspension pulley (displacing this pulley medially produces internal rotation). The weight needed is 3 kg on average.

The upper body should not be elevated too much since this causes flexion of the hip that can rapidly become resistant to correction by rehabilitation therapy.

Tolerance of the Steinmann pin is excellent, allowing traction for over two months.

Other types of traction for acetabular fractures
(fig 5B)

Transcondylar traction puts no stress on the knee ligaments. However, if the traction is relatively distal, there is a high risk of adhesion of the capsule to the condyles, which limits flexion of the knee. If the pin travels through the synovial recesses along the condyles, there is a risk of infection. To avoid these complications, transcondylar traction should be used only for a short time (for instance, before surgery) or in patients with a contraindication to tibial traction. The Steinmann pin is inserted at the medial aspect of the limb, in the plane of and 1 to 2 cm above, the lateral tubercles of the condyles.

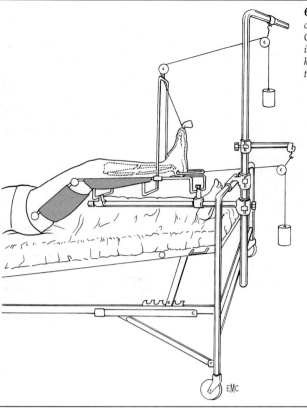

6 *Treatment of leg fractures by transcalcaneal traction with the Braun splint. Counter-traction by the weight of the body is achieved by raising the foot of the bed. A knitted sock can be used, if needed, to control equinus and rotation of the foot.*

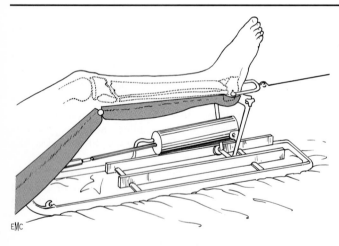

7 *Traction with early motion on a continuous passive motion splint of a fracture of the tibial plateaux.*

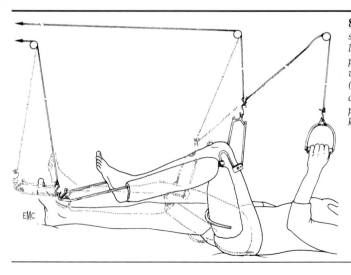

8 *Suspension allowing mobilisation after surgical treatment of a lower limb fracture. This is a suspension device that does not provide traction on the lower limb (i.e. the bed is horizontal). To facilitate flexion, the patient can pull on the hoop that supports the knee.*

Skeletal traction with a Kirschner wire in the calcaneus

INDICATIONS

Initial treatment of a leg fracture before internal fixation or orthopaedic treatment (cast, Sarmiento splint).

The goal of the traction is to align the bony fragments so that these become bonded to one another. The fracture can then be treated using conventional orthopaedic techniques (Boehler: immobilisation by a plaster spica after 3 to 6 weeks with no weight-bearing until radiographs show that the fracture is healed) or using the hydraulic system designed by Sarmiento (an adjusted leg device is set up after 10 to 20 days and allows walking with gradual weight-bearing).

TECHNIQUE *(fig 6)*

Counter-traction must be provided in a manner that does not cause injury to the popliteal fossa: devices derived from the Braun splint are used with the goal of keeping the limb in flexion, while the traction is applied through a pulley attached to the bed and counter-traction is provided by the weight of the body. The set-up is the same as above: the foot of the bed is raised to reduce pressure on the thigh; an outward-facing patella denotes antalgic external rotation of the thigh, which should be corrected by placing folded sheets under the buttock on the side of the injury.

The knee is flexed and the leg kept horizontal to eliminate tension on the gastrocnemius and hamstring muscles.

Traction through an anti-equinus sock is usually sufficient to control rotation of the segment under the fracture.

Traction and continuous passive motion in tibial plateau fractures *(fig 7)*

This therapeutic method is useful provided:

– the fracture can be reduced by traction (i.e. the lesions are due to separation rather than to central subsidence);

– the operative risk is high (skin lesions, comminution compromising the chances of successful internal fixation);

– the patient can tolerate prolonged dorsal decubitus (this method is not desirable in elderly patients).

All these conditions are only rarely present, and we usually treat tibial plateau fractures by internal fixation.

We use a combination of axial traction (to reduce the fragments) and early motorised continuous passive motion.

The lower limb is placed on a motorised splint. Traction is applied to the knee through a transcalcaneal nail held in place by a stirrup. A sock can be useful to control rotation. The motorised splint is used to keep the knee at 30° of flexion between mobilisation sessions of which there are two or three each day. Each session lasts two hours; the range of flexion-extension is increased from 0-45° initially to 0-90° after the tenth day. A weight of 3 kg is usually sufficient, and the traction is continued until bonding of the fragments is obtained, i.e. from six to eight weeks. Weight-bearing is allowed only at the third month.

As with all traction treatments, particularly in patients with articular fractures, follow-up radiographs should be obtained to check the quality of the reduction.

Postoperative suspension of lower limb fractures
(fig 8)

In some surgically-treated fractures, particularly articular fractures (supra-condylar and intercondylar fractures of the femur, tibial plateau fractures), early active or passive rehabilitation is useful. This can be facilitated by suspending the lower limb to decrease the pull of gravity. Furthermore, the suspension raises the limb, decreasing the risk of trophic disorders. We use a suspension sling with a leg splint and a crural splint. The sling is articulated at the knee. Suspension is with 5 kg at the knee and 3 kg at the foot. A traction handle can be placed on the upper hoop and used by the patient to facilitate flexion of the limb *(fig 8)*. This device does not provide traction: there is no need to tilt the bed or to use a pulley at the foot of the bed (this would prevent raising of the leg splint). It does not counteract rotation of the segment under the fracture as do the traction-suspension devices described above; this means that the device can be used only after surgery. It is the rigidity of the internal fixation material that controls the rotations. A useful alternative is the motorised splint which both suspends the limb and mobilises the knee.

References

[1] Langlais F, Lambotte JC. Tractions et suspensions (membre inférieur, membre supérieur, rachis). *Encycl Méd Chir* (Éditions Scientifiques et Médicales Elsevier SAS, Paris), Techniques chirurgicales - Orthopédie-Traumatologie, 44-010, 1996 : 1-8

[2] Steward JD. Traction treatment of fractures. In : Bentley G, Greer R eds. Robb and Smith Operative Surgery, Orthopaedics. London : Butterworth 1993 : 123-144

Extracorporeal shock waves in orthopaedics

M Krismer
R Biedermann

Abstract. – *This chapter presents the current knowledge, as presented in the literature, on extracorporeal shock wave therapy for musculoskeletal conditions. It starts with a brief description of the principles and modes of application of extracorporeal shock wave therapy. As shock wave therapy is not currently a widely accepted form of treatment, importance was attached to the principal indications and outcomes of therapy as presented in the literature. Controversial studies are also mentioned to show the existing discussion about this form of therapy. We have tried to present an overview with emphasis on well-designed studies in the literature.*

Keywords: extracorporeal shock waves, bone healing, calcifying tendinitis of the shoulder, lateral epicondylitis, heel spur, plantar fasciitis, cement removal.

Introduction

Extracorporeal shock wave therapy (ESWT) was used for the first time about 20 years ago for disintegration of stones in urolithiasis. It has now become the gold standard for the primary treatment of this condition. It was subsequently applied to biliary or salivary stones. More than a decade ago, the technique was also adopted to treat various musculoskeletal disorders, for which it rapidly came into routine use, mainly in central European countries. In 1996, the number of shock wave therapies performed for orthopaedic indications in Germany had already come close to the number of shock wave therapies used for urolithiasis (66,000 versus 70,000).

Specific devices have now been developed for the following orthopaedic indications: enthesopathies (tennis elbow, tendopathies at the shoulder, calcaneal spurs), pain in soft tissues in proximity to bones, tendopathies with extra-osseous calcification and nonunion of fractures. For the latter indication, shock wave therapy has even been referred to as the treatment of first choice [7]. Other indications are not yet established, although some authors are engaged in studies on the use of ESWT for cement removal in total hip revision arthroplasty, as well as the treatment of avascular necrosis of the femoral head, osteochondrosis dissecans and still other conditions.

Technical aspects

The shock wave is a single-impulse acoustic wave with a high initial amplitude and a short length (positive pressure amplitude), followed by a longer negative tensile wave. The shock wave is generated by a piezoelectric, electromagnetic or electrohydraulic source, focused by an acoustic lens or reflector shield and applied to the body via a water-filled balloon and contact gel. This sound wave will be transformed into mechanical forces at the boundary of tissues with different rigidities by two main effects:

– the positive pressure and the short rise cause high tension and direct mechanical effects at the interfaces;

– the tensile part of the shock wave lowers the pressure and is responsible for an indirect mechanical effect via cavitation [34].

This effect was first described by Delius et al in 1995 [5].

For targeting, lithotripters are usually equipped with an X-ray C-arm that can be revolved around the shock wave focus as indicated by the cross-hair on the X-ray monitor, and/or an ultrasound localisation system. The power at the focus point is defined as the energy flux density (EFD) per impulse and measured in millijoules per square millimetre (mJ/mm^2). For older devices, the energy flux density is not defined and the energy level of shock waves is specified in kilovolt (kV), the level of output voltage. The latter values cannot be converted in a directly proportional manner. The existence of different devices with non-comparable specifications and levels of energy make a comparison of the present studies difficult. Rompe and co-workers defined a concept for graduation of energy levels for the different orthopaedic indications: low-energy (EFD: 0.08 mJ/mm^2), medium-energy (EFD: 0.28 mJ/mm^2) and high-energy shock waves with an EFD of 0.6 mJ/mm^2 [21, 24]. Medium- and high-energy therapies generally require regional or general anaesthesia, whereas application of low-energy shock waves can be carried out under local anaesthesia in most cases. Practical application of shock waves is uncomplicated; the handling of the different devices varies and is therefore not addressed in detail.

Contraindications and side effects

The effect of shock waves is reported to be directly related to the number and energy density of the shock waves applied. Kaulesar Sukul and co-workers

Martin Krismer, M.D., Professor.
Rainer Biedermann, M.D.
Department of Orthopaedics, University of Innsbruck, Anichstrasse 35, A–6020 Innsbruck, Austria.

demonstrated the possibility to produce dose-related (micro) fractures and bone chips peeled from cortical bone [11]. After direct exposure of organs to shock waves, complications such as small bowel perforations, kidney and liver damage, as well as intra-abdominal or intrapulmonal bleeding may occur. Other authors have advised about growth disturbance subsequent to application of shock waves to an epiphysis. However, when these contraindications are taken into account and the technique is carried out correctly, extracorporeal shock wave therapy for orthopaedic disorders has been demonstrated to have only minor complications, such as superficial haematomas or transient blood pressure elevations [32]. Absolute contraindications to shock wave therapy include coagulopathies, anticoagulant treatment and pregnancy. Application of shock waves in the thoracic region, lung or growth plate, or close to nervous or vascular structures, must be avoided. The presence of malignancy or infection is considered as a relative or absolute contraindication depending on different studies; in fact, the effect of shock waves on malignant or infected tissues is unknown and is still under investigation.

Indications

DELAYED UNION AND NON-UNION OF FRACTURES

■ *Mode of action of shock waves on bone healing*

Kaulesar Sukul et al [11] demonstrated a linear relationship between the energy level of shock waves applied to bone specimens of rabbit femurs and tibiae and the severity of the resulting cortical bone defects. The higher the power setting, the more severe the resulting cortical changes. With an energy flux density of $0.54\,\mathrm{mJ/mm^2}$, gross cortical changes were detected, such as bone chips peeled from cortex.

Delius et al [5] applied 1,500 shock waves at 27.5 kV to the right femur of nineteen rabbits. Initially, diffuse haemorrhages, haematomas and foci of fractured and displaced bony trabeculae were noted, but no cortical changes were evidenced. In the further course, there was intense apposition of new cortical bone resulting in considerable cortical thickening, while trabecular remodelling was only minor. Cavitation was postulated as the major mechanism of shock wave damage to bone.

In a dog model, Wang and co-workers detected histologically a significant increase in cortical bone formation after shock wave application, compared with a control group [36]. In an in vitro study on cultivated human cancellous bone cells, a decrease in cell survival after shock wave application, depending on the number and intensity of

impulses, was demonstrated. Between the 3rd and 8th day, proliferation increased significantly in the surviving cells. As a consequence, a medium-term cell stimulating effect after shock wave application was postulated [14]. Another research group indicated a membrane hyperpolarisation and activation of osteogenesis in human bone marrow stromal cells in vitro, after application of 500 impulses of low- to medium-energy shock waves of $0.16\,\mathrm{mJ/mm^2}$, and suggested that physical shock waves promote bone cell differentiation toward the osteogenic lineage [37].

■ *Mode of application of shock waves*

A number of authors have used high energy shock wave therapy for treatment of nonunions. Energy levels were chosen between 18 to 28 kV or $> 0.6\,\mathrm{mJ/mm^2}$ and the number of shock waves applied was usually between 2,000 and 6,000 impulses, depending on the diameter of the bone. As a variety of differing devices were used, dosages cannot be compared between the studies.

■ *Outcome of therapy*

The first experiments to investigate the osteogenetic potential of shock waves were performed in 1986 [8]. After inflicting fractures to the left humeri of forty Sprague-Dawley rats through digital pressure, 100 shock waves with either 14 kV or 18 kV were applied. Fourteen of these rats served as a control group. X-ray readings revealed radiological signs of faster healing in the treated groups in comparison to the control group; therefore, enhanced fracture healing as a result of treatment with extracorporeal shock waves was suggested. In another model using two randomised groups of five dogs, each with segmental resection of the distal radius, one treatment group with application of 4,000 shock waves of 0.54 $\mathrm{mJ/mm^2}$ and one control group, radiographically observable union was reached in all animals in the treatment group within twelve weeks. In the control group, four dogs had persistent nonunion after the same time interval, as reported by Johannes et al [10].

Valchanou and Michailov [35] presented the first clinical results in 1991. They treated eighty-two delayed unions or nonunions at a mean time of 20.2 months after fracture with 1,000 to 4,000 shock waves. The healing rate was reported to be 85.4%, but the study was poorly controlled. Schleberger and Senge found that shock waves induce callus formation in three out of four cases of pseudarthrosis [29]. Radiological union of ununited fractures after extracorporeal shock wave therapy, at a mean of 3.3 (two to nine) months after the initial trauma, was seen in 52% of fifty-eight patients by the research group of Rompe et al [21, 24]. They applied

3,000 impulses at an energy level of 0.6 $\mathrm{mJ/mm^2}$. Failures were especially encountered with the atrophic type of nonunion. Beutler et al reported a success rate of 41% in 27 nonunions of long bones six months after application of shock waves with an MFL 5000® lithotripter [2]. Radiological union was seen within three months in most of the 11 patients that healed. In a more recent study, bony consolidation was found in 31 out of 43 cases (72%) of nonunion of at least nine months duration [25]. Other authors reported a rate of bony union of 40% at three months, and 60.9% at six months [28]. A retrospective study on 73 delayed unions and nonunions was performed by the present authors. Concordant with the literature, union was achieved in 56% of patients with nonunions; better results were achieved for the hypertrophic type of nonunion (62% versus 50% for the atrophic type of nonunion). Patients treated twice did not show a higher rate of bony union (56%). In contrast to this, the group of patients with delayed unions did show a higher and earlier rate of union (93%) (unpublished data).

■ *Controversial studies*

Only a few authors have mentioned the critical aspects in the evaluation of ESWT [9, 21, 24]. No beneficial effect in acute fracture repair was reported by two research groups. Augat and co-workers could not detect any significant differences after shock wave application to a fractured ovine tibia in comparison to the untreated control group [1]. Forriol et al [6] performed drill holes and window osteotomies on the tibiae of thirty-seven lambs and exposed the bony lesions to shock waves up to 1.2 $\mathrm{mJ/mm^2}$ EFD. Three weeks later, specimens of the bone were examined histologically and radiographically. No effect was noted on the periosteal surface and only some new trabecular bone were seen on the endosteal surface; this research group therefore considered it unlikely that shock waves were able to promote healing in nonunion.

■ *Concluding assessment*

The majority of publications have postulated positive effects of extracorporeal shock waves in initiating or enhancing fracture healing. In any case, they also conclude that stabilisation of the fracture is an essential condition for the success of the therapy. So far, no controlled prospective randomised clinical trial has been published that would demonstrate the effectiveness of ESWT for the treatment of nonunions in comparison to the natural history of union. Despite promising results in the literature, only a study with a prospective, controlled design will bring definitive knowledge about the benefit of shock wave therapy for this indication. Such studies have now been initiated and results will hopefully be available in the near future.

CALCIFYING TENDONITIS OF THE SHOULDER

■ *Mode of action and side effects*

The mechanism of action remains unknown. It is assumed to consist in mechanical disintegration followed by resorption of the calcific deposit in the tendon or its breakthrough into the adjacent subacromial bursa, and reactive hypervascularisation. An instant mechanical effect on the calcifying deposits is suggested as unlikely, and the absorption of the deposits is believed to be induced through a cellular clearing function [20]. Shock waves lead to focal damage inducing tissue changes. Investigations on rabbit Achilles tendons have shown dose-dependent changes in the tendon and paratendon. Low- and medium-energy shock waves (up to 0.28 mJ/mm^2) led only to transient swelling and minor inflammatory changes. High-energy therapy (0.6 mJ/mm^2) caused fibrinoid necrosis, fibrosis and infiltration of inflammatory cells. As a consequence, it was suggested that high-energy shock waves not be used clinically in the treatment of tendon disorders [23]. On the other hand, no cases of damage to the rotator cuff, cartilage or bone were observed on radiographs, ultrasonographs or MRI scans in a subsequent clinical study, after application of 3,000 impulses at an EFD of 0.6 mJ/mm^2 [27].

■ *Mode of application of shock waves*

For targeting, the shock wave device should be equipped with an X-ray intensifier with a cross-hair on the monitor. Local anaesthesia is required for this form of therapy. In an experimental study, it was shown that between 2,000 and 3,000 impulses at an energy level of 0.42 mJ/mm^2 are required for disintegration of a stone implanted in a pig shoulder. Nevertheless, two sessions with at least 1,500 impulses and an energy of 0.28-0.3 mJ/mm^2 were recommended [20]. Almost all clinical studies were performed with medium-energy shock waves (EFD = 0.28 mJ/mm^2).

■ *Outcome of therapy*

Some authors reported good clinical results and frequent elimination of the deposits in the radiographs after low-dose therapy. Better results with complete disintegration of the deposit in 62.5% of the patients were reported to occur at an energy level of 0.28 mJ/mm^2 [26]. In a controlled prospective study, good clinical results and radiological disappearance or disintegration of the calcium deposits up to 77% were reported after two sessions with an interval of one week, with 3,000 impulses delivered at each session at an EFD of 0.3 mJ/mm^2, compared with low-energy therapy and a single therapy strategy. No correlation between the size of calcifications and effectiveness of shock wave was found [16].

■ *Concluding assessment*

Medium-energy extracorporeal shock-wave therapy is reported to be effective in chronic calcifying tendonitis of the shoulder. It should be considered before surgery, due to its non-invasiveness, when conservative therapy has failed for at least six months. Because of the benign natural history of smaller calcifications, it is advisable to restrict the indication of ESWT to a calcification with a minimum size of 10 to 15 mm.

LATERAL EPICONDYLITIS

■ *Mode of action of shock waves for enthesopathies and pain in soft tissue*

The precise mode for the analgesic action of ESWT is not known. The initial analgesic effect may be caused by an altered or increased cell membrane permeability leading to the inability of nociceptors to generate a potential which is needed to evoke a pain signal response. The gate control mechanism postulates that activation of afferent nociceptors (mechanoreceptors) leads to a presynaptic inhibition of pain transmission in the medulla. Other theories are based on activation of inhibitory neurons and long-term repression of pain via local hyperstimulation. So far, no secured explanation for this long-term analgesic effect has been established.

■ *Mode of application of shock waves*

Almost all studies were performed following low-energy principles of shock waves ($\approx$ 0.08 mJ/mm^2 or 14 kV). Localisation can be performed with an X-ray intensifier or ultrasound device.

■ *Outcome of therapy*

With a few exceptions, most studies report a long-lasting analgesic effect after shock wave application in tennis elbow. Nevertheless, as they were designed without a control group, a placebo effect could not be excluded. So far, only the research group of Rompe has published the results of a controlled, prospective study of 100 patients. Significant decrease of pain and improvement of function after treatment, in comparison to the placebo group, were seen with good or excellent outcome in 48% and an acceptable result in 42% after 24 weeks [22]. However, in a critical overview of the literature, it was estimated that the effect of shock waves in tennis elbow may have been overestimated due to the methodological insufficiency of the published studies, and it was concluded that, at present, the efficiency of this therapy can be neither confirmed nor excluded [3].

■ *Concluding assessment*

Considering the non-invasive character and low rate of complications of extracorporeal shock wave therapy, it seems to be a treatment alternative for chronic lateral epicondylitis refractory to other forms of conservative therapy, before surgical intervention.

HEEL SPUR AND PLANTAR FASCIITIS

■ *Mode of action – see "Lateral epicondylitis" above*

■ *Mode of application of shock waves*

Shock wave targeting can either be performed with an X-ray intensifier or ultrasound device. Positive results have been reported under low- to medium-energy regimes (0.08 to 0.3 mJ/mm^2, or 14 to 18 kV).

■ *Outcome of therapy*

Comparable with chronic tennis elbow, studies reporting on the efficiency of shock wave therapy for chronic plantar fasciitis showed positive results with improvement in pain and function, but these studies usually lacked a control group and their study design was deficient. A Cochrane review showed limited evidence for the effectiveness of low energy extracorporeal shock wave therapy in reducing night pain, resting pain and pressure pain in the short term (12 weeks), but only English language reports were considered [4]. A prospective study of similar design as for the tennis elbow (see above), suggesting better outcome in the therapy group, was presented in German by Rompe et al in 1997 [21, 24]. In a randomised, double-blind evaluation of the efficacy of ESWT for this disorder, including 302 patients, 56% of the ESWT patients had a successful result when compared with the patients treated with a placebo, three months after one treatment with 1,500 shocks at an 18 kV power setting. This study was accepted by the American Food and Drug Administration, which resulted in approval of the specific shock wave device for this indication in October 2000 [19].

■ *Concluding assessment*

Extracorporeal shock wave therapy has been shown to be effective for chronic plantar fasciitis and should be considered before any surgical option.

OTHER INDICATIONS

■ *Cement removal in revision of total hip arthroplasty*

Several studies have been reported on the effect of shock waves on femoral prostheses and cement removal. Although some authors found no changes in stability of the prosthesis and only minor morphological changes of the bone cement, most studies suggest a facilitation of cement removal after high-energy shock wave application. Faster extraction time and a reduced amount of residual cement inside the bone surface has been reported [12]. Microfractures, loose bodies and widening were seen at the bone-cement interface [38]. Although concomitant cortical microfractures have been reported, exposure to shock waves was suggested to have only a minimal or insignificant effect on whole bone strength in an experimental study [33]. Following application of shock waves on bone cement, a reduction of fracture toughness of the cement was reported [15]. However, only microscopic lesions were seen after shock wave application on the frontal surface of discs of bone cement, smaller than the pores normally present in bone cement when applied clinically [31]. Extracorporeal shock waves might have the potential to facilitate cement removal in revision total joint surgery; however, their clinical value is still to be evaluated [18].

■ *Avascular necrosis of the femoral head*

Very few studies have been conducted so far. Improvement in pain and an increase of the Harris hip score one year after high-energy shock wave therapy in the early stages of femoral head necrosis was reported by the research group of Ludwig et al [17].

■ *Non-calcifying shoulder problems*

Several uncontrolled studies have suggested that extracorporeal shock wave therapy is an effective treatment for non-calcifying tendonitis of the supraspinatus. In a prospective randomised study, improvement of function and reduction of pain were noted, but no difference between the two groups was described. Therefore, the authors did not recommend ESWT for the treatment of tendinitis of the supraspinatus [30].

■ *Medial epicondylitis*

Only few data are available on the effect of ESWT for this indication, despite wide clinical use. A comparative study of 30 patients has shown a significantly worse outcome than for identically treated patients with chronic tennis elbow; medial epicondylitis was thus considered a questionable indication for shock wave therapy [13].

■ *Others*

It has been suggested to use ESWT to enhance osseo-integration of non-cemented hip prostheses through induced osteogenesis [7]. Attempts have been made to use ESWT for the treatment of osteochondrosis dissecans, Köhler's, Perthes' or Osgood-Schlatter's disease, patellar tendonitis, trochanteric bursitis, Achilles tendonitis and reversal of heterotopic bone formation in the early stages. However, to the authors' knowledge, no substantial data have been published so far.

Conclusion

Prospective, randomised studies have been published for plantar fasciitis and calcifying tendonitis of the shoulder, presenting extracorporeal shock waves as an effective form of therapy for these indications. Promising results have been reported for lateral epicondylitis and delayed union or nonunion of fractures, but the efficiency may still be questioned until supported by prospective controlled randomised studies. At this point, the efficiency of shock wave therapy for the other indications mentioned has not been established.

References

[1] Augat P, Claes L, Suger G. In vivo effect of shock-waves on the healing of fractured bone. *Clin Biomech* 1995 ; 10 : 374-378

[2] Beutler S, Regel G, Machtens S, Weinberg AM, Kremeike I, Jonas U et al. Extracorporeal shock wave therapy for delayed union of long bone fractures – preliminary results of a prospective cohort study. *Unfallchirurg* 1999 ; 102 : 839-847

[3] Böddeker I, Haake M. Die extrakorporale Stobwellenthera-pie zur Behandlung der Epicondylitis humeri radialis. Ein aktueller Überblick. *Orthopäde* 2000 ; 29 : 463-469

[4] Crawford F, Atkins D, Edwards J. Interventions for treating plantar heel pain. *Cochrane Database Syst Rev* 2000 ; 3 : CD000416

[5] Delius M, Draenert K, Al Diek Y, Draenert Y. Biological effects of shock waves: in vivo effect of high energy pulses on rabbit bone. *Ultrasound Med Biol* 1995 ; 21 : 1219-1225

[6] Forriol F, Solchaga L, Moreno JL, Canadell J. The effect of shock waves on mature and healing cortical bone. *Int Orthop* 1994 ; 18 : 325-329

[7] Haupt G. Use of extracorporeal shock waves in the treat-ment of pseudarthrosis, tendinopathy and other orthope-dic diseases. *J Urol* 1997 ; 158 : 4-11

[8] Haupt G, Haupt A, Ekkernkamp A, Gerety B, Chvapil M. Influence of shock waves on fracture healing. *Urology* 1992 ; 39 : 529-532

[9] Heller KD, Niethard FU. Der Einsatz der extrakorporellen Stobwellentherapie in der Orthopädie - eine Metaanalyse. *Z Orthop Ihre Grenzgeb* 1998 ; 136 : 390-401

[10] Johannes EJ, Dinesh M, Kaulesar Sukul DM, Matura E. High-energy shock waves for the treatment of nonunions: an experiment on dogs. *J Surg Res* 1994 ; 57 : 246-252

[11] Kaulesar Sukul DM, Johannes EJ, Pierik EG, Van Eijck GJ, Kristelijn MJ. The effect of high energy shock waves focused on cortical bone: an in vitro study. *J Surg Res* 1993 ; 54 : 46-51

[12] Kim JK, Park JB, Weinstein JN, Marsh JL, Kim YS, Loening SA. Effect of shock wave treatment on femoral prosthesis and cement removal. *Biomed Mater Eng* 1994 ; 4 : 451-461

[13] Krischek O, Hopf C, Nafe B, Rompe JD. Shock-wave therapy for tennis and golfer's elbow: 1 year follow-up. *Arch Orthop Trauma Surg* 1999 ; 119 : 62-66

[14] Kusnierczak D, Brocai DR, Vettel U, Loew M. Der Einflub der extrakorporalen Stobwellenapplikation (ESWA) auf das biologische Verhalten von Knochenzellen in vitro. *Z Orthop* 2000 ; 138 : 29-33

[15] Lewis G. Effect of lithotriptor treatment on the fracture toughness of acrylic bone cement. *Biomaterials* 1992 ; 13 : 225-229

[16] Loew M, Daecke W, Kusnierczak D, Rahmanzadeh M, Ewer-beck V. Shock wave therapy is effective for chronic calci-fying tendinitis of the shoulder. *J Bone Joint Surg Br* 1999 ; 81 : 863-867

[17] Ludwig J, Lauber S, Lauber HJ, Dreisilker U, Raedel R, Hotz-inger H. High-energy shock wave treatment of femoral head necrosis in adults. *Clin Orthop* 2001 ; 387 : 119-126

[18] Magee FP, Gruen TW, Mobley T. The Lithotriptor and its potential use in the revision of total hip arthroplasty. *Clin Orthop* 2001 ; 387 : 4-7

[19] Ogden JA, Alvarez R, Levitt R, Cross GL, Marlow M. Shock wave therapy for chronic proximal plantar fasciitis. *Clin Orthop* 2001 ; 387 : 47-59

[20] Perlick L, Korth O, Wallny T, Wagner U, Hesse A, Schmitt O. Die Desintegrationswirkung der Stobwellen bei der extrakorporalen Stobwellenbehandlung der Tendinosis calcarea: ein in vitro Modell. *Z Orthop* 1999 ; 137 : 10-16

[21] Rompe JD, Eysel P, Hopf C, Vogel J, Küllmer K. Extrakorpo-rale Stobwellenapplikation bei gestörter Knochenheilung. Eine kritische Bestandsaufnahme. *Unfallchirurg* 1997 ; 100 : 845-849

[22] Rompe JD, Hope C, Kullmer K, Heine J, Burger R. Analgesic effect of extracorporeal shock-wave therapy on chronic tennis elbow. *J Bone Joint Surg Br* 1996 ; 78 : 233-237

[23] Rompe JD, Kirkpatrick CJ, Küllmer K, Schwitalle M, Krischek O. Dose-related effects of shock waves on rabbit tendo Achillis. A sonographic and histological study. *J Bone Joint Surg Br* 1998 ; 80 : 546-552

[24] Rompe JD, Küllmer K, Vogel J, Eckardt A, Wahlmann U, Eysel P et al. Extrakorporelle Stosswellentherapie. Experi-mentelle Grundlagen, Klinischer Einsatz. *Orthopade* 1997 ; 26 : 215-228

[25] Rompe JD, Rosendahl T, Schöllner C, Theis C. High-energy extracorporeal shock wave treatment of nonunions. *Clin Orthop* 2001 ; 387 : 102-111

[26] Rompe JD, Rumler F, Hopf C, Nafe B, Heine J. Extracorpo-real shock wave therapy for calcifying tendinitis of the shoulder. *Clin Orthop* 1995 ; 321 : 196-201

[27] Rompe JD, Zoellner J, Nafe B. Shock wave therapy versus conventional surgery in the treatment of calcifying tendi-nitis of the shoulder. *Clin Orthop* 2001 ; 387 : 72-82

[28] Schaden W, Fischer A, Sailler A. Extracorporeal shock wave therapy of nonunion or delayed osseous union. *Clin Orthop* 2001 ; 387 : 90-94

[29] Schleberger R, Senge T. Non-invasive treatment of long-bone pseudarthrosis by shock waves (ESWL). *Arch Orthop Trauma Surg* 1992 ; 111 : 224-227

[30] Schmitt J, Haake M, Tosch A, Hildebrand R, Deike B, Griss P. Low-energy extracorporeal shock-wave treatment (ESWT) for tendinitis of the shoulder. A prospective, randomised study. *J Bone Joint Surg Br* 2001 ; 83 : 873-876

[31] Schreurs BW, Bierkens AF, Huiskes R, Hendrikx AJ, Slooff TJ. The effect of the extracorporeal shock wave lithotriptor on bone cement. *J Biomed Mater Res* 1991 ; 25 : 157-164

[32] Sistermann R, Katthagen BD. Komplikationen, Nebenwir-kungen und Kontraindikationen der Anwendung von mittel- und hoch-energetischen extrakorporellen Stos-swellen im orthopädischen Bereich. *Z Orthop* 1998 ; 136 : 175-181

[33] Stranne SK, Callaghan JJ, Cocks FH, Weinert JL, Seaber AV, Myers BS. Would revision arthroplasty be facilitated by extracorporeal shock wave lithotripsy? *Clin Orthop* 1990 ; 287 : 252-258

[34] Thiel M. Application of shock waves in medicine. *Clin Orthop* 2001 ; 387 : 18-21

[35] Valchanov VD, Michailov P. High energy shock waves in the treatment of delayed and nonunion of fractures. *Int Orthop* 1991; 15 : 181-184

[36] Wang CJ, Chen HS, Chen CE, Yang KD. Treatment of nonu-nions of long bone fractures with shock waves. *Clin Orthop* 2001 ; 387 : 95-101

[37] Wang FS, Wang CJ, Huang HJ, Chung H, Chen RF, Yang KD. Physical shock wave mediates membrane hyperpolarisa-tion and Ras activation for osteogenesis in human bone marrow stromal cells. *Biochem Biophys Res Commun* 2001 ; 287 : 648-655

[38] Weinstein JN, Oster DM, Park JB, Park SH, Loening S. The effect of the extracorporeal shock wave Lithotriptor on the bone-cement interface in dogs. *Clin Orthop* 1988 ; 235 : 261-367

Index
Volume 1 - General knowledge
Surgical Techniques in Orthopaedics and Traumatology